Dietary Phosphorus: Health, Nutrition, and Regulatory Aspects

Dietary Phosphorus: Health, Nutrition, and Regulatory Aspects

Edited by
Jaime Uribarri
Mona S. Calvo

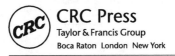

CRC Press
Taylor & Francis Group
Boca Raton London New York

CRC Press is an imprint of the
Taylor & Francis Group, an **informa** business

CRC Press
Taylor & Francis Group
6000 Broken Sound Parkway NW, Suite 300
Boca Raton, FL 33487-2742

© 2018 by Taylor & Francis Group, LLC
CRC Press is an imprint of Taylor & Francis Group, an Informa business

No claim to original U.S. Government works

Printed on acid-free paper

International Standard Book Number-13: 978-1-4987-0696-4 (Hardback)

This book contains information obtained from authentic and highly regarded sources. Reasonable efforts have been made to publish reliable data and information, but the author and publisher cannot assume responsibility for the validity of all materials or the consequences of their use. The authors and publishers have attempted to trace the copyright holders of all material reproduced in this publication and apologize to copyright holders if permission to publish in this form has not been obtained. If any copyright material has not been acknowledged please write and let us know so we may rectify in any future reprint.

Except as permitted under U.S. Copyright Law, no part of this book may be reprinted, reproduced, transmitted, or utilized in any form by any electronic, mechanical, or other means, now known or hereafter invented, including photocopying, microfilming, and recording, or in any information storage or retrieval system, without written permission from the publishers.

For permission to photocopy or use material electronically from this work, please access www.copyright.com (http://www.copyright.com/) or contact the Copyright Clearance Center, Inc. (CCC), 222 Rosewood Drive, Danvers, MA 01923, 978-750-8400. CCC is a not-for-profit organization that provides licenses and registration for a variety of users. For organizations that have been granted a photocopy license by the CCC, a separate system of payment has been arranged.

Trademark Notice: Product or corporate names may be trademarks or registered trademarks, and are used only for identification and explanation without intent to infringe.

Library of Congress Cataloging-in-Publication Data

Names: Uribarri, Jaime, editor. | Calvo, Mona, editor.
Title: Dietary phosphorus : health, nutrition, and regulatory aspects / Jaime
Uribarri and Mona Calvo, editors.
Description: Boca Raton : CRC Press, 2018. | Includes bibliographical references.
Identifiers: LCCN 2017015227 | ISBN 9781498706964 (hardback : alk. paper)
Subjects: LCSH: Food--Phosphorus content. | Phosphorus.
Classification: LCC TX553.P45 D54 2018 | DDC 613.2/85--dc23
LC record available at https://lccn.loc.gov/2017015227

Visit the Taylor & Francis Web site at
http://www.taylorandfrancis.com

and the CRC Press Web site at
http://www.crcpress.com

Contents

Preface...ix
Editor Bios xi
Contributors xiii

SECTION I   Health Issues Associated with Dietary Phosphorus Intake

Chapter 1   Overview of Chronic Health Risks Associated with Phosphorus Excess....................3

Swati Mehta and Jaime Uribarri

Chapter 2   Preclinical Evidence of the Nonskeletal Adverse Health Effects of High Dietary Phosphorus 13

George R. Beck, Jr.

Chapter 3   Clinical and Preclinical Evidence of the Skeletal and Vascular Adverse Health Effects of High Dietary Phosphorus 31

Jorge B. Cannata-Andía, Pablo Román-García, Natalia Carrillo-López, and Adriana S. Dusso

Chapter 4   Associations between Phosphorus Intake and Mortality 45

Andrea Galassi, Denis Fouque, and Mario Cozzolino

Chapter 5   Phosphorus Intake and Whole-Body Phosphorus Homeostasis 63

Jaime Uribarri and Man S. Oh

Chapter 6   Endocrine Regulation of Phosphate Homeostasis.. 71

Marta Christov and Harald Jüppner

Chapter 7   Dietary Phosphorus Intake and Kidney Function.. 83

Lili Chan and Jaime Uribarri

Chapter 8   Dietary Phosphorus Intake and Cardiotoxicity.. 93

Sven-Jean Tan and Nigel D. Toussaint

Chapter 9   The Relationship between Phosphorus Intake and Blood Pressure 111

Melissa M. Melough and Alex R. Chang

vi Contents

Chapter 10 Phosphorus Intake Contribution to Dietary Acid–Base Balance
and Bone Health 125

Tanis R. Fenton and David A. Hanley

Chapter 11 Dietary Phosphorus Regulation of Vitamin D Metabolism in the Kidneys 141

Adriana S. Dusso, M. Vittoria Arcidiacono, Natalia Carrillo-López,
and Jorge B. Cannata-Andía

SECTION II Dietary Phosphorus Intake and Nutritional Needs

Chapter 12 Phosphorus: An Essential Nutrient for Bone Health Throughout Life 155

Jean-Philippe Bonjour

Chapter 13 Dietary Phosphate Needs in Early Life and Adolescence....................................... 167

Alicia M. Diaz-Thomas, Russell W. Chesney, and Craig B. Langman

Chapter 14 Overview of Phosphorus-Wasting Diseases and Need for Phosphorus
Supplements 185

Carolyn M. Macica

Chapter 15 Phosphate and Calcium Stone Formation 201

Hans-Göran Tiselius

Chapter 16 Impact of Socioeconomic Factors on Phosphorus Balance 213

Orlando M. Gutiérrez

Chapter 17 Bioavailability of Phosphorus 221

Suvi T. Itkonen, Heini J. Karp, and Christel J. E. Lamberg-Allardt

Chapter 18 Special Nutritional Needs of Chronic Kidney and End-Stage Renal Disease
Patients: Rationale for the Use of Plant-Based Diets 235

Ranjani N. Moorthi and Sharon M. Moe

SECTION III Food and Environmental Use and Regulation of Phosphorus

Chapter 19 The Regulatory Aspects of Phosphorus Intake: Dietary Guidelines and Labeling.... 249

Mona S. Calvo and Susan J. Whiting

Contents

Chapter 20 Dietary Guidelines for Safe Levels of Phosphorus Intake in North America and Europe 267

Susan J. Whiting and Mona S. Calvo

Chapter 21 Phosphorus Food Additive Use in the European Union 279

Ray J. Winger

Chapter 22 A European Perspective: Questionable Safety of Current Phosphorus Intakes in the General Healthy and Chronic Kidney Disease Populations 313

Kai M. Hahn, Markus Ketteler, and Eberhard Ritz

Chapter 23 Save the P(ee)! The Challenges of Phosphorus Sustainability and Emerging Solutions 327

James J. Elser, Neng Ion Chan, Jessica R. Corman, and Jared Stolzfus

Chapter 24 The Effects of Changing Global Food Choices on Human Health and a Sustainable Supply of Phosphorus 341

Charles J. Ferro

Index 353

Preface

Phosphorus is an essential nutrient serving as a component of the cell membranes, the endocellular and external support components, cell energy cycles, and the molecules and enzymes that encode and regulate all genetic and synthetic information, as well as a multitude of other metabolic pathways critical to all life forms—both plant and animal. Indeed, life cannot exist without a sustained source of phosphorus; yet in Western nations, we waste a great deal of this nonrenewable nutrient as it passes from farm to fork, through human and animal food consumption and ultimately excretion and loss to the environment. This book deals with three important features of the prevailing cycle of human phosphorus use that is emerging as potentially damaging to human and environmental health. In each of the 24 chapters, the expert contributing authors take a closer look at specific aspects of these features, which concern the serious life-threatening disease consequences of excessive phosphorus intake in vulnerable groups, the never-ending need to secure adequate phosphorus intake over all stages of life, and the negative and disruptive influence of human activities involving the use of phosphorus in food production. Many believe these activities have led to agricultural mismanagement of the environment and unconstrained, widespread use of phosphorus in agricultural food production and the processing of food.

Experts in a variety of scientific and medical fields have come together in this book to carefully examine how higher consumption levels of this essential nutrient, phosphorus, which are beyond an individual's physiologic requirements, affect higher serum phosphorus concentrations shown to be significantly associated with a high incidence of morbidity and mortality in North America and Europe. Nephrologists and renal dietitians involved in the care of chronic kidney disease (CKD) patients have long been aware of the serious health risks associated with the body's retention of dietary phosphorus as the decline in renal function progresses with the inability to restrict phosphorus intake. Much of what is known about the damaging effects of elevated serum phosphorus and its link to bone, cardiovascular, and even the progression of kidney disease itself stems from studies focusing on dietary phosphorus intake in CKD. For a growing number of older individuals with failing kidneys—an estimated 26 million in America alone—total phosphorus intake must be delicately balanced between what the body needs for maintenance and the inability to efficiently excrete phosphorus. This is an increasingly difficult balance to maintain given the current high levels of phosphorus in processed foods and limited label information identifying the phosphorus content. The typical Western diet is high in natural sources of phosphorus such as red meat and added phosphorus in the form of inorganic phosphate salts whose use is widespread in industrialized countries to improve taste and other desirable qualities. Mounting evidence stresses the need for mandatory labeling of the phosphorus content of foods to assist in the management of renal disease and the prevention of disease progression. What is an even more compelling reason to label the phosphorus content of foods concerns findings from recent large epidemiological studies suggesting significant associations between mild elevations of serum phosphorus within the normal range and cardiovascular disease risk and increased all-cause mortality in the general healthy population without evidence of impaired kidney function.

The many disease conditions and possible mechanisms of action through which high intakes of phosphorus may bring about increased morbidity and mortality are addressed in the first two sections of this book. More and more studies show dietary phosphorus intakes in excess of the nutrient needs of the healthy population may significantly disrupt the hormonal regulation of phosphorus, calcium, and vitamin D. The disrupted hormonal balance when phosphorus accumulates in serum and the adverse health effects of this hormone dysregulation involving parathyroid hormone, bone-derived fibroblast growth factor-23, and the active form of vitamin D, 1-25-dihydroxyvitamin D, are discussed in detail in several chapters. Other chapters address the increased need of dietary phosphorus due to inborn errors of metabolism or natural nutrient demands of growth or aging. The great variability in the rate and efficiency of phosphorus absorption from different food sources and how application of these differences in bioavailability may enable the effective use of plant-rich dietary patterns to lower dietary phosphorus intake in CKD and dialysis patients are also addressed.

The third section of the book takes a closer look at the dietary guidelines that identify how much phosphorus the general Canadian, American, and European Union populations need to consume each day, how much is actually consumed, how foods are labeled for the general public to know if they are consuming enough based on these dietary guidelines, and how our current dietary patterns and methods of food processing affect the actual amount of phosphorus consumed. Chapters in this section explain the widespread use of phosphate-containing food additives on both continents, the concerns brought about by their use in an endless variety of foods, the existence of reasonable evidence for health risks from seemingly unlimited use of these phosphate additives in food, and most important, how all of these affect the environment and our ability to sustain sources of phosphorus. In North America and now in Europe, there is growing evidence that our dominant and preferred dietary patterns or food choices, methods of food processing, and agricultural practices waste and permanently lose phosphorus at various points in the production and consumption of food. Such loss to the environment is now creating problems by polluting our rivers, lakes, and oceans with phosphorus, causing algal overgrowth and fish die-offs. There clearly is a phosphorus dilemma facing the human and environmental health of Western nations, and the contents of this book will hopefully bring these issues to light for the sake of future generations.

Jaime Uribarri, MD
Mona S. Calvo, PhD

Editor Bios

Jaime Uribarri, MD Dr. Jaime Uribarri is a physician and clinical investigator. He was born in Chile and received his medical degree from the University of Chile School of Medicine, Santiago, Chile. He did all his postgraduate training in the United States. He has been in The Icahn School of Medicine at Mount Sinai, New York, since 1990, where he is currently Professor of Medicine and Director of the Renal Clinic and the Home Dialysis Program at the Mount Sinai Hospital.

In parallel with his clinical activities, Dr. Uribarri has been very active in clinical investigation for the past 30 years. His main areas of research have been on acid–base and fluid and electrolyte disorders, as well as nutrition in chronic kidney disease and diabetic patients. He was one of the first to bring attention to the important role of food-derived advanced glycation end products (AGEs) in chronic diseases in humans. He has published over 150 peer-reviewed papers and written many chapters in books. He has lectured extensively on these research topics in New York City, as well as in national and international meetings. He serves as an ad hoc referee for numerous nutrition, medical, and other scientific journals, and he is an active member of several health organizations and professional associations, including The American Society of Nephrology, The American Society of Nutrition, The International Society of Nephrology, The New York Academy of Sciences, and The Maillard Society.

Mona S. Calvo, PhD After earning a doctorate in Nutritional Sciences from the University of Illinois, Champaign-Urbana, Dr. Calvo pursued postdoctoral studies in the Endocrine Research Unit of the Mayo Clinic in Rochester, Minnesota. Recently retired from the Food and Drug Administration (FDA) after 28 years, her former position and title was that of Expert Regulatory Review Scientist and Research Principal Investigator at the FDA's Center for Food Safety and Applied Nutrition. Her current and past research interests focus on dietary influences on the hormonal regulation of calcium, phosphorus, and vitamin D and their impact on bone and kidney disease and other chronic diseases of public health significance. These research interests have been the topics for over 150 peer-reviewed manuscripts, book chapters, government reports/guidelines, FDA regulations, and abstracts presented at national and international meetings. She serves as an Associate Editor for *Public Health Nutrition*; an ad hoc referee for numerous nutrition, medical, and other scientific journals; and is a member of the Endocrine Society, American Society for Nutrition, the Nutrition Society (UK), and the American Society for Bone and Mineral Research and serves as a member of the advisory board for ODIN (an organization that seeks food-based solutions for optimal vitamin D nutrition and healthy through the life cycle), which seeks food-based solutions for optimal vitamin D nutrition and health through the life cycle.

Contributors

M. Vittoria Arcidiacono, PhD
Department of Morphology
Surgery and Experimental Medicine and
 LTTA Centre
University of Ferrara
Ferrara, Italy

George R. Beck, Jr., PhD
Division of Endocrinology
Department of Medicine
Emory University School of Medicine
Atlanta, Georgia

Jean-Philippe Bonjour, MD
Division of Bone Diseases
University Hospital
Geneva, Switzerland

Mona S. Calvo, PhD
Retired, Expert Regulatory Review Scientist
Center for Food Safety and Applied Nutrition
FDA
Laurel, Maryland

Jorge B. Cannata-Andía, MD, PhD
Bone and Mineral Research Unit
Hospital Universitario Central de Asturias
Asturias, Spain

Natalia Carrillo-López, PhD
Bone and Mineral Research Unit
Hospital Universitario Central de Asturias
Asturias, Spain

Lili Chan, MD
The Icahn School of Medicine at Mount Sinai
New York, NY

Neng Iong Chan
School of Life Sciences
Arizona State University
Tempe, Arizona

Alex R. Chang, MD
Nephrology
Geisinger Medical Center
Danville, Pennsylvania

Russell W. Chesney, MD (deceased)
Pediatrics
The University of Tennessee Health
 Science Center
Memphis, Tennessee

Marta Christov, MD, PhD
Department of Medicine
New York Medical College
Valhalla, New York

Jessica R. Corman, PhD
Center for Limnology
University of Wisconsin
Madison, Wisconsin

Mario Cozzolino, MD, PhD
Renal Unit
San Paolo Hospital Milan
Department of Health and Science
University of Milan
Milan, Italy

Alicia M. Diaz-Thomas, MD
Pediatrics
The University of Tennessee Health
 Science Center
Memphis, Tennessee

Adriana S. Dusso, PhD
Bone and Mineral Research Unit
Hospital Universitario Central de Asturias
Asturias, Spain

James J. Elser, PhD
School of Life Sciences
Arizona State University
Tempe, Arizona

Tanis R. Fenton, PhD
Department of Community Health Sciences
Alberta Children's Hospital Research Institute
O'Brien Institute for Public Health
Cumming School of Medicine
University of Calgary
Calgary, Alberta, Canada

Charles J. Ferro, MD
Nephrology
Queen Elizabeth Hospital and University of
Birmingham
Birmingham, United Kingdom

Denis Fouque, MD, PhD
Service de Néphrologie-Dialyse-Nutrition
Centre Hospitalier LYON-SUD
Lyon, France

Andrea Galassi, MD
Renal and Dialysis Unit
ASST Monza
Desio, Italy

Orlando M. Gutiérrez, MD
University of Alabama at Birmingham
Birmingham, Alabama

Kai M. Hahn, MD
Nephrologische Gemeinschaftspraxis/Dialyse
Dortmund, Germany

David A. Hanley, MD
Medical Director
Grace Osteoporosis Centre, Professor
Division of Endocrinology and Metabolism
University of Calgary
Calgary, Alberta, Canada

Suvi T. Itkonen, PhD
Department of Food and Environmental
Sciences
University of Helsinki
Helsinki, Finland

Harald Jüppner, MD
Professor of Pediatrics
Massachusetts General Hospital
Harvard University
Boston, Massachusetts

Heini J. Karp, PhD
Hyvinkää Hospital
The Hospital District of Helsinki and Uusimaa
Hyvinkää, Finland

Markus Ketteler, MD
Department of Medicine II: Nephrology
Klinikum Coburg GmbH
Coburg, Germany

Christel J. E. Lamberg-Allardt, PhD
Professor and Head
Department of Food and Environmental
Sciences
University of Helsinki
Helsinki, Finland

Craig B. Langman, MD
Pediatrics
Feinberg School of Medicine
Northwestern University
Chicago, Illinois

Carolyn M. Macica, PhD
Department of Medical Sciences
Frank Netter School of Medicine at Quinnipiac
University
North Haven, Conneticut

Swati Mehta, MD
Assistant Professor of Medicine
Division of Nephrology and Hypertension
Albany Medical Center
Albany, New York

Melissa M. Melough, RD
Department of Nutritional Sciences
University of Connecticut
Mansfield, Connecticut

Sharon M. Moe, MD
Professor of Medicine, Director
Division of Nephrology
Department of Medicine
Indiana University School of Medicine
Indianapolis, Indiana

Ranjani N. Moorthi, MD
Department of Medicine
Indiana University School of Medicine
Indianapolis, Indiana

Man S. Oh, MD
Professor of Medicine
SUNY Downstate Medical Center
Brooklyn, New York

Eberhard Ritz, MD
Department of Nephrology
Ruprecht-Karls-University Heidelberg
Heidelberg, Germany

Contributors

Pablo Román-García, PhD
Bone and Mineral Research Unit
Hospital Universitario Central de Asturias
Asturias, Spain

Jared Stoltzfus
School of Sustainability
Arizona State University
Tempe, Arizona

Sven-Jean Tan, MBBS, FRACP, PhD
Department of Nephrology
The Royal Melbourne Hospital
Parkville, Victoria, Australia

Hans-Göran Tiselius, MD
Division of Urology
Department of Clinical Science
Intervention and Technology
Karolinska Institutet
Stockholm, Sweden

Nigel D. Toussaint, MBBS, FRACP, PhD
Department of Nephrology
The Royal Melbourne Hospital
Parkville, Victoria, Australia

Jaime Uribarri, MD
Professor of Medicine
The Icahn School of Medicine at Mount Sinai
New York City, New York

Susan J. Whiting, PhD
Professor of Nutrition and Dietetics
College of Pharmacy and Nutrition
University of Saskatchewan
Saskatoon, Saskatchewan, Canada

Ray J. Winger, PhD
Managing Director
Inside Foods Limited
London, United Kingdom

Section I

Health Issues Associated with Dietary Phosphorus Intake

1 Overview of Chronic Health Risks Associated with Phosphorus Excess

Swati Mehta and Jaime Uribarri

CONTENTS

Abstract 3
Bullet Points 3
1.1 Introduction 4
1.2 Chronic Health Risks Associated with Phosphorus Excess 4
    1.2.1 Progression of Chronic Kidney Disease 4
    1.2.2 Mineral Bone Disease and Soft Tissue Calcifications 4
    1.2.3 Cardiovascular Disease 5
    1.2.4 Mortality 7
    1.2.5 Increased Anemia Risk 7
    1.2.6 Increased Cancer Risk 8
1.3 Conclusions 8
References 8

ABSTRACT

Although phosphorus is an essential nutrient, in excess it could be linked to tissue damage by a variety of mechanisms resulting from either direct precipitation with calcium or secondary to excess of hormonal factors involved in its endocrine regulation, specifically the secretion and action of fibroblast growth factor 23 and parathyroid hormone. This excess phosphorus has been associated with disordered mineral metabolism, vascular calcifications, cardiovascular disease, chronic kidney disease, and bone loss. This chapter explores many of chronic health risks that have been associated with excess phosphorus in patients with chronic kidney disease, as well as in healthy individuals.

BULLET POINTS

- Although phosphorus is an essential nutrient, its excess can produce chronic disease through a variety of mechanisms.
- Excess phosphorus was originally thought to be important only in chronic kidney disease patients, but newer information suggests it cannot be ignored even for people with normal kidney function.
- For many decades excess phosphorus has been recognized as an important factor in inducing bone mineral disease and soft tissue calcifications.
- Nowadays, excess phosphorus has also been strongly associated with cardiovascular disease and all-cause mortality.
- Recently, attention has been called to even less recognized potential associations with excess phosphorus, including cancer.

1.1 INTRODUCTION

Recently, there has been growing epidemiological evidence linking higher serum phosphate concentrations to cardiovascular disease (CVD), and this association is not only seen in the chronic kidney disease (CKD) population, but it has also been identified in the general population. Although phosphorus is an essential nutrient, its excess could be linked to tissue damage by a variety of mechanisms, some of which are normally involved in endocrine regulation of extracellular phosphate, including parathyroid hormone (PTH) and fibroblast growth factor 23 (FGF23). Moreover, there is increasing concern regarding the growing consumption in most modern societies of foods whose processing includes phosphate additives. Both animal and clinical studies have shown that a diet high in phosphorus can induce secondary hyperparathyroidism, bone loss, and FGF23 release from bone, and both PTH and FGF23 are thought to have pathogenic cardiovascular effects. Even a potential association between excess phosphorus in the diet and cancer has recently been suspected. The focus of this chapter is to discuss in depth the many chronic health risks associated with excess dietary phosphorus both in CKD patients and in the healthy population.

1.2 CHRONIC HEALTH RISKS ASSOCIATED WITH PHOSPHORUS EXCESS

1.2.1 PROGRESSION OF CHRONIC KIDNEY DISEASE

It has been shown that hyperphosphatemia is associated with rapid progression of established CKD (Voormolen et al. 2007) and development of end-stage renal disease (ESRD) (Schwarz et al. 2006). This could be in part explained by development of vascular calcifications induced by elevated phosphorus levels (Ferro et al. 2009). Hyperphosphatemia may directly stimulate arterial calcification via upregulation of core binding factor a-1 in vascular smooth muscle cells (Moe & Chen 2008). Higher calcium–phosphorus product is also associated with more progressive CKD, supporting the hypothesis that tissue calcification (nephrocalcinosis) may be the underlying mechanism. Another proposed mechanism is a role of intracellular phosphate level on podocyte function; for example, transgenic overexpression of type III P (i) transporter Pit-1 in rats induced phosphate-dependent podocyte injury and damage to the glomerular barrier, which resulted in the progression of glomerular sclerosis in the kidney (Sekiguchi et al. 2011).

A prospective study conducted on 2269 participants free of CKD showed that serum phosphate level in the upper-normal range at baseline was associated with doubling in the risk of developing incident CKD and ESRD (O'Seaghdha et al. 2011). Restriction of protein and phosphorus intake early in the course of renal failure has been shown to delay progression of renal failure, presumably not only by prevention of hyperfiltration and histologic lesions in surviving lesions, but also by prevention of secondary hyperparathyroidism and maintenance of a normal calcium–phosphate product (Maschio et al. 1982). FGF23 levels that increase in parallel with deterioration of renal function, along with an increase in serum phosphorus and PTH concentrations, have also been shown to be an independent predictor of progression of renal disease in patients with nondiabetic CKD (Fliser et al. 2007).

1.2.2 MINERAL BONE DISEASE AND SOFT TISSUE CALCIFICATIONS

Whereas the level of free calcium in blood is normally the principal determinant of PTH secretion, disturbances in phosphate metabolism and calcitriol also play an important role in development of secondary hyperparathyroidism during the course of CKD. In advanced CKD hyperphosphatemia stimulates PTH secretion directly and indirectly by inducing hypocalcemia, skeletal resistance to PTH, and low levels of calcitriol.

Hyperphosphatemia has direct effects on the parathyroid gland to increase PTH secretion and parathyroid cell growth (Naveh-Many et al. 1995; Denda, Finch, and Slatopolsky 1996). A study in experimental animals with advanced renal failure demonstrated that dietary phosphorus restriction to normalize plasma phosphate concentration lowered the plasma PTH concentrations from 130 to 35 pg/mL (Slatopolsky et al. 1996). This occurred without changes in plasma calcium or calcitriol concentration. Parathyroid size also decreased in these animals, suggesting that hyperphosphatemia stimulates parathyroid growth directly in renal failure (Naveh-Many et al. 1995). These observations may be applicable to humans as well; one study showed that hyperplastic parathyroid tissue obtained from patients with renal failure exposed in vitro to high phosphate concentrations increased prepro-PTH mRNA and enhanced PTH secretion (Almaden et al. 1998). Clinically, hyperparathyroidism is associated with the development of osteitis fibrosa cystica. In this form of bone disease there is increased osteoclast and osteoblast activity along with peritrabecular fibrosis. This high bone turnover disease can manifest clinically as nonspecific aches and pains in bones and joints such as lower back, hips, and legs. Pain around joints may also be caused by acute periarthritis, which is associated with periarticular deposition of calcium phosphate crystals. Radiologically, the disease may be suggested by subperiosteal bone resorption, which can be detected in hands, clavicles, and pelvis. Skull radiographs may show focal areas of radiolucency and a ground glass appearance, an appearance known as pepper pot skull. More rarely, brown tumors—focal collections of giant cells—are seen, as well demarcated radiolucent zones in long bones, clavicles, and digits.

Calcific uremic arteriolopathy (CUA), or calciphylaxis, is an uncommon lesion characterized by calcification of small arterioles that occurs most commonly, although not exclusively, in ESRD patients. The clinical incidence of this disorder appears to have been increasing recently. Hyperparathyroidism, active vitamin D administration, hyperphosphatemia, and elevated calcium–phosphate product are all implicated in the pathogenesis of CUA (Ahmed et al. 2001). The histologic analysis of calcified tissue also suggests that the calcification is associated with increased expression of osteopontin by smooth muscle cells. Clinical manifestations include violaceous, painful, plaque-like subcutaneous nodules, which progress to ischemic/necrotic ulcers with eschars that often become superinfected. Lesions classically develop on areas with greatest adiposity, including abdomen, buttock, and thigh (Bhambri and Del Rosso 2008).

1.2.3 Cardiovascular Disease

High serum phosphate levels have been linked to higher rates of cardiovascular events or CVD-related mortality in CKD patients (Voormolen et al. 2007; Kestenbaum et al. 2005), in patients on hemodialysis (Block et al. 1998), and in the general population (Dhingra et al. 2007). Various studies have shown that higher phosphate levels are independently associated with stroke, fatal and non-fatal myocardial infarction (Tonelli et al. 2005), and congestive heart failure (Tonelli et al. 2005).

One of the potential mechanisms leading to increased CVD is direct vascular calcification (Sigrist et al. 2007). This calcification can occur in either intima or media of blood vessels and will lead to decreased arterial wall elasticity and impeded blood flow, which can result in myocardial infarction and stroke.

Vascular calcification can be induced in rat models by high-phosphate diets (El-Abbadi et al. 2009) and could also be induced in other experimental settings by causing hyperphosphatemia either by genetic deletion of klotho or FGF23 (Shimada et al. 2004; Hu et al. 2011). High phosphate concentrations stimulated apoptosis of vascular smooth muscle cells and caused overt calcification (Shroff et al. 2010); when human vascular smooth muscle cells were incubated in high-phosphate–containing media they underwent transition to a mineralizing phenotype (Jono et al. 2000). It has also been shown that deletion of NaPi-2a normalized serum phosphate levels and reversed calcification in klotho-deficient mice that initially exhibited severe hyperphosphatemia (Razzaque 2009). The role of FGF23 in vascular calcification has not been studied as extensively as that of phosphate. Studies in vitro indicate that FGF23 does not potentiate calcification in human vascular smooth muscle cells or mouse aortic rings under normal or high-phosphate conditions, nor does it potentiate intracellular uptake of phosphate even in vascular smooth muscle cells incubated with soluble klotho (Scialla et al. 2013).

Data from epidemiological studies further support high serum phosphate as a risk factor for vascular calcification in humans. In a community-based cohort of individuals with CKD and no clinically apparent CVD, higher serum phosphate concentrations within normal laboratory ranges were associated with a statistically greater prevalence of coronary artery, descending thoracic aorta, and mitral valve calcification. These associations were independent of traditional atherosclerosis risk factors, estimated kidney function, and measured dietary variables (Adeney et al. 2009). An association of high serum phosphate levels with valvular calcification and sclerosis (Linefsky et al. 2011) has also been shown, and these anatomical changes have been linked with functional measures of calcification such as increased peripheral arterial stiffness indicated by ankle brachial pressure index score greater than 1.30 (Kendrick et al. 2010). There have been conflicting results regarding the role of FGF23 levels and vascular calcification, but one of the larger vascular calcification studies with approximately 1500 participants with CKD stage 2 to 4 reported that higher serum phosphate, but not FGF23 levels, were associated with increased prevalence and severity of coronary artery calcification, independent of traditional CVD risk factors (Scialla et al. 2013). This finding was consistent with the in vitro data and strongly favors elevated serum levels of phosphate, but not FGF23, as a major risk factor for vascular calcification in CKD.

Another possible mechanism leading to increased cardiovascular events is related to endothelial dysfunction and atherosclerosis (Ruan et al. 2010). Animal studies suggest that high intracellular phosphorus induces endothelial cell dysfunction by various mechanisms, which cause apoptosis (Di Marco et al. 2008), stimulate production of reactive oxygen species (Di Marco et al. 2013), and impair secretion of nitric oxide in response to acetylcholine and inhibits angiogenic behavior (Di Marco et al. 2013). The majority of these effects could be blocked by inhibiting the cellular uptake of phosphorus (Di Marco et al. 2008). These animal studies are further supported by observational studies in humans, which show increased extent of coronary and carotid atherosclerosis with higher serum phosphate levels. One major prospective study done on 3015 healthy young adults showed that baseline serum phosphate levels >1.26 mmol/L (normal range 0.74–1.52 mmol/L) were associated with an increased risk of atherosclerosis, assessed by computed tomography (CT) scans 15 years later (Foley et al. 2009).

To date, there are limited data to determine whether or not an elevation in FGF23 levels clearly precedes the development of atherosclerosis or is simply a marker of established disease (Voigt et al. 2010). In a small observational study of patients with CKD patients stages 3 to 4, but without CVD or diabetes mellitus, higher levels of FGF23 were independently associated with decreased flow-mediated dilatation, which is a noninvasive clinical measure of endothelial function (Yilmaz et al. 2010). Lower FGF23 levels have also been associated with increased endothelium-dependent and endothelium-independent vasodilatation in individuals older than 70 years, most of whom had normal kidney function (Mirza et al. 2009a). Some evidence also suggests that manipulation of dietary phosphorus intake to decrease circulating levels of phosphate or FGF23 may affect cardiovascular risk factors. In a study of 11 healthy adult men, a high-phosphate meal substantially lowered flow-mediated dilatation within 2 hours, compared with a low-phosphate meal. In patients with CKD, lowering of serum phosphate and FGF23 levels, accomplished by 8 weeks of treatment with the phosphate-binding agent, sevelamer, improved flow-mediated dilatation (Yilmaz et al. 2012), but there were different results when a different phosphate binder—calcium acetate—was used. The benefits associated with sevelamer treatment might be due to its more effective lowering of FGF23 or phosphate levels, other pleiotropic effects, or a combination thereof. Therefore more studies are needed to investigate the exact mechanisms underlying how phosphorus homeostasis alters endothelial function and the relative contributions of its many components, including dietary phosphorus intake, serum phosphate levels, FGF23, 1,25(OH)D, PTH, klotho, and perhaps other currently undiscovered factors.

Left ventricular hypertrophy is an established predictor of cardiovascular mortality and all-cause mortality in different patient populations, including CKD (Shlipak et al. 2005). It has been shown

Overview of Chronic Health Risks Associated with Phosphorus Excess

that high phosphorus intake was associated with increased left ventricular mass in a population of healthy individuals (Yamamoto et al. 2013), and as mentioned earlier, increase in dietary phosphorus induces a significant increase in FGF23 (Antoniucci, Yamashita, and Portale 2006). Increasing concentrations of FGF23 stimulate hypertrophic growth of cultured neonatal rat ventricular myocytes and activate the transcription of genes involved in pathological cardiac hypertrophy in animal models (Faul et al. 2011). In clinical studies, high FGF23 levels at baseline are associated with increased left ventricular mass and increased prevalence of left ventricular hypertrophy independent of kidney function or in patients with CKD (Gutierrez et al. 2009; Mirza et al. 2009b; Faul et al. 2011). An association of high phosphate levels and ventricular hypertrophy has also been shown in clinical studies. An observational study in 208 patients with stage 2 to 4 CKD showed that high serum phosphate is associated with increased left ventricular mass in both men and women (Chue et al. 2012). Also, higher serum levels of phosphate are associated with increased prevalence of left ventricular hypertrophy independent of kidney function in a wide variety of settings (Dhingra et al. 2010; Gutierrez et al. 2009). However, these studies have not measured levels of FGF23. Therefore, there is a possibility that undetermined elevation of FGF23 levels could explain the association of high phosphate levels and ventricular hypertrophy and increased ventricular mass. Also high serum phosphate levels can lead to left ventricular hypertrophy indirectly by increasing left ventricular pressure overload, causing reduced vascular compliance and valvular heart diseases as a result of vascular calcification (Adeney et al. 2009; Linefsky et al. 2011).

1.2.4 Mortality

As mentioned earlier, hyperphosphatemia is associated with increased cardiovascular and all-cause mortality in patients with CKD (Kestenbaum et al. 2005) and on chronic hemodialysis (Ganesh et al. 2001). A national study conducted on 7096 hemodialysis patients showed that patients with a serum phosphate level above 6.5 mg/dL had higher mortality, and this risk was independent of intact PTH (Block et al. 1998). Similarly, observational studies on patients with CKD not yet on hemodialysis have also shown that elevated serum phosphate is independently associated with increased mortality risk. A possible mechanism explaining this association could be vascular calcification (Goodman et al. 2000; Raggi et al. 2002). Phosphate excess may also affect mortality by increasing circulating levels of PTH. Indeed, clinical studies on chronic hemodialysis patients have documented an association between excess PTH and all-cause mortality (Ganesh et al. 2001). Excess FGF23 has also been associated with increased mortality in CKD patients. More recently, researchers in South Korea concluded in a study done on 92,756 individuals at three tertiary centers with a mean follow-up of 75 months that higher serum phosphate level predicts increased mortality among men, but not in women, with normal kidney function, a very interesting finding (Yoo et al. 2016).

1.2.5 Increased Anemia Risk

An association between hyperphosphatemia and anemia has been suggested for CKD and ESRD patients. Erythropoietin deficiency, inflammation, and oxidative stress have been implicated as potential factors linking the phosphate levels and anemia. High serum phosphate leads to higher polyamines production, which can function as uremic toxins inhibiting erythropoiesis (Kovesdy et al. 2011). Moreover, high PTH and FGF23 seen in CKD and ESRD may play a role by directly inhibiting erythropoiesis (Rao, Shih, and Mohini 1993; Sim et al. 2010). Moreover, a recent study on 155,974 adult individuals showed that an increment of 0.5 mg/dL in phosphorus level was associated with a significant 16% increased risk for moderate anemia, not only in patients with mild CKD but also in patients with normal kidney function. The authors postulated that FGF23, induced by high phosphate, might have a role in the mechanism underlying the association between hyperphosphatemia and anemia (Tran et al. 2016).

1.2.6 Increased Cancer Risk

Inorganic phosphates used in food processing have been identified as a potential cancer-modifying factor, mostly through in vitro cell-based studies and in vivo murine cancer models (Camalier et al. 2013). High phosphorus concentrations in cell cultures have been shown to directly activate specific metabolic pathways that promote cell transformation and tumorigenesis in skin and lungs (Camalier et al. 2010, 2013; Jin et al. 2007, 2009). Moreover, inorganic phosphate consumption has been shown to regulate osteopontin, which in turn can induce cancer cell–mediated angiogenesis that would enhance tumor growth (Beck and Knecht 2003).

Recently, several epidemiological studies suggest an association between inorganic phosphate and cancer risks. In a recent 24-year follow-up study of the association between phosphate intake and advanced stage and high-grade prostate cancer, an independent associated increased risk of advanced stage and high-grade disease 0 to 8 years after exposure was reported (Wilson et al. 2015).

1.3 CONCLUSIONS

Hyperphosphatemia appears to be a major cause of morbidity and mortality in patients with CKD or ESRD, and these risks might also be extended to the general population. Efforts should be made to timely recognize the health risks associated with phosphorus excess in order to implement preventive and treatment therapies for the same.

REFERENCES

Adeney, K. L., D. S. Siscovick, J. H. Ix, S. L. Seliger, M. G. Shlipak, N. S. Jenny, and B. R. Kestenbaum. 2009. Association of serum phosphate with vascular and valvular calcification in moderate CKD. *J Am Soc Nephrol* 20 (2):381–7. doi:10.1681/ASN.2008040349.

Ahmed, S., K. D. O'Neill, A. F. Hood, A. P. Evan, and S. M. Moe. 2001. Calciphylaxis is associated with hyperphosphatemia and increased osteopontin expression by vascular smooth muscle cells. *Am J Kidney Dis* 37 (6):1267–76.

Almaden, Y., A. Hernandez, V. Torregrosa, A. Canalejo, L. Sabate, L. Fernandez Cruz, J. M. Campistol, A. Torres, and M. Rodriguez. 1998. High phosphate level directly stimulates parathyroid hormone secretion and synthesis by human parathyroid tissue in vitro. *J Am Soc Nephrol* 9 (10):1845–52.

Antoniucci, D. M., T. Yamashita, and A. A. Portale. 2006. Dietary phosphorus regulates serum fibroblast growth factor-23 concentrations in healthy men. *J Clin Endocrinol Metab* 91 (8):3144–9. doi:10.1210/jc.2006-0021.

Beck, G. R., Jr. and N. Knecht. 2003. Osteopontin regulation by inorganic phosphate is ERK1/2-, protein kinase C-, and proteasome-dependent. *J Biol Chem* 278 (43):41921–9. doi:10.1074/jbc.M304470200.

Bhambri, A. and J. Q. Del Rosso. 2008. Calciphylaxis: A review. *J Clin Aesthet Dermatol* 1 (2):38–41.

Block, G. A., T. E. Hulbert-Shearon, N. W. Levin, and F. K. Port. 1998. Association of serum phosphorus and calcium x phosphate product with mortality risk in chronic hemodialysis patients: A national study. *Am J Kidney Dis* 31 (4):607–17.

Camalier, C. E., M. Yi, L. R. Yu, B. L. Hood, K. A. Conrads, Y. J. Lee, Y. Lin, L. M. Garneys, G. F. Bouloux, M. R. Young, T. D. Veenstra, R. M. Stephens, N. H. Colburn, T. P. Conrads, and G. R. Beck, Jr. 2013. An integrated understanding of the physiological response to elevated extracellular phosphate. *J Cell Physiol* 228 (7):1536–50. doi:10.1002/jcp.24312.

Camalier, C. E., M. R. Young, G. Bobe, C. M. Perella, N. H. Colburn, and G. R. Beck, Jr. 2010. Elevated phosphate activates N-ras and promotes cell transformation and skin tumorigenesis. *Cancer Prev Res (Phila)* 3 (3):359–70. doi:10.1158/1940-6207.CAPR-09-0068.

Chue, C. D., N. C. Edwards, W. E. Moody, R. P. Steeds, J. N. Townend, and C. J. Ferro. 2012. Serum phosphate is associated with left ventricular mass in patients with chronic kidney disease: A cardiac magnetic resonance study. *Heart* 98 (3):219–24. doi:10.1136/heartjnl-2011-300570.

Denda, M., J. Finch, and E. Slatopolsky. 1996. Phosphorus accelerates the development of parathyroid hyperplasia and secondary hyperparathyroidism in rats with renal failure. *Am J Kidney Dis* 28 (4):596–602.

Dhingra, R., P. Gona, E. J. Benjamin, T. J. Wang, J. Aragam, R. B. D'Agostino, Sr., W. B. Kannel, and R. S. Vasan. 2010. Relations of serum phosphorus levels to echocardiographic left ventricular mass and incidence of heart failure in the community. *Eur J Heart Fail* 12 (8):812–8. doi:10.1093/eurjhf/hfq106.

Overview of Chronic Health Risks Associated with Phosphorus Excess

Dhingra, R., L. M. Sullivan, C. S. Fox, T. J. Wang, R. B. D'Agostino, Sr., J. M. Gaziano, and R. S. Vasan. 2007. Relations of serum phosphorus and calcium levels to the incidence of cardiovascular disease in the community. *Arch Intern Med* 167 (9):879–85. doi:10.1001/archinte.167.9.879.

Di Marco, G. S., M. Hausberg, U. Hillebrand, P. Rustemeyer, W. Wittkowski, D. Lang, and H. Pavenstadt. 2008. Increased inorganic phosphate induces human endothelial cell apoptosis in vitro. *Am J Physiol Renal Physiol* 294 (6):F1381–7. doi:10.1152/ajprenal.00003.2008.

Di Marco, G. S., M. Konig, C. Stock, A. Wiesinger, U. Hillebrand, S. Reiermann, S. Reuter, S. Amler, G. Kohler, F. Buck, M. Fobker, P. Kumpers, H. Oberleithner, M. Hausberg, D. Lang, H. Pavenstadt, and M. Brand. 2013. High phosphate directly affects endothelial function by downregulating annexin II. *Kidney Int* 83 (2):213–22. doi:10.1038/ki.2012.300.

El-Abbadi, M. M., A. S. Pai, E. M. Leaf, H. Y. Yang, B. A. Bartley, K. K. Quan, C. M. Ingalls, H. W. Liao, and C. M. Giachelli. 2009. Phosphate feeding induces arterial medial calcification in uremic mice: Role of serum phosphorus, fibroblast growth factor-23, and osteopontin. *Kidney Int* 75 (12):1297–307. doi:10.1038/ki.2009.83.

Faul, C., A. P. Amaral, B. Oskouei, M. C. Hu, A. Sloan, T. Isakova, O. M. Gutierrez, R. Aguillon-Prada, J. Lincoln, J. M. Hare, P. Mundel, A. Morales, J. Scialla, M. Fischer, E. Z. Soliman, J. Chen, A. S. Go, S. E. Rosas, L. Nessel, R. R. Townsend, H. I. Feldman, M. St John Sutton, A. Ojo, C. Gadegbeku, G. S. Di Marco, S. Reuter, D. Kentrup, K. Tiemann, M. Brand, J. A. Hill, O. W. Moe, O. M. Kuro, J. W. Kusek, M. G. Keane, and M. Wolf. 2011. FGF23 induces left ventricular hypertrophy. *J Clin Invest* 121 (11):4393–408. doi:10.1172/JCI46122.

Ferro, C. J., C. D. Chue, R. P. Steeds, and J. N. Townend. 2009. Is lowering phosphate exposure the key to preventing arterial stiffening with age? *Heart* 95 (21):1770–2. doi:10.1136/hrt.2008.162594.

Fliser, D., B. Kollerits, U. Neyer, D. P. Ankerst, K. Lhotta, A. Lingenhel, E. Ritz, F. Kronenberg, MMKD Study Group, E. Kuen, P. Konig, G. Kraatz, J. F. Mann, G. A. Muller, H. Kohler, and P. Riegler. 2007. Fibroblast growth factor 23 (FGF23) predicts progression of chronic kidney disease: The Mild to Moderate Kidney Disease (MMKD) Study. *J Am Soc Nephrol* 18 (9):2600–8. doi:10.1681/ASN.2006080936.

Foley, R. N., A. J. Collins, C. A. Herzog, A. Ishani, and P. A. Kalra. 2009. Serum phosphorus levels associate with coronary atherosclerosis in young adults. *J Am Soc Nephrol* 20 (2):397–404. doi:10.1681/ASN.2008020141.

Ganesh, S. K., A. G. Stack, N. W. Levin, T. Hulbert-Shearon, and F. K. Port. 2001. Association of elevated serum PO(4), Ca x PO(4) product, and parathyroid hormone with cardiac mortality risk in chronic hemodialysis patients. *J Am Soc Nephrol* 12 (10):2131–8.

Goodman, W. G., J. Goldin, B. D. Kuizon, C. Yoon, B. Gales, D. Sider, Y. Wang, J. Chung, A. Emerick, L. Greaser, R. M. Elashoff, and I. B. Salusky. 2000. Coronary-artery calcification in young adults with end-stage renal disease who are undergoing dialysis. *N Engl J Med* 342 (20):1478–83. doi:10.1056/NEJM200005183422003.

Gutierrez, O. M., J. L. Januzzi, T. Isakova, K. Laliberte, K. Smith, G. Collerone, A. Sarwar, U. Hoffmann, E. Coglianese, R. Christenson, T. J. Wang, C. deFilippi, and M. Wolf. 2009. Fibroblast growth factor 23 and left ventricular hypertrophy in chronic kidney disease. *Circulation* 119 (19):2545–52. doi:10.1161/CIRCULATIONAHA.108.844506.

Hu, M. C., M. Shi, J. Zhang, H. Quinones, C. Griffith, M. Kuro-o, and O. W. Moe. 2011. Klotho deficiency causes vascular calcification in chronic kidney disease. *J Am Soc Nephrol* 22 (1):124–36. doi:10.1681/ASN.2009121311.

Jin, H., S. H. Chang, C. X. Xu, J. Y. Shin, Y. S. Chung, S. J. Park, Y. S. Lee, G. H. An, K. H. Lee, and M. H. Cho. 2007. High dietary inorganic phosphate affects lung through altering protein translation, cell cycle, and angiogenesis in developing mice. *Toxicol Sci* 100 (1):215–23. doi:10.1093/toxsci/kfm202.

Jin, H., C. X. Xu, H. T. Lim, S. J. Park, J. Y. Shin, Y. S. Chung, S. C. Park, S. H. Chang, H. J. Youn, K. H. Lee, Y. S. Lee, Y. C. Ha, C. H. Chae, G. R. Beck, Jr., and M. H. Cho. 2009. High dietary inorganic phosphate increases lung tumorigenesis and alters Akt signaling. *Am J Respir Crit Care Med* 179 (1):59–68. doi:10.1164/rccm.200802-306OC.

Jono, S., M. D. McKee, C. E. Murry, A. Shioi, Y. Nishizawa, K. Mori, H. Morii, and C. M. Giachelli. 2000. Phosphate regulation of vascular smooth muscle cell calcification. *Circ Res* 87 (7):E10–7.

Kendrick, J., J. H. Ix, G. Targher, G. Smits, and M. Chonchol. 2010. Relation of serum phosphorus levels to ankle brachial pressure index (from the Third National Health and Nutrition Examination Survey). *Am J Cardiol* 106 (4):564–8. doi:10.1016/j.amjcard.2010.03.070.

Kestenbaum, B., J. N. Sampson, K. D. Rudser, D. J. Patterson, S. L. Seliger, B. Young, D. J. Sherrard, and D. L. Andress. 2005. Serum phosphate levels and mortality risk among people with chronic kidney disease. *J Am Soc Nephrol* 16 (2):520–8. doi:10.1681/ASN.2004070602.

Kovesdy, C. P., I. Mucsi, M. E. Czira, A. Rudas, A. Ujszaszi, L. Rosivall, S. J. Kim, M. Wolf, and M. Z. Molnar. 2011. Association of serum phosphorus level with anemia in kidney transplant recipients. *Transplantation* 91 (8):875–82. doi:10.1097/TP.0b013e3182111edf.

Linefsky, J. P., K. D. O'Brien, R. Katz, I. H. de Boer, E. Barasch, N. S. Jenny, D. S. Siscovick, and B. Kestenbaum. 2011. Association of serum phosphate levels with aortic valve sclerosis and annular calcification: The cardiovascular health study. *J Am Coll Cardiol* 58 (3):291–7. doi:10.1016/j.jacc.2010.11.073.

Maschio, G., L. Oldrizzi, N. Tessitore, A. D'Angelo, E. Valvo, A. Lupo, C. Loschiavo, A. Fabris, L. Gammaro, C. Rugiu, and G. Panzetta. 1982. Effects of dietary protein and phosphorus restriction on the progression of early renal failure. *Kidney Int* 22 (4):371–6.

Mirza, M. A., A. Larsson, L. Lind, and T. E. Larsson. 2009a. Circulating fibroblast growth factor-23 is associated with vascular dysfunction in the community. *Atherosclerosis* 205 (2):385–90. doi:10.1016/j.atherosclerosis.2009.01.001.

Mirza, M. A., A. Larsson, H. Melhus, L. Lind, and T. E. Larsson. 2009b. Serum intact FGF23 associate with left ventricular mass, hypertrophy and geometry in an elderly population. *Atherosclerosis* 207 (2):546–51. doi:10.1016/j.atherosclerosis.2009.05.013.

Moe, S. M. and N. X. Chen. 2008. Mechanisms of vascular calcification in chronic kidney disease. *J Am Soc Nephrol* 19 (2):213–6. doi:10.1681/ASN.2007080854.

Naveh-Many, T., R. Rahamimov, N. Livni, and J. Silver. 1995. Parathyroid cell proliferation in normal and chronic renal failure rats. *The effects of calcium, phosphate, and vitamin D. J Clin Invest* 96 (4):1786–93. doi:10.1172/JCI118224.

O'Seaghdha, C. M., S. J. Hwang, P. Muntner, M. L. Melamed, and C. S. Fox. 2011. Serum phosphorus predicts incident chronic kidney disease and end-stage renal disease. *Nephrol Dial Transplant* 26 (9):2885–90. doi:10.1093/ndt/gfq808.

Raggi, P., A. Boulay, S. Chasan-Taber, N. Amin, M. Dillon, S. K. Burke, and G. M. Chertow. 2002. Cardiac calcification in adult hemodialysis patients. *A link between end-stage renal disease and cardiovascular disease? J Am Coll Cardiol* 39 (4):695–701.

Rao, D. S., M. S. Shih, and R. Mohini. 1993. Effect of serum parathyroid hormone and bone marrow fibrosis on the response to erythropoietin in uremia. *N Engl J Med* 328 (3):171–5. doi:10.1056/NEJM199301213280304.

Razzaque, M. S. 2009. The FGF23-Klotho axis: Endocrine regulation of phosphate homeostasis. *Nat Rev Endocrinol* 5 (11):611–9. doi:10.1038/nrendo.2009.196.

Ruan, L., W. Chen, S. R. Srinivasan, J. Xu, A. Toprak, and G. S. Berenson. 2010. Relation of serum phosphorus levels to carotid intima-media thickness in asymptomatic young adults (from the Bogalusa Heart Study). *Am J Cardiol* 106 (6):793–7. doi:10.1016/j.amjcard.2010.05.004.

Schwarz, S., B. K. Trivedi, K. Kalantar-Zadeh, and C. P. Kovesdy. 2006. Association of disorders in mineral metabolism with progression of chronic kidney disease. *Clin J Am Soc Nephrol* 1 (4):825–31. doi:10.2215/CJN.02101205.

Scialla, J. J., W. L. Lau, M. P. Reilly, T. Isakova, H. Y. Yang, M. H. Crouthamel, N. W. Chavkin, M. Rahman, P. Wahl, A. P. Amaral, T. Hamano, S. R. Master, L. Nessel, B. Chai, D. Xie, R. R. Kallem, J. Chen, J. P. Lash, J. W. Kusek, M. J. Budoff, C. M. Giachelli, M. Wolf, and Investigators Chronic Renal Insufficiency Cohort Study. 2013. Fibroblast growth factor 23 is not associated with and does not induce arterial calcification. *Kidney Int* 83 (6):1159–68. doi:10.1038/ki.2013.3.

Sekiguchi, S., A. Suzuki, S. Asano, K. Nishiwaki-Yasuda, M. Shibata, S. Nagao, N. Yamamoto, M. Matsuyama, Y. Sato, K. Yan, E. Yaoita, and M. Itoh. 2011. Phosphate overload induces podocyte injury via type III Na-dependent phosphate transporter. *Am J Physiol Renal Physiol* 300 (4):F848–56. doi:10.1152/ajprenal.00334.2010.

Shimada, T., M. Kakitani, Y. Yamazaki, H. Hasegawa, Y. Takeuchi, T. Fujita, S. Fukumoto, K. Tomizuka, and T. Yamashita. 2004. Targeted ablation of Fgf23 demonstrates an essential physiological role of FGF23 in phosphate and vitamin D metabolism. *J Clin Invest* 113 (4):561–8. doi:10.1172/JCI19081.

Shlipak, M. G., L. F. Fried, M. Cushman, T. A. Manolio, D. Peterson, C. Stehman-Breen, A. Bleyer, A. Newman, D. Siscovick, and B. Psaty. 2005. Cardiovascular mortality risk in chronic kidney disease: Comparison of traditional and novel risk factors. *JAMA* 293 (14):1737–45. doi:10.1001/jama.293.14.1737.

Shroff, R. C., R. McNair, J. N. Skepper, N. Figg, L. J. Schurgers, L. Deanfield, L. Rees, and C. M. Shanahan. 2010. Chronic mineral dysregulation promotes vascular smooth muscle cell adaptation and extracellular matrix calcification. *J Am Soc Nephrol* 21 (1):103–12. doi:10.1681/ASN.2009060640.

Sigrist, M. K., M. W. Taal, P. Bungay, and C. W. McIntyre. 2007. Progressive vascular calcification over 2 years is associated with arterial stiffening and increased mortality in patients with stages 4 and 5 chronic kidney disease. *Clin J Am Soc Nephrol* 2 (6):1241–8. doi:10.2215/CJN.02190507.

Sim, J. J., P. T. Lac, I. L. Liu, S. O. Meguerditchian, V. A. Kumar, D. A. Kujubu, and S. A. Rasgon. 2010. Vitamin D deficiency and anemia: A cross-sectional study. *Ann Hematol* 89 (5):447–52. doi:10.1007/s00277-009-0850-3.

Slatopolsky, E., J. Finch, M. Denda, C. Ritter, M. Zhong, A. Dusso, P. N. MacDonald, and A. J. Brown. 1996. Phosphorus restriction prevents parathyroid gland growth. High phosphorus directly stimulates PTH secretion in vitro. *J Clin Invest* 97 (11):2534–40. doi:10.1172/JCI118701.

Tonelli, M., F. Sacks, M. Pfeffer, Z. Gao, G. Curhan, and Cholesterol And Investigators Recurrent Events Trial. 2005. Relation between serum phosphate level and cardiovascular event rate in people with coronary disease. *Circulation* 112 (17):2627–33. doi:10.1161/CIRCULATIONAHA.105.553198.

Tran, L., M. Batech, C. M. Rhee, E. Streja, K. Kalantar-Zadeh, S. J. Jacobsen, and J. J. Sim. 2016. Serum phosphorus and association with anemia among a large diverse population with and without chronic kidney disease. *Nephrol Dial Transplant* 31 (4):636–45. doi:10.1093/ndt/gfv297.

Voigt, M., D. C. Fischer, M. Rimpau, W. Schareck, and D. Haffner. 2010. Fibroblast growth factor (FGF)-23 and fetuin-A in calcified carotid atheroma. *Histopathology* 56 (6):775–88. doi:10.1111/j.1365-2559.2010.03547.x.

Voormolen, N., M. Noordzij, D. C. Grootendorst, I. Beetz, Y. W. Sijpkens, J. G. van Manen, E. W. Boeschoten, R. M. Huisman, R. T. Krediet, F. W. Dekker, and PREPARE study group. 2007. High plasma phosphate as a risk factor for decline in renal function and mortality in pre-dialysis patients. *Nephrol Dial Transplant* 22 (10):2909–16. doi:10.1093/ndt/gfm286.

Wilson, K. M., I. M. Shui, L. A. Mucci, and E. Giovannucci. 2015. Calcium and phosphorus intake and prostate cancer risk: A 24-y follow-up study. *Am J Clin Nutr* 101 (1):173–83. doi:10.3945/ajcn.114.088716.

Yamamoto, K. T., C. Robinson-Cohen, M. C. de Oliveira, A. Kostina, J. A. Nettleton, J. H. Ix, H. Nguyen, J. Eng, J. A. Lima, D. S. Siscovick, N. S. Weiss, and B. Kestenbaum. 2013. Dietary phosphorus is associated with greater left ventricular mass. *Kidney Int* 83 (4):707–14. doi:10.1038/ki.2012.303.

Yilmaz, M. I., A. Sonmez, M. Saglam, H. Yaman, S. Kilic, E. Demirkaya, T. Eyileten, K. Caglar, Y. Oguz, A. Vural, M. Yenicesu, and C. Zoccali. 2010. FGF-23 and vascular dysfunction in patients with stage 3 and 4 chronic kidney disease. *Kidney Int* 78 (7):679–85. doi:10.1038/ki.2010.194.

Yilmaz, M. I., A. Sonmez, M. Saglam, H. Yaman, S. Kilic, T. Eyileten, K. Caglar, Y. Oguz, A. Vural, M. Yenicesu, F. Mallamaci, and C. Zoccali. 2012. Comparison of calcium acetate and sevelamer on vascular function and fibroblast growth factor 23 in CKD patients: A randomized clinical trial. *Am J Kidney Dis* 59 (2):177–85. doi:10.1053/j.ajkd.2011.11.007.

Yoo, K. D., S. Kang, Y. Choi, S. H. Yang, N. J. Heo, H. J. Chin, K. H. Oh, K. W. Joo, Y. S. Kim, and H. Lee. 2016. Sex, Age, and the Association of Serum Phosphorus With All-Cause Mortality in Adults With Normal Kidney Function. *Am J Kidney Dis* 67 (1):79–88. doi:10.1053/j.ajkd.2015.06.027.

2 Preclinical Evidence of the Nonskeletal Adverse Health Effects of High Dietary Phosphorus

George R. Beck, Jr.

CONTENTS

Abstract 13
Bullet Points 14
2.1 Cancer, Diet, and Phosphorus Consumption 14
    2.1.1 The Significance of Diet to Cancer 14
    2.1.2 Dietary Inorganic Phosphate and Cancer 14
    2.1.3 Preclinical Models of Cancer 15
2.2 Preclinical Evidence for a Modulating Effect of Phosphorus Consumption on Cancer 16
    2.2.1 Cell-Based Models Identify Increased Pi Availability as a Risk Factor for Cancer 16
    2.2.2 Dietary Pi Consumption and Carcinogen-Induced Skin Cancer 16
    2.2.3 Dietary Pi Consumption and Oncogene-Induced Lung Cancer 17
    2.2.4 Relevance to Humans 17
    2.2.5 Dietary Pi as a Modulator of Cancer Initiation and Progression 18
2.3 Cell Autonomous Effects of Phosphorus Availability on Cell Growth and Transformation 18
    2.3.1 Pi Availability and Cell Growth 18
    2.3.2 Increased Pi Availability Alters the Cellular and Molecular Phenotype 19
    2.3.3 Cell Transport and Sensing of Pi 19
    2.3.4 Slc20a1 and Cell Proliferation 20
    2.3.5 Slc34a2: A Novel Cancer Therapeutic Target 20
2.4 Phosphorus-Responsive Endocrine, Paracrine, and Autocrine Factors and Cancer 20
    2.4.1 Dietary Pi-Responsive Endocrine Factors 20
    2.4.2 Vitamin D 21
    2.4.3 FGF23 21
    2.4.4 Klotho 21
    2.4.5 Osteopontin 22
2.5 Conclusions 22
Acknowledgments 23
References 23

ABSTRACT

Complex diseases such as cancer are influenced by numerous risk factors, including genetic makeup, environmental stresses, and lifestyle choices such as diet. These risk factors combine to alter cellular and molecular function, ranging from uncontrolled proliferation to evading programmed cell death to invasion and migration, ultimately resulting in the myriad of negative health consequences that define cancer. Lifestyle choices such as diet represent risk factors that can be reasonably controlled and manipulated for disease prevention and general health benefit. However, identifying and understanding the contribution of individual components of the human diet to health and pathological conditions represents a tremendous challenge, particularly in the context of a disease such as cancer, which can arise in most tissues and has a multitude of underlying etiologies. One dietary component that has recently gained attention as a potential cancer-modifying factor is inorganic phosphate (Pi), which is highly abundant in the Western diet. Cell-based studies have identified Pi as a factor that can alter cell behavior, including proliferation, metabolism, and migration, through direct effects on cellular and molecular functions, as well as changes in the micro and macro environment. Pi therefore represents a dietary element that has the potential to influence multiple facets of cancer etiology and progression. Indeed, recent studies utilizing murine cancer models have identified a diet high in Pi as a contributing risk factor for cancer initiation and progression relative to a reduced Pi diet. This chapter will discuss the modulating effects of dietary Pi consumption on cancer evaluated using preclinical models and will consider the potential mechanisms by which cancer might be influenced by varying Pi consumption, including cell autonomous, autocrine, paracrine, and endocrine effects.

BULLET POINTS

- Preclinical cancer models suggest that dietary phosphorus influences tumor promotion and progression, although the mechanisms remain to be defined.
- A number of dietary phosphorus responsive circulating factors such as osteopontin, vitamin D, and klotho have been linked to cancer modulation.
- Extracellular phosphorus availability alters the growth properties of cells through specific signal transduction pathways and changes in gene expression.
- The sodium-dependent phosphate transporters Slc20a1 and Slc34a2 have been identified to regulate cell growth and proliferation and are overexpressed in a number of human cancers.
- Modulation of dietary phosphorus consumption may represent a novel cancer prevention strategy.

2.1 CANCER, DIET, AND PHOSPHORUS CONSUMPTION

2.1.1 THE SIGNIFICANCE OF DIET TO CANCER

The development of cancer, generally defined as uncontrolled cell growth and survival, is a complex multistage process often involving a combination of mutational events produced and influenced by a partially understood combination of genetic, environmental, and lifestyle components. Cells have evolved mechanisms to cope with mutational events, and therefore whether a given genetic mutation(s) ultimately produces a cancerous cell can be influenced by factors such as nutrient availability and nutrient-responsive growth factors and cytokines (Hanahan and Weinberg 2000). Studies evaluating the effects of human migration on the incidence of cancer suggest that lifestyle factors such as diet can have a profound influence on prevalence (reviewed in [Newberne and Conner 1988]). A general estimate of the potential contribution of diet to cancer ranges from 10% to 70% (Doll and Peto 1981), and therefore nutritional intervention represents a risk factor that can be relatively easily modulated for cancer prevention, postdisease mitigation and/or recovery, and general health benefits (Afman and Muller 2006; Go, Butrum, and Wong 2003).

2.1.2 DIETARY INORGANIC PHOSPHATE AND CANCER

One particular nutritional element that is gaining attention as a potential modulator of health and disease is phosphorus, often in the dietary form of inorganic phosphate (Pi). Pi is highly abundant in the human diet and particularly in the Western diet, and due in part to the increased consumption of processed foods, as discussed in Chapters 19 and 20, the amount of Pi in the American diet far exceeds individual requirements for most age and sex groups, and some evidence suggests intake levels continue to rise and may soon approach the upper level of safe intake (UL) in a growing segment of the US population (Calvo 1993; Calvo and Park 1996). To date, most micronutrients have been investigated for negative health effects due to diet insufficiency and not excess, as is the case for Pi, creating a relatively unique circumstance in nutritional cancer research. There is a growing appreciation that increases in dietary Pi consumption and/or serum phosphorus levels, even in the context of normal renal function, influence age-associated disease progression, as seen with bone metabolism (Calvo 1993; Kemi, Karkkainen, and Lamberg-Allardt 2006; Huttunen et al. 2007; Draper, Sie, and Bergan 1972; Gutierrez et al. 2015) and cardiovascular function (Giachelli 2009; Onufrak et al. 2008; Dhingra et al. 2007; Ferro et al. 2009) (reviewed in [Uribarri and Calvo 2013]). As discussed herein, studies now suggest a possible link between excessive Pi consumption and cancer (Camalier et al. 2010; Jin et al. 2009; Wulaningsih et al. 2013; Wilson et al. 2015). Although the potential mechanisms are still under investigation, cell-based studies suggest that changes in Pi availability can alter a number of cell functions associated with cancer initiation and progression, as discussed in detail herein. Moreover, a diet high in Pi can alter serum phosphorus and calcium levels, which result in changes in paracrine and endocrine factors such as osteopontin, fibroblast growth factor 23 (FGF23), and klotho, which have been linked to various aspects of cancer development and progression. Pi therefore possesses the characteristics of a nutritional factor that might represent a modulator of cancer initiation and progression and as such be harnessed for cancer prevention.

2.1.3 Preclinical Models of Cancer

Understanding the contribution of individual components of the human diet to health and disease represents a tremendous challenge, particularly to a multifaceted disease such as cancer. The combinations of mutations and abnormalities that lead to a cancerous cell are often decades in the making,

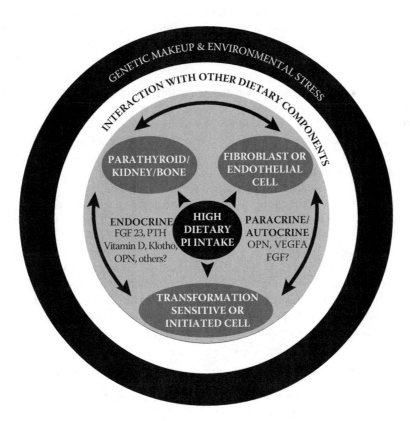

FIGURE 2.1 Potential mechanisms by which high dietary phosphorus consumption might influence the initiation or progression of complex diseases such as cancer.

and dietary habits as well as environmental factors can change dramatically in that period of time. This is further complicated by a poorly understood and vast array of potential interactions between individual nutrients that might vary from diet to diet and also likely change over time, and all in the context that the net effect of a given nutrient on a cell is also likely influenced by genetic makeup. Consequently, assessing and assigning a link between an individual dietary component and a disease such as cancer represents a significant challenge. Preclinical animal models, although not always perfect with regard to human relevance, offer a means to assess individual dietary components in the context of developing disease in a controlled environment. Mice are particularly well suited for cancer studies in that the disease can be developed relatively rapidly, on the order of weeks and months, as opposed to years or decades, as in other species, and they can be genetically engineered, providing mechanistic insight into etiology (Cheon and Orsulic 2011). Cancer in mice can be initiated by application of a carcinogen or environmental stress that results in somatic mutations, or it can be driven by transgenic modification of the mouse with an activated oncogene or knockout of tumor suppressor. A distinct advantage of these models for nutritional studies is that the diets the mice are fed are strictly defined and portions can be tightly controlled. This chapter will consider studies that have utilized such mouse models to investigate the potential role of dietary Pi in modulating cancer initiation and progression, as well as address the potential underlying mechanisms (Figure 2.1).

2.2 PRECLINICAL EVIDENCE FOR A MODULATING EFFECT OF PHOSPHORUS CONSUMPTION ON CANCER

2.2.1 CELL-BASED MODELS IDENTIFY INCREASED PI AVAILABILITY AS A RISK FACTOR FOR CANCER

Preclinical cancer studies are often time consuming and costly, and therefore agents that are being investigated for either cancer prevention or promotion properties are often first examined in cell-based models that measure transformation, the progression of a cell toward uncontrolled growth, and resistance to death. Early studies using the NIH3T3 focus formation assay established Pi as a required nutrient in the regulation and stimulation of transformation (Rubin and Chu 1984; Rubin and Sanui 1977). A more recent study has demonstrated that Pi is not only required, but that excess Pi can promote transformation. This study utilized the transformation-sensitive epidermal keratinocyte cell line JB6, which when treated with various tumor promoters such as TPA (12-O-tetradecanoylphorbol-13-acetate) responds with anchorage-independent growth in soft agar and tumorigenicity (Colburn et al. 1979). This model is considered an excellent one to investigate the promoting effects of an agent on the process of transformation (reviewed in [Dhar, Young, and Colburn 2002; Abel et al. 2009]) because the cellular and molecular events required for transformation in this model are well defined (reviewed in [Dhar et al. 2004]), and the in vitro response has been validated as representative of in vivo events using the two-stage skin carcinogenesis model (Young, Yang, and Colburn 2003). The JB6 cell model was used to demonstrate that small increases in available Pi, 1 to 2 mM, in addition to the 1 mM in the medium, resulted in a significant increase in JB6 cell proliferation (Camalier et al. 2010). Further, the ability of 12-O-Tetradecanoylphorbol-13-acetate (TPA) to induce anchorage-independent growth (transformation) in soft agar was significantly augmented by increasing Pi in the medium (Camalier et al. 2010). Taken together, these results identified that increased Pi availability is sufficient to promote cell growth as well as anchorage-independent growth in cell models, indicative of cell transformation toward a cancerous phenotype in preclinical models.

2.2.2 DIETARY PI CONSUMPTION AND CARCINOGEN-INDUCED SKIN CANCER

The two-stage skin carcinogenesis model induces papilloma (tumor) formation through treatment of the skin of mice with a carcinogen (DMBA; 7,12-dimethylbenz[a]anthracene), followed by weekly treatment with a tumor promoter, such as TPA. Papilloma formation occurs between 10 and 20 weeks after treatment initiation (Slaga et al. 1996). This cancer model was used in combination with diets

Preclinical Evidence of the Nonskeletal Adverse Health Effects of High Dietary Phosphorus   17

that contained high Pi (1.2%) or low Pi (0.2%) levels, approximating 1800 mg/day or 500 mg/day intake, respectively, in humans. The diets contained equal amounts of calcium (0.6%) and were isocaloric. Nineteen weeks after carcinogen initiation papilloma number, multiplicity, and size were recorded. The mice on the high-Pi diet were not statically different in weight compared to the low-Pi diet but did exhibit a significant increase in serum Pi and decrease in serum calcium (Camalier et al. 2010). The mice fed the high-Pi diet developed twice as many papillomas as mice fed the low-Pi diet, and these papillomas developed at an earlier time point and were initially larger (Camalier et al. 2010). The data therefore demonstrated that a high-Pi diet alters both initiation and progression of carcinogen-induced tumorigenesis. These mice also had significantly elevated serum parathyroid hormone (PTH) and osteopontin (OPN), a secreted cytokine-like factor associated with bone metabolism, cardiovascular calcification, kidney disease, and cancer (Sodek, Ganss, and McKee 2000; Wai and Kuo 2008). Therefore, in addition to the direct and autocrine effects of Pi on cell transformation identified in cell-based assays, this study identified the possibility that Pi-responsive paracrine and endocrine factors might influence the cancer phenotype.

2.2.3 DIETARY PI CONSUMPTION AND ONCOGENE-INDUCED LUNG CANCER

A preclinical cancer model that represents an example of oncogene-driven tumorigenesis is the K-ras^{LA1} model of spontaneous lung cancer (Johnson et al. 2001). These genetically modified mice develop lung cancer due to a latent transgene that is susceptible to spontaneous recombination resulting in an activated K-ras (G12D) allele and production of a constitutively active protein (Johnson et al. 2001). The lung cancer that develops in these mice progresses through a series of morphological stages from mild hyperplasia/dysplasia to adenoma to overt carcinoma and is thought to reasonably represent the events that occur in many human lung cancers. This oncogene-driven model has also been used to study the potential role of dietary Pi in tumor development and progression. In this study, K-ras^{LA1} mice, at 5 weeks of age, were fed a diet with either normal Pi levels (0.5%) or high Pi levels (1.0%) (~750 and 1500 mg/day intake) for 4 weeks (Jin et al. 2009). Measurement of animal weight identified no significant differences between the diet groups; however, a significant increase in serum Pi in the mice fed a high-Pi diet was determined. Analyses of the lungs revealed a significant increase in the total number of tumors, as well as tumor size, with an increase in both small (<1.5 mm diameter) and large tumors (>1.5 mm) (Jin et al. 2009). Histological analyses of the lungs identified significantly increased proliferation as measured by proliferating cell nuclear antigen (PCNA) labeling index in mice on the high-Pi diet. The results therefore suggested that the high-Pi diet influenced both the initiation of tumor formation and tumor growth and progression. Interestingly, the same K-ras^{LA1} mouse model was used with a very low-Pi diet (0.1%) and identified an increase in lung tumor number relative to the control Pi diet (0.5%) (Xu et al. 2010). The results suggest the possibility of a U-shaped safety curve regarding Pi intake and risk of tumorigenesis in the presence of an activating oncogenic mutation.

2.2.4 RELEVANCE TO HUMANS

Although preclinical animal models have identified potentially significant consequences of a long-term diet high in Pi on cancer initiation and progression, data from humans are lacking. Based in part on the mouse cancer studies noted earlier, the association between serum Pi and risk of cancer was recently analyzed in a population-based observational assessment of the Swedish Apolipoprotein Mortality Risk (AMORIS) study (Wulaningsih et al. 2013). Multivariate Cox proportional hazard regression analyses found no overall correlation between serum phosphorus with cancer risk; however, a statistical correlation was identified with cancer from specific tissues (Wulaningsih et al. 2013). Increasing serum phosphorus quartiles in men correlated with increased risk of pancreatic, lung, thyroid, bone, and "other" cancers and an association with liver and gallbladder only in the highest quartile. In women high serum phosphorus was correlated with increased risk of esophageal, lung, and nonmelanoma skin cancer and an association with stomach and bone cancer only in the highest quartile (Wulaningsih et al. 2013). Additionally, a recent 24-year follow-up in the Health Professionals Study used Cox proportional hazards modeling to assess the association between Pi and calcium intake and prostate cancer (Wilson et al. 2015). The study identified Pi intake as associated with increased risk of poorly differentiated and clinically advanced-stage prostate cancer, independent of calcium intake (Wilson et al. 2015). Although these are only associative studies and additional studies focused specifically on Pi consumption are sorely needed, they are some of the first to provide an epidemiological link between dietary Pi intake and serum phosphorus levels with cancer in humans.

2.2.5 DIETARY PI AS A MODULATOR OF CANCER INITIATION AND PROGRESSION

To date, these relatively limited preclinical mouse models and human studies collectively support a role for dietary Pi consumption as a modulator of cancer initiation and progression. The two different preclinical mouse models of cancer were driven individually by a carcinogen or oncogene and in two different tissues, skin and lung, suggesting the possibility that modulating dietary Pi may represent a means to influence cancer originating in varying tissues. Further, it should be noted that the amount of Pi in the diets used in the mouse studies is considered "high" by the Food and Drug Administration (FDA), but actually represents a range that is close to a normal level of consumption for the Western-style diet, and therefore the studies might be viewed as a reduced-Pi diet being preventative as opposed to a high-Pi diet being promotive. Because of the difficulties in assigning specific effects of individual dietary components to specific biological outcomes, a consideration of mechanism of action is important. Defining mechanism of action not only increases confidence in the link between nutrient and disease, but might also provide additional therapeutic targets or options for disease treatment. In this regard, there is a growing literature on the direct cell autonomous effects of Pi on cell function as well as autocrine, paracrine, and endocrine effects, which provide insight into the potential mechanism(s) by which dietary Pi might influence cancer.

2.3 CELL AUTONOMOUS EFFECTS OF PHOSPHORUS AVAILABILITY ON CELL GROWTH AND TRANSFORMATION

2.3.1 PI AVAILABILITY AND CELL GROWTH

One mechanism by which increased dietary Pi consumption and the resulting changes in serum Pi might alter cancer initiation and progression is through direct effects on cells. Cancer is in large part driven by cell growth, and a number of cell-based studies have demonstrated that the availability of Pi influences cell growth properties. Pi was identified over four decades ago as a limiting nutrient in the proliferation of Swiss 3T3 fibroblast-like cells (Holley and Kiernan 1974; Weber and Edlin 1971; Hilborn 1976). Further, contact-inhibited 3T3 cells respond to serum stimulation with a rapid increase in Pi transport (Cunningham and Pardee 1969; Barsh, Greenberg, and Cunningham 1977; de Asua, Rozengurt, and Dulbecco 1974). Whereas the earlier studies identified Pi as a required nutrient for cell growth, other studies suggest that excess Pi, added to culture medium already sufficient in Pi, can actively drive cell proliferation (Chang et al. 2006; Conrads et al. 2005; Cunningham and Pardee 1969; Roussanne et al. 2001; Engstrom and Zetterberg 1983; Camalier et al. 2010). Cancer cell growth is often associated with the need for increased nutrient supply, and two recent cell culture studies have demonstrated that increased Pi availability stimulated cell migration and angiogenesis through both direct and autocrine/paracrine signaling (Rangrez et al. 2012; Lin et al. 2015a). Based on the requirement of Pi for numerous critical cell functions, it is consistent that rapidly dividing cells would have an increased need for Pi, and this is supported by in vivo studies that have found increased Pi uptake and retention in tumors relative to the corresponding normal tissue controls (Elser et al. 2007; Thomas, Harrington, and Bovington 1958; Jones, Chaikoff, and Lawrence 1940). However, not all studies have found a positive correlation between Pi levels and cell growth. A number of studies have found an increase in apoptosis in certain cell types,

Preclinical Evidence of the Nonskeletal Adverse Health Effects of High Dietary Phosphorus   **19**

including cancer cells, and under certain culture conditions (Meleti, Shapiro, and Adams 2000; Rahabi-Layachi et al. 2015; Di Marco et al. 2008; Zhong et al. 2011; Sapio et al. 2015; Spina et al. 2013). Whether this is a result of culture conditions or differences in cell types still remains to be determined. Collectively, the results identify Pi as a nutrient that can be manipulated to control cell growth, particularly in rapidly dividing cells.

2.3.2 INCREASED PI AVAILABILITY ALTERS THE CELLULAR AND MOLECULAR PHENOTYPE

The idea that Pi availability can directly alter cell behavior is further supported by studies identifying specific genes responsive to changes in extracellular Pi. To date, hundreds of genes have been identified that are temporally upregulated or downregulated by increased extracellular Pi in varying cell types (Beck, Zerler, and Moran 2000; Jono et al. 2000; Beck and Knecht 2003; Beck, Moran, and Knecht 2003; Foster et al. 2006; Camalier et al. 2010; Chang et al. 2006; Camalier et al. 2013). The intracellular mechanisms, in part, involve the stimulation of specific intracellular signaling pathways. Elevated extracellular Pi has been demonstrated to regulate signaling pathways and proteins, including the mitogen activated protein kinase (MAPK)–Erk1/2 (Beck and Knecht 2003; Chang et al. 2006; Jin et al. 2006; Julien et al. 2009; Wittrant et al. 2009; Yamazaki et al. 2010; Camalier et al. 2013), AKT (Chang et al. 2006), N-Ras, c-Raf (Camalier et al. 2010; Chang et al. 2006; Kimata et al. 2010), and PKC (Beck and Knecht 2003). Elevated extracellular Pi has also been demonstrated to increase intracellular signaling molecules such as nitric oxide (Teixeira et al. 2001), reactive oxygen species (Takeda et al. 2006), and the generation of adenosine triphosphate (ATP) through increased oxidative phosphorylation (Camalier et al. 2013). Although all of the aforementioned studies have been performed in cell culture, a recent microarray analysis of kidneys from mice on high (1.2%) or low (0.3%) Pi diets for 24 days identified increased expression of genes such as osteopontin (*spp1*), Timp1, c-fos (*Fos*), and Egr1, among others, in the high-Pi-diet mice (Suyama et al. 2012). These genes in particular have been previously identified as Pi induced in cell culture studies (Beck, Moran, and Knecht 2003; Camalier et al. 2013; Rutherford et al. 2006) and therefore support the possibility of cell autonomous Pi-regulated effects in vivo in response to changing Pi consumption. Although the initiating membrane event has yet to be fully elucidated, cell-based studies have identified the specific requirement of Pi transporters and FGF receptor for the intracellular signaling response generated by elevated Pi (Camalier et al. 2013; Suzuki et al. 2000; Yamazaki et al. 2010; Kimata et al. 2010).

2.3.3 CELL TRANSPORT AND SENSING OF PI

Cells regulate, and possibly sense, Pi levels primarily through a family of sodium-dependent phosphate transporters (reviewed in [Biber, Hernando, and Forster 2013]). Type II transporters (current nomenclature Slc34a1-3) are thought to be responsible mainly for absorption in the intestine and resorption in the kidney (reviewed in [Tenenhouse 2007]), although recent data suggest the possibility of a more diverse function (Lundquist, Murer, and Biber 2007). Type III transporters (current nomenclature Slc20a1-2) are expressed more ubiquitously, but evidence suggests important roles in calcifying tissues (reviewed in [Collins, Bai, and Ghishan 2004]). Although the potential role(s) of Pi transporters as active regulators of cell function, as opposed to the more "housekeeping" transport functions, are not fully understood, cell culture studies have linked changes in extracellular Pi concentrations to changes in cell behavior in numerous cell types of varying function (Beck 2003; Mansfield et al. 2001; Fujita et al. 2001; Julien et al. 2007; Foster et al. 2006; Kanatani et al. 2003; Yates et al. 1991; Mozar et al. 2007; Camalier et al. 2010; Chang et al. 2006; Roussanne et al. 2001; Jono et al. 2000). The requirement of Pi for cell functions related to proliferation positions the Pi transporters as potential modulators of cell growth, and in fact, two specific transporters, Slc20a1 and Slc34a2, have been linked to modulation of cell behavior related to the cancer phenotype.

2.3.4 Slc20a1 and Cell Proliferation

Functional studies have identified the requirement specifically of Slc20a1 (*Pit1, Glvr-1*) for Pi-induced changes in cell behavior (Li, Yang, and Giachelli 2006; Suzuki et al. 2006; Yoshiko et al. 2007; Kimata et al. 2010), including proliferation, transformation, and tumor growth. Using RNA interference in HeLa and HepG2 cells, Slc20a1 (Pit1) depletion reduced cell proliferation, delayed cell cycle, and impaired mitosis and cytokinesis (Beck et al. 2009). In the same study, a mouse xenograft model was used to assess the effects of Slc20a1 knockdown on HeLa cell growth. The results identified a significant decrease in the resulting tumor size in the Slc20a1 knockdown cells relative to control (Beck et al. 2009). This group further provided evidence that the effect on cell proliferation was specific to Slc20a1 and not shared by the related Slc20a2 (*Pit2, Ram-1*) Pi transporter and that modulation of cell proliferation by Slc20a1 is independent from its transport function. In a similar study, knockdown of Slc20a1 (Pit1) with shRNA resulted in decreased proliferation and transformation as measured using the NIH3T3 soft agar assay, whereas overexpression of the transporter increased proliferation of NIH3T3 and pre-osteoblast MC3T3-E1 cells (Byskov et al. 2012). With regard to human cancer, gene expression profiling studies have identified Slc20a1 as more highly expressed in cervical cancer patients who do not respond to therapy (Harima et al. 2004), in pancreatic cancer cell lines (Cao et al. 2004), and has been associated with BRCA2 mutations in breast cancer (Walker et al. 2008). Taken together, the mostly cell-based assays have identified Slc20a1 as a potential regulator of increased cell growth in the context of cancer and underscore the potential direct role of Pi transport/sensing in influencing cell behavior.

2.3.5 Slc34a2: A Novel Cancer Therapeutic Target

The type-II cotransporter, Slc34a2 (*NAPI-IIb, NaPi-3b, NPTIIb*), has also been identified as a potential novel cancer therapeutic target. Studies have identified increased RNA and protein levels of Slc34a2 in the lungs of mice consuming a high-Pi diet (Jin et al. 2007, 2009), which was correlated with increased expression in human lung cancer cells exposed to elevated Pi (Chang et al. 2006). Slc34a2 has also been linked to cancer in humans as overexpressed in ovarian cancer (Rangel et al. 2003; Shyian et al. 2011), papillary thyroid cancers (Kim et al. 2010), and breast cancer samples, although an association with overall survival was not identified (Chen et al. 2010). Knockdown of Slc34a2 in the lungs of mice predisposed to lung cancer through spontaneous K-*ras* mutation (K-*ras*[LA1] mice) resulted in suppressed lung cancer growth and decreased cancer cell proliferation and angiogenesis while increasing apoptosis (Hong et al. 2013). A recent study used an antibody–drug conjugate (ADC) approach to selectively deliver a cytotoxic drug to ovarian and non-small cell lung cancer cells, which highly express Slc34a2. This study utilized an antibody recognizing SLC34A2 to deliver the ADC in rat and monkey tumor xenograph models and demonstrated significant antitumor activity, with an acceptable safety profile (Lin et al. 2015b). These results generally demonstrated that targeting Slc34a2 is an effective new therapy for lung and ovarian cancers. Collectively, these results identify the specific Pi transporter Slc34a2 as a novel cancer therapeutic target with regard to both function and as a cell surface marker.

2.4 PHOSPHORUS-RESPONSIVE ENDOCRINE, PARACRINE, AND AUTOCRINE FACTORS AND CANCER

2.4.1 Dietary Pi-Responsive Endocrine Factors

In addition to the direct effects of Pi on cell function discussed previously, a number of dietary Pi-responsive secreted and circulating factors might also influence the cancer phenotype. Increased dietary Pi consumption increases circulating levels of FGF23, PTH, and the cytokine-like factor OPN (Antoniucci, Yamashita, and Portale 2006; Burnett et al. 2006; Ferrari, Bonjour, and Rizzoli 2005; Camalier et al. 2010; Portale, Halloran, and Morris 1989; Portale et al. 1986; Reiss et al. 1970; Karkkainen

Preclinical Evidence of the Nonskeletal Adverse Health Effects of High Dietary Phosphorus **21**

and Lamberg-Allardt 1996; Calvo, Kumar, and Heath 1990; Gutierrez et al. 2015), and circulating levels of 1,25-dihydroxyvitamin D and klotho have been demonstrated to decrease in rodents and humans, at least temporarily (Portale et al. 1986; Gray et al. 1977; Maierhofer, Gray, and Lemann 1984; Portale, Halloran, and Morris 1989; Hughes et al. 1975). Although PTH has not been currently linked to cancers in preclinical models, other dietary Pi-responsive circulating factors have and therefore could influence disease initiation and/or progression in response to increased Pi consumption, although a direct link to dietary intake has yet to be established.

2.4.2 Vitamin D

A number of in vitro and in vivo studies have demonstrated the property of vitamin D to promote growth inhibition and differentiation in numerous cell types and tissues as well as cancerous cells (reviewed in [Giovannucci 1998]). Vitamin D insufficiency is common, and many epidemiological studies have investigated the possible inverse correlation of serum vitamin D and cancer risk with inconsistent outcomes (Tuohimaa 2008). A recent analysis of the NHANES III (Third National Health and Nutritional Examination Survey) participants did not support the hypothesis that serum 25(OH)D levels are associated with reduced cancer mortality (Freedman et al. 2010). However, a number of preclinical animal studies, using carcinogen- or oncogene-induced cancer, do support a role of vitamin D deficiency as a contributing factor in the disease, as well as the supplementation of vitamin D in the prevention or reduction of disease (reviewed in [Feldman et al. 2014]). Together, the role of vitamin D deficiency as a risk factor for cancer and vitamin D supplementation as a therapeutic option remains controversial.

2.4.3 FGF23

There is strong evidence for a role of FGF signaling and FGF receptors in cancer initiation and progression (Turner and Grose 2010); however, only recently has a causal association between FGF23 with cancer been identified. Feng et al. have demonstrated that exogenously added FGF23 enhanced proliferation, invasion, and anchorage-independent growth of prostate cancer cell lines in culture (Feng et al. 2015). These investigators also probed the potential role of FGF23 as an autocrine regulator of prostate cancer cell growth using a subcutaneous xenograft model. Knockdown of FGF23 in prostate cancer cells resulted in a decrease in tumor volume and weight (Feng et al. 2015), suggesting a role as a promoting autocrine factor. Additionally, recent evidence suggests the possibility that FGF23 may be a biomarker for ovarian and colorectal cancers (Tebben et al. 2005; Jacobs et al. 2011). To date, the data are limited to one study and therefore will need to be confirmed in additional models; however, the idea that the phosphatonin FGF23 might alter cancer initiation or progression provides a potential novel link between nutrition and cancer modulation.

2.4.4 Klotho

Klotho is a membrane-bound protein predominantly expressed in the kidney and parathyroid gland (Urakawa et al. 2006) that acts as a coreceptor for FGF23, increasing affinity and subsequent signaling. Klotho has also been identified in a soluble form capable of acting in a paracrine manner (reviewed in [Kuro 2011]). A number of studies have recently linked this secreted/soluble form of klotho with cancer in both mice and humans (reviewed in [Zhou and Wang 2015]). Klotho has been suggested to act as a tumor suppressor through modulation of insulin-like growth factor 1 (IGF-1) and FGF pathways in breast cancer (Wolf et al. 2008), as well as decreasing reactive oxygen species and regulating autophagy (Shu et al. 2013; Xie et al. 2013a, b). Moreover, cell culture studies have linked klotho with growth inhibition of pancreatic cancer (Abramovitz et al. 2011) and melanoma cell growth (Camilli et al. 2011). Loss of klotho has been associated with epigenetic silencing in human cervical carcinoma (Lee et al. 2010), gastric (Wang et al. 2011), hepatocellular (Xie et al.

2013c), and colorectal cancers (Pan et al. 2011), and low klotho levels resulted in increased epithelial-to-mesenchymal transition in renal cell carcinoma (Zhu et al. 2013). Overexpression of klotho inhibited cell proliferation and motility and induced apoptosis in A549 lung cancer cells (Chen et al. 2012) and sensitized human lung cancer cells to cisplatin (Wang et al. 2013). In mice, klotho has been demonstrated to function as a secreted antagonist to Wnt signaling (Liu et al. 2007) and to inhibit transforming growth factor $\beta 1$ signaling–induced endothelial-to-mesenchyme transition and cancer metastasis (Doi et al. 2011). Collectively, these recent results identify klotho as an exciting and novel factor in suppressing cancer initiation and progression; however, more direct preclinical cancer studies are needed to clarify the response to both dietary Pi consumption and regulation of cell transformation and tumorigenesis.

2.4.5 OSTEOPONTIN

OPN (*Spp1, 2ar, eta-1*) is a circulating and highly responsive Pi-regulated gene/protein capable of regulating cancer cell behavior as an autocrine, paracrine, and endocrine factor. Cell culture studies have determined that elevated Pi strongly stimulated OPN expression from multiple cell types through specific signaling pathways (Beck and Knecht 2003; Beck, Moran, and Knecht 2003; Beck 2003; Beck, Zerler, and Moran 2000; Camalier et al. 2013; Conrads et al. 2005; Beck et al. 1998; Jono et al. 2000; Foster et al. 2006; Fatherazi et al. 2009; Sage et al. 2011; Chen et al. 2002; Kimata et al. 2010; Lin et al. 2015a). Further, a high-Pi diet has been demonstrated to increase circulating OPN levels in both mice and humans (Camalier et al. 2010; Gutierrez et al. 2015). OPN was originally identified as a marker of neoplastic transformation in 1979 by Senger and colleagues (Senger, Perruzzi, and Papadopoulos 1989), and overexpression of OPN is tightly linked to cancer and metastasis arising from most tissue types (reviewed in [Oates, Barraclough, and Rudland 1997; Rittling and Chambers 2004]). OPN can influence changes in cell behavior such as proliferation, cell survival, cytoskeletal organization, motility, and phagocytosis (Giachelli and Steitz 2000) and can also act as an immune-modulatory factor (Cantor and Shinohara 2009; Denhardt, Giachelli, and Rittling 2001; O'Regan, Hayden, and Berman 2000). OPN modulates cell function by acting as an endocrine, paracrine, or autocrine cytokine (reviewed in [El-Tanani et al. 2006; Denhardt, Giachelli, and Rittling 2001]) through its ability to bind multiple receptors such as CD44 and $\alpha\beta$-integrins (Bayless et al. 1998; Denhardt, Giachelli, and Rittling 2001). A cell based study in which breast cancer cells were grown in an elevated Pi medium (2 and 4 mM) identified OPN as a Pi-responsive secreted factor capable of increasing angiogenesis and thereby providing a potential means of recruiting blood supply to a growing tumor (Lin et al. 2015a). These results suggest an additional mechanism, through the stimulation of an autocrine/paracrine factor, by which Pi availability and Pi responsive factors might modulate the cancer cell behavior (Figure 2.1).

2.5 CONCLUSIONS

Preclinical animal models of tumor initiation and progression have identified dietary Pi as a modulator of cancer. The in vivo models have been complemented with mechanistic in vitro studies that suggest multiple mechanisms by which dietary Pi might influence cancer etiology, including cell autonomous, autocrine, paracrine, and/or endocrine signaling (Figure 2.1). Developing a complete understanding of the modulatory roles of dietary Pi on cancer, particularly in humans, will additionally require understanding how dietary Pi functions in the context of varying environmental stresses, including other dietary components, as well as genetic makeup in the prevention, initiation, or progression of the disease (Figure 2.1). Manipulation of the diet represents a cost-effective and easily achievable intervention for disease prevention or treatment; however, additional dietary Pi-focused studies are needed to determine whether Pi represents such a nutritional factor.

ACKNOWLEDGMENTS

Funding has been provided by grants from the National Cancer Institute (CA136716) and the Biomedical Laboratory Research & Development Service of the Veterans Administration Office of Research and Development (Award Number I01BX002363).

REFERENCES

Abel, E. L., J. M. Angel, K. Kiguchi, and J. DiGiovanni. 2009. Multi-stage chemical carcinogenesis in mouse skin: Fundamentals and applications. *Nat Protoc* no. 4 (9):1350–62. doi:10.1038/nprot.2009.120.

Abramovitz, L., T. Rubinek, H. Ligumsky, S. Bose, I. Barshack, C. Avivi, B. Kaufman, and I. Wolf. 2011. KL1 internal repeat mediates klotho tumor suppressor activities and inhibits bFGF and IGF-I signaling in pancreatic cancer. *Clin Cancer Res* no. 17 (13):4254–66. doi:10.1158/1078-0432.CCR-10-2749.

Afman, L. and M. Muller. 2006. Nutrigenomics: From molecular nutrition to prevention of disease. *J Am Diet Assoc* no. 106 (4):569–76.

Antoniucci, D. M., T. Yamashita, and A. A. Portale. 2006. Dietary phosphorus regulates serum fibroblast growth factor-23 concentrations in healthy men. *J Clin Endocrinol Metab* no. 91 (8):3144–9. doi:10.1210/jc.2006-0021.

Barsh, G. S., D. B. Greenberg, and D. D. Cunningham. 1977. Phosphate uptake and control of fibroblasts growth. *J Cell Physiol* no. 92 (1):115–28. doi:10.1002/jcp.1040920114.

Bayless, K. J., G. A. Meininger, J. M. Scholtz, and G. E. Davis. 1998. Osteopontin is a ligand for the alpha-4beta1 integrin. *J Cell Sci* no. 111 (Pt 9):1165–74.

Beck, G. R., Jr. 2003. Inorganic phosphate as a signaling molecule in osteoblast differentiation. *J Cell Biochem* no. 90 (2):234–43. doi:10.1002/jcb.10622.

Beck, G. R., Jr. and N. Knecht. 2003. Osteopontin regulation by inorganic phosphate is ERK1/2, protein kinase C-, and proteasome-dependent. *J Biol Chem* no. 278 (43):41921–9. doi:10.1074/jbc.M304470200.

Beck, L., C. Leroy, C. Salaun, G. Margall-Ducos, C. Desdouets, and G. Friedlander. 2009. Identification of a novel function of PiT1 critical for cell proliferation and independent of its phosphate transport activity. *J Biol Chem* no. 284 (45):31363–74. doi:10.1074/jbc.M109.053132.

Beck, G. R., Jr., E. Moran, and N. Knecht. 2003. Inorganic phosphate regulates multiple genes during osteoblast differentiation, including Nrf2. *Exp Cell Res* no. 288 (2):288–300.

Beck, G. R., Jr., E. C. Sullivan, E. Moran, and B. Zerler. 1998. Relationship between alkaline phosphatase levels, osteopontin expression, and mineralization in differentiating MC3T3-E1 osteoblasts. *J Cell Biochem* no. 68 (2):269–80.

Beck, G. R., Jr., B. Zerler. and E. Moran. 2000. Phosphate is a specific signal for induction of osteopontin gene expression. *Proc Natl Acad Sci U S A* no. 97 (15):8352–7. doi:10.1073/pnas.140021997.

Biber, J., N. Hernando, and I. Forster. 2013. Phosphate transporters and their function. *Annu Rev Physiol* no. 75:535–50. doi:10.1146/annurev-physiol-030212-183748.

Burnett, S. M., S. C. Gunawardene, F. R. Bringhurst, H. Juppner, H. Lee, and J. S. Finkelstein. 2006. Regulation of C-terminal and intact FGF-23 by dietary phosphate in men and women. *J Bone Miner Res* no. 21 (8):1187–96. doi:10.1359/jbmr.060507.

Byskov, K., N. Jensen, I. B. Kongsfelt, M. Wielsoe, L. E. Pedersen, C. Haldrup, and L. Pedersen. 2012. Regulation of cell proliferation and cell density by the inorganic phosphate transporter PiT1. *Cell Div* no. 7 (1):7. doi:10.1186/1747-1028-7-7.

Calvo, M. S. 1993. Dietary phosphorus, calcium metabolism and bone. *J Nutr* no. 123 (9):1627–33.

Calvo, M. S., R. Kumar, and H. Heath. 1990. Persistently elevated parathyroid hormone secretion and action in young women after four weeks of ingesting high phosphorus, low calcium diets. *J Clin Endocrinol Metab* no. 70 (5):1334–40.

Calvo, M. S. and Y. K. Park. 1996. Changing phosphorus content of the U.S. diet: Potential for adverse effects on bone. *J Nutr* no. 126 (4 Suppl):1168S–80S.

Camalier, C. E., M. Yi, L. R. Yu, B. L. Hood, K. A. Conrads, Y. J. Lee, Y. Lin, L. M. Garneys, G. F. Bouloux, M. R. Young, T. D. Veenstra, R. M. Stephens, N. H. Colburn, T. P. Conrads, and G. R. Beck, Jr. 2013. An integrated understanding of the physiological response to elevated extracellular phosphate. *J Cell Physiol* no. 228 (7):1536–50. doi:10.1002/jcp.24312.

Camalier, C. E., M. R. Young, G. Bobe, C. M. Perella, N. H. Colburn, and G. R. Beck, Jr. 2010. Elevated phosphate activates N-ras and promotes cell transformation and skin tumorigenesis. *Cancer Prev Res (Phila)* no. 3 (3):359–70. doi:10.1158/1940-6207.CAPR-09-0068.

Camilli, T. C., M. Xu, M. P. O'Connell, B. Chien, B. P. Frank, S. Subaran, F. E. Indig, P. J. Morin, S. M. Hewitt, and A. T. Weeraratna. 2011. Loss of Klotho during melanoma progression leads to increased filamin cleavage, increased Wnt5A expression, and enhanced melanoma cell motility. *Pigment Cell Melanoma Res* no. 24 (1):175–86. doi:10.1111/j.1755-148X.2010.00792.x.

Cantor, H. and M. L. Shinohara. 2009. Regulation of T-helper-cell lineage development by osteopontin: The inside story. *Nat Rev Immunol* no. 9 (2):137–41. doi:10.1038/nri2460.

Cao, D., S. R. Hustinx, G. Sui, P. Bala, N. Sato, S. Martin, A. Maitra, K. M. Murphy, J. L. Cameron, C. J. Yeo, S. E. Kern, M. Goggins, A. Pandey, and R. H. Hruban. 2004. Identification of novel highly expressed genes in pancreatic ductal adenocarcinomas through a bioinformatics analysis of expressed sequence tags. *Cancer Biol Ther* no. 3 (11):1081–9; discussion 1090–1.

Chang, S. H., K. N. Yu, Y. S. Lee, G. H. An, G. R. Beck, Jr., N.H. Colburn, K. H. Lee, and M. H. Cho. 2006. Elevated inorganic phosphate stimulates Akt-ERK1/2-Mnk1 signaling in human lung cells. *Am J Respir Cell Mol Biol* no. 35 (5):528–39.

Chen, D. R., S. Y. Chien, S. J. Kuo, Y. H. Teng, H. T. Tsai, J. H. Kuo, and J. G. Chung. 2010. SLC34A2 as a novel marker for diagnosis and targeted therapy of breast cancer. *Anticancer Res* no. 30 (10):4135–40.

Chen, B., X. Ma, S. Liu, W. Zhao, and J. Wu. 2012. Inhibition of lung cancer cells growth, motility and induction of apoptosis by Klotho, a novel secreted Wnt antagonist, in a dose-dependent manner. *Cancer Biol Ther* no. 13 (12):1221–8. doi:10.4161/cbt.21420.

Chen, N. X., K. D. O'Neill, D. Duan, and S. M. Moe. 2002. Phosphorus and uremic serum up-regulate osteopontin expression in vascular smooth muscle cells. *Kidney Int* no. 62 (5):1724–31. doi:10.1046/j.1523-1755 .2002.00625.x.

Cheon, D. J. and S. Orsulic. 2011. Mouse models of cancer. *Annu Rev Pathol* no. 6:95–119. doi:10.1146/ annurev.pathol.3.121806.154244.

Colburn, N. H., B. F. Former, K. A. Nelson, and S. H. Yuspa. 1979. Tumour promoter induces anchorage independence irreversibly. *Nature* no. 281 (5732):589–91.

Collins, J. F., L. Bai, and F. K. Ghishan. 2004. The SLC20 family of proteins: Dual functions as sodium-phosphate cotransporters and viral receptors. *Pflugers Arch* no. 447 (5):647–52.

Conrads, K. A., M. Yi, K. A. Simpson, D. A. Lucas, C. E. Camalier, L. R. Yu, T. D. Veenstra, R. M. Stephens, T. P. Conrads, and G. R. Beck, Jr. 2005. A combined proteome and microarray investigation of inorganic phosphate-induced pre-osteoblast cells. *Mol Cell Proteomics* no. 4 (9):1284–96. doi:10.1074/mcp. M500082-MCP200.

Cunningham, D. D. and A. B. Pardee. 1969. Transport changes rapidly initiated by serum addition to "contact inhibited" 3T3 cells. *Proc Natl Acad Sci U S A* no. 64 (3):1049–56.

de Asua, L. J., E. Rozengurt, and R. Dulbecco. 1974. Kinetics of early changes in phosphate and uridine transport and cyclic AMP levels stimulated by serum in density-inhibited 3T3 cells. *Proc Natl Acad Sci U S A* no. 71 (1):96–8.

Denhardt, D. T., C. M. Giachelli, and S. R. Rittling. 2001. Role of osteopontin in cellular signaling and toxicant injury. *Annu Rev Pharmacol Toxicol* no. 41:723–49. doi:10.1146/annurev.pharmtox.41.1.723.

Dhar, A., J. Hu, R. Reeves, L. M. Resar, and N. H. Colburn. 2004. Dominant-negative c-Jun (TAM67) target genes: HMGA1 is required for tumor promoter-induced transformation. *Oncogene* no. 23 (25):4466–76.

Dhar, A., M. R. Young, and N. H. Colburn. 2002. The role of AP-1, NF-kappaB and ROS/NOS in skin carcinogenesis: The JB6 model is predictive. *Mol Cell Biochem* no. 234–5 (1–2):185–93.

Dhingra, R., L. M. Sullivan, C. S. Fox, T. J. Wang, R. B. D'Agostino, Sr., J. M. Gaziano, and R. S. Vasan. 2007. Relations of serum phosphorus and calcium levels to the incidence of cardiovascular disease in the community. *Arch Intern Med* no. 167 (9):879–85.

Di Marco, G. S., M. Hausberg, U. Hillebrand, P. Rustemeyer, W. Wittkowski, D. Lang, and H. Pavenstadt. 2008. Increased inorganic phosphate induces human endothelial cell apoptosis in vitro. *Am J Physiol Renal Physiol* no. 294 (6):F1381–7. doi:10.1152/ajprenal.00003.2008.

Doi, S., Y. Zou, O. Togao, J. V. Pastor, G. B. John, L. Wang, K. Shiizaki, R. Gotschall, S. Schiavi, N. Yorioka, M. Takahashi, D. A. Boothman, and M. Kuro-o. 2011. Klotho inhibits transforming growth factor-beta1 (TGF-beta1) signaling and suppresses renal fibrosis and cancer metastasis in mice. *J Biol Chem* no. 286 (10):8655–65. doi:10.1074/jbc.M110.174037.

Doll, R. and R. Peto. 1981. The causes of cancer: Quantitative estimates of avoidable risks of cancer in the United States today. *J Natl Cancer Inst* no. 66 (6):1191–308.

Draper, H. H., T. L. Sie, and J. G. Bergan. 1972. Osteoporosis in aging rats induced by high phosphorus diets. *J Nutr* no. 102 (9):1133–41.

El-Tanani, M. K., F. C. Campbell, V. Kurisetty, D. Jin, M. McCann, and P. S. Rudland. 2006. The regulation and role of osteopontin in malignant transformation and cancer. *Cytokine Growth Factor Rev* no. 17 (6):463–74.

Elser, J. J., M. M. Kyle, M. S. Smith, and J. D. Nagy. 2007. Biological stoichiometry in human cancer. *PLOS ONE* no. 2 (10):e1028. doi:10.1371/journal.pone.0001028.

Engstrom, W. and A. Zetterberg. 1983. Phosphate and the regulation of DNA replication in normal and virus-transformed 3T3 cells. *Biochem J* no. 214 (3):695–702.

Fatherazi, S., D. Matsa-Dunn, B. L. Foster, R. B. Rutherford, M. J. Somerman, and R. B. Presland. 2009. Phosphate regulates osteopontin gene transcription. *J Dent Res* no. 88 (1):39–44. doi:10.1177/0022034508328072.

Feldman, D., A. V. Krishnan, S. Swami, E. Giovannucci, and B. J. Feldman. 2014. The role of vitamin D in reducing cancer risk and progression. *Nat Rev Cancer* no. 14 (5):342–57. doi:10.1038/nrc3691.

Feng, S., J. Wang, Y. Zhang, C. J. Creighton, and M. Ittmann. 2015. FGF23 promotes prostate cancer progression. *Oncotarget* no. 6 (19):17291–301.

Ferrari, S. L., J. P. Bonjour, and R. Rizzoli. 2005. Fibroblast growth factor-23 relationship to dietary phosphate and renal phosphate handling in healthy young men. *J Clin Endocrinol Metab* no. 90 (3):1519–24. doi:10.1210/jc.2004-1039.

Ferro, C. J., C. D. Chue, R. P. Steeds, and J. N. Townend. 2009. Is lowering phosphate exposure the key to preventing arterial stiffening with age? *Heart* no. 95 (21):1770–2.

Foster, B. L., F. H. Nociti, Jr., E. C. Swanson, D. Matsa-Dunn, J. E. Berry, C. J. Cupp, P. Zhang, and M. J. Somerman. 2006. Regulation of cementoblast gene expression by inorganic phosphate in vitro. *Calcif Tissue Int* no. 78 (2):103–12.

Freedman, D. M., A. C. Looker, C. C. Abnet, M. S. Linet, and B. I. Graubard. 2010. Serum 25-hydroxyvitamin D and cancer mortality in the NHANES III study (1988–2006). *Cancer Res* no. 70 (21):8587–97. doi:10.1158/0008-5472.CAN-10-1420.

Fujita, T., T. Meguro, N. Izumo, C. Yasutomi, R. Fukuyama, H. Nakamuta, and M. Koida. 2001. Phosphate stimulates differentiation and mineralization of the chondroprogenitor clone ATDC5. *Jpn J Pharmacol* no. 85 (3):278–81.

Giachelli, C. M. 2009. The emerging role of phosphate in vascular calcification. *Kidney Int* no. 75 (9):890–7.

Giachelli, C. M. and S. Steitz. 2000. Osteopontin: A versatile regulator of inflammation and biomineralization. *Matrix Biol* no. 19 (7):615–22.

Giovannucci, E. 1998. Dietary influences of 1,25(OH)2 vitamin D in relation to prostate cancer: A hypothesis. *Cancer Causes Control* no. 9 (6):567–82.

Go, V. L., R. R. Butrum, and D. A. Wong. 2003. Diet, nutrition, and cancer prevention: The postgenomic era. *J Nutr* no. 133 (11 Suppl 1):3830S–3836S.

Gray, R. W., D. R. Wilz, A. E. Caldas, and J. Lemann, Jr. 1977. The importance of phosphate in regulating plasma 1,25-(OH)2-vitamin D levels in humans: Studies in healthy subjects in calcium-stone formers and in patients with primary hyperparathyroidism. *J Clin Endocrinol Metab* no. 45 (2):299–306.

Gutierrez, O. M., A. Luzuriaga-McPherson, Y. Lin, L. C. Gilbert, S. W. Ha, and G. R. Beck, Jr. 2015. Impact of phosphorus-based food additives on bone and mineral metabolism. *J Clin Endocrinol Metab* no. 100 (11):4264–71. doi:10.1210/jc.2015-2279.

Hanahan, D. and R. A. Weinberg. 2000. The hallmarks of cancer. *Cell* no. 100 (1):57–70.

Harima, Y., A. Togashi, K. Horikoshi, M. Imamura, M. Sougawa, S. Sawada, T. Tsunoda, Y. Nakamura, and T. Katagiri. 2004. Prediction of outcome of advanced cervical cancer to thermoradiotherapy according to expression profiles of 35 genes selected by cDNA microarray analysis. *Int J Radiat Oncol Biol Phys* no. 60 (1):237–48. doi:10.1016/j.ijrobp.2004.02.047.

Hilborn, D. A. 1976. Serum stimulation of phosphate uptake into 3T3 cells. *J Cell Physiol* no. 87 (1):111–21.

Holley, R. W. and J. A. Kiernan. 1974. Control of the initiation of DNA synthesis in 3T3 cells: Low-molecular weight nutrients. *Proc Natl Acad Sci U S A* no. 71 (8):2942–5.

Hong, S. H., A. Minai-Tehrani, S. H. Chang, H. L. Jiang, S. Lee, A. Y. Lee, H. W. Seo, C. Chae, G. R. Beck, Jr., and M. H. Cho. 2013. Knockdown of the sodium-dependent phosphate co-transporter 2b (NPT2b) suppresses lung tumorigenesis. *PLOS ONE* no. 8 (10):e77121. doi:10.1371/journal.pone.0077121.

Hughes, M. R., P. F. Brumbaugh, M. R. Hussler, J. E. Wergedal, and D. J. Baylink. 1975. Regulation of serum 1alpha,25-dihydroxyvitamin D3 by calcium and phosphate in the rat. *Science* no. 190 (4214): 578–80.

Huttunen, M. M., I. Tillman, H. T. Viljakainen, J. Tuukkanen, Z. Peng, M. Pekkinen, and C. J. Lamberg-Allardt. 2007. High dietary phosphate intake reduces bone strength in the growing rat skeleton. *J Bone Miner Res* no. 22 (1):83–92. doi:10.1359/jbmr.061009.

Jacobs, E., M. E. Martinez, J. Buckmeier, P. Lance, M. May, and P. Jurutka. 2011. Circulating fibroblast growth factor-23 is associated with increased risk for metachronous colorectal adenoma. *J Carcinog* no. 10:3. doi:10.4103/1477–3163.76723.

Jin, H., S. H. Chang, C. X. Xu, J. Y. Shin, Y. S. Chung, S. J. Park, Y. S. Lee, G. H. An, K. H. Lee, and M. H. Cho. 2007. High dietary inorganic phosphate affects lung through altering protein translation, cell cycle, and angiogenesis in developing mice. *Toxicol Sci* no. 100 (1):215–23. doi:10.1093/toxsci/kfm202.

Jin, H., S. K. Hwang, K. Yu, H. K. Anderson, Y. S. Lee, K. H. Lee, A. C. Prats, D. Morello, G. R. Beck, Jr., and M. H. Cho. 2006. A high inorganic phosphate diet perturbs brain growth, alters Akt-ERK signaling, and results in changes in cap-dependent translation. *Toxicol Sci* no. 90 (1):221–9.

Jin, H., C. X. Xu, H. T. Lim, S. J. Park, J. Y. Shin, Y. S. Chung, S. C. Park, S. H. Chang, H. J. Youn, K. H. Lee, Y. S. Lee, Y. C. Ha, C. H. Chae, G. R. Beck, Jr., and M. H. Cho. 2009. High dietary inorganic phosphate increases lung tumorigenesis and alters Akt signaling. *Am J Respir Crit Care Med* no. 179 (1):59–68.

Johnson, L., K. Mercer, D. Greenbaum, R. T. Bronson, D. Crowley, D. A. Tuveson, and T. Jacks. 2001. Somatic activation of the K-ras oncogene causes early onset lung cancer in mice. *Nature* no. 410 (6832):1111–6.

Jones, H. B., I. L. Chaikoff, and J. H. Lawrence. 1940. Phosphorus metabolism of neoplastic tissues (mammary carcinoma, lymphoma, lymphosarcoma) as indicated by radioactive phosphorus. *Cancer Res* no. 40:243–250.

Jono, S., M. D. McKee, C. E. Murry, A. Shioi, Y. Nishizawa, K. Mori, H. Morii, and C. M. Giachelli. 2000. Phosphate regulation of vascular smooth muscle cell calcification. *Circ Res* no. 87 (7):E10–7.

Julien, M., S. Khoshniat, A. Lacreusette, M. Gatius, A. Bozec, E. F. Wagner, Y. Wittrant, M. Masson, P. Weiss, L. Beck, D. Magne, and J. Guicheux. 2009. Phosphate-dependent regulation of MGP in osteoblasts: Role of ERK1/2 and Fra-1. *J Bone Miner Res* no. 24 (11):1856–68. doi:10.1359/jbmr.090508.

Julien, M., D. Magne, M. Masson, M. Rolli-Derkinderen, O. Chassande, C. Cario-Toumaniantz, Y. Cherel, P. Weiss, and J. Guicheux. 2007. Phosphate stimulates matrix Gla protein expression in chondrocytes through the extracellular signal regulated kinase signaling pathway. *Endocrinology* no. 148 (2):530–7.

Kanatani, M., T. Sugimoto, J. Kano, M. Kanzawa, and K. Chihara. 2003. Effect of high phosphate concentration on osteoclast differentiation as well as bone-resorbing activity. *J Cell Physiol* no. 196 (1):180–9.

Karkkainen, M. and C. Lamberg-Allardt. 1996. An acute intake of phosphate increases parathyroid hormone secretion and inhibits bone formation in young women. *J Bone Miner Res* no. 11 (12):1905–12.

Kemi, V. E., M. U. Karkkainen, and C. J. Lamberg-Allardt. 2006. High phosphorus intakes acutely and negatively affect Ca and bone metabolism in a dose-dependent manner in healthy young females. *Br J Nutr* no. 96 (3):545–52.

Kim, H. S., H. Kim do, J. Y. Kim, N. H. Jeoung, I. K. Lee, J. G. Bong, and E. D. Jung. 2010. Microarray analysis of papillary thyroid cancers in Korean. *Korean J Intern Med* no. 25 (4):399–407. doi:10.3904/kjim.2010.25.4.399.

Kimata, M., T. Michigami, K. Tachikawa, T. Okada, T. Koshimizu, M. Yamazaki, M. Kogo, and K. Ozono. 2010. Signaling of extracellular inorganic phosphate up-regulates cyclin D1 expression in proliferating chondrocytes via the Na+/Pi cotransporter Pit-1 and Raf/MEK/ERK pathway. *Bone* no. 47 (5):938–47. doi:10.1016/j.bone.2010.08.006.

Kuro, O. M. 2011. Phosphate and Klotho. *Kidney Int Suppl* (121):S20–3. doi:10.1038/ki.2011.26.

Lee, J., D. J. Jeong, J. Kim, S. Lee, J. H. Park, B. Chang, S. I. Jung, L. Yi, Y. Han, Y. Yang, K. I. Kim, J. S. Lim, I. Yang, S. Jeon, D. H. Bae, C. J. Kim, and M. S. Lee. 2010. The anti-aging gene KLOTHO is a novel target for epigenetic silencing in human cervical carcinoma. *Mol Cancer* no. 9:109. doi:10.1186/1476-4598-9-109.

Li, X., H. Y. Yang, and C. M. Giachelli. 2006. Role of the sodium-dependent phosphate cotransporter, Pit-1, in vascular smooth muscle cell calcification. *Circ Res* no. 98 (7):905–12.

Lin, Y., K. E. McKinnon, S. W. Ha, and G. R. Beck, Jr. 2015a. Inorganic phosphate induces cancer cell mediated angiogenesis dependent on forkhead box protein C2 (FOXC2) regulated osteopontin expression. *Mol Carcinog* no. 54 (9):926–34. doi:10.1002/mc.22153.

Lin, K., B. Rubinfeld, C. Zhang, R. Firestein, E. Harstad, L. Roth, S. P. Tsai, M. Schutten, K. Xu, M. Hristopoulos, and P. Polakis. 2015b. Preclinical development of an Anti-NaPi2b (SLC34A2) antibody-drug conjugate as a therapeutic for non-small cell lung and ovarian cancers. *Clin Cancer Res* no. 21 (22):5139–50. doi:10.1158/1078-0432.CCR-14-3383.

Liu, H., M. M. Fergusson, R. M. Castilho, J. Liu, L. Cao, J. Chen, D. Malide, Rovira, II, D. Schimel, C. J. Kuo, J. S. Gutkind, P. M. Hwang, and T. Finkel. 2007. Augmented Wnt signaling in a mammalian model of accelerated aging. *Science* no. 317 (5839):803–6. doi:10.1126/science.1143578.

Lundquist, P., H. Murer, and J. Biber. 2007. Type II Na+-Pi cotransporters in osteoblast mineral formation: Regulation by inorganic phosphate. *Cell Physiol Biochem* no. 19 (1–4):43–56.

Maierhofer, W. J., R. W. Gray, and J. Lemann, Jr. 1984. Phosphate deprivation increases serum 1,25-(OH)2-vitamin D concentrations in healthy men. *Kidney Int* no. 25 (3):571–5.

Mansfield, K., C. C. Teixeira, C. S. Adams, and I. M. Shapiro. 2001. Phosphate ions mediate chondrocyte apoptosis through a plasma membrane transporter mechanism. *Bone* no. 28 (1):1–8.

Meleti, Z., I. M. Shapiro, and C. S. Adams. 2000. Inorganic phosphate induces apoptosis of osteoblast-like cells in culture. *Bone* no. 27 (3):359–66.

Mozar, A., N. Haren, M. Chasseraud, L. Louvet, C. Maziere, A. Wattel, R. Mentaverri, P. Morliere, S. Kamel, M. Brazier, J. C. Maziere, and Z. A. Massy. 2007. Phosphate inhibits RANKL induce NF-kappa B activation during the differentiation of monocytes-macrophages to osteoclast-like cells: Possible role in CKD-MBD. *Nephrol Dial Transplant* no. 22:139–140.

Newberne, P. M. and M. W. Conner. 1988. Dietary modifiers of cancer. *Prog Clin Biol Res* no. 259:105–29.

Oates, A. J., R. Barraclough, and P. S. Rudland. 1997. The role of osteopontin in tumorigenesis and metastasis. *Invasion Metastasis* no. 17 (1):1–15.

Onufrak, S. J., A. Bellasi, L. J. Shaw, C. A. Herzog, F. Cardarelli, P. W. Wilson, V. Vaccarino, and P. Raggi. 2008. Phosphorus levels are associated with subclinical atherosclerosis in the general population. *Atherosclerosis* no. 199 (2):424–31.

O'Regan, A. W., J. M. Hayden, and J. S. Berman. 2000. Osteopontin augments CD3-mediated interferon-gamma and CD40 ligand expression by T cells, which results in IL-12 production from peripheral blood mononuclear cells. *J Leukoc Biol* no. 68 (4):495–502.

Pan, J., J. Zhong, L. H. Gan, S. J. Chen, H. C. Jin, X. Wang, and L. J. Wang. 2011. Klotho, an anti-senescence related gene, is frequently inactivated through promoter hypermethylation in colorectal cancer. *Tumour Biol* no. 32 (4):729–35. doi:10.1007/s13277-011-0174-5.

Portale, A. A., B. P. Halloran, and R. C. Morris, Jr. 1989. Physiologic regulation of the serum concentration of 1,25-dihydroxyvitamin D by phosphorus in normal men. *J Clin Invest* no. 83 (5):1494–9. doi:10.1172/JCI114043.

Portale, A. A., B. P. Halloran, M. M. Murphy, and R. C. Morris, Jr. 1986. Oral intake of phosphorus can determine the serum concentration of 1,25-dihydroxyvitamin D by determining its production rate in humans. *J Clin Invest* no. 77 (1):7–12. doi:10.1172/JCI112304.

Rahabi-Layachi, H., R. Ourouda, A. Boullier, Z. A. Massy, and C. Amant. 2015. Distinct effects of inorganic phosphate on cell cycle and apoptosis in human vascular smooth muscle cells. *J Cell Physiol* no. 230 (2):347–55. doi:10.1002/jcp.24715.

Rangel, L. B., C. A. Sherman-Baust, R. P. Wernyj, D. R. Schwartz, K. R. Cho, and P. J. Morin. 2003. Characterization of novel human ovarian cancer-specific transcripts (HOSTs) identified by serial analysis of gene expression. *Oncogene* no. 22 (46):7225–32. doi:10.1038/sj.onc.1207008.

Rangrez, A. Y., E. M'Baya-Moutoula, V. Metzinger-Le Meuth, L. Henaut, M. S. Djelouat, J. Benchitrit, Z. A. Massy, and L. Metzinger. 2012. Inorganic phosphate accelerates the migration of vascular smooth muscle cells: Evidence for the involvement of miR-223. *PLOS ONE* no. 7 (10):e47807. doi:10.1371/journal.pone.0047807.

Reiss, E., J. M. Canterbury, M. A. Bercovitz, and E. L. Kaplan. 1970. The role of phosphate in the secretion of parathyroid hormone in man. *J Clin Invest* no. 49 (11):2146–9. doi:10.1172/JCI106432.

Rittling, S. R. and A. F. Chambers. 2004. Role of osteopontin in tumour progression. *Br J Cancer* no. 90 (10):1877–81.

Roussanne, M. C., M. Lieberherr, J. C. Souberbielle, E. Sarfati, T. Drueke, and A. Bourdeau. 2001. Human parathyroid cell proliferation in response to calcium, NPS R-467, calcitriol and phosphate. *Eur J Clin Invest* no. 31 (7):610–6.

Rubin, H. and B. M. Chu. 1984. Solute concentration effects on the expression of cellular heterogeneity of anchorage-independent growth among spontaneously transformed BALB/c3T3 cells. *In Vitro* no. 20 (7):585–96.

Rubin, H. and H. Sanui. 1977. Complexes of inorganic pyrophosphate, orthophosphate, and calcium as stimulants of 3T3 cell multiplication. *Proc Natl Acad Sci U S A* no. 74 (11):5026–30.

Rutherford, R. B., B. L. Foster, T. Bammler, R. P. Beyer, S. Sato, and M. J. Somerman. 2006. Extracellular phosphate alters cementoblast gene expression. *J Dent Res* no. 85 (6):505–9.

Sage, A. P., J. Lu, Y. Tintut, and L. L. Demer. 2011. Hyperphosphatemia-induced nanocrystals upregulate the expression of bone morphogenetic protein-2 and osteopontin genes in mouse smooth muscle cells in vitro. *Kidney Int* no. 79 (4):414–22. doi:10.1038/ki.2010.390.

Sapio, L., L. Sorvillo, M. Illiano, E. Chiosi, A. Spina, and S. Naviglio. 2015. Inorganic phosphate prevents Erk1/2 and Stat3 activation and improves sensitivity to doxorubicin of MDA-MB-231 breast cancer cells. *Molecules* no. 20 (9):15910–28. doi:10.3390/molecules200915910.

Senger, D. R., C. A. Perruzzi, and A. Papadopoulos. 1989. Elevated expression of secreted phosphoprotein I (osteopontin, 2ar) as a consequence of neoplastic transformation. *Anticancer Res* no. 9 (5):1291–9.

Shu, G., B. Xie, F. Ren, D. C. Liu, J. Zhou, Q. Li, J. Chen, L. Yuan, and J. Zhou. 2013. Restoration of klotho expression induces apoptosis and autophagy in hepatocellular carcinoma cells. *Cell Oncol (Dordr)* no. 36 (2):121–9. doi:10.1007/s13402-012-0118-0.

Shyian, M., V. Gryshkova, O. Kostianets, V. Gorshkov, Y. Gogolev, I. Goncharuk, S. Nespryadko, L. Vorobjova, V. Filonenko, and R. Kiyamova. 2011. Quantitative analysis of SLC34A2 expression in different types of ovarian tumors. *Exp Oncol* no. 33 (2):94–8.

Slaga, T. J., I. V. Budunova, I. B. Gimenez-Conti, and C. M. Aldaz. 1996. The mouse skin carcinogenesis model. *J Investig Dermatol Symp Proc* no. 1 (2):151–6.

Sodek, J., B. Ganss, and M. D. McKee. 2000. Osteopontin. *Crit Rev Oral Biol Med* no. 11 (3):279–303.

Spina, A., L. Sorvillo, F. Di Maiolo, A. Esposito, R. D'Auria, D. Di Gesto, E. Chiosi, and S. Naviglio. 2013. Inorganic phosphate enhances sensitivity of human osteosarcoma U2OS cells to doxorubicin via a p53-dependent pathway. *J Cell Physiol* no. 228 (1):198–206. doi:10.1002/jcp.24124.

Suyama, T., S. Okada, T. Ishijima, K. Iida, K. Abe, and Y. Nakai. 2012. High phosphorus diet-induced changes in NaPi-IIb phosphate transporter expression in the rat kidney: DNA microarray analysis. *PLOS ONE* no. 7 (1):e29483. doi:10.1371/journal.pone.0029483.

Suzuki, A., C. Ghayor, J. Guicheux, D. Magne, S. Quillard, A. Kakita, Y. Ono, Y. Miura, Y. Oiso, M. Itoh, and J. Caverzasio. 2006. Enhanced expression of the inorganic phosphate transporter Pit-1 is involved in BMP-2-induced matrix mineralization in osteoblast-like cells. *J Bone Miner Res* no. 21 (5):674–83.

Suzuki, A., G. Palmer, J. P. Bonjour, and J. Caverzasio. 2000. Stimulation of sodium-dependent phosphate transport and signaling mechanisms induced by basic fibroblast growth factor in MC3T3-E1 osteoblast-like cells. *J Bone Miner Res* no. 15 (1):95–102.

Takeda, E., Y. Taketani, K. Nashiki, M. Nomoto, E. Shuto, N. Sawada, H. Yamamoto, and M. Isshiki. 2006. A novel function of phosphate-mediated intracellular signal transduction pathways. *Adv Enzyme Regul* no. 46:154–61. doi:10.1016/j.advenzreg.2006.01.003.

Tebben, P. J., K. R. Kalli, W. A. Cliby, L. C. Hartmann, J. P. Grande, R. J. Singh, and R. Kumar. 2005. Elevated fibroblast growth factor 23 in women with malignant ovarian tumors. *Mayo Clin Proc* no. 80 (6):745–51. doi:10.1016/S0025-6196(11)61528-0.

Teixeira, C. C., K. Mansfield, C. Hertkorn, H. Ischiropoulos, and I. M. Shapiro. 2001. Phosphate-induced chondrocyte apoptosis is linked to nitric oxide generation. *Am J Physiol Cell Physiol* no. 281 (3):C833–9.

Tenenhouse, H. S. 2007. Phosphate transport: Molecular basis, regulation and pathophysiology. *J Steroid Biochem Mol Biol* no. 103 (3–5):572–7.

Thomas, C. I., H. Harrington, and M. S. Bovington. 1958. Uptake of radioactive phosphorus in experimental tumors. III. The biochemical fate of P32 in normal and neoplastic ocular tissue. *Cancer Res* no. 18 (9):1008–11.

Tuohimaa, P. 2008. Vitamin D, aging, and cancer. *Nutr Rev* no. 66 (10 Suppl 2):S147–52. doi:10.1111/j.1753-4887.2008.00095.x.

Turner, N. and R. Grose. 2010. Fibroblast growth factor signalling: From development to cancer. *Nat Rev Cancer* no. 10 (2):116–29. doi:10.1038/nrc2780.

Urakawa, I., Y. Yamazaki, T. Shimada, K. Iijima, H. Hasegawa, K. Okawa, T. Fujita, S. Fukumoto, and T. Yamashita. 2006. Klotho converts canonical FGF receptor into a specific receptor for FGF23. *Nature* no. 444 (7120):770–4. doi:10.1038/nature05315.

Uribarri, J. and M. S. Calvo. 2013. Dietary phosphorus excess: A risk factor in chronic bone, kidney, and cardiovascular disease? *Adv Nutr* no. 4 (5):542–4. doi:10.3945/an.113.004234.

Wai, P. Y. and P. C. Kuo. 2008. Osteopontin: Regulation in tumor metastasis. *Cancer Metastasis Rev* no. 27 (1):103–18.

Walker, L. C., N. Waddell, A. Ten Haaf, Investigators kConFab, S. Grimmond, and A. B. Spurdle. 2008. Use of expression data and the CGEMS genome-wide breast cancer association study to identify genes that may modify risk in BRCA1/2 mutation carriers. *Breast Cancer Res Treat* no. 112 (2):229–36. doi:10.1007/s10549-007-9848-5.

Wang, Y., L. Chen, G. Huang, D. He, J. He, W. Xu, C. Zou, F. Zong, Y. Li, B. Chen, S. Wu, W. Zhao, and J. Wu. 2013. Klotho sensitizes human lung cancer cell line to cisplatin via PI3k/Akt pathway. *PLOS ONE* no. 8 (2):e57391. doi:10.1371/journal.pone.0057391.

Wang, L., X. Wang, X. Wang, P. Jie, H. Lu, S. Zhang, X. Lin, E. K. Lam, Y. Cui, J. Yu, and H. Jin. 2011. Klotho is silenced through promoter hypermethylation in gastric cancer. *Am J Cancer Res* no. 1 (1):111–9.

Weber, M. J. and G. Edlin. 1971. Phosphate transport, nucleotide pools, and ribonucleic acid synthesis in growing and in density-inhibited 3T3 cells. *J Biol Chem* no. 246 (6):1828–33.

Wilson, K. M., I. M. Shui, L. A. Mucci, and E. Giovannucci. 2015. Calcium and phosphorus intake and prostate cancer risk: A 24-y follow-up study. *Am J Clin Nutr* no. 101 (1):173–83. doi:10.3945/ajcn.114.088716.

Wittrant, Y., A. Bourgine, S. Khoshniat, B. Alliot-Licht, M. Masson, M. Gatius, T. Rouillon, P. Weiss, L. Beck, and J. Guicheux. 2009. Inorganic phosphate regulates Glvr-1 and -2 expression: Role of calcium and ERK1/2. *Biochem Biophys Res Commun* no. 381 (2):259–63. doi:10.1016/j.bbrc.2009.02.034.

Wolf, I., S. Levanon-Cohen, S. Bose, H. Ligumsky, B. Sredni, H. Kanety, M. Kuro-o, B. Karlan, B. Kaufman, H. P. Koeffler, and T. Rubinek. 2008. Klotho: A tumor suppressor and a modulator of the IGF-1 and FGF pathways in human breast cancer. *Oncogene* no. 27 (56):7094–105. doi:10.1038/onc.2008.292.

Wulaningsih, W., K. Michaelsson, H. Garmo, N. Hammar, I. Jungner, G. Walldius, L. Holmberg, and M. Van Hemelrijck. 2013. Inorganic phosphate and the risk of cancer in the Swedish AMORIS study. *BMC Cancer* no. 13:257. doi:10.1186/1471-2407-13-257.

Xie, B., J. Chen, B. Liu, and J. Zhan. 2013a. Klotho acts as a tumor suppressor in cancers. *Pathol Oncol Res* no. 19 (4):611–7. doi:10.1007/s12253-013-9663-8.

Xie, B., J. Zhou, G. Shu, D. C. Liu, J. Zhou, J. Chen, and L. Yuan. 2013b. Restoration of klotho gene expression induces apoptosis and autophagy in gastric cancer cells: Tumor suppressive role of klotho in gastric cancer. *Cancer Cell Int* no. 13 (1):18. doi:10.1186/1475-2867-13-18.

Xie, B., J. Zhou, L. Yuan, F. Ren, D. C. Liu, Q. Li, and G. Shu. 2013c. Epigenetic silencing of Klotho expression correlates with poor prognosis of human hepatocellular carcinoma. *Hum Pathol* no. 44 (5):795–801. doi:10.1016/j.humpath.2012.07.023.

Xu, C. X., H. Jin, H. T. Lim, Y. C. Ha, C. H. Chae, G. H. An, K. H. Lee, and M. H. Cho. 2010. Low dietary inorganic phosphate stimulates lung tumorigenesis through altering protein translation and cell cycle in K-ras(LA1) mice. *Nutr Cancer* no. 62 (4):525–32. doi:10.1080/01635580903532432.

Yamazaki, M., K. Ozono, T. Okada, K. Tachikawa, H. Kondou, Y. Ohata, and T. Michigami. 2010. Both FGF23 and extracellular phosphate activate Raf/MEK/ERK pathway via FGF receptors in HEK293 cells. *J Cell Biochem* no. 111 (5):1210–21. doi:10.1002/jcb.22842.

Yates, A. J., R. O. Oreffo, K. Mayor, and G. R. Mundy. 1991. Inhibition of bone resorption by inorganic phosphate is mediated by both reduced osteoclast formation and decreased activity of mature osteoclasts. *J Bone Miner Res* no. 6 (5):473–8. doi:10.1002/jbmr.5650060508.

Yoshiko, Y., G. A. Candeliere, N. Maeda, and J. E. Aubin. 2007. Osteoblast autonomous Pi regulation via Pit1 plays a role in bone mineralization. *Mol Cell Biol* no. 27 (12):4465–74. doi:10.1128/MCB.00104-07.

Young, M. R., H. S. Yang, and N. H. Colburn. 2003. Promising molecular targets for cancer prevention: AP-1, NF-kappa B and Pdcd4. *Trends Mol Med* no. 9 (1):36–41.

Zhong, M., D. H. Carney, H. Jo, B. D. Boyan, and Z. Schwartz. 2011. Inorganic phosphate induces mammalian growth plate chondrocyte apoptosis in a mitochondrial pathway involving nitric oxide and JNK MAP kinase. *Calcif Tissue Int* no. 88 (2):96–108. doi:10.1007/s00223-010-9433-5.

Zhou, X. and X. Wang. 2015. Klotho: A novel biomarker for cancer. *J Cancer Res Clin Oncol* no. 141 (6):961–9. doi:10.1007/s00432-014-1788-y.

Zhu, Y., L. Xu, J. Zhang, W. Xu, Y. Liu, H. Yin, T. Lv, H. An, L. Liu, H. He, H. Zhang, J. Liu, J. Xu, and Z. Lin. 2013. Klotho suppresses tumor progression via inhibiting PI3K/Akt/GSK3beta/Snail signaling in renal cell carcinoma. *Cancer Sci* no. 104 (6):663–71. doi:10.1111/cas.12134.

3 Clinical and Preclinical Evidence of the Skeletal and Vascular Adverse Health Effects of High Dietary Phosphorus

Jorge B. Cannata-Andía, Pablo Román-García, Natalia Carrillo-López, and Adriana S. Dusso

CONTENTS

Abstract 31
Bullet Points 32
3.1 Introduction 32
3.2 Pathophysiology of Vascular Calcification 32
    3.2.1 Role of Phosphorus 33
    3.2.2 Role of PTH and Other Factors 34
3.3 Pathophysiology of Bone Fragility in CKD 35
    3.3.1 Role of Phosphorus 35
    3.3.2 Role of PTH and Other Factors 36
3.4 Vascular Calcification, Bone Health, and Survival: Lessons from Clinical and
    Preclinical Evidence 37
    3.4.1 Clinical Evidence 37
    3.4.2 Preclinical Evidence 37
3.5 Areas for Future Research 39
3.6 Conclusions 39
References 39

ABSTRACT

High dietary phosphorus and hyperphosphatemia contribute to impair skeletal and vascular health. Hyperphosphatemia activates signaling pathways that impair bone remodeling and mineralization and increase the propensity to vascular calcification. In bone, hyperphosphatemia increases the expression of inhibitors of the Wnt pathway and favors osteoblast and osteocyte apoptosis and, in the vessels, induces the differentiation of vascular smooth muscle cells from a vascular to an osteoblastic, bone-forming phenotype. The elevations in serum parathyroid hormone (PTH) induced by hyperphosphatemia favor bone resorption and could worsen vascular calcification.

These phosphorus/PTH interactions make it difficult to separate direct phosphorus actions on the bone/vasculature axis from those that are PTH driven. Phosphorus induction of fibroblast growth factor 23 (FGF23) could also reduce bone mass through FGF23-induced increases of Wnt inhibitors in bone.

Severe vascular calcification may induce reduced bone mass and propensity to fractures. The mechanisms involving the reciprocal adverse interactions between vascular calcification and loss of bone mass are not fully understood; however, they could involve the inhibition of the Wnt pathway to protect vessels, but with a deleterious consequence to bone.

This chapter presents the current understanding of the molecular and cellular mechanisms, as well as the yet unresolved basic and clinical controversies on the severe disturbances in the bone/vasculature axis induced by hyperphosphatemia. This knowledge is a mandatory first step to identify accurate biomarkers of subclinical disease and improve current therapeutic strategies.

BULLET POINTS

- Hyperphosphatemia contributes to worsen the prevalence and progression of vascular calcification as well as the decreases in bone mass favoring fragility fractures.
- Activation of the Wnt pathway, a requirement for proper skeletal remodeling and mineralization, is an important stimulus for vascular calcification.
- Vascular calcification, bone loss, and increased propensity for fractures are common findings in aging and chronic kidney disease, all independently associated with higher mortality.
- Novel therapeutic strategies directed to antagonize the elevations of Wnt inhibitors to allow more bone formation may worsen vascular health by promoting mineralization of the vessel wall.
- Calcified vessels may be a nonnegligible source of circulating Wnt pathway inhibitors, which could reduce Wnt activation in bone, impairing mineralization and reducing bone mass.

3.1 INTRODUCTION

Hyperphosphatemia is a systemic alteration causing a large number of multifaceted adverse consequences on mineral homeostasis and renal, bone, and vascular health in the general population, all of which are aggravated in the process of aging and even further in the course of chronic kidney disease (CKD) (Moe et al. 2006; Friedman 2005; Hruska et al. 2008).

Renal phosphorus retention, as a consequence of the renal impairment associated with ageing or CKD, imposes a wide range of hormonal adaptations in the parathyroid glands ($\Uparrow$PTH), in bone ($\Uparrow$ FGF23), and in the kidney ($\Downarrow$ 1,25 OH$_2$vit D$_3$ and α-klotho), which together with phosphorus, direct pro-aging actions to accelerate renal, bone, and cardiovascular damage (Roman-Garcia et al. 2009).

The study of the mechanisms and signals involved in the crosstalk between bone, the kidney, and the vasculature in CKD and of the strong association between impaired bone remodeling and the increased propensity to vascular calcification and cardiovascular disease and vice versa are issues of intensive research due to their high clinical relevance to improve the current therapeutic strategies used in the management of bone remodeling in osteoporosis, renal, and cardiovascular disorders.

This chapter will update the current understanding of the pathophysiology of the adverse impact of high phosphorus on the renal/bone/vasculature axis from a bench to bedside perspective.

3.2 PATHOPHYSIOLOGY OF VASCULAR CALCIFICATION

Vascular calcification is an active precipitation of calcium phosphate aggregates as a consequence of unstable supersaturation of the exchangeable calcium and phosphorus pools. This process involves a transition of the vascular smooth muscle cells (VSMCs) in the medial layer of the vessels away from their mesenchymal contractile functional phenotype to a secretory (also mesenchymal)

Evidence of the Skeletal and Vascular Adverse Health Effects 33

osteoblastic phenotype. These osteoblast-like cells express markers of bone formation and generate calcium–phosphorus deposits in the vasculature analogous to those mediating skeletal calcification (Shroff, Long, and Shanahan 2013). In addition to the acquisition of an osteoblastic phenotype by VSMC, vascular calcification results from the loss of vascular calcification inhibitors. In fact, calcification appears to be an adaptive process in response to pro-aging or uremic insults including: a) the loss of calcification inhibitors as osteopontin, matrix-Gla protein, fetuin A, or pyrophosphate (PPi) (Lomashvili et al. 2004; Ketteler et al. 2005; Moe et al. 2005), which inhibit hydroxyapatite formation, and b) osteoblastic VSMC differentiation by expressing skeletal transcription factors such as core-binding factor 1 (CBFA-1, also known as RUNX2), MSX2, and SOX9 (Ducy et al. 1997; Engelse et al. 2001), bone morphogenetic proteins (BMPs) such as BMP2 and BMP4, and bone-forming proteins such as tissue-nonspecific alkaline phosphatase (TNAP) and osteocalcin (Reynolds et al. 2004).

TNAP, expressed in osteoblast-like cells, hydrolyzes PPi and is a major determinant of hydroxyapatite formation in bone or vessels (O'Neill 2006). Osteocalcin, produced by osteoblasts and osteoblast-like cells, is stored in the mineralized matrix and currently used as a marker of bone activity. In its undercarboxylated circulating form osteocalcin is also a hormone capable of regulating energy metabolism, fertility, and brain development (Rached et al. 2010; Oury et al. 2013; Lee et al. 2007; Ducy et al. 1996). When overexpressed in VSMCs (using a viral strategy), osteocalcin locally shifts cells toward enhanced glucose uptake and stimulates calcification (Idelevich, Rais, and Monsonego-Ornan 2011).

The osteoblastic transition is followed by the osteoblast-like VSMC release of cell-derived matrix vesicles (Kapustin et al. 2011) that contain hydroxyapatite (Mathew et al. 2008) and finally the full loss of their muscular phenotype (Shen et al. 2011). As mineralization takes place, a macroscopic consequence in large- and medium-caliber arteries (Roman-Garcia et al. 2011) is an increase in stiffness, which enhances the relative risk of mortality in the general aging population and in CKD patients (Rodriguez Garcia et al. 2005; Muntner et al. 2013; Stubbs et al. 2007; Wilson et al. 2001).

3.2.1 Role of Phosphorus

The change in VSMC phenotype is driven by an increase in systemic and/or local factors that promote calcification and by a decrease in calcification inhibitors. Phosphorus load, a potent systemic promoter of calcification, is a common feature in CKD patients. Renal phosphorus retention associated with either age-dependent reductions in renal function or CKD progression is aggravated by the contribution of occidental diets rich in organic phosphorus or in food preservatives rich in inorganic phosphorus (Cannata-Andia and Naves-Diaz 2009). In fact, silencing the putative phosphorus channel, the sodium-dependent phosphorus cotransporter, Pit-1, inhibited phosphorus-stimulated mineralization of VSMCs (Li, Yang, and Giachelli 2006), indicating that vascular calcification can be regulated by the cellular uptake of phosphorus. Intracellular phosphorus increases hydrogen peroxide to directly activate the Akt pathway (Byon et al. 2008), which in turn, increases RUNX2, the transcription factor that drives the expression of the osteoblast transcriptome (Giachelli 2004) and stimulates the release of matrix vesicles. Thus, increased intracellular phosphorus stimulates VSMCs' transition to an osteoblastic phenotype.

Phosphorus also influences the levels of several microRNAs (miRNAs) critical for vascular health (Panizo et al. 2016). miRNAs are small (~22 nucleotides) noncoding, single-stranded RNAs that mediate posttranscriptional gene silencing by binding to sites of antisense complementarity in 3' untranslated regions of target messenger RNAs. In fact, in a rat model of uremia and high dietary phosphorus, decreased levels of miR-133b and miR-211 correlated with increased RUNX2 expression. In contrast, increased levels of miR-29b correlated with a decreased expression of osteoblast differentiation inhibitors (Panizo et al. 2016). More importantly, the cause–effect relationship between the expression of the identified miRNAs and the magnitude of calcification was corroborated using the silencing and overexpression of the previously mentioned specific miRNA in in vitro models of vascular calcification. Exposure of VSMCs to either uremic serum or high calcium and phosphorus media provided direct evidence of the role of miR-133b, miR-211, and miR-29b in the calcification of VSMC induced by high phosphorus (Panizo et al. 2016).

An additional role for high serum phosphorus and calcium in the initiation of vascular calcification may be to promote VSMC apoptosis (Panizo et al. 2016), because apoptotic bodies function similarly to matrix vesicles in heterotopic mineralization.

The established paradigm considers that vascular calcification is driven by intracellular increments in phosphorus, which is transported to the matrix in a hydroxyapatite form by calcifying VSMCs to ultimately produce mineralized foci in the vessels. In addition to this, it has been proposed that phosphorus can interact with calcium at physiological concentrations, forming calcium–phosphorus deposits in a passive physicochemical process that does not require any cellular activity (Villa-Bellosta and Sorribas 2009). The role of VSMCs in this case would be to inhibit hydroxyapatite formation with PPi, a potent inhibitor of hydroxyapatite formation, rather than forming it. Thus, in addition to the established paradigm, vascular calcification may also occur as a consequence of the loss of the ability of VSMC to inhibit mineralization. Furthermore, it has been suggested that these mineral deposits may induce the same transition to a bone-forming phenotype as that described for intracellular Pi-induced vascular calcification (Villa-Bellosta and Sorribas 2011). This suggests that in addition to the putative active mechanisms, calcium–phosphorus deposition combined with a decrease in PPi (O'Neill et al. 2011; Lomashvili, Khawandi, and O'Neill 2005) may collaborate in the calcifying response of the vasculature to high serum phosphorus (Villa-Bellosta and Egido 2015; Lomashvili et al. 2014).

3.2.2 Role of PTH and Other Factors

Two phosphaturic hormones that markedly increase in response to high phosphorus are PTH and FGF23, and both may independently contribute to the development and progression of vascular calcification (Yuan et al. 2011; Oliveira et al. 2010; Bellorin-Font et al. 1985).

The role of high PTH in vascular calcification is unclear. VSMCs express PTHR1, so they might be susceptible to regulation by PTH (Whitfield 2005). In CKD patients, high PTH levels are often associated with high calcification scores and increased risk for cardiovascular mortality (Coen et al. 2009; Naves-Diaz et al. 2011; Panichi et al. 2010; Tentori et al. 2008; Coen et al. 2007). However, a meta-analysis of factors related to vascular calcification and mortality has reinforced the role of inorganic phosphorus (Pi) as a cardiovascular risk factor but failed to identify any role for PTH (Palmer et al. 2011).

As proof of this controversy, preclinical murine models of atherosclerotic vascular calcification have demonstrated that whereas PTH fragment 1–34 inhibits calcification (Shao et al. 2003), PTH 7–84 appears to increase calcium deposition (Vattikuti and Towler 2004).

To discriminate the actions of PTH from those attributable to high phosphorus, several groups have developed experimental CKD models using parathyroidectomy (PTX) in addition to nephrectomy (NX) and high dietary phosphorus (HP) diets. In these models, the desired serum PTH levels are achieved through appropriate exogenous supplementation through a continuous PTH infusion by pellets or minipumps (Neves et al. 2004; Graciolli et al. 2009; Ferreira et al. 2013). In elegant studies by Neves et al. PTX+NX rats given high exogenous PTH presented large areas of vascular calcification regardless of the dietary phosphate intake. Instead, in PTX+NX rats receiving low PTH and high dietary phosphorus, VSMC also showed phenotypic changes toward an osteoblastic phenotype, as suggested by the upregulation of aortic RUNX2. In contrast to these findings, preliminary results from our group demonstrate that in the absence of elevated PTH, high dietary phosphorus has a lower potency to induce vascular calcification in experimental uremia, suggesting a synergistic adverse effect on the vasculature of high circulating PTH and phosphorus (Naves et al. 2013; Carrillo-Lopez et al. 2014).

Preclinical and clinical data show that serum levels of FGF23 increase early in CKD and may reflect an increased phosphorus load ahead of the development of hyperphosphatemia

Evidence of the Skeletal and Vascular Adverse Health Effects 35

(Fang et al. 2009). Although the early increases of FGF23 render beneficial effects reducing the phosphorus load, the exponentially high levels of circulating FGF23, mainly observed in advanced stages of CKD, are associated with adverse outcomes (Gutierrez et al. 2008) and with development and progression of cardiovascular disease (Faul et al. 2011), not only in CKD but also in the general population (Mirza et al. 2009).

FGF23 actions require its receptors FGFR1 or 3 (Lindberg et al. 2014) and its coreceptor, klotho, an anti-aging protein (Kuro-o et al. 1997) expressed mainly in the kidney but also in the parathyroid gland and the choroid plexus, to exert the effects. However, the exact role of this interaction is still not fully understood. There are conflicting reports as to vascular α-klotho content and protection from vascular calcification by FGF23/klotho signals and on the vascular health protection provided by soluble klotho.

Some studies demonstrate expression of klotho in the vasculature (Donate-Correa et al. 2013; Ritter et al. 2015) and a positive and independent association of FGF23 with aortic calcification, especially in early human CKD and in ex vivo and in vitro models (Nasrallah et al. 2010). On the contrary, many studies failed to detect arterial klotho (Jimbo et al. 2014; Kuro-o et al. 1997). In addition, despite the controversy on vascular klotho content and FGF23 actions, it has been conclusively demonstrated that renal klotho content does exert vascular protection. Indeed, specific ablation of renal klotho confers the same calcifying phenotype of the global α-klotho

null mice. Importantly, renal klotho content progressively declines in CKD, and this reduction is directly linked to vascular calcification (Hu et al. 2011), oxidative stress (Olauson and Larsson 2013), and multiple organ damage beyond the vasculature, including bone and the kidney.

The decrease of renal α-klotho impairs the phosphaturic action of FGF23, thereby stimulating the pro-aging actions of high serum phosphate, including its direct induction of vascular calcification. In addition, the decrease of renal α-klotho in the course of CKD contributes to a reduction of circulating and urinary levels of soluble klotho, a product of the cleavage of transmembrane α-klotho. Soluble klotho in the urinary space has phosphaturic properties by itself through the induction of the internalization of the NaPi2a cotransporter, thereby preventing renal phosphorus retention. The reduction of renal klotho also results in decreases in soluble klotho in the urinary space and, consequently, impaired phosphaturia and increased phosphate retention, thus enhancing hyperphosphatemia-driven pro-aging and procalcifying features.

3.3 PATHOPHYSIOLOGY OF BONE FRAGILITY IN CKD

In addition to the induction of an osteoblastic phenotype on VSMC, high serum phosphorus contributes to the link between abnormalities in bone turnover, bone fragility, and the increased propensity to vascular calcification. The next sections present the direct and indirect impact of serum phosphorus on bone homeostasis.

3.3.1 ROLE OF PHOSPHORUS

The evidence of direct effects of hyperphosphatemia on bone biology is scarce. Two studies examined the effect of a high phosphorus intake on bone properties. The first evaluated the impact of one single-day oral dose of phosphorus from 0 (placebo) to 250, 750, or 1500 mg, all given as meals to healthy young women (Kemi et al. 2006). The phosphorus doses affected serum PTH and markers of bone formation. Bone-specific alkaline phosphatase decreased, and the bone resorption marker, N-terminal telopeptide of collagen type I, increased in a dose-dependent manner. Interestingly, only the highest dose of phosphorus affected serum calcium concentration. Therefore, short-term increases in phosphorus intake have a dose-dependent adverse impact on bone metabolism.

The second study assessed how high dietary phosphorus influences bone mass in growing rats (Huttunen et al. 2007). After an eight-week intervention with control (Ca:P = 1:1) or high dietary phosphorus (Ca:P = 1:3) diets, rats receiving the high-phosphorus diet showed impaired growth and elevated serum PTH. Regarding bone properties, whereas osteoclast number, osteoblast perimeter, and mineral apposition rate increased, trabecular area and width decreased. Furthermore, the high-phosphorus intake also reduced femoral neck and tibial shaft mechanical properties. In conclusion, high dietary phosphorus reduced the bone quality of growing rats, misbalancing bone remodeling and possibly increasing bone fragility. A main limitation from these studies is that they cannot discriminate the effects of elevated phosphorus from those resulting from the elevated serum PTH.

To overcome this limitation, an experimental CKD model of adynamic bone disease (ABD) was developed by performing simultaneously parathyroidectomy and nephrectomy, together with dietary phosphorus manipulations. In rats fed high phosphorus, there was a decrease in bone mass (measured as bone volume) with increases in the Wnt inhibitors sclerostin (SOST) and DKK1, increased osteoblast and osteocyte apoptosis, and higher serum SOST in a PTH-independent manner (Sabbagh et al. 2012). This is a critical finding, as the impairment of the osteocyte Wnt/beta-catenin signaling pathway is a main determinant of the early abnormalities in bone health in CKD, as they occur even before elevations in serum PTH (Sabbagh et al. 2012), a recognized inhibitor of bone SOST. These results suggest that a high phosphorus intake adversely affects bone formation through a PTH-independent mechanism.

3.3.2 Role of PTH and Other Factors

The most potent systemic effects of high phosphate in bone are through the induction of increases in serum levels of PTH and FGF23, two hormones that promote phosphaturia targeting the same renal phosphate/sodium cotransporters. However, whereas FGF23 reduces the renal expression of NaPi2a and NaPi2c cotransporters, high PTH induces their internalization. In addition to this compensatory urinary phosphate wasting (Lanske and Razzaque 2014), FGF23 reduces renal calcitriol production through dual mechanisms: suppression of its renal synthesis by 1α-hydroxylase (CYP27B1) and induction of its degradation through the induction of CYP24A1, the enzyme responsible for the biological degradation of vitamin D metabolites. This tight control of renal calcitriol production prevents further intestinal calcium and phosphate absorption and the increases in bone resorption associated with an excess of circulating calcitriol. It is unclear how phosphate induces FGF23. The only certainty is that it does not involve transcriptional regulation.

Regarding phosphorus regulation of serum PTH, a seminal work by Almadén and collaborators (Almadén et al. 1996) in fresh rat parathyroid glands has demonstrated a direct and dose-dependent effect of increases in extracellular phosphorus on parathyroid hormone secretion. Continuously elevated PTH, as a consequence of a phosphate load, acts directly on osteoblasts to stimulate RANKL expression and reduce expression of OPG (Jilka et al. 2010; Huang et al. 2004), impairing bone remodeling by favoring bone resorption.

Different from the recognized bone resorptive effects of high serum PTH, until very recently, there was no evidence of a direct adverse effect of FGF23 on bone in vivo. Carrillo-López and collaborators have demonstrated that in advanced experimental CKD, the strong associations between high serum phosphate PTH and FGF23, and loss of cortical bone due to inhibition of Wnt/β-catenin could not be attributed to the increased PTH, but to FGF23 (Carrillo-Lopez et al. 2016). In fact, reproducing the uremic conditions in osteoblastic cells, the combination of FGF23 and soluble klotho was sufficient to markedly increase the Wnt inhibitors DKK1 and Srfp1 and inactivate the Wnt/β-catenin signals for appropriate bone formation (Carrillo-Lopez et al. 2016). Gene silencing experiments conclusively demonstrated that FGF23 induction of DKK1 was a main determinant of Wnt inhibition. The requirement of soluble klotho for FGF23 suppression of Wnt signals in bone differ from in vitro studies in cells of the osteoblast lineage, showing that supraphysiological FGF23 concentrations with no soluble klotho can act in an autocrine/paracrine form to suppress bone mineralization (Wang et al. 2008). Undoubtedly, the contribution of FGF23 actions, both soluble klotho dependent or independent, on the adverse impact on bone in the course of CKD cannot be easily addressed in these patients.

Evidence of the Skeletal and Vascular Adverse Health Effects   37

3.4 VASCULAR CALCIFICATION, BONE HEALTH, AND SURVIVAL: LESSONS FROM CLINICAL AND PRECLINICAL EVIDENCE

Vascular calcification and bone loss are two intimately related disorders that share causes and pathogenic mechanisms in which hyperphosphatemia (Cannata-Andia et al. 2011) plays an important role. Both disorders lead to increased cardiovascular disease and mortality rate. So far, the clinical and preclinical evidence briefly discussed next confirms the interest for the existing relationship between these two disorders.

3.4.1 CLINICAL EVIDENCE

Vascular calcification, bone loss, and increased propensity for fracture are common features of aging in the general population that are aggravated in the accelerated aging of CKD patients (Naves et al. 2008; Rodriguez-Garcia et al. 2009; Goldsmith et al. 2004; Cannata-Andia et al. 2006).

In fact, the results of the EPOS-EVOS studies, published in 2008, demonstrated that the degree and progression of vascular calcification was inversely correlated with bone mineral density and bone loss (Naves et al. 2008). In fact, after four years of follow-up, individuals with the most severe vascular calcification or with the greatest progression of vascular calcification showed the lowest bone mass and the highest incidence of new fragility fractures (Naves et al. 2008). Similar results were reported in dialysis patients with vascular calcification (large- and medium-caliber arteries) in whom the severity of the arterial calcification was associated with an increased risk for vertebral fractures (Rodriguez-Garcia et al. 2009). Furthermore, using bone histomorphometry, an inverse relationship between the severity of vascular calcification and bone turnover has been reported (Coen et al. 2009; London et al. 2008; Adragao et al. 2009), as well as between coronary calcification, vascular stiffness, and bone volume (Adragao et al. 2009).

In summary, the bulk of evidence strongly suggests that the prevalence and progression of vascular calcification are directly related to decreases in bone turnover and bone mass, which increase the propensity to osteoporotic fragility fractures.

In addition to the vascular–bone health impact on morbidity described earlier, there is a well-known impact on mortality rates (Rodriguez Garcia et al. 2005; Rodriguez-Garcia et al. 2009; London et al. 2003; Marco et al. 2003; Block et al. 2004; Stevens et al. 2004; Connolly et al. 2009). In fact, in the general population, the progression of aortic calcifications has been associated with higher mortality rates in men and with fragility bone fractures in women (Naves et al. 2008). Also in women undergoing dialysis, severe vascular calcifications (any localization) and vertebral fractures have been found to be associated with a higher risk of mortality. A two-year follow-up of this cohort showed a prevalence of vertebral fractures three times higher in the women who died during that period (58.8 vs. 19.3%) compared with the survivors.

Although the significant inverse correlation between aortic calcification and osteoporosis was reported more than 20 years ago (Frye et al. 1992), the pathogenic factors linking these two disorders are not fully understood. Possibly, the slow progress in this area can be attributed to the belief that vascular calcification and osteoporosis are nonmodifiable, age-dependent disorders. However, recent data support this association may not be just a consequence of aging (Rodriguez-Garcia et al. 2009; Naves et al. 2008), as biological links between vascular calcification and bone loss have emerged as pathogenic factors. In fact, vascular calcification and bone loss are influenced by several common risk factors. Also, most of the promoters and inhibitors of vascular calcification are involved in the biology of bone (Figure 3.1).

3.4.2 PRECLINICAL EVIDENCE

Studies in a rat model of CKD fed high dietary phosphorus have shown that the increase in aortic calcification was associated with decreases in bone mass. Microarray analysis of severely calcified areas showed overexpression of the family of secreted frizzled-related proteins (SFRPs)

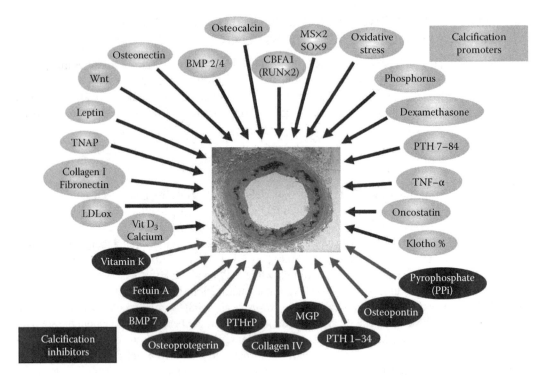

FIGURE 3.1 Promoters and inhibitors of vascular calcification (From Cannata-Andía, J. B. et al., *Nephrol Dial Transplant*, 26, 3429–36, 2011. With permission). TNAP, tissue-nonspecific alkaline phosphatase; LDLox, oxidized low-density lipoprotein; MGP, matrix GLA protein; PTHrP, parathyroid hormone-related protein; TNF-α, tumor necrosis factor-alpha; Vit D3, calcitriol.

(Roman-Garcia et al. 2010), a group of circulating Wnt protein inhibitors. Not only phosphorus load, but also experimental interstitial nephritis, has been associated with upregulation of SFRP4, SFRP2, and DDK1 in the vascular adventitia (Surendran et al. 2005).

As SFRPs, DKK1, and SOST are inhibitors of the canonical signaling Wnt pathway, which is required for skeletal development and bone mineralization (Holmen et al. 2004; Al-Aly et al. 2007; Towler et al. 2006), the increases of these Wnt inhibitors in areas of severe vascular calcification may reflect a defense response of the vascular wall to attenuate further mineralization.

Unfortunately, the likely negative price to pay for an excess of Wnt inhibitors in calcified arteries is that all these Wnt inhibitor proteins are secreted proteins. Thus, their increases in the circulation will not be restricted to local actions in the artery wall to reduce mineralization, but also in bone cells of the osteocyte/osteoblastic lineage, impairing mineralization and reducing bone mass.

This new and challenging hypothesis that calcified vessels may be a nonnegligible source of Wnt pathway inhibitors may help to explain why in the general population and in CKD patients progressive vascular calcification is associated with greater bone loss and bone fractures (Rodriguez-Garcia et al. 2009; Naves et al. 2008). However, it is important to stress that the role of the Wnt activators and inhibitors in the pathogenesis of vascular calcification and bone demineralization is complex and may vary in the course of CKD.

In fact, neutralization of DKK1 in CKD stage 2 mice by administration of a monoclonal antibody stimulated bone formation rates, corrected the osteodystrophy, and prevented CKD-stimulated vascular calcification (Fang et al. 2014). The systemic blockage of this Wnt inhibitor activated Wnt signals in bone and corrected bone abnormalities, but at the same time prevented vascular calcification and aortic expression of the osteoblastic factors, increased the expression of vascular smooth muscle proteins, and restored aortic expression of α-klotho.

Evidence of the Skeletal and Vascular Adverse Health Effects

Although strategies directed to activate the Wnt pathway through reducing circulating levels of Wnt inhibitors (anti-SOST or anti-Dkk1 antibodies) are smart and attractive approaches to improve bone mineralization and bone mass in conditions of normal renal function, the response in CKD seems to be heterogeneous and dependent on PTH levels (Moe et al. 2015). In fact, in a recent study on vascular calcification in a stable CKD model, mineral apposition rate and eroded perimeter—two parameters highly dependent on PTH—predicted aortic calcification (Neven et al. 2015). These experimental findings together with clinical and epidemiological evidence (Roman-Garcia et al. 2011; Wilson et al. 2001; Stubbs et al. 2007; Muntner et al. 2013; Rodriguez Garcia et al. 2005; Cannata-Andia and Naves-Diaz 2009; Li et al. 2006; Byon et al. 2008; Giachelli 2004; Panizo et al. 2016; Villa-Bellosta and Sorribas 2009, 2011; O'Neill et al. 2011; Lomashvili et al. 2005; Lomashvili et al. 2014; Villa-Bellosta and Egido 2015; Bellorin-Font et al. 1985; Oliveira et al. 2010; Yuan et al. 2011; Whitfield 2005; Coen et al. 2007, 2009; Cannata-Andia et al. 2011; Cannata-Andia et al. 2006; London et al. 2008) support the concept that in early stages of CKD, bone disorders affecting bone remodeling could trigger vascular calcification, suggesting an adverse bone-vessel interaction, which may act in either direction in the course of CKD.

3.5 AREAS FOR FUTURE RESEARCH

Despite the intensive clinical and preclinical research describing novel common components of the bone–vessel interactions and the abnormalities of this crosstalk in CKD that expedite bone and vascular aging, there are still important debated questions and unclear findings.

α-klotho was discovered in 1997, and the null (hypomorphic) *kl/kl* mouse shows an accelerated renal, skeletal, and vascular aging that resembles CKD. Indeed, CKD can be defined as a state of renal α-klotho deficiency. In addition to determining the efficacy for the phosphaturic actions of FGF23, thus preventing/attenuating the pro-aging effects of hyperphosphatemia, α-klotho exists in a soluble form that exerts protective actions in the vasculature and in bone through the regulation of the activity of calcium–potassium channels in addition to renal NaPi2a and c phosphorus cotransporters and antagonizing Wnt signaling. Despite the uncertainty about α-klotho expression in human aortas, it is clear that maintenance of renal α-klotho may preserve skeletal and vascular integrity.

3.6 CONCLUSIONS

In summary, in addition to the studies in progress designed to better understand the molecular effect of the promoters of vascular calcification in which phosphorus plays a key role, it is necessary to better delineate the mechanisms involving the interaction between high serum phosphorus, FGF23, klotho, and the Wnt pathway balance in the skeletal and vascular adverse health associated with aging.

REFERENCES

Adragao, T., J. Herberth, M. C. Monier-Faugere, A. J. Branscum, A. Ferreira, J. M. Frazao, J. Dias Curto, and H. H. Malluche. 2009. Low bone volume--a risk factor for coronary calcifications in hemodialysis patients. *Clin J Am Soc Nephrol* 4 (2):450–5. doi:10.2215/CJN.01870408.

Al-Aly, Z., J. S. Shao, C. F. Lai, E. Huang, J. Cai, A. Behrmann, S. L. Cheng, and D. A. Towler. 2007. Aortic Msx2-Wnt calcification cascade is regulated by TNF-alpha-dependent signals in diabetic Ldlr-/- mice. *Arterioscler Thromb Vasc Biol* 27 (12):2589–96. doi:10.1161/ATVBAHA.107.153668.

Almaden, Y., A. Canalejo, A. Hernandez, E. Ballesteros, S. Garcia-Navarro, A. Torres, and M. Rodriguez. 1996. Direct effect of phosphorus on PTH secretion from whole rat parathyroid glands in vitro. *J Bone Miner Res* 11 (7):970–6.

Bellorin-Font, E., J. Humpierres, J. R. Weisinger, C. L. Milanes, V. Sylva, and V. Paz-Martinez. 1985. Effect of metabolic acidosis on the PTH receptor-adenylate cyclase system of canine kidney. *Am J Physiol* 249 (4 Pt 2):F566–72.

Block, G. A., P. S. Klassen, J. M. Lazarus, N. Ofsthun, E. G. Lowrie, and G. M. Chertow. 2004. Mineral metabolism, mortality, and morbidity in maintenance hemodialysis. *J Am Soc Nephrol* 15 (8):2208–18.

Byon, C. H., A. Javed, Q. Dai, J. C. Kappes, T. L. Clemens, V. M. Darley-Usmar, J. M. McDonald, and Y. Chen. 2008. Oxidative stress induces vascular calcification through modulation of the osteogenic transcription factor Runx2 by AKT signaling. *J Biol Chem* 283 (22): 15319–27. doi:10.1074/jbc.M800021200.

Cannata-Andia, J. B. and M. Naves-Diaz. 2009. Phosphorus and survival: Key questions that need answers. *J Am Soc Nephrol* 20 (2):234–6. doi:10.1681/ASN.2008121277.

Cannata-Andia, J. B., M. Rodriguez-Garcia, N. Carrillo-Lopez, M. Naves-Diaz, and B. Diaz-Lopez. 2006. Vascular calcifications: Pathogenesis, management, and impact on clinical outcomes. *J Am Soc Nephrol* 17(12 Suppl 3): S267–73.

Cannata-Andia, J. B., P. Roman-Garcia, and K. Hruska. 2011. The connections between vascular calcification and bone health. *Nephrol Dial Transplant* 26 (11):3429–36. doi:10.1093/ndt/gfr591.

Carrillo-Lopez, N., S. Panizo, C. Alonso-Montes, P. Roman-Garcia, I. Rodriguez, C. Martinez-Salgado, A. S. Dusso, M. Naves, and J. B. Cannata-Andia. 2016. Direct inhibition of osteoblastic Wnt pathway by fibroblast growth factor 23 contributes to bone loss in chronic kidney disease. *Kidney Int* 90 (1):77–89. doi:10.1016/j.kint.2016.01.024.

Carrillo-Lopez, N., S. Panizo, P. Roman-Garcia, C. Alonso-Montes, G. Solache-Berrocal, M. Colinas-Rodriguez, A. Fernandez-Vazquez, N. Avello, J. B. Cannata-Andia, and M. Naves. 2014. Calcificación vascular y desmineralización ósea: Efecto de PTH independiente de fósforo. *Rev Osteoporos Metab Miner* 6 (3):7. doi:10.1016/j.kint.2016.01.024.

Coen, G., P. Ballanti, D. Mantella, M. Manni, B. Lippi, A. Pierantozzi, S. Di Giulio, L. Pellegrino, A. Romagnoli, G. Simonetti, and G. Splendiani. 2009. Bone turnover, osteopenia and vascular calcifications in hemodialysis patients. A histomorphometric and multislice CT study. *Am J Nephrol* 29 (3):145–52.

Coen, G., M. Manni, D. Mantella, A. Pierantozzi, A. Balducci, S. Condo, S. Digiulio, L. Yancovic, B. Lippi, S. Manca, M. Morosetti, L. Pellegrino, G. Simonetti, M. T. Gallucci, and G. Splendiani. 2007. Are PTH serum levels predictive of coronary calcifications in haemodialysis patients? *Nephrol Dial Transplant* 22 (11):3262–7.

Connolly, G. M., R. Cunningham, P. T. McNamee, I. S. Young, and A. P. Maxwell. 2009. Elevated serum phosphate predicts mortality in renal transplant recipients. *Transplantation* 87 (7):1040–4. doi:10.1097/10.1097/TP.0b013e31819cd122.

Donate-Correa, J., C. Mora-Fernandez, R. Martinez-Sanz, M. Muros-de-Fuentes, H. Perez, B. Meneses-Perez, V. Cazana-Perez, and J. F. Navarro-Gonzalez. 2013. Expression of FGF23/KLOTHO system in human vascular tissue. *Int J Cardiol* 165 (1): 179–83. doi:10.1016/j.ijcard.2011.08.850.

Ducy, P., C. Desbois, B. Boyce, G. Pinero, B. Story, C. Dunstan, E. Smith, J. Bonadio, S. Goldstein, C. Gundberg, A. Bradley, and G. Karsenty. 1996. Increased bone formation in osteocalcin-deficient mice. *Nature* 382 (6590):448–52. doi:10.1038/382448a0.

Ducy, P., R. Zhang, V. Geoffroy, A. L. Ridall, and G. Karsenty. 1997. Osf2/Cbfa1: A transcriptional activator of osteoblast differentiation. *Cell* 89 (5):747–54.

Engelse, M. A., J. M. Neele, A. L. Bronckers, H. Pannekoek, and C. J. de Vries. 2001. Vascular calcification: Expression patterns of the osteoblast-specific gene core binding factor alpha-1 and the protective factor matrix gla protein in human atherogenesis. *Cardiovasc Res* 52 (2):281–9.

Fang, Y., C. Ginsberg, M. Seifert, O. Agapova, T. Sugatani, T. C. Register, B. I. Freedman, M. C. Monier-Faugere, H. Malluche, and K. A. Hruska. 2014. CKD-induced wingless/integration1 inhibitors and phosphorus cause the CKD-mineral and bone disorder. *J Am Soc Nephrol* 25 (8):1760–73. doi:10.1681/ASN.2013080818.

Fang, Y., Y. Zhang, S. Mathew, J. Futhey, R. Lund, and K. Hruska. 2009. Early chronic kidney disease (CKD) stimulates vascular calcification (VC) and decreased bone formation rates prior to positive phosphate balance. *J Am Soc Nephrol 20 (36A):Free communication*.

Faul, C., A. P. Amaral, B. Oskouei, M. C. Hu, A. Sloan, T. Isakova, O. M. Gutierrez, R. Aguillon-Prada, J. Lincoln, J. M. Hare, P. Mundel, A. Morales, J. Scialla, M. Fischer, E. Z. Soliman, J. Chen, A. S. Go, S. E. Rosas, L. Nessel, R. R. Townsend, H. I. Feldman, M. St John Sutton, A. Ojo, C. Gadegbeku, G. S. Di Marco, S. Reuter, D. Kentrup, K. Tiemann, M. Brand, J. A. Hill, O. W. Moe, O. M. Kuro, J. W. Kusek, M. G. Keane, and M. Wolf. 2011. FGF23 induces left ventricular hypertrophy. *J Clin Invest* 121 (11):4393–408. doi:10.1172/JCI46122.

Ferreira, J. C., G. O. Ferrari, K. R. Neves, R. T. Cavallari, W. V. Dominguez, L. M. Dos Reis, F. G. Graciolli, E. C. Oliveira, S. Liu, Y. Sabbagh, V. Jorgetti, S. Schiavi, and R. M. Moyses. 2013. Effects of dietary phosphate on adynamic bone disease in rats with chronic kidney disease--role of sclerostin? *PLOS ONE* 8 (11):e79721. doi:10.1371/journal.pone.0079721.

Evidence of the Skeletal and Vascular Adverse Health Effects   **41**

Friedman, E. A. 2005. Consequences and management of hyperphosphatemia in patients with renal insufficiency. *Kidney Int Suppl* (95):S1–7. doi:10.1111/j.1523-1755.2005.09500.x

Frye, M. A., L. J. Melton, 3rd, S. C. Bryant, L. A. Fitzpatrick, H. W. Wahner, R. S. Schwartz, and B. L. Riggs. 1992. Osteoporosis and calcification of the aorta. *Bone Miner* 19 (2):185–94.

Giachelli, C. M. 2004. Vascular calcification mechanisms. *J Am Soc Nephrol* 15 (12):2959–64.

Goldsmith, D., E. Ritz, and A. Covic. 2004. Vascular calcification: A stiff challenge for the nephrologist: Does preventing bone disease cause arterial disease? *Kidney Int* 66 (4):1315–33.

Graciolli, F. G., K. R. Neves, L. M. dos Reis, R. G. Graciolli, I. L. Noronha, R. M. Moyses, and V. Jorgetti. 2009. Phosphorus overload and PTH induce aortic expression of Runx2 in experimental uraemia. *Nephrol Dial Transplant* 24 (5):1416–21.

Gutierrez, O. M., M. Mannstadt, T. Isakova, J. A. Rauh-Hain, H. Tamez, A. Shah, K. Smith, H. Lee, R. Thadhani, H. Juppner, and M. Wolf. 2008. Fibroblast growth factor 23 and mortality among patients undergoing hemodialysis. *N Engl J Med* 359 (6):584–92.

Holmen, S. L., T. A. Giambernardi, C. R. Zylstra, B. D. Buckner-Berghuis, J. H. Resau, J. F. Hess, V. Glatt, M. L. Bouxsein, M. Ai, M. L. Warman, and B. O. Williams. 2004. Decreased BMD and limb deformities in mice carrying mutations in both Lrp5 and Lrp6. *J Bone Miner Res* 19 (12):2033–40. doi:10.1359/JBMR.040907.

Hruska, K. A., S. Mathew, R. Lund, P. Qiu, and R. Pratt. 2008. Hyperphosphatemia of chronic kidney disease. *Kidney Int* 74 (2):148–57.

Hu, M. C., M. Shi, J. Zhang, H. Quinones, C. Griffith, M. Kuro-o, and O. W. Moe. 2011. Klotho deficiency causes vascular calcification in chronic kidney disease. *J Am Soc Nephrol* 22 (1):124–36. doi:10.1681/ASN.2009121311.

Huang, J. C., T. Sakata, L. L. Pfleger, M. Bencsik, B. P. Halloran, D. D. Bikle, and R. A. Nissenson. 2004. PTH differentially regulates expression of RANKL and OPG. *J Bone Miner Res* 19 (2):235–44.

Huttunen, M. M., I. Tillman, H. T. Viljakainen, J. Tuukkanen, Z. Peng, M. Pekkinen, and C. J. Lamberg-Allardt. 2007. High dietary phosphate intake reduces bone strength in the growing rat skeleton. *J Bone Miner Res* 22 (1):83–92. doi:10.1359/jbmr.061009.

Idelevich, A., Y. Rais, and E. Monsonego-Ornan. 2011. Bone Gla protein increases HIF-1alpha-dependent glucose metabolism and induces cartilage and vascular calcification. *Arterioscler Thromb Vasc Biol* 31 (9):e55–71. doi:10.1161/ATVBAHA.111.230904.

Jilka, R. L., C. A. O'Brien, S. M. Bartell, R. S. Weinstein, and S. C. Manolagas. 2010. Continuous elevation of PTH increases the number of osteoblasts via both osteoclast-dependent and -independent mechanisms. *J Bone Miner Res* 25 (11):2427–37. doi:10.1002/jbmr.145.

Jimbo, R., F. Kawakami-Mori, S. Mu, D. Hirohama, B. Majtan, Y. Shimizu, Y. Yatomi, S. Fukumoto, T. Fujita, and T. Shimosawa. 2014. Fibroblast growth factor 23 accelerates phosphate-induced vascular calcification in the absence of Klotho deficiency. *Kidney Int* 85 (5):1103–11. doi:10.1038/ki.2013.332.

Kapustin, A. N., J. D. Davies, J. L. Reynolds, R. McNair, G. T. Jones, A. Sidibe, L. J. Schurgers, J. N. Skepper, D. Proudfoot, M. Mayr, and C. M. Shanahan. 2011. Calcium regulates key components of vascular smooth muscle cell-derived matrix vesicles to enhance mineralization. *Circ Res* 109 (1):e1–12. doi:10.1161/CIRCRESAHA.110.238808.

Kemi, V. E., M. U. Karkkainen, and C. J. Lamberg-Allardt. 2006. High phosphorus intakes acutely and negatively affect Ca and bone metabolism in a dose-dependent manner in healthy young females. *Br J Nutr* 96 (3):545–52.

Ketteler, M., R. Westenfeld, G. Schlieper, V. Brandenburg, and J. Floege. 2005. "Missing" inhibitors of calcification: General aspects and implications in renal failure. *Pediatr Nephrol* 20 (3):383–8.

Kuro-o, M., Y. Matsumura, H. Aizawa, H. Kawaguchi, T. Suga, T. Utsugi, Y. Ohyama, M. Kurabayashi, T. Kaname, E. Kume, H. Iwasaki, A. Iida, T. Shiraki-Iida, S. Nishikawa, R. Nagai, and Y. I. Nabeshima. 1997. Mutation of the mouse klotho gene leads to a syndrome resembling ageing. *Nature* 390 (6655):45–51. doi:10.1038/36285.

Lanske, B. and M. S. Razzaque. 2014. Molecular interactions of FGF23 and PTH in phosphate regulation. *Kidney Int* 86 (6):1072–4. doi:10.1038/ki.2014.316.

Lee, N. K., H. Sowa, E. Hinoi, M. Ferron, J. D. Ahn, C. Confavreux, R. Dacquin, P. J. Mee, M. D. McKee, D. Y. Jung, Z. Zhang, J. K. Kim, F. Mauvais-Jarvis, P. Ducy, and G. Karsenty. 2007. Endocrine regulation of energy metabolism by the skeleton. *Cell* 130 (3):456–69. doi:10.1016/j.cell.2007.05.047.

Li, X., H. Y. Yang, and C. M. Giachelli. 2006. Role of the sodium-dependent phosphate cotransporter, Pit-1, in vascular smooth muscle cell calcification. *Circ Res* 98 (7):905–12.

Lindberg, K., R. Amin, O. W. Moe, M. C. Hu, R. G. Erben, A. Ostman Wernerson, B. Lanske, H. Olauson, and T. E. Larsson. 2014. The kidney is the principal organ mediating klotho effects. *J Am Soc Nephrol* 25 (10):2169–75. doi:10.1681/ASN.2013111209.

Lomashvili, K. A., S. Cobbs, R. A. Hennigar, K. I. Hardcastle, and W. C. O'Neill. 2004. Phosphate-induced vascular calcification: Role of pyrophosphate and osteopontin. *J Am Soc Nephrol* 15 (6):1392–401.

Lomashvili, K. A., W. Khawandi, and W. C. O'Neill. 2005. Reduced plasma pyrophosphate levels in hemodialysis patients. *J Am Soc Nephrol* 16 (8):2495–500. doi:10.1681/ASN.2004080694.

Lomashvili, K. A., S. Narisawa, J. L. Millan, and W. C. O'Neill. 2014. Vascular calcification is dependent on plasma levels of pyrophosphate. *Kidney Int* 85 (6):1351–6. doi:10.1038/ki.2013.521.

London, G. M., A. P. Guerin, S. J. Marchais, F. Metivier, B. Pannier, and H. Adda. 2003. Arterial media calcification in end-stage renal disease: Impact on all-cause and cardiovascular mortality. *Nephrol Dial Transplant* 18 (9):1731–40.

London, G. M., S. J. Marchais, A. P. Guerin, P. Boutouyrie, F. Metivier, and M. C. de Vernejoul. 2008. Association of bone activity, calcium load, aortic stiffness, and calcifications in ESRD. *J Am Soc Nephrol* 19 (9):1827–35.

Marco, M. P., L. Craver, A. Betriu, M. Belart, J. Fibla, and E. Fernandez. 2003. Higher impact of mineral metabolism on cardiovascular mortality in a European hemodialysis population. *Kidney Int Suppl* (85):S111–4.doi:10.1046/j.1523-1755.63.s85.26.x.

Mathew, S., K. S. Tustison, T. Sugatani, L. R. Chaudhary, L. Rifas, and K. A. Hruska. 2008. The mechanism of phosphorus as a cardiovascular risk factor in CKD. *J Am Soc Nephrol* 19 (6):1092–105.

Mirza, M. A., A. Larsson, L. Lind, and T. E. Larsson. 2009. Circulating fibroblast growth factor-23 is associated with vascular dysfunction in the community. *Atherosclerosis* 205 (2):385–90.

Moe, S. M., N. X. Chen, C. L. Newman, J. M. Organ, M. Kneissel, I. Kramer, V. H. Gattone, 2nd, and M. R. Allen. 2015. Anti-sclerostin antibody treatment in a rat model of progressive renal osteodystrophy. *J Bone Miner Res* 30 (3):499–509. doi:10.1002/jbmr.2372.

Moe, S., T. Drueke, J. Cunningham, W. Goodman, K. Martin, K. Olgaard, S. Ott, S. Sprague, N. Lameire, and G. Eknoyan. 2006. Definition, evaluation, and classification of renal osteodystrophy: A position statement from Kidney Disease: Improving Global Outcomes (KDIGO). *Kidney Int* 69 (11):1945–53.

Moe, S. M., M. Reslerova, M. Ketteler, K. O'Neill, D. Duan, J. Koczman, R. Westenfeld, W. Jahnen-Dechent, and N. X. Chen. 2005. Role of calcification inhibitors in the pathogenesis of vascular calcification in chronic kidney disease (CKD). *Kidney Int* 67 (6):2295–304.

Muntner, P., S. E. Judd, L. Gao, O. M. Gutierrez, D. V. Rizk, W. McClellan, M. Cushman, and D. G. Warnock. 2013. Cardiovascular risk factors in CKD associate with both ESRD and mortality. *J Am Soc Nephrol* 24 (7):1159–65. doi:10.1681/ASN.2012070642.

Nasrallah, M. M., A. R. El-Shehaby, M. M. Salem, N. A. Osman, E. El Sheikh, and U. A. Sharaf El Din. 2010. Fibroblast growth factor-23 (FGF-23) is independently correlated to aortic calcification in haemodialysis patients. *Nephrol Dial Transplant* 25 (8):2679–85.

Naves-Diaz, M., J. Passlick-Deetjen, A. Guinsburg, C. Marelli, J. L. Fernandez-Martin, D. Rodriguez-Puyol, and J. B. Cannata-Andia. 2011. Calcium, phosphorus, PTH and death rates in a large sample of dialysis patients from Latin America. The CORES Study. *Nephrol Dial Transplant* 26 (6):1938–47. doi:10.1093/ndt/gfq304.

Naves, M., N. Carrillo-Lopez, A. Rodriguez-Rebollar, S. Panizo, N. Avello, S. Braga, and J. B. Cannata-Andia. 2013. Efecto del fósforo y PTH en la inducción de calcificación vascular ¿Qué factor contribuye en mayor medida? *Nefrologia* 33 (2):45. doi:10.1016/j.kint.2016.01.024.

Naves, M., M. Rodriguez-Garcia, J. B. Diaz-Lopez, C. Gomez-Alonso, and J. B. Cannata-Andia. 2008. Progression of vascular calcifications is associated with greater bone loss and increased bone fractures. *Osteoporos Int* 19 (8):1161–6. doi:10.1007/s00198-007-0539-1.

Neven, E., R. Bashir-Dar, G. Dams, G. J. Behets, M. Verhulst, M. Elseviers, and P. C. D'Haese. 2015. Disturbances in bone largely predict aortic calcification in an alternative rat model developed to study both vascular and bone pathology in chronic kidney disease. *J Bone Miner Res* 30 (12):2313–24. doi:10.1002/jbmr.2585.

Neves, K. R., F. G. Graciolli, L. M. dos Reis, C. A. Pasqualucci, R. M. Moyses, and V. Jorgetti. 2004. Adverse effects of hyperphosphatemia on myocardial hypertrophy, renal function, and bone in rats with renal failure. *Kidney Int* 66 (6):2237–44.

O'Neill, W. C. 2006. Pyrophosphate, alkaline phosphatase, and vascular calcification. *Circ Res* 99 (2):e2. doi:10.1161/01.RES.0000234909.24367.a9.

O'Neill, W. C., K. A. Lomashvili, H. H. Malluche, M. C. Faugere, and B. L. Riser. 2011. Treatment with pyrophosphate inhibits uremic vascular calcification. *Kidney Int* 79 (5):512–7. doi:10.1038/ki.2010.461.

Olauson, H. and T. E. Larsson. 2013. FGF23 and Klotho in chronic kidney disease. *Curr Opin Nephrol Hypertens* 22 (4):397–404. doi:10.1097/MNH.0b013e32836213ee.

Oliveira, R. B., A. L. Cancela, F. G. Graciolli, L. M. Dos Reis, S. A. Draibe, L. Cuppari, A. B. Carvalho, V. Jorgetti, M. E. Canziani, and R. M. Moyses. 2010. Early control of PTH and FGF23 in normophosphatemic CKD patients: A new target in CKD-MBD therapy? *Clin J Am Soc Nephrol* 5 (2):286–91. doi:10.2215/CJN.05420709.

Oury, F., L. Khrimian, C. A. Denny, A. Gardin, A. Chamouni, N. Goeden, Y. Y. Huang, H. Lee, P. Srinivas, X. B. Gao, S. Suyama, T. Langer, J. J. Mann, T. L. Horvath, A. Bonnin, and G. Karsenty. 2013. Maternal and offspring pools of osteocalcin influence brain development and functions. *Cell* 155 (1):228–41. doi:10.1016/j.cell.2013.08.042.

Palmer, S. C., A. Hayen, P. Macaskill, F. Pellegrini, J. C. Craig, G. J. Elder, and G. F. Strippoli. 2011. Serum levels of phosphorus, parathyroid hormone, and calcium and risks of death and cardiovascular disease in individuals with chronic kidney disease: A systematic review and meta-analysis. *Jama* 305 (11):1119–27. doi:10.1001/jama.2011.308.

Panichi, V., R. Bigazzi, S. Paoletti, E. Mantuano, S. Beati, V. Marchetti, G. Bernabini, G. Grazi, R. Giust, A. Rosati, M. Migliori, A. Pasquariello, E. Panicucci, G. Barsotti, and A. Bellasi. 2010. Impact of calcium, phosphate, PTH abnormalities and management on mortality in hemodialysis: Results from the RISCAVID study. *J Nephrol* 23 (5):556–62. doi:4962795E-4F53-48ED-B47E-A3CF5020D130 [pii].

Panizo, S., M. Naves-Diaz, N. Carrillo-Lopez, L. Martinez-Arias, J. L. Fernandez-Martin, M. P. Ruiz-Torres, J. B. Cannata-Andia, and I. Rodriguez. 2016. MicroRNAs 29b, 133b, and 211 regulate vascular smooth muscle calcification mediated by high phosphorus. *J Am Soc Nephrol* 27 (3):824–34. doi:10.1681/ASN.2014050520.

Rached, M. T., A. Kode, B. C. Silva, D. Y. Jung, S. Gray, H. Ong, J. H. Paik, R. A. DePinho, J. K. Kim, G. Karsenty, and S. Kousteni. 2010. FoxO1 expression in osteoblasts regulates glucose homeostasis through regulation of osteocalcin in mice. *J Clin Invest* 120 (1):357–68. doi:10.1172/JCI39901.

Reynolds, J. L., A. J. Joannides, J. N. Skepper, R. McNair, L. J. Schurgers, D. Proudfoot, W. Jahnen-Dechent, P. L. Weissberg, and C. M. Shanahan. 2004. Human vascular smooth muscle cells undergo vesicle-mediated calcification in response to changes in extracellular calcium and phosphate concentrations: A potential mechanism for accelerated vascular calcification in ESRD. *J Am Soc Nephrol* 15 (11):2857–67.

Ritter, C. S., S. Zhang, J. Delmez, J. L. Finch, and E. Slatopolsky. 2015. Differential expression and regulation of Klotho by paricalcitol in the kidney, parathyroid, and aorta of uremic rats. *Kidney Int* 87 (6):1141–52. doi:10.1038/ki.2015.22.

Rodriguez-Garcia, M., C. Gomez-Alonso, M. Naves-Diaz, J. B. Diaz-Lopez, C. Diaz-Corte, and J. B. Cannata-Andia. 2009. Vascular calcifications, vertebral fractures and mortality in haemodialysis patients. *Nephrol Dial Transplant* 24 (1):239–46. doi:10.1093/ndt/gfn466.

Rodriguez Garcia, M., M. Naves Diaz, and J. B. Cannata Andia. 2005. Bone metabolism, vascular calcifications and mortality: Associations beyond mere coincidence. *J Nephrol* 18 (4):458–63.

Roman-Garcia, P., N. Carrillo-Lopez, and J. B. Cannata-Andia. 2009. Pathogenesis of bone and mineral related disorders in chronic kidney disease: Key role of hyperphosphatemia. *J Ren Care* 35 (Suppl 1):34–8. doi:10.1111/j.1755-6686.2009.00050.x

Roman-Garcia, P., N. Carrillo-Lopez, J. L. Fernandez-Martin, M. Naves-Diaz, M. P. Ruiz-Torres, and J. B. Cannata-Andia. 2010. High phosphorus diet induces vascular calcification, a related decrease in bone mass and changes in the aortic gene expression. *Bone* 46 (1):121–8. doi:S8756-3282(09)01915-2 [pii] 10.1016/j.bone.2009.09.006.

Roman-Garcia, P., M. Rodriguez-Garcia, I. Cabezas-Rodriguez, S. Lopez-Ongil, B. Diaz-Lopez, and J. B. Cannata-Andia. 2011. Vascular calcification in patients with chronic kidney disease: Types, clinical impact and pathogenesis. *Med Princ Pract* 20 (3): 203–12. doi:10.1159/000323434.

Sabbagh, Y., F. G. Graciolli, S. O'Brien, W. Tang, L. M. dos Reis, S. Ryan, L. Phillips, J. Boulanger, W. Song, C. Bracken, S. Liu, S. Ledbetter, P. Dechow, M. E. Canziani, A. B. Carvalho, V. Jorgetti, R. M. Moyses, and S. C. Schiavi. 2012. Repression of osteocyte Wnt/beta-catenin signaling is an early event in the progression of renal osteodystrophy. *J Bone Miner Res* 27 (8):1757–72. doi:10.1002/jbmr.1630.

Shao, J. S., S. L. Cheng, N. Charlton-Kachigian, A. P. Loewy, and D. A. Towler. 2003. Teriparatide (human parathyroid hormone (1–34)) inhibits osteogenic vascular calcification in diabetic low density lipoprotein receptor-deficient mice. *J Biol Chem* 278 (50):50195–202. doi:10.1074/jbc.M308825200.

Shen, J., M. Yang, H. Jiang, D. Ju, J. P. Zheng, Z. Xu, T. D. Liao, and L. Li. 2011. Arterial injury promotes medial chondrogenesis in Sm22 knockout mice. *Cardiovasc Res* 90 (1):28–37. doi:10.1093/cvr/cvq378.

Shroff, R., D. A. Long, and C. Shanahan. 2013. Mechanistic insights into vascular calcification in CKD. *J Am Soc Nephrol* 24 (2):179–89. doi:10.1681/ASN.2011121191.

Stevens, L. A., O. Djurdjev, S. Cardew, E. C. Cameron, and A. Levin. 2004. Calcium, phosphate, and parathyroid hormone levels in combination and as a function of dialysis duration predict mortality: Evidence for the complexity of the association between mineral metabolism and outcomes. *J Am Soc Nephrol* 15 (3):770–9.

Stubbs, J. R., S. Liu, W. Tang, J. Zhou, Y. Wang, X. Yao, and L. D. Quarles. 2007. Role of hyperphosphatemia and 1,25-dihydroxyvitamin D in vascular calcification and mortality in fibroblastic growth factor 23 null mice. *J Am Soc Nephrol* 18 (7):2116–24.

Surendran, K., S. Schiavi, and K. A. Hruska. 2005. Wnt-dependent beta-catenin signaling is activated after unilateral ureteral obstruction, and recombinant secreted frizzled-related protein 4 alters the progression of renal fibrosis. *J Am Soc Nephrol* 16 (8):2373–84.

Tentori, F., M. J. Blayney, J. M. Albert, B. W. Gillespie, P. G. Kerr, J. Bommer, E. W. Young, T. Akizawa, T. Akiba, R. L. Pisoni, B. M. Robinson, and F. K. Port. 2008. Mortality risk for dialysis patients with different levels of serum calcium, phosphorus, and PTH: The Dialysis Outcomes and Practice Patterns Study (DOPPS). *Am J Kidney Dis* 52 (3):519–30.

Towler, D. A., J. S. Shao, S. L. Cheng, J. M. Pingsterhaus, and A. P. Loewy. 2006. Osteogenic regulation of vascular calcification. *Ann N Y Acad Sci* 1068:327–33. doi:10.1196/annals.1346.036.

Vattikuti, R. and D. A. Towler. 2004. Osteogenic regulation of vascular calcification: An early perspective. *Am J Physiol Endocrinol Metab* 286 (5):E686–96.

Villa-Bellosta, R. and J. Egido. 2015. Phosphate, pyrophosphate, and vascular calcification: A question of balance. *Eur Heart J*. [Epub ahead of print] doi:10.1093/eurheartj/ehv605.

Villa-Bellosta, R. and V. Sorribas. 2009. Phosphonoformic acid prevents vascular smooth muscle cell calcification by inhibiting calcium-phosphate deposition. *Arterioscler Thromb Vasc Biol* 29 (5):761–6. doi:10.1161/ATVBAHA.108.183384.

Villa-Bellosta, R. and V. Sorribas. 2011. On the osteogenic expression induced by calcium/phosphate deposition. *Kidney Int* 79 (8):921; author reply 921. doi:10.1038/ki.2010.561.

Wang, H., Y. Yoshiko, R. Yamamoto, T. Minamizaki, K. Kozai, K. Tanne, J. E. Aubin, and N. Maeda. 2008. Overexpression of fibroblast growth factor 23 suppresses osteoblast differentiation and matrix mineralization in vitro. *J Bone Miner Res* 23 (6):939–48. doi:10.1359/jbmr.080220.

Whitfield, J. F. 2005. Osteogenic PTHs and vascular ossification-Is there a danger for osteoporotics? *J Cell Biochem* 95 (3):437–44. doi:10.1002/jcb.20424.

Wilson, P. W., L. I. Kauppila, C. J. O'Donnell, D. P. Kiel, M. Hannan, J. M. Polak, and L. A. Cupples. 2001. Abdominal aortic calcific deposits are an important predictor of vascular morbidity and mortality. *Circulation* 103 (11):1529–34.

Yuan, Q., T. Sato, M. Densmore, H. Saito, C. Schuler, R. G. Erben, and B. Lanske. 2011. FGF-23/Klotho signaling is not essential for the phosphaturic and anabolic functions of PTH. *J Bone Miner Res* 26 (9):2026–35. doi:10.1002/jbmr.433.

4 Associations between Phosphorus Intake and Mortality

Andrea Galassi, Denis Fouque, and Mario Cozzolino

CONTENTS

Abstract 45
Bullet Points 45
4.1 Introduction 46
4.2 Phosphate Homeostasis in Humans: Nutritional Intake, Intestinal Absorption, and Renal Excretion 47
4.3 Assessing Nutritional P Intake and P Balance: A Tough Goal in Research and Clinical Practice 50
4.4 Phosphate and Mortality: Mechanisms 55
4.5 Phosphate Intake and Mortality: Observational Studies 55
4.6 Conclusions 59
References 59

ABSTRACT

A direct and independent association between serum phosphate (P) levels and mortality has been reported. Higher circulating P concentrations, although still within the normal range, have been associated with unfavorable outcomes in normal subjects, as well as in predialysis renal cohorts. Experimental data support the notion that P overload may decrease survival expectancy, directly inducing vascular, skeletal, and renal aging. Phosphorus balance results from the interplay of dietary intake, intestinal absorption, glomerular filtration, and tubular reabsorption of phosphorus (TRP), as well as hormonal factors. The accurate estimation of P balance, however, is hampered by several methodological weaknesses and becomes critical when renal function declines. The present chapter critically discusses the physiology of P metabolism in humans, then deals with uncertainties regarding dietary P intake and P balance assessment, and finally addresses more recent data on P intake and mortality extending from the general population to dialysis cohorts.

BULLET POINTS

- Although phosphate (P) is a crucial element for life, both elevated and reduced serum P levels are associated with unfavorable outcomes in humans.
- Regulation of the P pool depends on homeostatic balance between nutritional intake, intestinal absorption, and renal excretion; decline of glomerular filtration rate exposes chronic kidney disease (CKD) patients to a considerable risk of positive P balance whenever the reduction of filtered P is not compensated by reduction of its tubular absorption.
- The assessment of nutritional P intake and P balance remains a tough goal in clinical practice. Serum P represents less than 1% of the total body P and is considered a weak marker

of both P intake and P balance; 24-hour urinary P excretion is accepted as an alternative and reliable estimate of net intestinal P uptake, although with potential imprecision in advanced CKD patients.

- A direct association between P intake and mortality is supported by a small number of observational studies, but with still inconsistent results.
- Although the impact of P load on survival remains a hot topic for contemporary medicine, current evidence is still insufficient to recommend targets of nutritional P intake and of serum P levels different from those proposed by the current guidelines.

4.1 INTRODUCTION

Phosphorus (P) is an essential element for life, being indispensable for energetic and mineral metabolism. However, both elevated and reduced serum P levels are associated with unfavorable outcomes. Clinical consequences of sustained hypophosphatemia may be relevant, as suggested by severe cellular and organ dysfunction observed in patients affected by inherited disorders of P metabolism [1]. On the other hand, hyperphosphatemia is accepted as a late consequence of advanced kidney disease, starting with a glomerular filtration rate (GFR) lower than 30 mL/min [2–5]. High circulating P levels were repeatedly linked to reduced survival in observational studies conducted among dialysis cohorts [6,7]. A direct and independent association between P levels and adverse outcomes was even reported in normophosphatemic renal patients, including those with GFR greater than 30 mL/min [8–11], as well as in the general population [12–15]. Observational data showed that predialysis and dialysis patients receiving oral P binders were exposed to lower mortality risk compared to controls [16–18]. Furthermore, high P load induced short lifespan in knock-out animal models [19], which was counteracted by decreased dietary P intake [20,21]. Experimental and epidemiological research has shed light in the same direction, suggesting how increased P concentrations may be primarily responsible for poor clinical outcomes by triggering and sustaining the chronic kidney disease and mineral bone disorder (CKD-MBD) syndrome, characterized by vascular aging and altered mineral metabolism [2].

Although the best target of circulating P level to improve survival has never been tested in randomized controlled trials, the aforementioned data suggest that flexible thresholds of P concentration exist in human organisms, beyond which P may elicit unsafe actions in addition to those considered indispensable for life. The committees of Kidney Disease Improving Global Outcomes (KDIGO) [22] and the National Institute for Health and Care Excellence (NICE) [23] have recently provided low graded suggestions to counteract the progressive increase of serum P levels with nutritional therapy and oral P binders, starting from GFR lower than 45 mL/min/1.73 m^2 and 30 mL/min/1.73 m^2, respectively.

Regulation of the P pool in humans depends on homeostatic *balance* between nutritional intake, intestinal absorption, and renal excretion [2]. Notably, the *distribution* of P concentrations is highly heterogeneous between body compartments and strictly regulated by hormonal assets. Both the net *balance* and the compartmental *distribution* of P are consequently expected to modulate the transition from homeostatic to maladaptive or pathologic actions of P. Consequently, nutritional intake, renal excretion, and hormonal asset appear as fundamental modulators of the ratio between safe and unsafe effects elicited by P in humans. From this perspective, controlling dietary P intake may represent the easiest way to affect P balance through preventive and therapeutic interventions.

The two following issues hamper the investigation of links between P intake and hard endpoints: (1) uncertainties on how to reliably assess the nutritional P intake and the net P balance on the long run and (2) disagreement on the most reliable marker of P load across different ranges of GFR. Thus, treating the link between P intake and mortality will require a cautious roadmap, starting with P balance in normal and renal patients, then moving to sources of nutritional P and the mechanism of P toxicity, and only after dealing with observational and intervention studies on the topic.

4.2 PHOSPHATE HOMEOSTASIS IN HUMANS: NUTRITIONAL INTAKE, INTESTINAL ABSORPTION, AND RENAL EXCRETION

A 70-kg healthy man commonly stores 700 mg of P, mainly distributed as hydroxyapatite in skeletal tissues (85%) and to a lesser extent in intracellular space (14%) as organic P (nucleic acid, adenosine triphosphate [ATP], phospholipids, creatine phosphate, and phosphoproteins) (Figure 4.1). Circulating P represents less than 1% of the total body P and is therefore a weak marker of the body P pool and its compartmental distribution [3].

Nutrients are the main source of P in humans. About 60% of dietary P is absorbed in the intestine as inorganic P, which can rise up to 80% in the presence of high circulating levels of calcitriol. P absorption takes place in the small intestine by passive paracellular diffusion, regulated by electrochemical gradient, and by active transport elicited by luminal sodium P cotransporters type 2b (NPT2b) and type 2c (NPT2b) [24]. Intestinal P uptake is mainly influenced by (1) vitamin D activity, (2) the amount of P present in the diet, (3) bioavailability of P, and (4) the presence of P binders [25]. At the same time serum P, circulating unbound to albumin, is continuously cleared by glomerular filtration, potentially leading to continuous P loss with unrelenting negative balance if a net balance was not ensured by TRP (Figure 4.2). In normal subjects, under homeostatic conditions, about 75% and 10% of the filtered P are reabsorbed in the proximal convoluted tubule by 3Na-HPO4

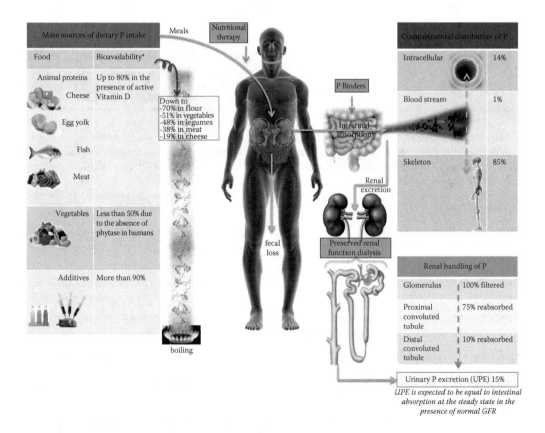

FIGURE 4.1 (See color insert.) Phosphate homeostasis. P homeostasis depends on the nutritional intake of P, its intestinal absorption, compartmental distribution, and renal excretion. Nutrition, P binders, and preservation of renal function (and dialysis for ESRD patients) represent the current interventions to affect P balance in humans. Intestinal absorption depends on the bioavailability of nutritional P, presence of P binders in the gut lumen, cooking methods, and levels of active vitamin D.

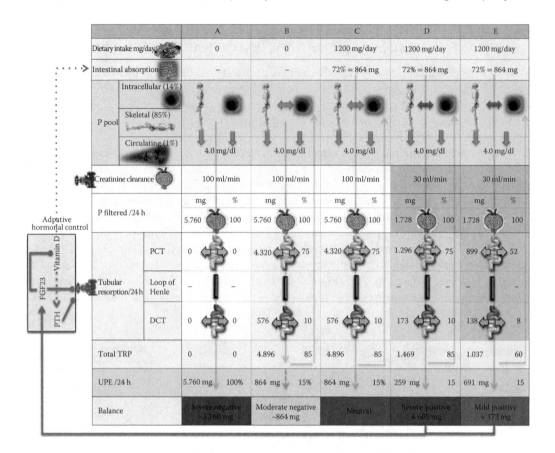

FIGURE 4.2 (See color insert.) Teaching simulation of P balance, according to nutritional intake, serum levels, glomerular filtration rate, and tubular handling of P. The simulation intends to simplify the variation of P balance according to changes in nutritional intake, serum levels, and glomerular filtration, particularly stressing the active regulatory effect elicited by tubular handling. For simplification, P serum levels are assumed as constant during 24 hours. Positive P balance activates a hormonal adaptive cascade pivoted by FGF23. Five sequential models are summarized.

MODEL A. Assuming null dietary intake of P, constant serum P levels of 4.0 mg/dL and normal CrCl of 100 mL/min with null TRP, 5760 mg of P are expected to be cleared and excreted over 24 hours, leading to a severely negative P balance (−5760 mg/24 hours).

MODEL B. Adding to Model A a TRP of 85%, 4.896 mg of P are expected to be reabsorbed, considerably reducing UPE from 5760 mg to 864 mg over 24 hours, leading to a smoldered negative P balance (−864 mg/day).

MODEL C. The achievement of a neutral balance (steady state) is expected after adding to Model B dietary P intake of 1200 mg/day, with a 72% intestinal absorption (864 mg of P absorbed/day).

MODEL D. Switching the scenario of Model C into CKD stage 4 (CrCl 30 mL/min) without modified TRP values, the amount of P cleared by glomerular filtration and reabsorbed by renal tubules is expected to fall 1728 mg and 1469 mg over 24 hours, respectively, leading to a considerable reduction of UPE (259 mg/24 hours) and a severe positive balance (+605 mg/day).

MODEL E. Reducing TRP from 85% to 60% is expected to reduce P reabsorbed by renal tubules from 1469 to 1037 mg, leading to increased UPE from 259 mg to 691 mg over 24 hours and a smoldering positive P balance (from +605 mg to 173 mg per day).

ABBREVIATIONS CrCl: creatinine clearance, DCT: distal convoluted tubule, FGF23: fibroblast growth factor 23, P: phosphate, PCT: proximal convoluted tubule, PTH: parathyroid hormone, TRP: tubular resorption of P, UPE: urinary P excretion, Line with end dotted: inhibitory effect, Arrows: activator effect.

cotransporter type 2a (NPT2a) [26] and in the distal convoluted tubule, respectively [3], with only 15% of the filtered P being excreted in urine. Thus, tubular handling is a leading guarantor of P equilibrium, actively responding to variations of nutritional intake, intestinal absorption, and GFR under strict hormonal regulation [26,27]. An intestinal–glomerular feedback has also been postulated [28]. Based on these physiological considerations, the 24-hour urinary P excretion (UPE) is generally considered equivalent to daily intestinal absorption (not intake) of P in normal subjects at the steady state [29,30] (Figure 4.2).

A positive P balance may result from the combination of one or more of the following factors: excessive nutritional intake, uncontrolled intestinal absorption, and insufficient renal excretion (Figure 4.2). The reduction of GFR at levels still higher than 60 mL/min may hamper the renal excretion of P, requiring the compensatory reduction of TRP, pivoted by fibroblast growth factor 23 (FGF23) [2,4]. Assuming the maintenance of common nutritional intake and unchanged intestinal absorption of P, progressive reduction of GFR toward end-stage renal disease (ESRD) may become too pronounced to be counteracted by inhibited TRP, leading to inexorable positive P balance [2,4,5]. Phosphaturic response to a certain nutritional P load can be even subjected to individual predisposition [31–35], leading to a heterogeneous risk profile of positive P balance with relative clinical consequences. Dialysis patients are prone to severe risk of P overload due to the minimal or null amount of renal excretion and the limited P clearance elicited by current dialysis techniques [2].

Although medical interventions are still far from optimizing the renal and dialysis clearance of P [2], nutritional P intake appears a more accessible target for preventive and therapeutic strategies. Any intervention focused on P intake should not be restricted to the whole amount of P delivered with meals, but rather include the form of nutritional P (animal, vegetable, or additive) and cooking methods, both of which are able to influence nutritional P bioavailability [2] (Figure 4.1). In Western countries dietary P content ranges from 1600 mg/day in adult men to 1000 mg/day in adult women, despite the Recommended Dietary Allowance suggesting 700 mg of daily P intake [2,12]. Animal proteins constitute the main source of dietary P, with a 60% bioavailability and an estimated average of 14 mg of P per g of proteins in a common mixed diet [36–38]. On the other hand, bioavailability of P of plant origin (as phytate) is less pronounced due to the lack of phytase in humans (<50%), limiting the degradation of phytate to intestinal flora metabolism or to nonenzymatic hydrolysis reaction [39]. Main natural sources of P are represented by cheese (220–700 mg/100 g), egg yolk (586 mg/100 g), and fish (190–290 mg/100 g) [40]. The choice of proteins with a lower P-to-protein ratio is crucial whenever reducing P intake to assure sufficient protein delivery [2,41]. Another significant source of nutritional P is represented by food additives as inorganic phosphate salts, which are almost entirely absorbed by the intestinal tract (>90%) [42]. The widespread adoption of additives in soft drinks and low-quality processed foods, together with poor labeling of P-containing preservatives, leads to considerable risk of "hidden" P load, especially in subjects of low socioeconomic strata [2,42–44].

Cooking manipulation modulates the effective dietary P burden. Although boiling is considered a poor technique due to the loss of minerals, it is now a well-accepted method to reduce the content of P in animal and vegetable foods without a corresponding loss of proteins [45,46]. Boiling is capable of reducing the content of P up to 70% in flour, 51% in vegetables, 48% in legumes, 38% in meat, and 19% in cheese [45] (Figure 4.1).

Controlling P intake is a unique target of nutritional intervention in renal patients, commonly exposed to increased risk of P overload in conjunction with GFR reduction. Nutritional P load can be easily counteracted in predialysis patients by reducing protein intake to 0.8 to 0.6 g/kg/day [47] as suggested by the current guidelines [22]. However, the higher recommended protein intake (1.2 g/kg/day) exposes dialysis patients to a considerable risk of nutritional P overload [48], if not accompanied by careful selection of proteins with an adequate P-to-protein ratio, avoidance of additive-enriched foods, and preference of adequate cooking methods [2].

4.3 ASSESSING NUTRITIONAL P INTAKE AND P BALANCE: A TOUGH GOAL IN RESEARCH AND CLINICAL PRACTICE

Several methodological weaknesses limit seriously the assessment of nutritional P intake and P balance in clinical practice (Figure 4.3). An accurate estimation of P balance requires four steps: (1) assessment of P amount present in food; (2) controlled amount of food delivered, with consequent estimation of the P amount ingested with meals; (3) stool collection to compute the mass of nutritional P absorbed by the intestinal tract; and (4) assessment of P and creatinine renal excretion in 24-hour urine collection (and/or in dialysate) to finally estimate the balance.

Although a similar approach is partially achievable only for research purposes in small and short intervention studies [49–57], it is difficult—if not impossible—to perpetuate this in large trials with long follow-up required to test the impact of nutritional therapy on hard endpoints. Thus, nutritional data collected from large cohorts are biased by problems in the estimation of P intake, often limited to baseline prescribed phosphate dose [58], dietary records validated on precoded menu books [59], dietary questionnaire [37], 24-hour dietary recall [60,61], and 1-month food frequency questionnaire [60].

Assessing 24-hour UPE is considered an alternative and reliable estimate of net intestinal P uptake [29,30]. However, its reliability is limited to the period of urine collection, generally confined to the study baseline and to further control visits, rather than representing the averaged nutritional P load during the entire length of follow-up (Figure 4.3). Furthermore, assuming that a direct correspondence between 24-hour UPE and intestinal absorption of P is maintained also in renal cohorts, especially at GFR lower than 30 mL/min, would imply that the exact amount of dietary P absorbed by the intestine is always excreted in urine also in CKD stage 4 to 5 patients, leading to the jarring assumption that a neutral P balance is always guaranteed in advanced CKD, which contradicts the common observation of increased serum P levels in CKD stages 4 to 5 [2–4] (Figure 4.2). However, this would not imply that CKD patients with higher but stable P cannot be in neutral P balance, but rather that a) even a minimum excess of dietary P absorbed by the intestine than the P excreted in the urine may lead to a slow but consistent positive P balance and b) UPE may negatively approximate the real dietary P absorbed in advanced CKD patients. Data from the Modification of Diet in Renal Disease (MDRD) clearly showed that patients with lower GFR (13–24 mL/min/1.73 m^2) experienced a progressive increase in serum P levels compared to patients with higher GFR (25–55 mL/min/1.73 m^2) despite the lower UPE, consequent to reduced P intake with a low-and very-low-protein diet (350–700 mg/day and 280–630 mg/day of P, respectively) [62]. Sigrist et al. randomized 18 CKD patients (GFR 15–60 mL/min) and 12 healthy controls to three interventions: (1) high P diet (2.000 mg/day), (2) low P diet (750 mg/day), and (3) low P diet plus aluminum hydroxide 500 mg thrice daily at meals [63]. Significant interaction between CKD status and the effect of P intake on absolute change of UPE and FGF23 was detected [63]. Phelps et al. have recently observed that at steady states of reduced GFR, serum P is determined by both the influx into extracellular space and TRP [33,34]. Notably, their conclusion was derived by fasting specimens of blood and urine in the morning, assuming that P homeostasis should be evaluated during the brief period required to create an aliquot of urine, although not being representative of the continuous variations that occurred during 24 hours [33,34]. However it can be argued that tubular handling of P may elicit a deep impact on P balance at reduced GFR, limiting the reliability of 24-hour UPE alone as a good marker of intestinal P absorption in those patients (Figure 4.2). Furthermore, observational data proposed a strong impact on mortality elicited by tubular sensitivity to the phosphaturic action of FGF23, represented by the FGF23/TRP ratio [32].

Caution should also be given while dealing with serum P as a marker of dietary P intake and P balance (Figure 4.3). Among 15,513 patients enrolled in the Third National Health and Nutrition Examination Survey (NHANES III), dietary P intake assessed by 24-hour dietary recall was poorly associated with serum P (0.03 mg/dL higher serum P for each 500 mg greater intake of P) only in subjects with GFR greater than 60 mL/min [60]. A weak association between dietary P and circulating

Associations between Phosphorus Intake and Mortality

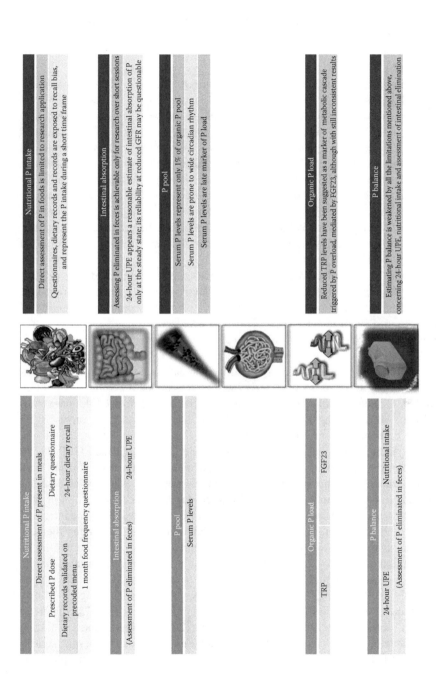

FIGURE 4.3 (See color insert.) Assessment of P balance: Methods and weaknesses. Techniques available to assess P balance are reported in green boxes (orange boxes report the methods limited to research application). Weaknesses of techniques are briefly described in red boxes.

ABBREVIATIONS FGF23: fibroblast growth factor 23, P: phosphate, TRP: tubular resorption of P, UPE: urinary P excretion.

P levels was observed among 1,105 CKD patients from the same cohort, with a 0.009 mg/dL increase of serum P for each 100 mg increase of daily P intake [64]. A nonsignificant 0.03 mg/dL higher serum P concentration was similarly reported for each 300 mg/day greater UPE in the Heart and Soul Study ($p = 0.07$) [30]. Furthermore, a single sample poorly represents the circadian fluctuations of serum P levels, characterized by a nadir around 11:00 AM and to further peaks at 04:00 PM and 01:00 to 03:00 AM [50]. In the NHANES III study serum P levels were descriptively higher when assessed in the afternoon, in the evening, and at a nonfasting state [60], compared to the morning and fasting sessions [65].

Concerns exist about the quantity of P intake variation required to induce detectable modification of mean circulating P levels within a short period (Table 4.1). Reduction of P intake from 1500 mg to less than 500 mg was associated with 40% reduction of circulating P levels and descriptive mitigation of diurnal peaks in healthy men, detectable after one day and even more pronounced after 10 days of diet modification [50]. Notably, serum P levels assessed at 8:00 were unchanged after the first 24 hours of diet restriction [50]. Doubling P intake to 3000 mg for 10 days led to a 14% increase of the 24-hour mean P levels without significant variations in the fasting morning levels and with an exaggerated early afternoon peak [50]. Increased serum P levels were similarly observed after switching P intake from 850 mg to 2880 mg for 36 hours [53]. On the contrary, a milder increase of dietary P intake (from 1556 mg/day to 2071 mg/day) did not induce any detectable change in serum P level, assessed by serial blood draws for 24 hours after two weeks of diet modification in 19 healthy volunteers [51].

Circulating P levels may also be modulated by gender [35,60], age [35,66], and race [60,67]. However, the observational source of data does not allow any conclusion about an active influence elicited by age, gender, and race on P balance and about their interaction with the reliability of serum P levels as a marker of P balance within specific patient categories.

Serum P was insensible to fixed doses of oral P binders and diet intervention in predialysis CKD patients in the short term, despite a significant reduction of UPE (Table 4.2). Isakova et al. randomly assigned 16 normophosphatemic CKD stage 3 to 4 patients to controlled diet intervention for two weeks (1500 mg versus 750 mg of P) associated with lanthanum carbonate 1 g thrice daily versus placebo [55]. Of note, circulating P and FGF23 levels were unchanged despite significant reduction of 24-hour UPE in patients undergoing a low P diet (249 ± 213 mg versus 702 ± 262 mg) and lanthanum carbonate (from 710 ± 192 mg at baseline to 267 ± 140 mg at the end of follow-up) [55]. Thirty-nine normophosphatemic CKD patients (mean estimated GFR 37.8 ± 11.0 mL/min) were randomized to nutritional intervention (ad libitum diet versus 900 mg of P intake), alternatively associated with placebo versus lanthanum carbonate 1000 mg thrice daily for 3 months [56]. Difference in daily P intake, estimated by three-day food records, was lower than 500 mg between the study arms [56]. Although 3 g of lanthanum were expected to reduce intestinal P absorption by 405 mg [49], the difference in 24-hour UPE between patients receiving the controlled diet and active lanthanum was lower than expected, compared to those allocated to placebo plus similar diet intervention (544 ± 294 mg versus 757 ± 371 at study end) [56]. Notably, serum P levels and TRP were insensible to study interventions independently from the widely ranged reduction of FGF23 levels (35% ± 32%) [56]. Eighteen normophosphatemic CKD stage 3 patients received controlled P intake lower than 700 mg for 28 days plus lanthanum carbonate 750 mg thrice weekly for four additional weeks [54]. UPE was assessed in the 12-hour urine sampled at fasting night time [54]. Consistent with previous results, serum P concentration did not vary despite significant reduction of UPE and FGF23 levels [54]. Oliveira et al. randomized 40 normophosphatemic CKD stage 3 to 4 patients to calcium carbonate versus sevelamer carbonate at escalating doses for six weeks (up to 5.3 g and 6.4 g of calcium carbonate and sevelamer, respectively) [57]. Patients were instructed to maintain a constant P intake of approximately 600 mg/day. Phosphate levels remained unchanged, although they were accompanied by a reduction of 24-hour UPE, serum FGF23 levels, and fractional excretion of P [57]. Despite the aforementioned results, repeated evidence showed that significant reduction of serum P levels could be achieved in CKD patients by

TABLE 4.1

Principal Studies Investigating Variations of Serum P after Controlled Interventions on Dietary P Intake

Study	Subjects	Kidney Function	P Diet Intervention	Follow-up	Main Results
Portale et al. (1987) [50]	6 healthy men	NA	• 1500 mg/day/70 Kg for 9 days • 500 mg/day plus aluminum hydroxide for 10 days • 3000 mg/day for 10 days	29 days	• 40% reduction of serum P levels after 10 days of P restriction • 14% increase in 24 hours mean serum P after 10 days of P supplementation
Vervloet et al. (2011) [53]	18 healthy subjects	CrCl 125 + 27 mL/min	• 850 mg/day for 3 days • 1 week interval • 2880 mg/day for 3 days	13 days	• No change in serum P after P restriction • Increased serum P from 1.10 + 0.09 mmol/L to maximum of 1.32 mmol/L after high dietary intake
Kremsdof 2013 [51]	19 healthy volunteers	eGFR > 60 mL/min/1.73 m^2	• 1156 + 271 mg/day for 13 days • 2071 + 346 mg/day for 14 days • 1622 + 442 mg/day for 101–115 days	14 weeks	• No change in serum P levels observed after diet modification

Note: Studies are presented as principal author's name and year of publication; eGFR = estimated glomerular filtration rate; P = phosphorus.

TABLE 4.2

Principal Studies Investigating the Effect of P Binders at Fixed Doses Plus Controlled Diet on Serum P Levels Among Predialysis CKD Patients

Study Subjects	Design	Kidney Function	Diet Intervention	P Binders	Follow-up	Main Results
Isakova et al. (2011) [55] 16 CKD stage 3–4 patients with normal serum P	Randomized controlled trial (2 × 2 factorial design)	eGFR 40 + 12 mL/ min/1.73 m^2	1.500 mg/day versus 750 mg/day	placebo versus lanthanum carbonate 1000 mg three times a day	2 weeks	• no difference in serum P levels between groups • FGF23 increased with 1.500 mg diet plus placebo • significant reduction of UPE with 750 mg P diet compared with 1.500 mg diet • significant reduction in UPE with lanthanum, although similar to placebo
Isakova et al. (2013) [56] 39 CKD stage 3–4 patients normal serum P	Randomized, single-blinded, placebo-controlled trial (2 × 2 factorial design)	eGFR 37.8 + 11.0 mL/min/1.73 m^2	ad libitum versus 900 mg/day	placebo versus lanthanum carbonate 1000 mg three times a day	3 months	• no difference in serum P levels between groups • modest decline in UPE with 900 mg diet plus placebo (−13% + 23%) and with lanthanum (−19% + 24%) • wide-ranging reduction of FGF23 with 900 mg diet plus lanthanum (−35% + 32%) • TRP unchanged
Gonzalez Parra et al. (2011) [54] 18 CKD stage 3 patients normal serum P	Prospective longitudinal open-label	CrCl 42.08 mL/ min (95% CI 35.6–48.5)	< 700 mg/day from animal protein for the whole study period	none for 4 weeks lanthanum carbonate 750 mg three times a day for the next 4 weeks	8 weeks	• no difference in serum P levels between groups • significant reduction of UPE, FGF23 and increase of TRP with addition of lanthanum
Oliveira et al. (2009) [57] 40 CKD stage 3–4 patients normal serum P	Randomized open-label controlled trial	CrCl 34 + 15.89 mL/min	615 + 63 mg/ day	sevelamer 800 mg 1.6 g/day then doubled every week up to 4.2 and 6.4 g/day versus calcium acetate 1.32 g/day then doubled every weeks up to 2.664 and 5.28 g/day	8 weeks	• no difference in serum P levels between groups • significant reduction of UPE • significant reduction of FGF23 only in sevelamer arm

Note: Studies are presented as principal author's name, year of publication, and reference followed by the characteristics of participants.

Follow-up data are expressed as mean or median values as reported in published studies.

CrCl = creatinine clearance; eGFR = estimated glomerular filtration rate; FGF23 = fibroblast growth factor 23; P = phosphorus; TRP = tubular reabsorption of phosphorus; UPE = urinary phosphorus excretion.

Associations between Phosphorus Intake and Mortality 55

administering oral P binders at escalating doses, properly titrated to reduce serum P levels toward a specific target [68,69].

In conclusion, assessing P load remains challenging in clinical practice (Figure 4.3). Hypophosphatemia and hyperphosphatemia are well-accepted markers of the contracted and expanded P pool, respectively. Variations of P intake greater than 1000 mg/day repeatedly induced acute modification of serum P levels in normal subjects. On the contrary, phosphatemia was insensible to lower modification of nutritional P intake in predialysis CKD patients within a few weeks. Thus, the best method to do an early estimate of small changes in P balance among normophosphatemic CKD patients remains an unsolved issue. It can be argued that small modification of dietary intake, intestinal absorption, and renal handling can affect the P pool and circulating P levels on the long run, with a significant interaction with both GFR and the tubular sensitivity to hormonal adaptive response (Figure 4.3). A current hot topic in the field is the search for a coveted surrogate marker sufficiently reliable to provide an accurate signal of P overload and of its toxic activity in still-normophosphatemic subjects. FGF23 and TRP have been proposed in this regard, although with still inconsistent results [47,54–57,68].

4.4 PHOSPHATE AND MORTALITY: MECHANISMS

Detailed mechanisms linking P to poor outcomes will be examined in chapters focused on P intake and cardiac–bone disease. It is herein sufficient to summarize that P overload may negatively affect survival by accelerating vascular, skeletal, and renal aging through the following pathways (Figure 4.4): (1) activation of CKD-MBD syndrome pivoted by FGF23 [2]; (2) endothelial dysfunction [70] and vascular calcification [2]; (3) oxidative stress; (4) left ventricular hypertrophy sustained by high FGF23 levels close to the downregulation of its coreceptor klotho [71]; and (5) glomerular damage [72] with worsening of proteinuria and GFR, associated with an impaired response to renin–angiotensin–aldosterone system inhibitors [73].

4.5 PHOSPHATE INTAKE AND MORTALITY: OBSERVATIONAL STUDIES

Although a large body of literature has investigated the link between serum P levels and mortality [6–15], the association between P intake and survival was addressed only by a small number of observational studies without any dedicated randomized controlled trial leading to discrepant results (Table 4.3). Among 9686 normal subjects from the NHANES III study, one unit logarithm increase of P consumption over 1400 mg/day was associated with adjusted 89% increased risk of all-cause mortality, without significant risk at P intake below 1400 mg/day [61]. Palomino et al. investigated the association between survival and baseline 24-hour UPE among 880 patients with stable cardiovascular disease and normal renal function from the Heart and Soul Study [30]. UPE greater than 748 mg/day compared to UPE lower than 500 mg/day was associated with a 44% risk reduction of all-cause mortality, although it lost significance after multivariate adjustment [30]. Furthermore, a 17% independent risk reduction for cardiovascular disease was observed for each 300 mg/day higher UPE [30]. Adherence to a Mediterranean diet was directly associated with a lower P intake (1.3 g/day versus 1.6 g/day, respectively) among 506 CKD men from the Uppsala Longitudinal Study of Adult Men cohort (estimated GFR <60 mL/min/1.73 m^2) [59]. During a 9.9-year follow-up, all-cause mortality risk was reduced by 52% and 58% in mildly and highly adherent compared to poorly adherent subjects, respectively ($p = 0.005$) [59]. Finally, higher dietary P intake, assessed by the Block Food Frequency Questionnaire, was independently associated with a 137% risk reduction for 5-year mortality among 224 hemodialysis patients [37].

Despite the aforementioned positive results, negative and even opposite data have also been published. Among 1105 CKD adults from the NHANES III cohort (eGFR 49.3 ± 9.5 mL/min 1.73 m^2), the highest compared to the lowest P intake (1.478 ± 28 mg/day versus 531 ± 11 mg/day, respectively) was not independently associated with mortality risk during a 6.5-year follow-up [HR1.07

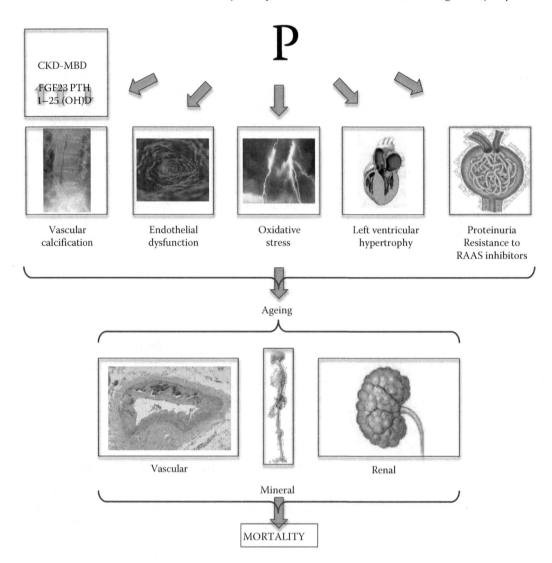

FIGURE 4.4 (See color insert.) Mechanisms linking P to mortality.

ABBREVIATIONS CKD-MBD: chronic kidney disease and mineral bone disorder, FGF23: fibroblast growth factor 23, P: phosphate, PTH: parathyroid hormone, RAAS: renin–angiotensin–aldosterone system.

(95% CI 0.67–1.70)] [64]. Selamet et al. investigated the association between baseline 24-hour UPE and hard endpoints among 795 patients from the MDRD Study A and Study B cohorts [29]. Higher UPE was not associated with ESRD and all-cause, cardiovascular, and noncardiovascular mortality [29]. Low prescribed dietary P intake (PDP) was not associated with reduced mortality risk in a post-hoc analysis among 1751 hemodialysis patients from the HEMO study [58]. Compared to P intake lower than 870 mg/day, PDP of 1000 to 2000 mg/day and no restricted diet were associated with a 27% and 29% reduction of all-cause mortality [HR 0.73 (95% CI 0.54–0.97) and 0.71 (95% CI 0.55–0.92), respectively] [58]. Notably, results of this post-hoc analysis may be biased by the lack of data concerning the widespread adoption of oral P binders within the HEMO study [58].

Oral phosphorus binders represent another strategy to counteract nutritional P load [2]. Unfortunately head-to-head comparison between P binders and placebo on hard endpoints has never been tested in dedicated randomized controlled trials. Scientific debate is still open about the opportunity to control dietary P load by P binders in normophosphatemic CKD patients [5]. Observational

TABLE 4.3

Principal Studies Investigating the Association between Dietary P Intake and Intestinal P Absorption and Mortality

Study	Subjects	Design	Kidney Function	Assessment of Dietary P	Follow-up	Main Results
Chang et al. (2014) [61]	9686 adults from NHANES III, without CKD, CVD, diabetes or cancer	Observational	-	24-hour dietary recall (*dietary P intake*)	14.7 years	Higher P intake associated with increased all-cause mortality risk [HR 1.89 (95% CI 1.03–3.46)] in subjects with P intake > 1400 mg/day
Palomino et al. (2013) [30]	880 patients from Heart and Soul Study with stable CVD and without CKD	Observational	eGFR 71 + 2 mL/min/ 1.73 m²	24-hour UPE (*intestinal absorption of P*)	7.4 years	17% lower risk of CVD events for each 300 mg higher UPE
Huang et al. (2013) [59]	1110 Swedish men from the ULSAM study	Observational	604 non CKD subjects [(eGFR 69.3 mL/ min/1.73 m² IQR 64.0–77.0)] 506 CKD patients [(eGFR 51.9 mL/ min/1.73 m² IQR 46.3–56.6)]	7-day dietary record based on validated precoded menu (*dietary P intake*) Mediterranean Diet Score (*adherence to Mediterranean diet*)	9.9 years	Higher P intake associated with high compared to low adherence to Mediterranean diet (1.6 mg/day [IQR 1.2–2.8)] versus 1.3 (IQR 1.0,1.8), respectively] All-cause mortality risk reduced by 52% and 58% in subjects with medium and high adherence to Mediterranean diet, respectively (p for trend = 0.005)
Noori et al. (2010) [37]	224 maintenance hemodialysis patients from the NIED study	Observational	ESRD	Block Food Frequency Questionnaire (*dietary P intake*)	5 years	Third tertile of dietary P intake associated with higher mortality risk [HR 2.37 (95% CI 1.01–6.32)]

(Continued)

TABLE 4.3 *(Continued)*

Principal Studies Investigating the Association between Dietary P Intake and Intestinal P Absorption and Mortality

Study	Subjects	Design	Kidney Function	Assessment of Dietary P	Follow-up	Main Results
Murtaugh et al. (2012) [64]	1105 CKD patients from the NHANES III	Observational	eGFR 49.3 + 9.5 mL/min/1.73 m^2	24-hour dietary recall (dietary P intake)	6.5 years	No association between mortality and highest versus lowest P intake (1478 + 28 mg/day versus 531 + 11 mg/day) [HR 1.07 (95% CI 0.67–1.70)]
Selamet et al. (2016) [29]	795 CKD stage 3–5 patients from the MDRD study	Post-hoc analysis of a randomized, multicenter clinical trial	Iothalamate GFR 33 + 12 mL/min	24-hour UPE *(intestinal absorption of P)* 3 day food record *(dietary P intake)*	16 years	No association between dietary P intake and all-cause, cardiovascular and noncardiovascular mortality
Lynch et al. (2011) [58]	1751 hemodialysis patients from the HEMO study	Post-hoc analysis of a randomized controlled trial	ESRD	Dietary recall converted into dietary intake data by Nutritionist IV program *(dietary P intake)* Diet prescribed by study dietitian to keep protein intake > 1 g/kg/day	2.3 years	Low prescribed P intake was not associated with lower mortality risk High prescribed P intake (1000–2000 mg/day) and no-restriction groups with significant reduction of all-cause mortality [HR 0.73 (95% CI 0.54–0.97) and HR 0.71 (95% CI 0.55–0.92)]

Note: Studies are presented as principal author's name, year of publication, and reference.

Follow-up data are expressed as mean or median values as reported in published studies.

CrCl = creatinine clearance; eGFR = estimated glomerular filtration rate; FGF23 = fibroblast growth factor-23; P = phosphorus; UPE = urinary phosphorus excretion; CI = confidence interval; ESRD = end-stage renal disease; IQR = interquartile range; HEMO = Hemodialysis Study; MDRD = Modification of Diet in Renal Disease Study; NHANES = National Health and Nutrition Examination Survey; NIED = National Institutes of Health-funded Nutritional and Inflammatory Evaluation in Dialysis Study.

Associations between Phosphorus Intake and Mortality 59

data reported an almost 30% reduction of mortality risk in predialysis [16] and dialysis patients [17] receiving P binders compared to those untreated, independently from the class of binder prescribed. Many expectations are placed on the ongoing ANSWER [74] and COMBINE [75] trials, comparing the effect of sevelamer [74] and lanthanum carbonate and/or nicotinamide [75] against placebo on surrogate outcomes as proteinuria [74], mineral metabolism, and markers of cardiovascular and renal damage [75] in predialysis CKD patients.

4.6 CONCLUSIONS

The impact of P load on survival remains a hot topic for contemporary medicine. Improving the knowledge about P balance and its potential toxicity sounds challenging yet indispensable to reduce the risks in the general population and improve the care of renal patients. Although both hypophosphatemia and hyperphosphatemia have been related to poor outcomes, uncertainties persist about the negative impact elicited by incremental P balance on normophosphatemic individuals in the general population and, especially, in predialysis CKD cohorts. Further insights are urgently needed to bridge the gaps still existing within and between the notions of pathophysiology and epidemiology. In addition, a holistic approach to nutrition should never be abandoned, always considering P as a crucial, but not unique, element of the diet close to calories, proteins, carbohydrates, and other elements. While waiting for dedicated randomized controlled trials, available evidence is mainly observational and still insufficient to recommend any different intervention from those proposed by the current guidelines.

REFERENCES

1. Wagner CA, Rubio-Aliaga I, Hernando N. Genetic disease of renal phosphate handling. *Nephrol Dial Transplant* 2014;29:iv45–iv54.
2. Galassi A, Cupisti A, Santoro A et al. Phosphate balance in ESRD: Diet dialysis and binders against the low evident masked pool. *J Nephrol* 2015;28:415–29.
3. Uribarri J. Phosphorus homeostasis in normal health and chronic kidney disease patients with special emphasis on dietary phosphorus intake. *Semin Dial* 2007;20:295–301.
4. Isakova T, Wahl P, Vargas GS et al. Fibrobalst growth factor 23 is elevated before parathyroid hormone and phosphate in chronic kidney disease. *Kidney Int* 2011;79:1370–8.
5. Bellasi A. Pro: Should phosphate binders be used in chronic kidney disease stage 3-4? *Nephrol Dial Transplant* 2016;31:184–8.
6. Block GA, Klassen PS, Lazarus JM et al. Mineral metabolism, mortality and morbidity in mineral maintenance hemodialysis. *J Am Soc Nephrol* 2004;15:2208–18.
7. Kalantar-Zadeh K, Kuwae N, Regidor DL et al. Survival predictability of time-varying indicators of bone disease in maintenance hemodialysis patients. *Kidney Int* 2006;70:771–80.
8. Bellasi A, Mandreoli M, Baldrati L et al. Chronic kidney disease progression and outcome according to serum phosphorus in mild-to-moderate kidney dysfunction. *Clin J Am Soc Nephrol* 2011;6:883–91.
9. Kestenbaum B, Sampson JN, Rudser KD et al. Serum phosphate levels and mortality risk among people with chronic kidney disease. *J Am Soc Nephrol* 2005;16:520–8.
10. Menon V, Greene T, Pereira AA et al. Relationship of phosphorus and calcium-phosphorus product with mortality in CKD. *Am J Kidney Dis* 2005;46:455–63.
11. Kovesdy CP, Ahmadzadeh S, Anderson JE et al. Secondary hyperparathyroidism is associated with higher mortality in men with moderate to severe chronic kidney disease. *Kidney Int* 2008;73:1296–302.
12. Dhingra R, Sullivan LM, Fox CS et al. Relations of serum phosphorus and calcium levels to the incidence of cardiovascular disease in the community. *Arch Intern Med* 2007;167(9):879–85.
13. Onufrak SJ, Bellasi A, Shaw LJ et al. Phosphorus levels are associated with subclinical atherosclerosis in the general population. *Atherosclerosis* 2008;199(2):424–31.
14. Foley RN, Collins AJ, Ishani A et al. Calcium-phosphate levels and cardiovascular disease in community-dwelling adults: The Atherosclerosis Risk in Communities (ARIC) Study. *Am Heart J* 2008;156:556–63.
15. Linefsky JP, O'Brien KD, Katz R et al. Association of phosphate levels with aortic valve sclerosis and anular calcification. *J Am Coll Cardiol* 2011;58:291–7.

16. Kovesdy CP, Kuchmak O, Lu JL et al. Outcomes associated with phosphorus binders in men with non-dialysis-dependent CKD. *Am J Kidney Dis* 2010;56:842–51.
17. Isakova T, Gutierrez OM, Chang Y et al. Phosphorus binders and survival on hemodialysis. *J Am Soc Npehrol* 2009;20:388–96.
18. Cannata-Andia JB, Fernandez-Martin JL, Locatelli F et al. Use of phosphate-binding agents is associated with a lower risk of mortality. *Kidney Int* 2013;84:998–1008.
19. Kuro-o M. Klotho and aging. *Biochim Biophys Acta* 2009;1790:1049–58.
20. Razzaque MS, Sitara D, Taguchi T et al. Premature aging-like phenotype in fibroblast growth factor 23 null mice is a vitamin D-mediated process. *FASEB J* 2006;20:720–2.
21. Stubbs JR, Liu S, Tang W et al. Role of hyperphosphatemia and 1,25-dihydroxyvitamin D in vascular calcification and mortality in fibroblastic growth factor 23 null mice. *J Am Soc Nephrol* 2007;18:2116–24.
22. Kidney Disease: Improving Global Outcomes (KDIGO) CKD Work Group. KDIGO 2012 clinical practice guideline for the evaluation and management of chronic kidney disease. *Kidney Int Suppl* 2013;3:1–150.
23. National Institute for Health and Care Excellence (NICE), 2013 Hyperphosphatemia in chronic kidney disease. Disponibile su guidance.nice.orguk/cg157
24. Allen LH, Wood RJ Calcium and phosphorus in modern nutrition. In: Shils ME, Olson JA, Shike M (eds.) *Health and Disease*, 8th edn. Philadelphia, PA: Lea & Febiger, 1994, 144–63.
25. Ramirez JA, Emmett M, White MG et al. The absorption of dietary phosphorus and calcium in hemodialysis patients. *Kidney Int* 1986;30:753–95.
26. Tenenhouse HS. Regulation of phosphate homeostasis by the type IIaNa/phosphate cotransporter. *Ann Rev Nutr* 2005;25:197–214.
27. Bernd TJ, Schiavi S, Kumar R et al. "Phosphatonins" and the regulation of phosphorus homeostasis. *Am J Physiol Renal Physiol* 2005;189:F1170–F82.
28. Marks J, Debnam E, Unwin RJ. Phosphate homeostasis and the renal-gastrointestinal axis. *Am J Physiol Renal Physiol* 2010;299:F285–F96.
29. Selamet U, Tighiouart H, Sarnak MJ et al. Relationship of dietary phosphate intake with risk of end-stage renal disease and mortality in chronic kidney disease stages 3-5: The Modification of Diet in Renal Disease Study. *Kidney Int* 2016;89;176–84.
30. Palomino HL, Rifkin DE, Anderson C et al. 24-hour urine phosphorus excretion and mortality and cardiovascular events. *Clin J Am Soc Nephrol* 2013;8:1202–13.
31. Yoda K, Imanishi Y, Yoda M et al. Impaired response of FGF-23 to oral phosphate in patients with type 2 diabetes: A possible mechanism of atherosclerosis. *J Clin Endocrinol Metab* 2012;97:1737–44.
32. Dominguez JR, Shlipak MG, Whooley MA et al. Fractional excretion of phosphorus modifies the association between fibroblast growth factor-23 and outcomes. *J Am Soc Nephrol* 2013;24:647–54.
33. Phelps KR, Mason DL. Parameters of phosphorus homeostasis at normal and reduced GFR: Theoretical considerations. *Clin Nephrol* 2015;83:167–76.
34. Phelps KR, Mason DL, Stote KS. Parameters of phosphorus homeostasis at normal and reduced GFR: Empiric observations. *Clin Nephrol* 2015;83:28–17.
35. Cirillo M, Ciacci C, De Santo NG. Age, renal tubular phosphate reabsorption, and serum phosphate levels in adults. *N Engl J Med* 2008;359:864–6.
36. Boaz M, Smetana S. Regression equation predicts dietary phosphorus intake from estimate of dietary protein intake. *J Am Diet Assoc* 1996;96:1268–70.
37. Noori N, Kalantar-Zadeh K, Kovesdy CP et al. Association of dietary phosphorus intake and phosphorus to protein ratio with mortality in hemodialysis patients. *Clin J Am Soc Nephrol* 2010;5:683–92.
38. Cupisti A, D'Alessandro C. The impact of known and unknown dietary components to phosphorus intake. *G Ital Nefrol* 2011;28:278–88.
39. Bohn L, Meyer AS, Rasmussen SK. Phytate: Impact on environment and human nutrition—A challenge for molecular breeding. *J Zhejiang Univ Sci B* 2008; 9:165–91.
40. Cupisti A, Kalantar-Zadeh K. Management of natural and added dietary phosphorus burden in kidney disease. *Semin Nephrol* 2013;33:180–90.
41. D'Alessandro C, Piccoli GB, Cupisti A. The "phosphorus pyramid" a visual tool for dietary phosphate management in dialysis and CKD patients. *BMC Nephrol* 2015;16:9.
42. Sherman RA, Mehta O. Dietary phosphorus in dialysis patients: Potential impact of processed meat, poultry, and fish products as protein sources. *Am J Kidney Dis* 2009;54:18–23.
43. León JB, Sullivan CM, Sehgal AR. The prevalence of phosphorus-containing food additives in top-selling foods in grocery stores. *J Ren Nutr* 2013;23:265–70.
44. Gutiérrez OM, Anderson C, Isakova T. Low socioeconomic status associates with higher serum phosphate irrespective of race. *J Am Soc Nephrol* 2010;21:1953–60.

45. Jones WL. Demineralization of a wide variety of foods for the renal patient. *J Ren Nutr* 2011;11:90–6.
46. Cupisti A, Comar F, Benini O et al. Effect of boiling on dietary phosphate and nitrogen intake. *J Ren Nutr* 2006;16:36–40.
47. Cozzolino M, Bruschetta E, Cusi D et al. Phosphate handling in CKD-MBD from stage 3 to dialysis and the three strengths of lanthanum carbonate. *Expert Opin Pharmacother* 2012;13:2337–53.
48. KDOQI. KDOQI clinical practice guidelines and clinical practice. Recommendations for diabetes and chronic kidney disease. *Am J Kidney Dis* 2007;49:S12–S154.
49. Martin P, Wang P, Robinson A et al. Comparison of dietary phosphate absorption after single doses of lanthanum carbonate and sevelamer carbonate in healthy volunteers: A balance study. *Am J Kidney Dis* 2011;57:700–6.
50. Portale AA, Halloran BP, Morris RC. Dietary intake of phosphorus modulates the circadian rhythm in serum concentration of phosphorus. *J Cin Invest* 1987;80:1147–54.
51. Kremsdof RA, Hoofnagle AN, Kratz M et al. Effects of a high-protein diet on regulation of phosphorus homeostasis. *J Clin Endocrin Metab* 2013;98:1207–13.
52. Goto S, Kentaro N, Kono K et al. Dietary phosphorus restriction by a standard low-protein diet decreased serum fibroblast growth factor 23 levels in patients with early and advanced stage chronic kidney disease. *Clin Exp Nephrol* 2014;18:925–31.
53. Vervloet MG, van Ittersum FJ, Buttler RM et al. Effects of dietary phosphate and calcium intake on fibroblast growth factor-23. *Clin J Am Soc Nephrol* 2011;6:383–9.
54. Gonzalez-Parra E, Gonzalez-Casaus ML, Galan A et al. Lanthanum carbonate reduces FGF23 in chronic kidney disease stage 3 patients. *Nephrol Dial Transplant* 2011;26:2567–71.
55. Isakova T, Gutierrez OM, Smith K et al. Pilot study of dietary phosphorus restriction and phosphorus binders to target fibroblast growth factor 23 in patients with chronic kidney disease. *Nephrol Dial Transplant* 2011;26:584–91.
56. Isakova T, Barchi-Chung A, Enfield G et al. Effects of dietary phosphate restriction and phosphate binders on FGF23 levels in CKD. *Clin J Am Soc Nephrol* 2013;8:1009–18.
57. Oliveira RB, Cancela ALE, Graciolli FG et al. Early control of PTH and FGF23 in normophosphatemic CKD patients: A new target in CKD-MBD therapy? *Clin J am Soc Nephrol* 2010;5:286–91.
58. Lynch KE, Lynch R, Curhan GC et al. Prescribed dietary phosphate restriction and survival amon hemodialysis patients. *Clin J Am Soc Nephrol* 2011;6:620–9.
59. Huang X, Jimenez-Moleon JJJ, Lindholm B et al. Mediterranean diet, kidney function and mortality in men with CKD. *Clin J Am Soc Nephrol* 2013;8:1548–55.
60. de Boer IH, Rue TC, Ketsenbaum B. Serum phosphorus in the third national health and nutrition examination survey (NHANES III). *Am J Kidney Dis* 2009;53:399–407.
61. Chang AR, Lazo M, Appel JL et al. High dietary phosphorus intake is associated with all-cause mortality: Results from the NHANES III. *Am J Clin Nutr* 2014;99:320–7. (erratum *Am J Clin Nutr* 105:1021-3.)
62. Newsome B, Ix JH, Tighiouart H et al. Effect of protein restriction on serum and urine phosphate in the modification of diet in renal disease (MDRD) study. *Am J Kidney Dis* 2013;61:1045–6.
63. Sigrist M, Tang M, Beaulieau M et al. Responsiveness of FGF-23 and mineral metabolism to altered dietary phosphate intake in chronic kidney disease (CKD): Results of a randomized trial. *Nephrol Dial Transplant* 2013;28:161–9.
64. Murtaugh MA, Filipowicz R, Baird BC et al. Dietary phosphorus intake and mortality in moderate chronic kidney disease: NHANES III. *Nephrol Dial Transplant* 2012;27:990–6.
65. Chang AR, Grams ME. Serum phosphorus and mortality in the Third National Health and Nutrition Examination Survey (NHANES III): Effect modification by fasting. *Am J Kidney Dis* 2014;64:567–73.
66. Cirillo M, Botta G, Chiricone D et al. Gloemrular filatrtion rate and serum phosphate: An inverse relationship diluted by age. *Nephrol Dial Transplant* 2009;24:2123–31.
67. Scialla JJ, Parekh RS, Eustace JA et al. Race, mineral homeostasis and mortality in patients with end-stage renal disease on dialysis. *Am J Nephrol* 2015;42:25–34.
68. Yilmaz MI, Sonmez A, Saglam M et al. Comparison of calcium acetate and sevelamer on vascular function and fibroblast growth factor 23 in CKD patients: A randomized clinical trial. *Am J Kidney Dis* 2012;59:177–85.
69. Block GA, Wheeler DC, Persky MS et al. Effects of phosphate binders in moderate CKD. *J Am Soc Nephrol* 2012;23:1407–15.
70. Shuto E, Taketani Y, Tanaka R et al. Dietary phosphorus acutely impairs endothelial function. *J Am Soc Nephrol* 2009;20:1504–12.
71. Hu MC, Shi M, Cho HJ et al. Klotho and phosphate are modulators of pathologic uremic cardiac remodeling. *J Am Soc Nephrol* 2015;26:1290–302.

72. Sekiguchi S, Suzuki A, Asano S et al. Phosphate overload induces podocyte injury via type III Na-dependent phosphate transporte. *Am J Physiol Renal Physiol* 2011;300:F848–56.
73. Zoccali C, Ruggenenti P, Perna A et al. Phosphate may promote CKD progression and attenuate renoprotective effect of ACE inhibition. *J Am Soc Nephrol* 2011;22:1923–30.
74. Sevelamer in Proteinuric CKD (ANSWER, 2013). https://clinicaltrials.gov/ct2/show/NCT01968759
75. The COMBINE Study: The CKD Optimal Management with Binders and NicotinamidE (COMBINE, 2014). http://clinicaltrials.gov/ct2/show/record/NCT02258074

5 Phosphorus Intake and Whole-Body Phosphorus Homeostasis

Jaime Uribarri and Man S. Oh

CONTENTS

Abstract 63
Bullet Points 63
5.1 Introduction 64
5.2 Body Phosphorus Homeostasis 64
5.3 Conclusions 69
References 69

ABSTRACT

The total phosphorus content in an average 70-kg healthy man is about 700 g, of which about 90% is located in bone and teeth, mostly in the form of calcium phosphate hydroxyapatite. An important clinical question regarding phosphorus homeostasis is how to define total body excess or deficiency. Unfortunately, we do not have a simple/easy clinical parameter to assess body phosphorus content except for serum phosphate, but the phosphate content in circulation represents a minute portion of the total body phosphorus content. Using serum phosphate as a marker of total phosphate content may be misleading, particularly in the short term, when acute changes of phosphorus between body compartments may move serum phosphate levels in directions unrelated to the total body phosphorus balance. Short-term balance studies may also be misleading because it may take weeks before a stable phosphorus balance is obtained. Although healthy subjects with normal renal function will eventually reach phosphorus balance without substantial phosphorus retention, most anuric patients on maintenance traditional dialysis are constantly retaining phosphorus. The actual phosphorus balance in patients with advanced chronic kidney disease is much more difficult to define than that of those on dialysis treatment. This chapter will attempt to address these issues in detail.

BULLET POINTS

- Acutely, fasting serum phosphate is an unreliable marker of total body phosphorus balance.
- Because calcium phosphate deposits in the bone mostly as hydroxyapatite at a weight ratio of 400:186, movements of each mineral between bone and extracellular space will affect calcium more than phosphorus when considered on a milligram-for-milligram basis.
- Although bone represents a potential site for large stores of calcium and phosphorus, there is no evidence that the bone content of calcium and phosphate is increased in subjects with end-stage renal disease who are in a sustained positive balance of calcium and phosphate. Thus prolonged positive balance of these minerals is inevitably accompanied by extraskeletal calcifications.
- One should be very suspicious of short-term balances studies showing significant imbalances for either phosphorus or calcium.

- Phosphorus in the bone and soft tissues appears to deposit only with calcium, but calcium can also deposit with other minerals, such as carbonate.

5.1 INTRODUCTION

Desirable homeostatic endpoints for phosphorus include maintenance of an external balance to prevent total body phosphorus excess or deficiency, as well as maintenance of an internal balance of phosphorus between the different compartments. Over the past few decades the clinical practice of nephrology has shown that defects in phosphorus balance are the main contributing factors to the metabolic bone and cardiovascular disease seen in chronic kidney disease (CKD) patients (Block et al.1998; Kestenbaum et al. 2005). More recently, the concept of toxicity of phosphorus, when ingested in large amounts, even in the absence of kidney disease, has been suggested by epidemiologic data (Dhingra et al. 2007; Chang et al. 2014). Therefore it becomes very important to be able to assess whole-body phosphorus homeostasis. An important clinical question is how to define whether there is total body excess or deficiency. This chapter will attempt to address these issues.

5.2 BODY PHOSPHORUS HOMEOSTASIS

The total phosphorus content in a 70-kg man is about 700 g. Approximately 90% of this phosphorus (Mitchell, Hamilton, Steggerda 1945) is in the bone and teeth, mostly in the form of calcium phosphate hydroxyapatite, $Ca_{10}(PO_4)_6(OH)_2$), 10% in soft tissues, and far less than 1% in the extracellular space. Most intracellular phosphorus is present as part of organic molecules such as creatine phosphate, adenosine triphosphate (ATP), nucleic acids, phospholipids, and phosphoproteins, and therefore it is unlikely to participate in significant accumulation of inorganic phosphate for long periods in the absence of increased cell mass. Therefore the main potential stores for excess body phosphorus are bone and teeth and extraosseous calcifications.

Body phosphorus homeostasis results from the interplay of intestinal absorption of dietary phosphate, renal phosphate reabsorption and excretion, and the exchange of phosphate between extracellular and bone and intracellular storage pools (Figure 5.1).

The kidneys play a major role in maintaining phosphorus homeostasis by matching urinary excretion (output) to net intestinal (gastrointestinal [GI]) absorption (input). On a usual mixed American diet of 1400 mg the net GI absorption adds about 900 mg of phosphorus to the extracellular fluid each day. As healthy adults age, they will have a slightly negative calcium and phosphorus balance because of progressive bone loss, which could potentially represent an extra source of urinary calcium and of urinary phosphate. However, because the bone mineral is mostly hydroxyapatite, which has a calcium-to-phosphorus ratio of 400:186 (each apatite contains 10 molecules of calcium with an atomic weight of 40 [40 × 10 = 400] for 6 molecules of phosphorus with an atomic weight of 31 [6 × 31 = 186]), every 100 mg of calcium lost from bone is accompanied by a loss of 46 mg of phosphorus, which represents only 1/20 of the daily balance of phosphorus. Although total bone Ca-to-P ratio is somewhat higher, 2.2:2.3, because Ca also exists as Ca carbonate, the daily contribution of habitual bone loss to urinary phosphate is insignificant, and a 24-hr urinary phosphate excretion will be almost equal to the net GI absorption of phosphate. This is true independent of the influence of whatever renal mechanisms or hormonal factors exist to influence phosphate balance. Although transient discrepancies between intake and output are frequently present, eventually balance has to be reached in order for the organism to survive, as prolonged substantial imbalance is incompatible with life for most electrolytes, including phosphate.

Because most of the body phosphorus is in bone (90%) complexed with calcium-forming hydroxyapatite, there is a relatively large space to accumulate phosphorus over prolonged periods without immediate dire consequences, except for increase in bone density. However, there is no evidence that bone content of calcium and phosphate is increased in uremic patients. On the other hand, there is ample evidence for accumulation of calcium and phosphate in soft tissues, heart valves, and vascular walls, leading to local calcifications that will produce significant tissue damage. These extra

Phosphorus Intake and Whole-Body Phosphorus Homeostasis

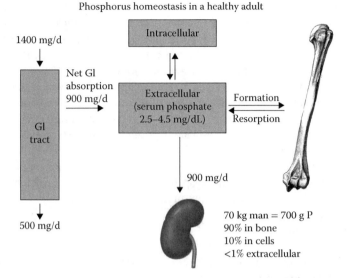

FIGURE 5.1 Phosphorus homeostasis in the healthy adult.

osseous calcifications are not always in the form of hydroxyapatite, as in the bone, but may also be in the form of carbonate apatite or amorphous calcium phosphate (Cofan et al. 1999; Smith 2016). The calcium phosphorus weight ratio in carbonate apatite, for example, is about 1.7, which is lower than that of hydroxyapatite at 2.15, as described earlier. Although phosphate can also be retained in the cells without calcium, this amount is limited over the long term and by the total cell mass. Therefore when phosphate is retained in a substantial amount in the body, it must be in precipitation with calcium in the form of hydroxyapatite, carbonate apatite, or other calcium phosphate crystals. In bone, phosphate deposits mostly with calcium, but a smaller percentage can combine with magnesium, and a portion of calcium can also be deposited without phosphate as calcium carbonate due to the local presence of carbonate (Pellegrino and Biltz 1965; Kaye et al. 1970). Table 5.1, adapted from Pellegrino and Biltz (1965), gives an idea of the respective amounts of calcium, phosphorus, and carbonate in human bone with a total bone mass taken as 4459.9 g (Smith 2016). Of interest, in CKD there is a relatively decreased content of carbonate in relation to phosphate in bone (Pellegrino and Biltz 1965; Kaye et al. 1970).

Deposition of calcium and phosphate, either in bone or extraskeletal tissues, always removes more calcium than phosphate from the extracellular space because both elements are deposited as minerals with a high Ca:P ratio, for example, as hydroxyapatite with a ratio of 2.15, calcium apatite

TABLE 5.1
Mean Mineral Composition of Human Bone

Mineral	Grams
Calcium	1146.20
Phosphate[a]	1539.32
Carbonate	258.30

Source: Adapted from Pellegrino ED and Biltz RM, *Medicine* 44:397–418, 1965.

[a] Although the weight of phosphorus expressed as elemental phosphorus is less than that of calcium at the ratio of 400:186, phosphorus exists in the form of $PO_4^=$ with a molecular weight o0f 95. Hence phosphate weighs more than calcium in bone. Furthermore, the actual weight of bone includes the weight of bone matrix.

as 1.7, etc. An uncorrected positive phosphorus balance of as little as 200 mg per day will lead to accumulation of phosphorus in the body of 73 g per year, which is approximately 10% of the total body P content (about 700 g). If we assume deposition as hydroxyapatite, this will necessarily lead to the simultaneous accumulation of 430 mg/day of calcium (or 157 g/year). If the retention is in the form of carbonate apatite, calcium retained will be 340 mg/day (or 124 g/year), both of which will have to be reflected in increased soft tissue/vascular calcification because there is no evidence of increased calcium and phosphate content in bone of uremic patients. Retention of such massive amounts of calcium and phosphate happens in healthy subjects only during rapid bone growth.

Another unavoidable consequence of phosphate deposition as hydroxyapatite is sequestration of alkali in bone, which in the case noted earlier would lead to a daily removal of alkali from the extracellular space of about 9.5 mEq (mmol), and is tantamount to the same amount of acid added to the extracellular space (1 mmol of calcium hydroxyapatite contains 10 mmol of calcium and 9.2 mmol or mEq of alkali, and therefore 413 mg of calcium in the example would contain 9.5 mmol of alkali) (Oh 1991). In other words, although some positive phosphorus balance can be present over relatively short periods, a long-term imbalance does not occur in healthy subjects because of excellent renal regulation.

A key question is how long will it take to reach phosphorus balance? The answer will vary depending on the presence or absence of good renal function. It is possible that prolonged imbalances of different magnitudes are common in end-stage renal disease (ESRD) patients on maintenance dialysis. Perhaps those patients with a substantial positive balance of phosphate for a prolonged period are the ones who develop massive tumoral calcinosis and severe vascular calcification, resulting in various complications and ultimate death, whereas those who are able to achieve phosphate balance maintain better health.

These concepts challenge findings in many short-term phosphorus and calcium balance studies reported in the literature. For example, a recent study of CKD patients concluded that patients developed a markedly positive calcium balance of 500 mg per day when treated with oral calcium carbonate, in the absence of positive phosphate balance (Hill et al. 2012). As discussed previously, it is theoretically possible to retain calcium without phosphate if calcium is deposited as calcium carbonate in bone, but it is unlikely that the discrepancy would remain for many years. Another balance study in six patients with CKD stages 3 or 4 exposed to a 2000 mg/day calcium diet for nine days showed a positive calcium balance of about 759 mg/day, but again such massive retention cannot be sustained over many years: increased body calcium of 277 g in one year! (Spiegel, Brady 2012). Therefore these findings most likely reflect the short duration of the studies, and the data cannot be interpolated for a long duration.

At present, the only parameter available in clinical practice to assess total body phosphorus status is plasma phosphate concentration, but the phosphate content of blood represents only a minute portion of total body phosphorus content. The assumption is made that high serum phosphate represents an increased phosphate content and low serum phosphate is a decreased phosphate content, which is generally true. Acutely, however, this may not be the case because acute shifts of phosphate between body compartments may affect transiently serum phosphate levels without affecting total body phosphorus content. For example, acute alkalemia or insulin administration causes hypophosphatemia by an intracellular shift of phosphate without affecting the total body phosphate content. Fortunately, disorders of transcellular phosphate shifts are transient in nature, so when sustained hyperphosphatemia and hypophosphatemia are present, there is in fact a correlation between serum levels and total body phosphorus. In anuric ESRD patients undergoing dialysis, the situation is quite different because fasting serum phosphate has a better correlation with total body phosphorus content.

As mentioned earlier, fasting serum phosphate levels may not always reflect well the body phosphorus stores or the GI absorption of phosphorus. In subjects with healthy kidneys an excess oral load of phosphorus will produce only a transient elevation of serum phosphate with rapid elimination of the excess phosphorus in the urine that brings down the serum phosphate to baseline in a few hours.

Moreover, there is a significant circadian variation and gender differences in serum phosphate levels unrelated to phosphorus balance.

In contrast to serum phosphate, a 24-hr urine phosphate excretion, although not commonly done clinically, would be the best test to estimate net intestinal phosphorus absorption under the assumption that the individual is in net zero external balance (input equals output). In a person with normal renal function, a 24-hour urine phosphate excretion probably reflects quite accurately the daily intestinal absorption of phosphate because substantial phosphate retention in the body fluids will result in substantial increase in serum phosphate, unless phosphate is deposited in tissues, which is possible only if calcium is also deposited. For example, retention in the body fluid of one third (300 mg) of daily phosphate absorption (900 mg) would increase serum phosphate by almost 2 mg/dL (300 mg/16 liters = 19 mg/L= 1.9 mg/dL), assuming no deposition with calcium. Moreover, the amount of phosphate that can be deposited with calcium is very limited because the daily absorption of calcium in a normal person is usually less than 200 mg. Even assuming (practically impossible) that this entire amount of calcium absorbed in a day is deposited along with phosphate as hydroxyapatite, it would result in the deposition of a mere 93 mg of phosphate.

Extrapolation from net GI absorption to actual intake of phosphorus is more complicated because it would depend on the phosphorus bioavailability of the specific foods being ingested, a quite variable parameter, depending on a number of other factors.

Bioavailability of food phosphorus varies among different foods depending on whether the food is of animal or plant origin, how much calcium is present in the food, and whether phosphorus is given in a liquid form without a solid food matrix. For example, Moe et al. (2011) fed two groups of CKD patients with the same amount of protein and total phosphorus, and one group received a vegetarian diet, whereas the other group received meat-derived protein. In the vegetarian group only about 52% of the dietary phosphorus was absorbed, whereas in the meat-derived protein group 70% of the phosphorus was absorbed, based on the results of the 24-hr urine phosphate excretion. Lewis et al. (1989) demonstrated a 10% decrease in the intestinal absorption of phosphorus by simply changing the oral intake of calcium from about 100 mg/d to about 1600 mg/day with a constant phosphorus intake of about 1271 mg/d in eight healthy adults. This situation becomes even more compounded with the increasing use of sodium salts of phosphate in modern food processing because phosphate as sodium or potassium salt is much more easily absorbed than phosphorus contained in natural foods. For example, Relman et al. demonstrated complete recovery in the urine of sodium phosphate added to a liquid diet in two subjects (Relman et al. 1961). Of interest, when a group of hemodialysis patients were instructed to avoid processed foods containing inorganic phosphate salts, their serum phosphate levels came down by 0.6 mg/dL compared to the control group of patients who were not instructed to follow the dietary restriction (Sullivan et al. 2009).

Although it seems clear that subjects with normal kidney function are in phosphorus balance and that this state is achieved over a relatively short period of weeks or months, it is also clear that anuric dialysis patients may be in constant phosphorus retention, which explains their high prevalence of vascular calcifications, tumoral calcinosis, and calciphylaxis (Cofan et al. 1999; Smith 2016; Nigwekar et al. 2015). Much more complicated and uncertain, however, is the situation in CKD patients not on dialysis, who may or may not be in phosphorus balance depending on their specific net GI phosphorus absorption and residual renal function. For example, let's consider a man with CKD stage IV (estimated glomerular filtration rate [GFR] = 25 mL/min = 36 liters/day) who is consuming an average mixed diet containing 1400 mg P/day and not being treated with oral phosphate binders. Therefore his daily input of phosphorus from the GI tract is about 900 mg, which needs to be excreted in the urine to allow him to be in phosphorus balance. If his serum phosphate concentration is 4 mg/dL (40 mg/L), his daily filtered load of phosphorus will be 1440 mg (40 × 36). At that level of GFR his fractional excretion of phosphorus may be about 50% (Gutierrez et al. 2005) and his daily urinary excretion of phosphorus will be 720 mg. Because he gets 900 mg from GI uptake and can only excrete 720 mg in the urine, this man must retain about 180 mg of phosphorus per day and some amount of calcium to accompany it depending on the kind of crystal formed. Again, as per our previous analysis, retention of 180 mg of phosphate would require daily retention of about 400 mg of calcium when they are deposited as calcium hydroxyapatite and perhaps slightly less if deposited in other forms. Decreased intestinal absorption of calcium is an early manifestation of CKD (Hill et al. 2012; Spiegel and Brady 2012; Coburn et al. 1973; Hsu 1997), and a patient with stage 4 CKD, unless treated with a massive amount of calcium, would not absorb 400 mg of calcium per day. As a consequence, in the absence of sufficient calcium supply from the intestine, excess phosphorus retention could only be possible if there is a supply of calcium from the bone because retention of phosphate in circulation has a limited capacity. Therefore, it is likely that daily substantial retention of phosphate is possible only in those subjects who have large amounts of calcium available to deposit with phosphorus, which essentially means CKD patients who are on a large calcium intake and vitamin D supplement or a constant supply of calcium from bone. The latter could happen in response to secondary hyperparathyroidism, but at the expense of decreased bone density over time.

How to explain then the progressive decline in urinary phosphate excretion described in CKD patients in view of these considerations? For example, in a study of 1836 subjects with different degrees of renal function, the mean difference in 24-hr urine phosphate excretion between CKD stage 1 and 4 was 400 mg/day (Craver et al. 2007). In another study of 3879 CKD patients the mean difference of daily urinary phosphate excretion between stages 1 and 4 was about 200 mg/day (Isakova et al. 2011). Therefore, these patients were either ingesting less phosphorus (no data on dietary intake are provided) or they were in positive phosphorus balance, retaining an amount determined by the difference between their net GI phosphorus absorption and the daily urinary excretion of phosphorus. If we assume that the change in 400 mg/day of urinary phosphate excretion as CKD advances (Craver et al. 2007) reflects actual retention, one will expect 146 g of positive balance per year, or a 25% of increase in bone phosphorus content! If this retention were to occur in the form of hydroxyapatite, a simultaneous retention of 860 mg calcium/day (314 g per year) would be required. Is this greatly positive phosphorus balance possible in the absence of obvious increase bone density in CKD? The only other place will be in soft tissue where an occasional tumoral calcinosis (Cofan et al. 1999; Smith 2016) can accommodate a large amount of calcium phosphate salts or in heart valves or arterial walls (Cofan et al. 1999; Smith 2016). Data from the literature provide estimates of the average calcium content in atherosclerotic plaques at about 194 mg Ca/cm^3 (Moselewski et al. 2005). The aorta, with a length of 80 cm, diameter of 3 cm, and thickness of 2 mm, will have a maximal wall volume of 150.72 cm^3 (Kronzon and Tunick 2006); the total body arterial tree reportedly has a maximal total surface of about 1000 cm^2 (Aird 2005), and if we assume an arterial wall thickness of about 1 mm, the arterial tree can provide another 100 cm^3. If we add the arteriolar tree with a total surface area up to 4000 cm^2 (Isakova et al. 2011) and a thickness of about 30 microns, we may end up with an approximate total arterial wall volume of about 263 cm^3 and therefore the potential to store 50,968 mg of calcium (Kronzon and Tunick 2006). Because most studies showed that hydroxyapatite is the main calcium salt present in calcified plaques, this would provide 23,706 mg of stored phosphorus, a substantial amount. This is even without considering the potential calcification of the heart valves, where a significant amount of mineral could be deposited. In other words, extraskeletal calcifications, which are observed clinically in CKD patients, could theoretically provide a significant space to store retained phosphorus in this population. A main problem with the previous analysis, however, is the need to have simultaneous availability of calcium to precipitate phosphate. Clearly, the likelihood of absorbing 860 mg of calcium daily from the GI tract is very low, and therefore calcium needed to precipitate retained phosphorus could only come from bone in the form of calcium carbonate, but there is also a limit to calcium carbonate supply. Indeed, the total amount of calcium carbonate in bone is about 258 g or 258,000 mg (Table 5.1). The consumption of half of the calcium carbonate store (129,000 mg) as calcium hydroxyapatite at the rate of 400 mg of Ca per day will take 322 days. If these conditions to supply calcium are not met and serum phosphate does not actually increase, the only reasonable conclusion would be the existence of a neutral phosphorus balance simply reflecting decreased dietary phosphorus intake and under these conditions a 24-hr urine phosphorus excretion will be a good reflection of the net

Phosphorus Intake and Whole-Body Phosphorus Homeostasis 69

GI absorption of phosphorus. It is likely that every step of GFR decline would produce a minimal increase in serum phosphate that increases Ca × P product enough to induce extraskeletal calcification and therefore phosphorus retention. In this scenario, phosphorus balance will eventually have to be reached, but at the expense of some amount of phosphorus being retained in soft tissues and/or increasing serum phosphate level.

5.3 CONCLUSIONS

Unfortunately, we do not have a simple or easy clinical tool to assess body phosphorus balance except for serum phosphate, which represents only a minute portion of the total body phosphorus content. The clinical use of serum phosphate as a marker of total phosphate content, however, may be misleading at times, particularly when isolated serum phosphate values are used. Although bone represents a site for large stores of calcium and phosphorus, bone content of calcium and phosphate is not increased in renal failure. Thus, sustained prolonged positive balance of these minerals occurs only with the development of extraskeletal calcifications. Precipitation of phosphorus in soft tissues requires a large supply of calcium that may not be easily available given the limited GI absorption of calcium in CKD; the latter may be compensated by calcium removal from bone in the form of calcium carbonate mediated by secondary hyperparathyroidism of CKD. On the other hand, calcium released from bone as calcium hydroxyapatite cannot be used to precipitate the retained phosphate, because calcium released from bone in that form is already accompanied by phosphate.

REFERENCES

Aird WC. 2005. Spatial and temporal dynamics of the endothelium. *J Thromb Haemost* 3:1392–1406.
Block GA et al. 1998. Association of serum phosphate and calcium x phosphate product with mortality risk in chronic hemodialysis patients: A national study. *Am J Kidney Dis* 31:607–617.
Chang AR et al. 2014. High dietary phosphate is associated with all-cause mortality: Results from NHANES III. *Am J Clin Nutr* 99:230–237.
Coburn JW, Koppel MH, Brickman AS. 1973. Study of intestinal absorption of calcium in patients with renal failure. *Kidney Int* 3:264–272.
Cofan F et al. 1999. Uremic tumoral calcinosis in patients receiving longterm hemodialysis therapy. *J Rheumatol* 26:379–385.
Craver et al. 2007. Mineral metabolism parameters throughout chronic kidney disease stages 1–5; achievement of K/DOQI guidelines. *Nephrol Dial Transplant* 22:1171–1176.
Dhingra R et al. 2007. Relations of serum phosphorus and calcium levels to the incidence of cardiovascular disease in the community. *Arch Intern Med* 167:879–885.
Gutierrez O et al. 2005. Fibroblast growth factor-23 mitigates hyperphosphatemia but accentuates calcitriol deficiency in chronic kidney disease. *J Am Soc Nephrol* 16:2205–2215.
Hill KM et al. 2012. Oral calcium carbonate affects calcium but not phosphorus balance in stage 3-4 chronic kidney disease. *Kidney Int* 83:959.
Hsu CH. 1997. Are we mismanaging calcium and phosphate metabolism in renal failure? *Am J Kidney Dis* 29:641–649.
Isakova T et al. 2011. Fibroblast growth factor 23 is elevated before parathyroid hormone and phosphate in chronic kidney disease. *Kidney Int* 79:1370–1378.
Kaye M, Frueh AJ, Silverman M. 1970. A study of vertebral bone powder from patients with chronic renal failure. *J Clin Invest* 49:442–453.
Kestenbaum B et al. 2005. Serum phosphate levels and mortality risk among people with chronic kidney disease. *J Am Soc Nephrol* 16:520–528.
Kronzon I, Tunick PA. 2006. Aortic atherosclerotic disease and stroke. *Circulation* 114:63–75.
Lewis NM et al. 1989. Calcium supplements and milk: Effects on acid-base balance and on retention of calcium, magnesium, and phosphorus. *Am J Clin Nutr* 49:527–533.
Mitchell HH, Hamilton TS, Steggerda FR. 1945. The chemical composition of the adult human body and its bearing on the biochemistry of growth. *J Biol Chem* 158:625–637.
Moe SM et al. 2011. Vegetarian compared with meat dietary protein source and phosphorus homeostasis in chronic kidney disease. *Clin J Am Soc Nephrol* 6:257–264.

Moselewski F et al. 2005. Calcium concentration of individual coronary calcified plaques as measured by multidetector row computed tomography. *Circulation* 111:3236–3241.

Nigwekar SU et al. 2015. Calciphylaxis: Risk factors, diagnosis and treatment. *Am J Kidney Dis* 66:133–146.

Oh MS. 1991. Irrelevance of bone buffering in chronic metabolic acidosis. *Nephron* 59:7–10.

Pellegrino ED, Biltz RM. 1965. The composition of human bone in uremia. *Medicine* 44:397–418.

Relman AS, Lennon EJ, Lemann J, Jr. 1961. Endogenous production of fixed acid and the measurement of the net balance of acid in normal subjects. *J Clin Invest* 40:1621–1630.

Smith ER. 2016. Vascular calcification in uremia: New-age concepts about an old-age problem. *Methods Mol Biol* 1397:175–208.

Spiegel DM, Brady K. 2012. Calcium balance in normal individuals and in patients with chronic kidney disease on low- and high-calcium diets. *Kidney Int* 81:1116–1122.

Sullivan C et al. 2009. Effect of food additives on hyperphosphatemia among patients with end-stage-renal-disease: A randomized controlled diet. *JAMA* 301:629–635.

6 Endocrine Regulation of Phosphate Homeostasis

Marta Christov and Harald Jüppner

CONTENTS

Abstract 71
Bullet Points 71
6.1　Introduction 71
6.2　Phosphate Homeostasis 72
6.3　FGF23 and PTH: The Primary Phosphate-Regulating Hormones 72
6.4　Hormonal Feedback of Phosphate Regulation 74
6.5　Lessons from Genetic Disorders of FGF23 75
6.6　Additional Regulators of FGF23 76
6.7　FGF23 and PTH in CKD 77
6.8　Can Endocrine Regulators of Phosphate Be Manipulated? 77
6.9　Conclusions 78
References 79

ABSTRACT

Phosphate regulation involves the complex interplay of at least three hormones: fibroblast growth factor 23 (FGF23), parathyroid hormone (PTH), and calcitriol (1,25D). Together they affect phosphate absorption in the gut, in the kidneys, and more generally bone turnover, which may release or store excess phosphate. This endocrine system responds slowly to changes in phosphate levels, and the precise molecular mechanisms of the response are still poorly understood. The phosphate endocrine axis is misregulated in patients with kidney disease, and altered levels of all of the key players have been associated with increased morbidity and mortality in this population. Despite great interest in controlling the levels of FGF23 and phosphate in kidney disease patients, the ideal modality has still not been found.

BULLET POINTS

- FGF23 and PTH both control phosphate excretion in the kidneys by regulating phosphate transporter abundance.
- Hormonal feedback in the control of phosphate excretion occurs more rapidly for PTH but takes longer for FGF23.
- Insights from genetic disorders highlight the importance of protein modification and processing in the production of FGF23 as an active hormone.
- FGF23 is a sensitive biomarker of abnormal kidney function.
- Elevations of FGF23 occur early during the course of chronic kidney disease, and these are associated with kidney disease progression, left ventricular hypertrophy, and mortality.

6.1　INTRODUCTION

Phosphate has numerous biological functions, which include the synthesis of nucleic acids and membrane lipids, protein modifications, energy metabolism, and second messenger formation. During evolution it has therefore been important to develop regulatory systems to conserve phosphate for essential biological functions as needed, especially during times of limited food supply. Together with calcium, phosphate is furthermore a critical component of bone. In contrast to the regulation of calcium homeostasis, the factors regulating phosphate levels remain incompletely understood. We will focus on two main endocrine regulators of phosphate homeostasis: fibroblast growth factor 23 (FGF23) and parathyroid hormone (PTH), which are part of a recently discovered hormonal bone–parathyroid–kidney axis. This endocrine system is modulated by 1,25(OH)$_2$ vitamin D (1,25D), calcium, phosphorus, and probably other factors, as regulation of FGF23 synthesis and secretion remains incompletely understood.

6.2 PHOSPHATE HOMEOSTASIS

The average adult on a Western diet ingests approximately 1.6 to 2 grams of phosphate a day [1]. Dietary phosphate is then absorbed in the intestine via both active and passive transport systems. Once inside the body, phosphate can be stored in bone, can contribute to circulating levels, or can be excreted in the urine or secreted into the intestine [2]. Only a very small fraction of total body phosphate stores (about 1%) is available in the circulation. At present, it is unclear if the hormonal systems regulating phosphate homeostasis respond to changes in circulating or total body stores. Circulating phosphate levels can be affected acutely by hormones such as insulin and catecholamines, as well as by blood pH [3,4]. For the purposes of this review, however, we will focus on the endocrine systems regulating phosphate homeostasis.

6.3 FGF23 AND PTH: THE PRIMARY PHOSPHATE-REGULATING HORMONES

PTH and FGF23 are the major regulators of phosphate homeostasis (reviewed in Bergwitz and Jüppner) [5] (Figure 6.1). Together with 1,25-dihydroxyvitamin D (1,25D) they form a complex feedback loop involving at least three endocrine organs: the bone, the parathyroid glands, and the

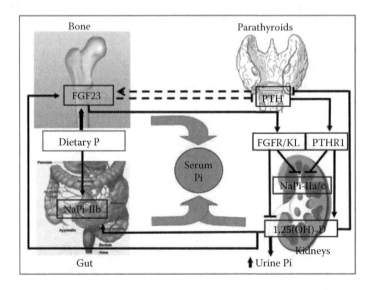

FIGURE 6.1 Interaction between endocrine regulators of serum phosphate levels. For details, see the text. PTH, parathyroid hormone; FGF23, fibroblast growth factor 23; PTHR1, PTH receptor 1; FGFR/KL, fibroblast growth factor receptor with co-receptor klotho; 1,25(OH)$_2$D, dihydroxyvitamin D. NaPi, sodium phosphate co-transporter. (Adapted from Bergwitz C, Jüppner H. *Annu Rev Med.*, 61, 91–104, 2010.)

Endocrine Regulation of Phosphate Homeostasis 73

kidneys. Although the intestine is the major entry site of phosphate into the body, the kidney plays a major role in the hormonal regulation of phosphate absorption and excretion.

The bone is both the main storage compartment of phosphate and the site of production of FGF23. Although FGF23 is likely the primary regulator of phosphate concentration, it is still unknown how osteocytes, the FGF23-producing cells, "measure" phosphate levels in the blood circulation. A dedicated phosphate "sensor," analogous to the calcium-sensing receptor, has not been identified so far and is unlikely to utilize a rapidly responding second-messenger system. Both animal and human experiments show that synthesis and secretion of FGF23 by osteocytes in bone is increased by 1,25D, dietary phosphate loading, and PTH [6,7] (Figure 6.1). However, with the possible exception of a rapid increase of FGF23 in response to a PTH challenge, these changes occur with a considerable delay [8]. Conversely, FGF23 inhibits the 1-alpha hydroxylase, stimulates the 24-hydroxylase, and reduces the secretion of PTH from the parathyroid glands [9].

PTH is the well-established regulator of extracellular calcium ion concentration that also regulates phosphate levels through its direct effects on the proximal tubular phosphate transporter and through its direct and indirect actions on FGF23 production (Figure 6.1). For example, mice with deletion of the PTH gene develop mild hyperphosphatemia and hypocalcemia, similar to patients with hypoparathyroidism [10]. Interestingly, however, FGF23 levels in these animals are not sufficiently elevated to normalize serum phosphate levels, suggesting that the hyperphosphatemia alone is not sufficient to increase FGF23 secretion in these animals. In fact, PTH and/or 1,25D may be needed to increase FGF23 production in response to hyperphosphatemia. Similarly, in the few patients with idiopathic hypoparathyroidism where this has been reported, FGF23 levels were found to be only slightly elevated in the setting of hyperphosphatemia [11], indicating that the osteocyte response to phosphate elevation was inadequate. In animals where the PTH receptor was deleted in long bones only but present in the axial skeleton, PTH treatment failed to increase circulating intact FGF23, levels suggesting that the PTH receptor is needed for FGF23 production [12]. Moreover, in FGF23-null mice, injection of PTH had phosphaturic and anabolic effects [13]. Thus, the data so far are inconclusive on the exact contribution of PTH to circulating FGF23 levels. This suggests that PTH deficiency or excess has independent effects on renal phosphate handling that may or may not be modulated by its effects on FGF23.

PTH and FGF23 converge their action on the renal phosphate cotransporters NaPi2a and NaPi2c (also known as NPT2a and NPT2c) (Figure 6.1). Thus, both hormonal phosphate regulators reduce expression and/or membrane abundance of the transporters, thereby increasing renal phosphate excretion. The importance of the two renal phosphate transporters as a crucial site of phosphate regulation is highlighted by studies in mice and humans with deficiencies in either NPT2a or NPT2c. Human homozygous or compound heterozygous mutations in the sodium-dependent phosphate transporters NPT2a and NPT2c lead to an increase in urinary phosphate excretion, independent of PTH and FGF23, resulting in hypophosphatemia and rickets/osteomalacia [14–17]. Note that rickets have been reported for patients with NPT2c mutations, whereas most patients with homozygous/compound heterozygous NPT2a mutations did not present with such growth plate abnormalities despite much more severe urinary phosphate wasting. However, the latter individuals presented with much more severe hypercalcemia due to increased 1,25D production [16] because hypophosphatemia is a major stimulus for the renal 1-alpha hydroxylase. As result of elevated 1,25D levels, intestinal calcium absorption is thought to be increased, leading to hypercalciuria and frequently nephrocalcinosis and/or kidney stones [15,18,19]. Similar observations, namely hypophosphatemia due to urinary phosphate wasting, are also made in some patients affected by Fanconi-Bickel syndrome, a disorder caused by homozygous mutations in the glucose transporter 2 GLUT2 (SLC2A2) that is expressed on the basolateral membrane of the proximal renal tubules [20]. Mice with homozygous deletion of this transporter in the kidney show only a small or no reduction in Npt2a expression, yet a major reduction in Npt2c expression, thus providing a plausible mechanism for the increase in urinary phosphate excretion and the resulting hypophosphatemia that is observed in some patients with Fanconi-Bickel syndrome.

Although both FGF23 and PTH increase urinary phosphate excretion by reducing proximal tubular expression of NPT2a and NPT2c, they have opposite effects on 1,25D levels, the biologically active form of vitamin D. FGF23 decreases expression of the renal 1-alpha hydroxylase, and it enhances expression of the 24-hydroxylase, thereby reducing the circulating levels of 1,25D through two mechanisms. In contrast, PTH increases the renal 1,25D production, thereby increasing indirectly the absorption of calcium and phosphate from the intestinal tract. PTH and 1,25D thus help maintain extracellular calcium concentration within normal limits, but both hormones also increase the extracellular phosphate concentration. Phosphate regulation therefore can be either independent of or intimately tied to calcium regulation.

6.4 HORMONAL FEEDBACK OF PHOSPHATE REGULATION

The existence of a gut phosphate-regulating hormone, or phosphatonin, has been hypothesized based on work in animals, where gavage of a phosphate load led within minutes to increased phosphate excretion by the kidneys, despite unchanged circulating phosphate levels [21]. However, as will be highlighted later, such a rapid hormonal system has not been found in humans. In fact, delivery of phosphate by intravenous infusion or via nasogastric (NG) tube requires at least 8 to 12 hrs before FGF23 increases.

The responsiveness of the phosphate-regulating endocrine system has been difficult to dissect. For example, injections of FGF23 protein into mice result in changes in signaling molecules in the kidneys within 10 minutes; however, changes in urinary phosphate levels and corresponding circulating phosphate levels do not occur until 8 to 12 hours later [22,23]. Remarkable experiments in humans have elegantly dissected the timing of these events (Figure 6.2) [24]. In this study, human volunteers were given a phosphate load over 36 hours, either as a continuous intravenous infusion of sodium phosphate or via a nasal tube placed into the duodenum; electrolytes and hormones were subsequently

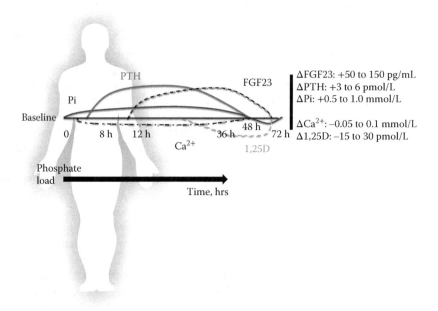

FIGURE 6.2 (See color insert.) Response of endocrine regulators to an intravenous or oral phosphate load over time in human volunteers. Graph represents change from baseline (not drawn to scale) illustrating the timing and magnitude of the homeostatic responses that are triggered by a high-dose phosphate challenge. The increase in serum phosphate level is sufficient to induce a small reduction in ionized calcium concentration that results in a robust increase in PTH level. The mild hyperphosphatemia is furthermore associated with an increase in FGF23 concentration that is followed by a decrease in 1,25(OH)2 vitamin D concentration. For further details, see reference. (Adapted from Scanni R et al., *J Am Soc Nephrol.*, 25, 2730–2739, 2014.)

Endocrine Regulation of Phosphate Homeostasis

monitored for up to three days. As shown in Figure 6.2, which is a rendering of one of the experimental protocols, PTH levels increased by eight hours after the start of phosphate loading, most likely secondary to the phosphate-induced decline in ionized calcium. Surprisingly, FGF23 levels did not increase until 12 hours after starting the phosphate load. This delayed response in FGF23 is consistent with animal data and suggests that the endocrine regulation of phosphate levels is much slower compared with calcium regulation. In addition, 1,25D levels decreased only after FGF23 levels started to rise, suggesting a causative effect. PTH levels increased at the same time that calcium levels decreased, which is consistent with the long-established role of calcium rather than phosphate in PTH regulation. Of note, the magnitudes for the changes in blood phosphate and calcium concentration were small, phosphate (+0.5 to 1 mmol/L) and calcium (−0.05 to 0.1 mmol/L), in comparison to the changes in PTH (+3 to 6 pmol/L) or FGF23 (+50 to 150 pg/mL). Thus, even small changes in mineral ion levels elicit prominent changes in the endocrine hormones that regulate them, PTH and FGF23.

6.5 LESSONS FROM GENETIC DISORDERS OF FGF23

Much of what we know about phosphate regulation, and especially FGF23 biology, has been learned by the molecular definition of rare human and animal genetic disorders.

Osteocytes are the primary cellular source of FGF23 after the fetal period [25]. Increased FGF23 production leading to hypophosphatemia and rickets occurs in several different monogenic disorders, and their molecular definition has helped to identify proteins that are expressed in bone cells and that decrease FGF23 production (Figure 6.3). Specifically, these include PHEX (phosphate-regulating gene with homologies to endopeptidases on the X chromosome), the gene mutated in patients with X-linked hypophosphatemia [26–28], as well as DMP1 (dentin matrix protein 1) [29,30], ENPP1 (ecto-nucleotide pyrophosphatase/phosphodiesterase 1) [31,32], FAM20c (family with sequence similarity 20, member 6) [33,34], and possibly ABCC6 (ATP-binding cassette subfamily C, member 6) [35] that are mutated in different forms of autosomal-recessive hypophosphatemia.

DMP1 is a bone matrix protein, and mutations in the gene encoding this protein lead to increased expression of FGF23 [29,30], suggesting that DMP1 normally represses FGF23 synthesis (Figure 6.3). Genetic studies of mice carrying both the *Dmp1* and *Fgf23* mutations suggest that *Fgf23* is epistatic to *Dmp1*, as the double mutants have a phenotype very similar to the *Fgf23* single-mutant animals [36]. Moreover, only the 57 kDa C-terminal fragment of DMP1 appears to be responsible for this regulatory role [37]. Furthermore, animals and humans carrying mutations in the PHEX gene also exhibit FGF23-dependent hypophosphatemia [27,38]. Thus, both DMP1 and PHEX are thought to be negative regulators of FGF23 (Figure 6.3), and they may affect FGF23 production via FGFR-dependent pathways [39,40].

FGF23, which belongs to the subfamily of endocrine FGFs, mediates its phosphate-regulating actions in the kidney through FGF receptors, most prominently the FGF receptor 1 (FGFR1). However, these actions require the transmembrane form of α-klotho (mKL), which acts as a coreceptor that enhances the binding affinity of FGF23 to different FGFRs [41,42]. Ablation of α-klotho in mice leads to severe hyperphosphatemia, elevated levels of 1,25D, hypercalcemia, soft tissue and vascular calcifications, accelerated aging, and premature death [43]. These findings are largely indistinguishable from those observed in murine FGF23 loss-of-function models [44,45] and in patients with homozygous inactivating mutations in FGF23 or UDP-N-acetyl-alpha-D-galactosamine: polypeptide N-acetylgalactosaminyl-transferase 3 (GALNT3) [46–48] (Figure 6.3). The latter enzyme is involved in O-glycosylation at FGF23 threonine residue 178, that is, a post-translational modification that is required for limiting cleavage at amino acid residues 176 to 179, namely the RXXR site that is mutated in patients with autosomal-dominant hypophosphatemia (ADHR) [49].

Fam20c, a secreted kinase and, when mutated, the cause of Raine syndrome, a lethal osteosclerotic bone dysplasia, was shown to be necessary for the phosphorylation of many secreted proteins involved in biomineralization [50]. Mice with deletion of Fam20c develop rickets and osteomalacia, rather than osteosclerosis, due to elevated FGF23 levels [34], and later Fam20c was shown to phosphorylate FGF23 in vitro [51] and in vivo, a process that regulates its O-glycosylation [33,51] (Figure 6.3).

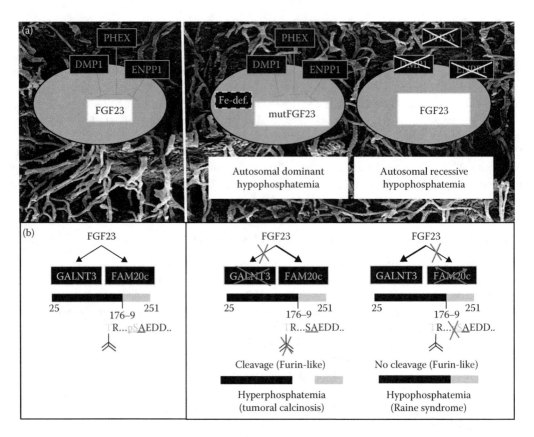

FIGURE 6.3 (See color insert.) Factors regulating FGF23 synthesis. FGF23 production in bone by osteocytes (background image in 3) is regulated by a number of other genes through unclear mechanisms. Panel (a): PHEX, DMP1, and ENPP1 appear to reduce FGF23 production (left) because homozygous loss-of-function mutations in PHEX, DMP1, and ENPP1 cause autosomal-recessive FGF23-dependent forms of hypophosphatemia (right). Heterozygous mutations at the RXXR cleavage site in FGF23 (mutFGF23) cause an autosomal-dominant form of hypophosphatemia that becomes particularly apparent when iron deficiency increases FGF23 synthesis through largely unknown mechanisms (middle). Panel (b): FGF23 undergoes O-glycosylation at T178 and phosphorylation at S180 (left). Loss-of-function mutations in the enzymes affecting the amount of post-translational processing of FGF23, namely GALNT3 and FAM20c, lead to hyperphosphatemia and hypophosphatemia, respectively (middle and right).

With few exceptions, it remains largely unknown, however, whether and how the different phosphate-regulating proteins interact with each other. Furthermore, it is almost certain that additional molecules contribute to these regulatory events and that genetic studies will continue to be of pivotal importance to identify genes encoding novel regulators of phosphate homeostasis. For example, in a cohort of 46 patients with familial hypophosphatemia, sequence analysis identified mutations in the exons encoding PHEX in 27 patients; in the exons encoding FGF23 in only 1 patient; and no exonic mutations in either *PHEX*, *FGF23*, or *DMP1* were identified in 18 patients [52]. Unless intronic mutations are responsible for urinary phosphate wasting in these unresolved patients, these findings indicate that additional as yet unknown genetic defects can cause hereditary hypophosphatemia disorders and that the definition of the underlying genetic defect will result in the definition of novel phosphate-regulating molecules.

6.6 ADDITIONAL REGULATORS OF FGF23

An additional aspect of FGF23 regulation involves its cleavage during periods of iron deficiency. Initially observed in humans affected by ADHR due to FGF23 mutations that render the peptide

Endocrine Regulation of Phosphate Homeostasis

resistant to cleavage at the RXXR site [53] and subsequently in mice carrying one of the ADHR mutations [54], it has become apparent that iron deficiency has a major role in FGF23 synthesis and its degradation. Thus reduced iron levels increase FGF23 mRNA not only in ADHR mice, but also in wild-type animals [54]. However, wild-type mice can readily cleave the intact, biologically active FGF23 into biologically inactive fragments, as determined by elevated levels of C-terminal FGF23 fragments, yet normal levels of the intact hormone. In contrast, cleavage cannot occur at the RXXR site if mutated as in ADHR mice or humans, thus leading to elevated levels of intact FGF23 and consequently hypophosphatemia. Similar findings were recently observed in females with heavy menstrual bleeding, who revealed readily detectable increases in C-terminal FGF23, but not intact FGF23, and consequently no increase in urinary phosphate excretion [55]. Acute inflammation, through a pathway similar to iron deficiency, also can increase FGF23 production and cleavage [56].

6.7 FGF23 AND PTH IN CKD

As outlined earlier, FGF23 levels are elevated in several genetic disorders that efficiently enhance urinary phosphate excretion leading to hypophosphatemia and rickets/osteomalacia; however, these elevations are small by comparison to the major increases in plasma FGF23 levels that can occur in patients with CKD. Already in CKD stages 2 to 3 circulating FGF23 levels are increased, indicating that FGF23 levels are a sensitive biomarker of an abnormal regulation of phosphate homeostasis, and hence kidney function [57–59]. During the later CKD stages, FGF23 levels can be increased by more than thousand-fold, and these vastly elevated levels are associated with CKD progression and in patients treated by dialysis with an increase in left ventricular hypertrophy and early mortality [26,60]. Unlike the immunoreactive PTH in CKD patients, which comprises mainly C-terminal fragments, FGF23 is largely intact in CKD stage 5. In fact, even in the earlier stages of CKD, surprisingly low levels of FGF23 fragments are observed [61,62]. Consequently, the large quantities of FGF23 circulating in CKD patients are biologically active and may exert unwarranted "off target" effects [63].

Death from cardiovascular causes is the leading contributor to the early mortality of patients with kidney disease. Given the epidemiological data linking elevated FGF23 levels with mortality and heart failure, a direct effect of FGF23 on the cardiovascular system was hypothesized. Consistent with this conclusion, recent studies have shown that FGF23 directly causes myocyte hypertrophy in vitro and leads to cardiac hypertrophy in vivo in mice via signaling through FGFR4 [64,65]. These actions occur despite the absence of the coreceptor klotho, and thus occur independently of the role of FG23 and the regulation of phosphate homeostasis. FGFR4 inhibition might provide a way to interfere with the off-target effects of FGF23, for example, on the heart, without affecting phosphate regulation.

The data regarding direct effects of FGF23 on the vasculature are more complex. It does not appear to be associated with increased vascular calcification by cross-sectional human studies or to cause increased vascular calcification in vitro [66]. However, FGF23 did appear to affect vasorelaxation, leading to impaired vessel function in mice, which is consistent with cross-sectional human observations [67,68].

6.8 CAN ENDOCRINE REGULATORS OF PHOSPHATE BE MANIPULATED?

Given the deleterious effects of both elevated phosphate levels and, independently, FGF23 and PTH on cardiovascular mortality, there is a lot of interest in finding ways to lower either phosphate and/or its regulators, especially in the chronic kidney disease (CKD) patient population (Table 6.1). Reduction of dietary intake by altering food choices (vegetarian versus meat based) [69], avoidance of foods high in phosphate such as colas and processed foods, or use of high-dose binders in the gut can be effective but is usually insufficient in the CKD population [70]. Partly, this is due to the contribution of paracellular phosphate uptake and increased NaPi2b expression in settings of

TABLE 6.1
Potential Avenues to Modulate Phosphate/FGF23

	Target	Effect	Side Effect
Vegetarian diet	Phosphate absorption gut	Lower phosphate, decrease FGF23 level	May be difficult to accept
Oral phosphate binders	Phosphate absorption gut	Lower phosphate, decrease FGF23 level[a]	Large pill burden
NaPi2a inhibitors	*Phosphate reabsorption kidney*	*Lower phosphate, decrease FGF23 level*	*Fanconi-type syndrome*
NaPi2b inhibitors	Phosphate absorption gut	Lower phosphate, decrease FGF23 level	Paradoxical increased absorption
FGF23 antibody	*FGF23 protein*	*Lower FGF23 bioactivity*	*Increased phosphate*
Treat iron deficiency	FGF23 production or cleavage	Lower FGF23 levels (some formulations increase levels of bioactive FGF23)[b]	Low phosphate with certain formulations
FGF23 cleavage inhibitors	*FGF23 production*	*Hypophosphatemia*	*Rickets/osteomalacia*

Note: Interventions in italics are hypothesized based on animal data or genetic data in animals/humans. For references, please see text.

[a] Compared with calcium acetate, sevelamer hydrochloride or carbonate, and lanthanum carbonate have been reported to variably reduce FGF23 levels, although not in all studies [69].

[b] Iron formulations such as ferric carboxymaltose, saccharated ferric oxide, and iron polymaltose have been shown to lead to increase in FGF23 levels, whereas formulations such as iron dextran do not [53].

phosphate restriction or oral phosphate binders [71]. Optimal therapy might need to include both phosphate restriction/oral phosphate binders and concurrent NaPi2b blockade [72]. Independent ways to interfere or reduce phosphate-regulating hormones have had unintended consequences. For example, efforts to lower PTH via suppression with 1,25D or analogs can lead to a severe reduction in bone turnover and thus an increase in serum phosphate (and FGF23). Additionally, efforts to interfere with FGF23 action via an FGF23 antibody in rats with CKD have led to severe hyperphosphatemia and accelerated death, which was to be expected because elevated FGF23 levels in early CKD stages serve to promote urinary phosphate excretion, thereby preventing calcifications in the vasculature and elsewhere [73].

Possible new avenues to lower FGF23 involve improving iron status, as iron deficiency can increase FGF23 production. In addition, interference with FGFR4, which was recently shown to mediate some of the "off-target" effects of FGF23, may allow for targeted suppression of deleterious effects without specifically affecting overall FGF23 levels [74]. The downside of such a strategy is that it addresses only one potential effect of FGF23, namely that on the cardiovascular system, and thus does not address possible other unwarranted effects of very high FGF23 levels, such as potential effects on hematopoiesis or peripheral vitamin D activation [75,76]. Further understanding of the cleavage mechanism, which regulates the level of active FGF23 in the circulation, will undoubtedly yield additional potential therapeutic targets for manipulating FGF23 levels.

6.9 CONCLUSIONS

Studying rare genetic disorders in humans and other mammals has provided important novel insights into the endocrine regulation of phosphate homeostasis. In 2001 FGF23 joined PTH as a key hormone affecting the kidney, bone, and gut handling of phosphate, both directly and through effects on 1,25D. Other genes affect locally FGF23 and PTH production, and our knowledge will continue to increase as more genetic disorders of hyperphosphatemia and hypophosphatemia are

Endocrine Regulation of Phosphate Homeostasis

molecularly defined. CKD is a condition where phosphate regulation is impaired. Thus FGF23 increases early during the course of kidney disease, and it likely serves as a biomarker of abnormal renal phosphate handling and kidney function. However, FGF23 also has major "off-target" effects in CKD patients. Understanding the contribution of phosphate to the abnormal regulation of FGF23 in this patient population and searching for ways to limit its increase will be a major challenge, which is likely to have significant clinical implications.

REFERENCES

1. Calvo MS, Moshfegh AJ, Tucker KL. Assessing the health impact of phosphorus in the food supply: Issues and considerations. *Adv Nutr.* 2014;5(1):104–113.
2. Peters J, Binswanger U. Calcium and inorganic phosphate secretion of rat ileum in vitro. Influence of uremia and 1,25 (OH)2D3 inhibition. *Res Exp Med (Berl).* 1988;188(2):139–149.
3. Kjeldsen SE, Moan A, Petrin J, Weder AB, Julius S. Effects of increased arterial epinephrine on insulin, glucose and phosphate. *Blood Press.* 1996;5(1):27–31.
4. Hoppe A, Metler M, Berndt TJ, Knox FG, Angielski S. Effect of respiratory alkalosis on renal phosphate excretion. *Am J Physiol.* 1982;243(5):F471–475.
5. Bergwitz C, Jüppner H. Regulation of phosphate homeostasis by PTH, vitamin D, and FGF23. *Annu Rev Med.* 2010;61:91–104.
6. Perwad F, Azam N, Zhang MY, Yamashita T, Tenenhouse HS, Portale AA. Dietary and serum phosphorus regulate fibroblast growth factor 23 expression and 1,25-dihydroxyvitamin D metabolism in mice. *Endocrinology.* 2005;146(12):5358–5364.
7. Burnett SM, Gunawardene SC, Bringhurst FR, Jüppner H, Lee H, Finkelstein JS. Regulation of C-terminal and intact FGF-23 by dietary phosphate in men and women. *J Bone Miner Res.* 2006;21(8):1187–1196.
8. Knab VM, Corbin B, Andrukhova O et al. Acute parathyroid hormone injection increases C-terminal, but not intact fibroblast growth factor 23 levels. *Endocrinology.* 2017;158(5):1–10.
9. Shimada T, Kakitani M, Yamazaki Y et al. Targeted ablation of Fgf23 demonstrates an essential physiological role of FGF23 in phosphate and vitamin D metabolism. *J Clin Invest.* 2004;113(4):561–568.
10. Bai X, Miao D, Goltzman D, Karaplis AC. Early lethality in Hyp mice with targeted deletion of Pth gene. *Endocrinology.* 2007;148(10):4974–4983.
11. Gupta A, Winer K, Econs MJ, Marx SJ, Collins MT. FGF-23 is elevated by chronic hyperphosphatemia. *J Clin Endocrinol Metab.* 2004;89(9):4489–4492.
12. Fan Y, Bi R, Densmore MJ et al. Parathyroid hormone 1 receptor is essential to induce FGF23 production and maintain systemic mineral ion homeostasis. *FASEB J.* 2016;30(1):428–440.
13. Yuan Q, Sitara D, Sato T et al. PTH ablation ameliorates the anomalies of Fgf23-deficient mice by suppressing the elevated vitamin D and calcium levels. *Endocrinology.* 2011;152(11):4053–4061.
14. Lorenz-Depiereux B, Benet-Pages A, Eckstein G et al. Hereditary hypophosphatemic rickets with hypercalciuria is caused by mutations in the sodium-phosphate cotransporter gene SLC34A3. *Am J Hum Genet.* 2006;78(2):193–201.
15. Bergwitz C, Roslin NM, Tieder M et al. SLC34A3 mutations in patients with hereditary hypophosphatemic rickets with hypercalciuria predict a key role for the sodium-phosphate cotransporter NaPi-IIc in maintaining phosphate homeostasis. *Am J Hum Genet.* 2006;78(2):179–192.
16. Schlingmann KP, Ruminska J, Kaufmann M et al. Autosomal-recessive mutations in SLC34A1 encoding sodium-phosphate cotransporter 2A cause idiopathic infantile hypercalcemia. *J Am Soc Nephrol.* 2015;27(2):604–614.
17. Magen D, Berger L, Coady MJ et al. A loss-of-function mutation in NaPi-IIa and renal Fanconi's syndrome. *N Engl J Med.* 2010;362(12):1102–1109.
18. Kremke B, Bergwitz C, Ahrens W et al. Hypophosphatemic rickets with hypercalciuria due to mutation in SLC34A3/NaPi-IIc can be masked by vitamin D deficiency and can be associated with renal calcifications. *Exp Clin Endocrinol Diabetes.* 2009;117(2):49–56.
19. Yu Y, Sanderson SR, Reyes M et al. Novel NaPi-IIc mutations causing HHRH and idiopathic hypercalciuria in several unrelated families: Long-term follow-up in one kindred. *Bone.* 2012;50(5):1100–1106.
20. Mannstadt M, Magen D, Segawa H et al. Fanconi-Bickel syndrome and autosomal recessive proximal tubulopathy with hypercalciuria (ARPTH) are allelic variants caused by GLUT2 mutations. *J Clin Endocrinol Metab.* 2012;97(10):E1978–1986.

21. Berndt T, Thomas LF, Craig TA et al. Evidence for a signaling axis by which intestinal phosphate rapidly modulates renal phosphate reabsorption. *Proc Natl Acad Sci U S A*. 2007;104(26):11085–11090.
22. Shimada T, Hasegawa H, Yamazaki Y et al. FGF-23 is a potent regulator of vitamin D metabolism and phosphate homeostasis. *J Bone Miner Res*. 2004;19(3):429–435.
23. Farrow EG, Davis SI, Summers LJ, White KE. Initial FGF23-mediated signaling occurs in the distal convoluted tubule. *J Am Soc Nephrol*. 2009;20(5):955–960.
24. Scanni R, von Rotz M, Jehle S, Hulter HN, Krapf R. The human response to acute enteral and parenteral phosphate loads. *J Am Soc Nephrol*. 2014;25(12):2730–2739.
25. Bonewald LF. The amazing osteocyte. *J Bone Miner Res*. 2011;26(2):229–238.
26. Jonsson KB, Zahradnik R, Larsson T et al. Fibroblast growth factor 23 in oncogenic osteomalacia and X-linked hypophosphatemia. *N Engl J Med*. 2003;348(17):1656–1663.
27. Yamazaki Y, Okazaki R, Shibata M et al. Increased circulatory level of biologically active full-length FGF-23 in patients with hypophosphatemic rickets/osteomalacia. *J Clin Endocrinol Metab*. 2002;87(11):4957–4960.
28. A gene (PEX) with homologies to endopeptidases is mutated in patients with X-linked hypophosphatemic rickets. The HYP Consortium. *Nat Genet*. 1995;11(2):130–136.
29. Feng JQ, Ward LM, Liu S et al. Loss of DMP1 causes rickets and osteomalacia and identifies a role for osteocytes in mineral metabolism. *Nat Genet*. 2006;38(11):1310–1315.
30. Lorenz-Depiereux B, Bastepe M, Benet-Pages A et al. DMP1 mutations in autosomal recessive hypophosphatemia implicate a bone matrix protein in the regulation of phosphate homeostasis. *Nat Genet*. 2006;38(11):1248–1250.
31. Mackenzie NC, Zhu D, Milne EM et al. Altered bone development and an increase in FGF-23 expression in Enpp1(-/-) mice. *PLOS ONE*. 2012;7(2):e32177.
32. Lorenz-Depiereux B, Schnabel D, Tiosano D, Hausler G, Strom TM. Loss-of-function ENPP1 mutations cause both generalized arterial calcification of infancy and autosomal-recessive hypophosphatemic rickets. *Am J Hum Genet*. 2010;86(2):267–272.
33. Tagliabracci VS, Engel JL, Wiley SE et al. Dynamic regulation of FGF23 by Fam20C phosphorylation, GalNAc-T3 glycosylation, and furin proteolysis. *Proc Natl Acad Sci U S A*. 2014;111(15):5520–5525.
34. Wang X, Wang S, Li C et al. Inactivation of a novel FGF23 regulator, FAM20C, leads to hypophosphatemic rickets in mice. *PLoS Genet*. 2012;8(5):e1002708.
35. Nitschke Y, Baujat G, Botschen U et al. Generalized arterial calcification of infancy and pseudo-xanthoma elasticum can be caused by mutations in either ENPP1 or ABCC6. *Am J Hum Genet*. 2012;90(1):25–39.
36. Lu Y, Yuan B, Qin C et al. The biological function of DMP-1 in osteocyte maturation is mediated by its 57-kDa C-terminal fragment. *J Bone Miner Res*. 2011;26(2):331–340.
37. Liu S, Zhou J, Tang W, Menard R, Feng JQ, Quarles LD. Pathogenic role of Fgf23 in Dmp1-null mice. *Am J Physiol Endocrinol Metab*. 2008;295(2):E254–261.
38. Liu S, Zhou J, Tang W, Jiang X, Rowe DW, Quarles LD. Pathogenic role of Fgf23 in Hyp mice. *Am J Physiol Endocrinol Metab*. 2006;291(1):E38–49.
39. Martin A, Liu S, David V et al. Bone proteins PHEX and DMP1 regulate fibroblastic growth factor Fgf23 expression in osteocytes through a common pathway involving FGF receptor (FGFR) signaling. *FASEB J*. 2011;25(8):2551–2562.
40. Wohrle S, Bonny O, Beluch N et al. FGF receptors control vitamin D and phosphate homeostasis by mediating renal FGF-23 signaling and regulating FGF-23 expression in bone. *J Bone Miner Res*. 2011;26(10):2486–2497.
41. Urakawa I, Yamazaki Y, Shimada T et al. Klotho converts canonical FGF receptor into a specific receptor for FGF23. *Nature*. 2006;444(7120):770–774.
42. Kurosu H, Ogawa Y, Miyoshi M et al. Regulation of fibroblast growth factor-23 signaling by klotho. *J Biol Chem*. 2006;281(10):6120–6123.
43. Kuro-o M, Matsumura Y, Aizawa H et al. Mutation of the mouse klotho gene leads to a syndrome resembling ageing. *Nature*. 1997;390(6655):45–51.
44. Shimada T, Kakitani M, Yamazaki Y et al. Targeted ablation of Fgf23 demonstrates an essential physiological role of FGF23 in phosphate and vitamin D metabolism. *J Clin Invest*. 2004;113(4):561–568.
45. Sitara D, Razzaque MS, Hesse M et al. Homozygous ablation of fibroblast growth factor-23 results in hyperphosphatemia and impaired skeletogenesis, and reverses hypophosphatemia in Phex-deficient mice. *Matrix Biol*. 2004;23:421–432.
46. Benet-Pages A, Orlik P, Strom TM, Lorenz-Depiereux B. An FGF23 missense mutation causes familial tumoral calcinosis with hyperphosphatemia. *Hum Mol Genet*. 2005;14(3):385–390.

Endocrine Regulation of Phosphate Homeostasis

47. White KE, Lorenz B, Evans WE, Meitinger T, Strom TM, Econs MJ. Molecular cloning of a novel human UDP-GalNAc: Polypeptide N-acetylgalactosaminyltransferase, GalNAc-T8, and analysis as a candidate autosomal dominant hypophosphatemic rickets (ADHR) gene. *Gene*. 2000;246(1–2):347–356.

48. Larsson T, Davis SI, Garringer HJ et al. Fibroblast growth factor-23 mutants causing familial tumoral calcinosis are differentially processed. *Endocrinology*. 2005;146(9):3883–3891.

49. White KE, Carn G, Lorenz-Depiereux B, Benet-Pages A, Strom TM, Econs MJ. Autosomal-dominant hypophosphatemic rickets (ADHR) mutations stabilize FGF-23. *Kidney Int*. 2001;60(6):2079–2086.

50. Tagliabracci VS, Engel JL, Wen J et al. Secreted kinase phosphorylates extracellular proteins that regulate biomineralization. *Science*. 2012;336(6085):1150–1153.

51. Lindberg I, Pang HW, Stains JP et al. FGF23 is endogenously phosphorylated in bone cells. *J Bone Miner Res*. 2015;30(3):449–454.

52. Ruppe MD, Brosnan PG, Au KS, Tran PX, Dominguez BW, Northrup H. Mutational analysis of PHEX, FGF23 and DMP1 in a cohort of patients with hypophosphatemic rickets. *Clin Endocrinol (Oxf)*. 2011;74(3):312–318.

53. Imel EA, Peacock M, Gray AK, Padgett LR, Hui SL, Econs MJ. Iron modifies plasma FGF23 differently in autosomal dominant hypophosphatemic rickets and healthy humans. *J Clin Endocrinol Metab*. 2011;96(11):3541–3549.

54. Farrow EG, Yu X, Summers LJ et al. Iron deficiency drives an autosomal dominant hypophosphatemic rickets (ADHR) phenotype in fibroblast growth factor-23 (Fgf23) knock-in mice. *Proc Natl Acad Sci U S A*. 2011;108(46):E1146–1155.

55. Wolf M, Koch TA, Bregman DB. Effects of iron deficiency anemia and its treatment on fibroblast growth factor 23 and phosphate homeostasis in women. *J Bone Miner Res*. 2013;28(8):1793–1803.

56. David V, Martin A, Isakova T et al. Inflammation and functional iron deficiency regulate fibroblast growth factor 23 production. *Kidney Int*. 2016;89(1):135–146.

57. Gutierrez O, Isakova T, Rhee E et al. Fibroblast growth factor-23 mitigates hyperphosphatemia but accentuates calcitriol deficiency in chronic kidney disease. *J Am Soc Nephrol*. 2005;16(7):2205–2215.

58. Portale AA, Wolf M, Jüppner H et al. Disordered FGF23 and mineral metabolism in children with CKD. *Clin J Am Soc Nephrol*. 2014;9(2):344–353.

59. van Husen M, Fischer AK, Lehnhardt A et al. Fibroblast growth factor 23 and bone metabolism in children with chronic kidney disease. *Kidney Int*. 2010;78(2):200–206.

60. Gutierrez OM, Mannstadt M, Isakova T et al. Fibroblast growth factor 23 and mortality among patients undergoing hemodialysis. *N Engl J Med*. 2008;359(6):584–592.

61. Shimada T, Urakawa I, Isakova T et al. Circulating fibroblast growth factor 23 in patients with end-stage renal disease treated by peritoneal dialysis is intact and biologically active. *J Clin Endocrinol Metab*. 2010;95(2):578–585.

62. Smith K, deFilippi C, Isakova T et al. Fibroblast growth factor 23, high-sensitivity cardiac troponin, and left ventricular hypertrophy in CKD. *Am J Kidney Dis*. 2013;61(1):67–73.

63. Jüppner H, Wolf M, Salusky IB. FGF-23: More than a regulator of renal phosphate handling? *J Bone Miner Res*. 2010;25(10):2091–2097.

64. Faul C, Amaral AP, Oskouei B et al. FGF23 induces left ventricular hypertrophy. *J Clin Invest*. 2011;121(11):4393–4408.

65. Grabner A, Amaral AP, Schramm K et al. Activation of cardiac fibroblast growth factor receptor 4 causes left ventricular hypertrophy. *Cell Metab*. 2015;22(6):1020–1032.

66. Scialla JJ, Lau WL, Reilly MP et al. Fibroblast growth factor 23 is not associated with and does not induce arterial calcification. *Kidney Int*. 2013;83(6):1159–1168.

67. Silswal N, Touchberry CD, Daniel DR et al. FGF23 directly impairs endothelium-dependent vasorelaxation by increasing superoxide levels and reducing nitric oxide bioavailability. *Am J Physiol Endocrinol Metab*. 2014;307(5):E426–436.

68. Mirza MA, Larsson A, Lind L, Larsson TE. Circulating fibroblast growth factor-23 is associated with vascular dysfunction in the community. *Atherosclerosis*. 2009;205(2):385–390.

69. Moe SM, Zidehsarai MP, Chambers MA et al. Vegetarian compared with meat dietary protein source and phosphorus homeostasis in chronic kidney disease. *Clin J Am Soc Nephrol*. 2011;6(2):257–264.

70. Finch JL, Lee DH, Liapis H et al. Phosphate restriction significantly reduces mortality in uremic rats with established vascular calcification. *Kidney Int*. 2013;84(6):1145–1153.

71. Schiavi SC, Tang W, Bracken C et al. Npt2b deletion attenuates hyperphosphatemia associated with CKD. *J Am Soc Nephrol*. 2012;23(10):1691–1700.

72. Isakova T, Ix JH, Sprague SM et al. Rationale and approaches to phosphate and fibroblast growth factor 23 reduction in CKD. *J Am Soc Nephrol*. 2015;26(10):2328–2339.

73. Shalhoub V, Shatzen EM, Ward SC et al. FGF23 neutralization improves chronic kidney disease-associated hyperparathyroidism yet increases mortality. *J Clin Invest*. 2012;122(7):2543–2553.
74. Di Marco GS, Reuter S, Kentrup D et al. Treatment of established left ventricular hypertrophy with fibroblast growth factor receptor blockade in an animal model of CKD. *Nephrol Dial Transplant*. 2014;29(11):2028–2035.
75. Coe LM, Madathil SV, Casu C, Lanske B, Rivella S, Sitara D. FGF-23 is a negative regulator of prenatal and postnatal erythropoiesis. *J Biol Chem*. 2014;289(14):9795–9810.
76. Bacchetta J, Sea JL, Chun RF et al. Fibroblast growth factor 23 inhibits extrarenal synthesis of 1,25-dihydroxyvitamin D in human monocytes. *J Bone Miner Res*. 2013;28(1):46–55.

7 Dietary Phosphorus Intake and Kidney Function

Lili Chan and Jaime Uribarri

CONTENTS

Abstract 83
Bullet Points 83
7.1 Introduction 84
7.2 Phosphorous Homeostasis 84
7.3 Serum Phosphate Measurements 85
7.4 Associations of Serum Phosphorus Levels with Outcomes in CKD and ESRD 85
7.5 Chronic Kidney Disease and Mineral and Bone Disorders 85
7.6 Fibroblast Growth Factor-23 86
7.7 Phosphorus and Progression of CKD 86
7.8 Cardiovascular Disease and Mortality 87
7.9 Serum Phosphate Monitoring 88
7.10 Treatment 88
7.11 Conclusions 89
References 89

ABSTRACT

Phosphorus is an essential mineral that is prevalent in a variety of foods. Additionally it is a common additive in processed foods, used as both a preservative and for flavor enhancement. Therefore, in the United States the average person's intake far exceeds the daily requirement. The human body has multiple mechanisms to maintain phosphorous homeostasis and prevent the excess phosphorous from causing complications.

However, once there is a breakdown in these mechanisms, such as in renal failure, there is mounting evidence of the systemic harm associated with elevated serum phosphorous levels. It has been known for a number of years that patients with renal failure and elevated serum phosphorous levels develop renal osteodystrophy, but newer evidence now reveals associations with left ventricular hypertrophy, cardiovascular disease, faster progression of chronic kidney disease, and increased mortality.

This chapter will attempt to describe the mechanism of phosphorous homeostasis and the consequences of elevated serum phosphorous levels in chronic kidney disease patients. Lastly, we will review the basics of treatments of hyperphosphatemia in these patients.

BULLET POINTS

- Phosphorous is present in abundance in many foods, and it is commonly used as an additive in food processing. In the United States, phosphorous intake generally exceeds the recommended daily allowance.
- Serum phosphate levels are controlled by parathyroid hormone (PTH), 1,25-hydroxyvitamin D3 (1,25(OH)$_2$D3), and fibroblast growth factor (FGF23) interacting with the kidneys, which maintain normal levels of serum phosphate in patients with normal renal function.

- Although a tendency toward phosphorous retention occurs with mild renal insufficiency, true fasting hyperphosphatemia does not become evident until advanced renal insufficiency.
- High serum phosphate levels are associated with abnormal bone mineralization, progression of chronic kidney disease, and increased cardiovascular disease and mortality.
- Serum phosphate levels should be monitored starting at stage 3 chronic kidney disease, with dietary restriction and phosphate binders the cornerstone of therapy.

7.1 INTRODUCTION

Phosphorus is an important mineral that is essential for energy production, cellular function, and bone mineralization. It is abundant in both animal and plant products. Phosphorus found in animal products such as meat and dairy is relatively easily absorbed because it is predominantly protein bound and proteins are easily digested. However in plant products, phosphorus is found mostly as phytic acid or phytate, and humans lack the necessary enzyme for degradation (Kalantar-Zadeh et al. 2010). Therefore, the bioavailability of plant-derived phosphorus is low.

Although phosphorus is naturally occurring in both animals and plants as organic phosphate, an inorganic phosphate form also exists, which is often used in processed foods for purposes such as flavor enhancement and as preservatives. Inorganic phosphate is much more easily absorbed (Bell et al. 1977). The U.S. daily recommended allowance is 700 mg/d; however, adults typically consume more than 1000 mg/day of phosphorus (Calvo and Uribarri 2013). The Food and Drug Administration (FDA) does not require that the phosphorus content in food be listed on labels. Even when it is listed, there is no way to distinguish between organic versus inorganic phosphorus. This lack of labeling makes dietary phosphorus restriction difficult. In addition, many of the studies on dietary phosphorus intake have utilized databases that do not necessarily include the phosphorus added during food processing, leading to a general underestimation of the amount of dietary phosphorus intake.

7.2 PHOSPHOROUS HOMEOSTASIS

Phosphorous homeostasis is carefully maintained by the interplay of gastrointestinal absorption, bone mineralization, and renal excretion. In people who have normal renal function, the excess dietary phosphorous will be handled by increased renal excretion; however, the excess becomes a problem in patients with chronic kidney disease (CKD).

Eighty-five percent of the phosphorous in humans is stored as bone and teeth, 14% in soft tissue, and the remaining less than 1% in extracellular space. Absorption of dietary phosphorous occurs in the small intestine via passive paracellular diffusion and actively across cell walls via sodium phosphate cotransporter type2B (Uribarri 2007). About 60% of dietary phosphorus of a mixed diet is usually absorbed, and the remainder comes out in the stool. This percentage, however, is highly variable depending on the kind of food, degree of phosphate added during food processing, relative amount of calcium in the diet, etc.

Phosphorous excretion is predominantly via the kidneys. It is filtered in the glomerulus, with 75% reabsorption in the proximal tubule, 10% in the distal tubule, and about 15% lost in urine. Two transporters have been identified that are responsible for renal tubular phosphate reabsorption: 3Na-HPO4 cotransporter type 2A (NaP-2A) and 3Na-HPO4 cotransporter type 2c (NaP-2c). NaP-2A is responsible for 70% of reabsorption, with 30% handled by NaP-2c. A small amount is reabsorbed by PiT-2 phosphate transporter (Blaine, Weinman, and Cunningham 2011). These transporters are located on the apical brush border membrane of renal proximal tubular cells.

Even though a tendency for phosphorus retention occurs early on in CKD, actual fasting hyperphosphatemia does not develop until advanced CKD. This is due to the complex interplay between phosphorus, parathyroid hormone (PTH), 1,25-hydroxyvitamin D3 (1,25(OH)2D3), and fibroblast growth factor (FGF23), hormones that help with phosphorus homeostasis. Figure 7.1 demonstrates how elevated phosphorous levels affect the body and how multiple factors control serum phosphate levels.

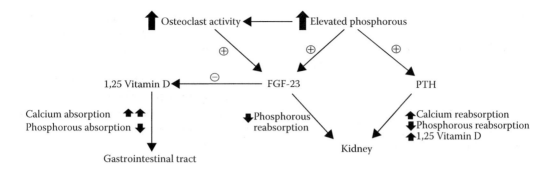

FIGURE 7.1 Homeostatic response to an increase of serum phosphate. Elevated serum phosphorous levels cause secretion of parathyroid hormone, which causes the kidney to increase calcium reabsorption, decrease phosphorous reabsorption, and increase 1,25 vitamin D. Because 1,25 vitamin D causes more calcium reabsorption than phosphorous reabsorption from the intestines, the net effect is a loss of phosphorous due to parathyroid hormone. Additionally elevated phosphorous levels increase fibroblast growth factor-23 (FGF23) levels directly and indirectly through increased osteoclast activity, which again increases phosphorous reabsorption in the kidney and decreases 1,25 vitamin D.

7.3 SERUM PHOSPHATE MEASUREMENTS

An isolated fasting serum phosphate level may not accurately represent total body phosphorus. As discussed earlier, the kidneys tend to eliminate rapidly an oral phosphorus load, and the serum phosphate will quickly normalize following an oral load. Additionally, serum phosphate has a circadian variation, peaking in late afternoon and with a smaller peak at midnight (Portale et al. 1989). Studies in end-stage renal disease (ESRD) patients seem to show a correlation between serum phosphorus level and dietary phosphorus intake, but this is not the case in patients with moderate CKD or in healthy subjects. Sullivan et al. (2009) demonstrated that their ESRD patients who started with a serum phosphorus level >5.5 mg/dL and received education on avoiding dietary phosphorus had a 0.6 mg/dL larger decline in serum phosphorus compared to those patients who did not receive the intervention.

7.4 ASSOCIATIONS OF SERUM PHOSPHORUS LEVELS WITH OUTCOMES IN CKD AND ESRD

Studies have demonstrated that increased serum phosphate is associated with increased mortality in both CKD and ESRD patients. Newer studies are now showing this to also be true in subjects with normal renal function. Elevated serum phosphate levels have also been linked with bone disease and progression of CKD.

7.5 CHRONIC KIDNEY DISEASE AND MINERAL AND BONE DISORDERS

The connection between phosphorus and bone disease has been well established in CKD. The traditional explanation has been that as phosphorous builds up in the body secondary to decreased renal excretion, parathyroid hormone (PTH) secretion increases. Serum phosphorus levels have been shown to independently increase PTH secretion (Kates et al. 1997). Kemi et al. (2009) evaluated 147 premenopausal women with normal renal function and found that patients with the highest dietary phosphate intake had higher PTH concentrations. The initial increase in PTH may help maintain bone health; however, with sustained high levels of PTH, bone mineral density declines (Takeda et al. 2014). PTH secretion works well to maintain normal serum phosphate levels, mostly by decreasing tubular reabsorption of phosphorus and therefore increasing its fractional urinary excretion. As renal function declines, however, phosphorous continues to build up, and more severe and sustained secondary hyperparathyroidism develops. Bone disease is common in CKD and is classically called renal osteodystrophy. Renal osteodystrophy encompasses multiple lesions, including osteitis fibrosa, osteomalacia, and adynamic bone disease.

Animal studies have shown that dietary restriction of phosphorous prevents the development of renal osteodystrophy. As early as the 1970s, dietary phosphorus restriction was shown to demonstrate a benefit on bone health (Maschio et al. 1980). Because a large source of dietary phosphorus is animal protein, dietary phosphorus restriction while maintaining acceptable protein intake is challenging in the CKD and ESRD populations.

7.6 FIBROBLAST GROWTH FACTOR-23

Recently, an increasing role for FGF23 in maintaining phosphorus balance is being recognized. High serum phosphate levels seem to stimulate the secretion of FGF23 by osteocytes. Studies have shown that serum FGF23 levels generally peak at eight hours post oral phosphate load (Burnett et al. 2006). FGF23 acts by binding to the FGF23 receptor and the coreceptor klotho in the kidney, which then downregulates the sodium-dependent phosphate transporters NaPi-2a and NaPi-2C, leading to phosphaturia. In addition to increasing phosphaturia, FGF23 inhibits CYP27B1 expression, which encodes for 25-hydroxyvitamin D3, 1 alpha hydroxylase, which is responsible for the conversion of 25(OH)2D3 to 1,25(OH)2D3. Because 1,25(OH)2D3 increases gastrointestinal (GI) absorption of calcium, its decreasing levels would decrease calcium absorption and potentially also phosphorus absorption that is bound to intraluminal calcium. In addition, FGF23 stimulates expression of CYP24A1, which encodes catabolic 1,25(OH)2D3 hydroxylase, leading to further reduction of 1,25(OH)2D3 levels.

FGF23 levels progressively increase with worsening renal failure and can reach 1000-fold above normal in ESRD patients. Elevated levels of FGF23 have been associated with increased cardiovascular disease, increased mortality, and increased renal disease progression. Gutiérrez et al. (2008) demonstrated in a prospective cohort of 10,044 hemodialysis patients that there is a strong correlation between elevated FGF23 levels and death, independent of serum phosphorus levels. In 2011, Faul et al. (2011) showed in mice models that elevations in FGF23 increased left ventricular hypertrophy (LVH). They also demonstrated a clinical association between high FGF23 levels and LVH, a clear risk factor for increased cardiac events.

In 2006, Antoniucci et al. (2006) subjected 13 healthy males to three different phosphorus intakes, 1500 mg/d, followed by 2300 mg/d, and lastly 625 mg/d over a period of four weeks. Patients on the 2300 mg/day intake had nonsignificant increase in their FGF23 concentration, but when phosphorus intake was restricted to the 625 mg/d, they had a significant drop in FGF23 levels. In 2010, Isakova et al. (2011) investigated the effect of dietary phosphorus modification on FGF23 levels in CKD patients. They randomized 16 normophosphatemic CKD stages 3 and 4 patients to high (1500 mg daily) vs. low (750 mg daily) phosphorus diets. They found that dietary phosphorus restriction combined with phosphate binders did not decrease serum phosphate or FGF23 levels. They did note that the patients who were on the high phosphorus diet and not on binders had the highest FGF23 levels. However, more recent studies in patients with CKD have demonstrated a drop in FGF23 in response to dietary phosphorus restriction. Sigrist et al. (2013) compared FGF23 levels in 18 normophosphatemic CKD subjects and 12 healthy controls. In their study, FGF23 levels changed in response to dietary phosphorus changes in both the CKD group and control group, without a change in serum phosphate levels.

7.7 PHOSPHORUS AND PROGRESSION OF CKD

Elevated phosphorous levels have been found to be associated with increased progression of CKD. This was first shown to be true in rat models. Neves et al. (2004) subjected 5/6 nephrectomized rats with parathyroidectomy to high-phosphorus diets vs. low-phosphorus diets. The rats fed

Dietary Phosphorus Intake and Kidney Function

high-phosphorus diets had myocardial hypertrophy, impaired renal function, and adverse effects of bone remodeling compared to those rats fed a low-phosphorus diet (Neves et al. 2004).

In 2006, Schwarz et al. (2006) reviewed 985 male Veterans Association patient records examining the relationship between serum phosphate and progression of CKD. In their study, 258 patients reached their composite endpoint of ESRD or doubling of serum creatinine. Patients who had the highest hazard ratios were those with higher serum phosphate, lower calcium, and higher calcium–phosphorus product. When the patients were grouped into quartiles of serum phosphate, the risk of their composite endpoint was increased with serum phosphate greater than 3.8 mg/dL, with the highest risk in those patients whose serum phosphate levels were greater than 4.3 mg/dL. Voormolen et al. (2007) confirmed this finding in a study of 547 incident predialysis patients with glomerular filtration rate (GFR) <20 mL/min/1.73 m^2. In this retrospective follow-up study, patients with higher phosphate levels had faster loss of renal function; the unadjusted analysis showed that each 1 mg/dL higher plasma phosphate was associated with 0.154 mL/min/month steeper slope of decline in renal function. When adjusted for known risk factors, the slope increased to 0.178 mL/min/month decline in renal function. The patients who started with normal phosphate and then developed elevated levels within 3 months of study entry had a relatively steeper decline in renal function. In contrast, those patients who entered the study with elevated serum phosphate levels that normalized by the end of the study had a trend toward improvement in their kidney function.

O'Seaghdha et al. (2011) looked at two study populations, 2269 non-CKD patients from the Framingham Heart Study (FHS) and 13,372 patients from the National Health and Nutrition Examination Survey (NHANES III). From the FHS study, they categorized participants based on their baseline phosphate levels, <2.5 mg/dL, 2.5 to 3.49 mg/dL, 3.5 to 3.99 mg/dL, and >4 mg/dL. Overall, 11.7% developed CKD, and those participants with phosphate levels >4 mg/dL had an increased risk of incident CKD with an odds ratio of 2.15. From the NHANES III study, participants were categorized as having phosphate levels either below or above 4 mg/dL. Eventually, 65 patients developed ESRD, and those patients with phosphorus levels >4 mg/dL had an increased relative risk of ESRD of 2.41.

The exact mechanism of CKD progression associated with increased phosphorus is unclear, but a potential mechanism is renal tissue calcification by calcium phosphate precipitation. Experimental models show a relationship between elevations in phosphorus and development of glomerulosclerosis. Sekiguchi et al. (2011) also demonstrated that phosphate overload induces podocyte injury. They used a transgenic mouse with overexpression of type III P_i transporter Pit1, which is ubiquitously expressed in all cells, and is important for the influx of phosphorus into cells. They found that overexpression of this transporter induced phosphate-dependent podocyte injury and damage to the glomerular barrier, resulting in glomerular sclerosis in the kidney.

As early as 1982, Maschio et al. (1982) showed that phosphorous restriction had some role in prevention of worsening renal function. He studied three different groups of patients, one group with serum creatinine levels of 1.55 to 2.7 mg/dL treated with phosphorus restriction, one group with creatinine levels of 2.99 to 5.4 mg/dL treated with phosphorus and protein restriction, and one group of 30 patients with all levels of CKD and no dietary restrictions. The patients with mild CKD and protein restriction had the least increase in serum creatinine over time.

7.8 CARDIOVASCULAR DISEASE AND MORTALITY

There is an approximate 20% annual mortality rate in hemodialysis patients in the United States. The risk of death and hospitalization is increased in those patients who have diabetes mellitus and underlying cardiovascular disease (CVD). Elevated serum phosphate levels have been linked with elevated rates of CVD. In 1998, Block et al. (1998), using the United States Renal Data System (USRDS) data, found that patients on hemodialysis with serum phosphate greater than 6.5 mg/dL had a higher relative risk of death compared with those who had serum phosphate levels between 2.7 and 6.5 mg/dL. In that study the higher the serum phosphate, the higher the risk; serum phosphate of 6.6 to 7.8 mg/dL had a relative risk of 13% compared to phosphate of 7.9 to 16.9 mg/dL with a relative risk of 34%. He later confirmed the same association between serum phosphate and mortality in another group of 40,538 hemodialysis patients (Block et al. 2004).

Chue et al. (2012) demonstrated that elevated serum phosphate levels are associated with changes in left ventricular mass in the CKD population. Sixty-two stage 2 to 4 CKD patients without known risk factors for LVH had cardiac magnetic resonance imaging (MRI) performed. Patients with serum phosphate levels greater than 3.7 mg/dL had a greater left ventricular mass index than those CKD patients with phosphate levels less than 3.7 mg/dL, 61 vs. 55 g/m^2. This finding has also been documented in hemodialysis patients (Strozecki et al. 2001; Patel et al. 2009). It has been well proven that LVH is associated with an increase in CVD, which may in part explain the connection between elevated serum phosphate and cardiovascular events and mortality.

The link between phosphorus and mortality in ESRD patients is clear; however, the association between elevated phosphate levels and mortality in CKD patients is not as robust. Mehrotra et al. (2013) reviewed a CKD population of 10,672 over a two-year follow-up period and did not find an increased risk for all-cause mortality when adjusted for confounders. These were patients with early-stage CKD, with serum creatinine averaging 1.3 mg/dL; maximum mean serum phosphate was 4.6 ± 0.05 mg/dL. However, in 2005, Kestenbaum et al. (2005) reviewed data from 6730 CKD patients and found that patients with serum phosphate levels >3.5 mg/dL had an increased risk for death. His study population was comparable to the study population in Mehrotra et al. (2013), except for a higher serum creatinine (mean serum creatinine level of 1.7 mg/dL). Each 1 mg/dL increase of serum phosphate was associated with a 44% increase in mortality risk in unadjusted analysis. When adjusted the association remained significant, but risk decreased to 23%.

Newer studies have found that the increase in mortality is not isolated to those with CKD. Yoo et al. (2016) described an increase in mortality in men with higher serum phosphate levels despite normal renal function.

The exact pathophysiology linking elevated serum phosphate and the increased risk of CVD and mortality is unclear. Among the most commonly proposed mechanism is an increase in vascular calcifications. Studies demonstrate that elevations in serum phosphate induce smooth muscle cells to transform into osteoblast-like cells, which then secrete matrix necessary for vascular calcification (Jono et al. 2000).

7.9 SERUM PHOSPHATE MONITORING

It has now become clear that serum phosphate levels require close monitoring, as high levels are associated with bone mineral disorders, progression of CKD, increase in cardiovascular events, and mortality. As per the 2009 Kidney Disease Improving Global Outcomes (KDIGO) initiative (Kidney Disease: Improving Global Outcomes [KDIGO] CKD-MBD Work Group 2009), recommendations in adult calcium, phosphorus, PTH, 25(OH)2D3, and alkaline phosphatase levels should be checked starting at CKD stage 3. In stage 3 CKD, calcium and phosphorus should be check every 6 to 12 months; PTH and 25(OH)2D3 will depend on level and CKD progression. In CKD stage 4, calcium and phosphorus should be checked every 3 to 6 months and PTH every 6 to 12 months. In CKD stage 5 calcium and phosphorus should be checked every 1 to 2 months, and PTH should be checked every 3 to 6 months. In CKD stages 3 to 5, the goal is to maintain serum phosphate levels within normal limits. And in CKD stage 5 on dialysis, the goal is to lower phosphate levels toward the reference range.

7.10 TREATMENT

A low-phosphorus diet and oral phosphate binders are the cornerstones of hyperphosphatemia treatment. Dialysis also decreases serum phosphorus; however, a typical dialysis treatment is usually insufficient to maintain normal serum phosphorus in a patient eating well. Serum phosphate levels plateau after two hours of dialysis and may actually rebound secondary to mobilization of

Dietary Phosphorus Intake and Kidney Function 89

intracellular phosphorus (Kalantar-Zadeh 2013). As previously discussed, it is very difficult to accurately determine the phosphorus content of the food that we eat. It is clear, however, in view of the growing evidence for the detriment of hyperphosphatemia that treatment should be instituted early with the use of dietary restriction and phosphorus binders.

Because much of the foods that are phosphorus rich are also protein rich, dietary phosphorus restriction necessitates a careful balance, as low protein intake may be associated with worsening mortality (Kovesdy and Kalantar-Zadeh 2009). Shinaberger et al. (2008) examined changes in phosphorus and normalized protein nitrogen appearance (nPNA) in 30,075 hemodialysis patients. They found that the patients with the best survival were those patients who had a decrease in their serum phosphate and an increase in nPNA. In the past, low-phosphorus diets have focused on low-protein diets; however, the current recommendations are to counsel patients on the different types of phosphorus in diets. Patients should be educated on avoidance of phosphorus additives, which are prevalent in cheap and processed foods.

Oral phosphorus binders are also commonly used in addition to dietary phosphorus restriction. Aluminum binders, which were commonly used in the past, are now generally restricted to short-term use out of concern for potential aluminum accumulation and toxicity. Calcium-based binders have recently also come under scrutiny due to concerns for increasing vascular calcification. Russo et al. (2014) randomized 113 patients on a phosphorus-restricted diet to either calcium-based binder or sevelamer. They found that in patients treated with calcium binders there was a significant increase in coronary artery calcification progression and higher risk of mortality and dialysis initiation. Ferric citrate is a new iron-based phosphate binder, which seems to have the same positive effect on phosphorus, calcium, and PTH as traditional binders without the concern for increased calcium overload and decreased GI side effects as other binders.

7.11 CONCLUSIONS

Although phosphorus is an essential mineral that is readily prevalent in most foods, hyperphosphatemia becomes a problem in the CKD population. It is linked with increased progression of CKD, bone disorders, cardiovascular events, and mortality. Treatment of hyperphosphatemia includes dietary control, phosphorus binders, and dialysis. More recent work suggests that the pathological links with phosphorus, well known in CKD patients for decades, may indeed also apply to the general population with normal kidney function.

REFERENCES

Antoniucci, D. M., T. Yamashita, and A. A. Portale. 2006. Dietary phosphorus regulates serum fibroblast growth factor-23 concentrations in healthy men. *Journal of Clinical Endocrinology and Metabolism* 91 (8): 3144–9. doi:10.1210/jc.2006-0021.

Bell, R. R., H. H. Draper, D. Y. Tzeng, H. K. Shin, and G. R. Schmidt. 1977. Physiological responses of human adults to foods containing phosphate additives. *The Journal of Nutrition* 107 (1): 42–50.

Blaine, J., E. J. Weinman, and R. Cunningham. 2011. The regulation of renal phosphate transport. *Advances in Chronic Kidney Disease* 18 (2): 77–84. doi:10.1053/j.ackd.2011.01.005.

Block, G. A., T. E. Hulbert-Shearon, N. W. Levin, and F. K. Port. 1998. Association of serum phosphorus and calcium X phosphate product with mortality risk in chronic hemodialysis patients: A national study. *American Journal of Kidney Diseases: The Official Journal of the National Kidney Foundation* 31 (4): 607–17. doi:10.1053/ajkd.1998.v31.pm9531176.

Block, G. A., P. S. Klassen, J. Michael Lazarus, N. Ofsthun, E. G. Lowrie, and G. M. Chertow. 2004. Mineral metabolism, mortality, and morbidity in maintenance hemodialysis. *Journal of the American Society of Nephrology: JASN* 15 (8): 2208–18. doi:10.1097/01.ASN.0000133041.27682.A2.

Burnett, S.-A.M., S. C. Gunawardene, F. Richard Bringhurst, H. Jüppner, H. Lee, and J. S. Finkelstein. 2006. Regulation of C-terminal and intact FGF-23 by dietary phosphate in men and women. *Journal of Bone and Mineral Research: The Official Journal of the American Society for Bone and Mineral Research* 21 (8): 1187–96. doi:10.1359/jbmr.060507.

Calvo, M. S. and J. Uribarri. 2013. Contributions to total phosphorus intake: All sources considered. *Seminars in Dialysis* 26 (1): 54–61. doi:10.1111/sdi.12042.

Chue, C. D., N. C. Edwards, W. E. Moody, R. P. Steeds, J. N. Townend, and C. J. Ferro. 2012. Serum phosphate is associated with left ventricular mass in patients with chronic kidney disease: A cardiac magnetic resonance study. *Heart* 98 (3): 219–24. doi:10.1136/heartjnl-2011-300570.

Faul, C., A. P. Amaral, B. Oskouei, M.-C. Hu, A. Sloan, T. Isakova, O. M. Gutiérrez et al. 2011. FGF23 induces left ventricular hypertrophy. *The Journal of Clinical Investigation* 121 (11): 4393–408. doi:10.1172/JCI46122.

Gutiérrez, O. M., M. Mannstadt, T. Isakova, J. A. Rauh-Hain, H. Tamez, A. Shah, K. Smith et al. 2008. Fibroblast growth factor 23 and mortality among patients undergoing hemodialysis. *The New England Journal of Medicine* 359 (6): 584–92. doi:10.1056/NEJMoa0706130.

Isakova, T., O. M. Gutirrez, K. Smith, M. Epstein, L. K. Keating, H. Jppner, and M. Wolf. 2011. Pilot study of dietary phosphorus restriction and phosphorus binders to target fibroblast growth factor 23 in patients with chronic kidney disease. *Nephrology Dialysis Transplantation* 26 (2): 584–91. doi:10.1093/ndt/gfq419.

Jono, S., M. D. McKee, C. E. Murry, A. Shioi, Y. Nishizawa, K. Mori, H. Morii et al. 2000. Phosphate regulation of vascular smooth muscle cell calcification. *Circulation Research* 87 (7): E10–7. doi:10.1161/01.RES.87.7.e10.

Kalantar-Zadeh, K. 2013. Patient education for phosphorus management in chronic kidney disease. *Patient Preference and Adherence* 7: 379–90. doi:10.2147/PPA.S43486.

Kalantar-Zadeh, K., L. Gutekunst, R. Mehrotra, C. P. Kovesdy, R. Bross, C. S Shinaberger, N. Noori et al. 2010. Understanding sources of dietary phosphorus in the treatment of patients with chronic kidney disease. *Clinical Journal of the American Society of Nephrology: CJASN* 5 (3): 519–30. doi:10.2215/CJN.06080809.

Kates, D. M., D. J. Sherrard, and D. L. Andress. 1997. Evidence that serum phosphate is independently associated with serum PTH in patients with chronic renal failure. *American Journal of Kidney Diseases: The Official Journal of the National Kidney Foundation* 30 (6): 809–13.

Kemi, V. E., H. J. Rita, M. U. M. Kärkkäinen, H. T. Viljakainen, M. M. Laaksonen, T. A. Outila, and C. J. E. Lamberg-Allardt. 2009. Habitual high phosphorus intakes and foods with phosphate additives negatively affect serum parathyroid hormone concentration: A cross-sectional study on healthy premenopausal women. *Public Health Nutrition* 12 (10): 1885–92. doi:10.1017/S1368980009004819.

Kestenbaum, B., J. N. Sampson, K. D. Rudser, D. J. Patterson, S. L. Seliger, B. Young, D. J. Sherrard, and D. L. Andress. 2005. Serum phosphate levels and mortality risk among people with chronic kidney disease. *Journal of the American Society of Nephrology: JASN* 16 (2): 520–28. doi:10.1681/ASN.2004070602.

Kidney Disease: Improving Global Outcomes (KDIGO) CKD-MBD Work Group. 2009. KDIGO clinical practice guideline for the diagnosis, evaluation, prevention, and treatment of Chronic Kidney Disease-Mineral and Bone Disorder (CKD-MBD). Kidney International. *Supplement* (113): S1–130. doi:10.1038/ki.2009.188.

Kovesdy, C. P. and K. Kalantar-Zadeh. 2009. Why is protein-energy wasting associated with mortality in chronic kidney disease? *Seminars in Nephrology* 29 (1): 3–14. doi:10.1016/j.semnephrol.2008.10.002.

Maschio, G., N. Tessitore, A. D'Angelo, E. Bonucci, A. Lupo, E. Valvo, C. Loschiavo et al. 1980. Early dietary phosphorus restriction and calcium supplementation in the prevention of renal osteodystrophy. *American Journal of Clinical Nutrition* 33 (7): 1546–54.

Maschio, G., L. Oldrizzi, N. Tessitore, A. D'Angelo, E. Valvo, A. Lupo, C. Loschiavo et al. 1982. Effects of dietary protein and phosphorus restriction on the progression of early renal failure. *Kidney International* 22 (4): 371–6. doi:10.1038/ki.1982.184.

Mehrotra, R., C. A. Peralta, S. C. Chen, S. Li, M. Sachs, A. Shah, K. Norris et al. 2013. No independent association of serum phosphorus with risk for death or progression to end-stage renal disease in a large screen for chronic kidney disease. *Kidney International* 84 (5): 989–97. doi:10.1038/ki.2013.145.

Neves, K. R., F. G. Graciolli, L. M. Dos Reis, C. A. Pasqualucci, R. M. Moysés, and V. Jorgetti. 2004. Adverse effects of hyperphosphatemia on myocardial hypertrophy, renal function, and bone in rats with renal failure. *Kidney International* 66 (6): 2237–44. doi:10.1111/j.1523-1755.2004.66013.x.

O'Seaghdha, C. M., S. J. Hwang, P. Muntner, M. L. Melamed, and C. S. Fox. 2011. Serum phosphorus predicts incident chronic kidney disease and end-stage renal disease. *Nephrology Dialysis Transplantation* 26 (9): 2885–90. doi:10.1093/ndt/gfq808.

Patel, R. K., S. Oliver, P. B. Mark, J. R. Powell, E. P. McQuarrie, J. P. Traynor, H. J. Dargie, and A. G. Jardine. 2009. Determinants of left ventricular mass and hypertrophy in hemodialysis patients assessed by cardiac magnetic resonance imaging. *Clinical Journal of the American Society of Nephrology: CJASN* 4 (9): 1477–83. doi:10.2215/CJN.03350509.

Portale, A. A., B. P. Halloran, and R. C. Morris. 1989. *Physiologic regulation of the serum concentration of 1,25-dihydroxyvitamin D by phosphorus in normal men. Journal of Clinical Investigation* 83 (5): 1494–9. doi:10.1172/JCI114043.

Russo, D., A. Bellasi, A. Pota, L. Russo, and B. Di Iorio. 2014. Effects of phosphorus-restricted diet and phosphate-binding therapy on outcomes in patients with chronic kidney disease. *Journal of Nephrology* 28 (1): 73–80. doi:10.1007/s40620-014-0071-2.

Schwarz, S., B. K. Trivedi, K. Kalantar-Zadeh, and C. P. Kovesdy. 2006. Association of disorders in mineral metabolism with progression of chronic kidney disease. *Clinical Journal of the American Society of Nephrology: CJASN* 1 (4): 825–31. doi:10.2215/CJN.02101205.

Sekiguchi, S., A. Suzuki, S. Asano, K. Nishiwaki-Yasuda, M. Shibata, S. Nagao, N. Yamamoto et al. 2011. Phosphate overload induces podocyte injury via type III Na-dependent phosphate transporter. American Journal of Physiology. *Renal Physiology* 300 (4): F848–56. doi:10.1152/ajprenal.00334.2010.

Shinaberger, C. S., S. Greenland, J. D. Kopple, D. Van Wyck, R. Mehrotra, C. P. Kovesdy, and K. Kalantar-Zadeh. 2008. Is controlling phosphorus by decreasing dietary protein intake beneficial or harmful in persons with chronic kidney disease? *American Journal of Clinical Nutrition* 88 (6): 1511–8. doi:10.3945/ajcn.2008.26665.

Sigrist, M., M. Tang, M. Beaulieu, G. Espino-Hernandez, L. Er, O. Djurdjev, and A. Levin. 2013. Responsiveness of FGF-23 and mineral metabolism to altered dietary phosphate intake in chronic kidney disease (CKD): Results of a randomized trial. *Nephrology Dialysis Transplantation* 28 (1): 161–9. doi:10.1093/ndt/gfs405.

Strozecki, P., A. Adamowicz, E. Nartowicz, G. Odrowaz-Sypniewska, Z. Wlodarczyk, and J. Manitius. 2001. Parathormon, calcium, phosphorus, and left ventricular structure and function in normotensive hemodialysis patients. *Ren Fail* 23 (1): 115–26. http://www.ncbi.nlm.nih.gov/pubmed/11256521.

Sullivan, C., S. S. Sayre, J. B. Leon, R. Machekano, T. E. Love, D. Porter, M. Marbury, and A. R. Sehgal. 2009. Effect of food additives on hyperphosphatemia among patients with end-stage renal disease: A randomized controlled trial. *JAMA: The Journal of the American Medical Association* 301 (6): 629–35. doi:10.1001/jama.2009.96.

Takeda, E., H. Yamamoto, H. Yamanaka-Okumura, and Y. Taketani. 2014. Increasing dietary phosphorus intake from food additives: Potential for negative impact on bone health. *Advances in Nutrition* 5 (1): 92–7. doi:10.3945/an.113.004002.Current.

Uribarri, J. 2007. Phosphorus homeostasis in normal health and in chronic kidney disease patients with special emphasis on dietary phosphorus intake. *Seminars in Dialysis* 20 (4): 295–301. doi:10.1111/j.1525-139X.2007.00309.x.

Voormolen, N., M. Noordzij, D. C. Grootendorst, I. Beetz, Y. W. Sijpkens, J. G. Van Manen, E. W. Boeschoten et al. 2007. High plasma phosphate as a risk factor for decline in renal function and mortality in predialysis patients. *Nephrology Dialysis Transplantation* 22 (10): 2909–16. doi:10.1093/ndt/gfm286.

Yoo, K. D., S. Kang, Y. Choi, S. H. Yang, N. J. Heo, H. J. Chin, K. H. Oh et al. 2016. Sex, age, and the association of serum phosphorus with all-cause mortality in adults with normal kidney function. *American Journal of Kidney Diseases* 67 (1): 79–88. doi:10.1053/j.ajkd.2015.06.027.

8 Dietary Phosphorus Intake and Cardiotoxicity

Sven-Jean Tan and Nigel D. Toussaint

CONTENTS

Abstract 93
Bullet Points 94
8.1   Introduction 94
8.2   Dietary Phosphorus 94
8.3   Serum Phosphorus: Associations with Mortality and Cardiovascular Outcomes 95
8.4   Urinary Phosphorus: Associations with Mortality and Cardiovascular Outcomes 96
8.5   Dietary Phosphorus Intake: Is Too Much Bad? 97
8.6   Intake and Mortality/Cardiovascular Outcomes 97
8.7   Intake with Fibroblast Growth Factor-23 100
8.8   Short-Term Dietary Phosphorus Interventions 100
8.9   Effect on Urinary Phosphorus Excretion 101
8.10 Effect on Serum Phosphorus Values 101
8.11 Effect on FGF23 Levels 102
8.12 Effect on Endothelial Function and Arterial Stiffness 102
8.13 Effect on Vascular Calcification 103
8.14 Phosphorus and Protein Consumption 103
8.15 Can Modifying Dietary Phosphorus Affect Outcomes? 104
8.16 Conclusions 105
References 105

ABSTRACT

Epidemiological studies show serum phosphorus levels are independently associated with all-cause and cardiovascular mortality in people with chronic kidney disease. Several observational studies have even reported associations between higher serum phosphorus levels within the normal reference range and cardiovascular events and mortality in people with normal kidney function. Serum phosphorus fulfils many criteria to be defined as a risk factor for cardiovascular disease. The association between serum phosphorus and dietary phosphorus intake, however, is only modest. Urinary excretion of phosphorus is often used as a measure of dietary phosphorus intake, and several observational studies have reported associations with urinary phosphorus and clinical outcomes but with conflicting results. Whether increased dietary phosphorus intake is harmful and associated with cardiovascular disease is unclear, and there are limited observational studies addressing this issue. There is also a paucity of interventional studies evaluating the role of manipulation of dietary phosphorus—either with restricted intake or reduction in absorption through the use of phosphorus binders—and clinical outcomes, especially cardiovascular disease. Disordered regulation of fibroblast growth factor-23 (FGF23) by high dietary phosphorus may be a key factor contributing to atherosclerosis and increased cardiovascular burden. This chapter outlines the current evidence linking phosphorus and adverse outcomes, focusing on associations between dietary phosphorus intake and cardiotoxicity.

BULLET POINTS

- Associations between serum phosphorus levels and adverse health outcomes, such as mortality and cardiovascular disease, are well reported in general-population cohorts and in subjects with chronic kidney disease; however, the relationship between dietary phosphorus intake and adverse outcomes is less clear.
- Dietary phosphorus may be the only modifiable source of phosphorus in humans, although better methods for assessment of dietary phosphorus intake are required.
- Urinary excretion of phosphorus can be used as a surrogate measure for dietary phosphorus intake, and observational studies have reported associations between adverse clinical outcomes and urinary phosphorus, although with conflicting results.
- Changes in fibroblast growth factor-23 (FGF23) through dietary phosphorus intake may be a mechanism to link increased cardiovascular disease with excess dietary phosphorus.
- Larger studies with more consistent assessment of dietary phosphorus are needed to evaluate the potential cardiotoxicity of increasing phosphorus intake.

8.1 INTRODUCTION

Phosphorus is required for many vital biological processes, and therefore phosphorus regulation is crucial in living organisms [1]. In some single-cell organisms a phosphorus-sensing mechanism has been identified [2], although in more complex life forms, the exact trigger or sensor for the intricate regulatory pathways of phosphorus is as yet unknown. Even so, serum phosphorus levels are tightly controlled. In health, the amount of phosphorus absorbed from the diet is equivalent to the amount excreted in the urine [1]. In a series of complex feedback mechanisms, a number of proteins act, directly or indirectly, to regulate the activity of key transporters to maintain phosphorus equilibrium, balancing supply (diet) and demand (cellular metabolism and bone mineralisation) [3]. These include active vitamin-D $(1,25(OH)_2D_3)$, parathyroid hormone (PTH), fibroblast growth factor-23 (FGF23), and its coreceptor klotho.

Associations between elevated serum phosphorus levels and mortality, as well as with cardiovascular disease (CVD), are well established in people with chronic kidney disease (CKD) [4,5]. Several large epidemiological studies report these associations also extend to the general population, where healthy subjects with serum phosphorus values in the highest quartile of the normal range have significantly increased risk of cardiovascular (CV) events and developing CKD [6–10]. Although dietary phosphorus seems the only modifiable source, the associations between dietary phosphorus and adverse outcomes are less clear. This chapter will outline current evidence linking phosphorus and adverse outcomes, focusing on associations between dietary phosphorus intake and CV outcomes.

8.2 DIETARY PHOSPHORUS

The typical Western diet has relatively high phosphorus content, primarily in the form of meat and dairy products. The dietary phosphorus intake in an average individual in the United States is augmented further with increasingly widespread use of phosphorus-containing additives in processed foods and fast foods [11]. More concerning is the ease with which phosphorus is readily absorbed from these additives, compared with foods that are naturally high in phosphorus content. There is also inadequate acknowledgement by food labels of phosphorus-containing additives [12]. A recent publication provided insight into a historical average U.S. dietary phosphorus intake, indicating >80% of the population consumed >700 mg of phosphorus per day, the recommended daily allowance (RDA), and ~35% consumed >1400 mg/d (more than twice the RDA) [13]. Interestingly, those who consumed more were more likely to be younger, more active, and more often male [13]. Given the convenience of fast foods and processed foods and the increasing reliance on such food preparations, it is plausible the average Western daily dietary phosphorus intake has increased even further since the recording of this dietary information.

Dietary Phosphorus Intake and Cardiotoxicity

In considering the impact of dietary phosphorus intake on health outcomes, several methods have been reported to estimate dietary phosphorus intake. Estimations are needed, as true direct measurement of human dietary phosphorus intake or absorption is technically challenging. Questionnaires, both participant administered and trained interviewer administered; prospective (single day or multiple day) dietary records; and retrospective dietary recall on food consumption are methods of reported intake estimations. Although these methods provide substantial information, some inadequacies have been identified. Food frequency questionnaires (FFQs) have been found to underestimate or overestimate intake compared to dietary recall or dietary records, although nutritional intake calculated from either method is closely correlated [14–17]. As such, these tools are commonly used to assess phosphorus intake and its impact on health outcomes.

Given the potential confounding that may be introduced from an assessment of dietary phosphorus intake, associations with serum phosphorus levels and adverse health outcomes have been more commonly reported. Serum phosphorus is relatively consistent and an easy and reliable measure to perform in a standard biochemistry laboratory. Consequently, the ability to extrapolate measurement of dietary phosphorus intake from serum levels would be appealing. The link between serum phosphorus and dietary phosphorus intake, however, is not a strong and consistent relationship. The largest observational study assessing this relationship, involving over 15,000 participants (NHANES III), recorded 24-hour dietary recall and found a weak but statistically significant association between serum phosphorus levels with dietary phosphorus intake [18]. Although this seems insufficient evidence to consider serum phosphorus as a reliable marker of dietary intake, many smaller intensive interventional studies demonstrate more convincingly that dietary phosphorus loading results in an increase in serum phosphorus levels. This is the case when measuring serum levels either at peak levels in the mid to late afternoon or over a 24-hour period to capture the diurnal variation seen with serum phosphorus [19–23]. These findings have been reported in healthy subjects as well as those with CKD [19].

Measurements of urine phosphorus may provide a more consistent assessment of dietary phosphorus intake, or at least dietary phosphorus absorption, as dietary phosphorus absorption is equivalent to phosphorus excretion in steady state. Urinary phosphorus excretion (UPE), as measured by a 24-hour urine collection, is considered a reliable marker of intestinal phosphorus absorption [24]. Fractional excretion of phosphorus (FePi), in contrast, is an indicator of renal phosphorus excretion relative to the concurrent serum phosphorus [25]. Hence, changes in 24-hour UPE and/or FePi may be more informative measures than serum phosphorus for understanding imbalances in phosphate homeostasis and may serve as more useful surrogate markers in clinical practice [26,27].

Evidently, certain limitations are present in the assessment of dietary phosphorus intake. Therefore, in understanding the potential role excess dietary phosphorus intake may play in contributing to increased CV events and mortality, an appreciation of the associations between both serum and urinary phosphorus levels with such outcomes is needed.

8.3 SERUM PHOSPHORUS: ASSOCIATIONS WITH MORTALITY AND CARDIOVASCULAR OUTCOMES

Over the last decade, there has been an increasing awareness of the independent association between increasing serum phosphorus levels and adverse outcomes. Several large epidemiological studies have evaluated this relationship in the general population, and more studies with modest-sized cohorts have substantiated these associations in the CKD population [28] as phosphorus control is progressively dysregulated with worsening kidney function.

Observational studies report a significant linear relationship between higher serum phosphorus studies and all-cause mortality, with hazard ratios (HRs) between 1.23 and 1.27 [28–32]. In the largest study of 4127 participants with prior myocardial infarction from the Cholesterol and Recurrent Events (CARE) study, post hoc analysis revealed HR of 1.27 (95% CI 1.02–1.58) per 1 mg/dL increase in serum phosphorus [29]. In those with CKD, a large meta-analysis, including 13 studies with 92,345 subjects, indicated an 18% increased risk in death per 1 mg/dL increase in serum phosphorus [33]. Smaller studies in kidney transplant recipients have also reported similar associations between high phosphorus levels and higher mortality risk, although these findings have not been consistent [28,32].

Measureable cardiac outcomes in relation to serum phosphorus that have been studied in both the general population and those with CKD include left ventricular hypertrophy (LVH), heart failure, and coronary artery calcification (CAC). Two large prospective studies in the general population with follow-up periods spanning up to two decades provide persuasive evidence of the strong association between serum phosphorus and CV outcomes [6–9].

The Framingham Offspring Study, with 3,368 participants without CKD or CVD, followed for 20 years (median 16.1 years), demonstrated an increase in CV events with an HR of 1.31 (95% CI 1.05–1.63) per 1 mg/dL increase in serum phosphorus. This was a composite of all CV events, including heart attacks, angina, stroke, peripheral vascular disease, and heart failure [6]. Assessing individuals in the same cohort in a cross-sectional nature, elevated serum phosphorus levels correlated with increased left ventricular mass, and longitudinally every 1 mg/dL increase in serum phosphorus was associated with 1.74-fold risk of heart failure (95% CI 1.28–3.40) [7].

Similarly, the Coronary Artery Risk Development in Young Adults (CARDIA) study, which recruited over 4000 healthy young adults followed at prespecified intervals up to 15 years, also reported an association between serum phosphorus and CV outcomes [8,9]. Echocardiography after five-year follow-up showed baseline serum phosphorus levels were associated with LVH, with an odds ratio (OR) of 1.27 (95% CI 1.09–1.47) per standard deviation of serum phosphorus [8]. Of those who returned for the 15-year follow-up examination, 3015 participants underwent computed tomography, and serum phosphorus was significantly associated with CAC, OR 1.17 (95% CI 1.01–1.34) per every 0.5 mg/dL increase in phosphorus [9].

Post hoc analysis of the CARE study (individuals with preexisting cardiac history) also described a graded relationship between higher serum phosphorus levels, with increased risk of incident heart failure and myocardial infarction [29]. In those with CKD, the relationship was even stronger. In the largest single-center prospective study involving 1203 CKD patients, the Chronic Renal Insufficiency Standards Implementation Study (CRISIS) observed within a shorter time frame (mean follow-up of 1051 days) a 50% increase in CV mortality (HR 1.5, 95% CI 1.2–2.0) for every 1 mg/dL increase in phosphorus, where CVD was inclusive of prior heart attack, coronary bypass surgery, coronary angioplasty, stroke, angina, and peripheral vascular disease [31]. Two smaller studies of CKD participants also reported an increased risk of vascular calcification within the coronary arteries and cardiac valves and greater left ventricular mass with higher serum phosphorus levels [34,35].

Cohesively, these data highlight a robust relationship between elevated serum phosphorus levels and poorer outcomes, namely all-cause mortality and CVD, and this seems to be the case for those with prior CVD, known CKD, and the general population.

8.4 URINARY PHOSPHORUS: ASSOCIATIONS WITH MORTALITY AND CARDIOVASCULAR OUTCOMES

Measurement of urinary phosphorus is often considered to be reliable in assessing dietary phosphorus absorption, and UPE has been used in various studies to determine the effect on absorption from phosphorus-lowering interventions, including dietary modification and phosphorus binder administration [22,23,36–38].

Measurements of urinary phosphorus, both total 24-hour UPE and FePi, have been evaluated with regard to associations between phosphorus excretion and mortality and CV outcomes [24,25]. The findings, however, are arguably less convincing than data related to serum phosphorus. Dominguez et al. reported no association between spot urine FePi and all-cause or CV mortality in

Dietary Phosphorus Intake and Cardiotoxicity

1325 community-dwelling older men followed up for a median period of 9.3 years [25]. In another study, higher UPE, measured using 24-hour urine collection in a U.S. population cohort, was associated with a lower risk of CV events. This study, with 880 participants followed for a median of 7.4 years, also showed a nonsignificant association between UPE and mortality [24]. Prevalent CVD was a prerequisite, and notably no association between serum phosphorus and CV events was seen. This may explain the inverse relationship between UPE and CV events and suggest other factors contributing to UPE in various settings that are beyond the scope of this discussion [24].

The inherent difficulty in trying to draw any conclusions from these studies is the inability to standardize measurements used. In the first study, a spot urine collection was performed, whereas in the second a 24-hour urine collection was undertaken. Further, the drawback of these studies relate to generalizability, as both were gender biased, with the first specifically studying males and in the second over 80% of the participants were male [24,25]. These limitations reduce the applicability of results to the wider community but also restrict our interpretation of the findings with respect to the relationship between urinary phosphorus measurements and dietary phosphorus intake.

8.5 DIETARY PHOSPHORUS INTAKE: IS TOO MUCH BAD?

Associations between phosphorus and CV events thus far have been compelling for serum phosphorus levels and less convincing with urinary phosphorus values. Remembering that phosphorus homeostasis is complex and involves incompletely understood pathways, there are other unknown factors still to be considered in evaluation of the data. In examining the existing literature on dietary phosphorus intake and clinical endpoints, differences in various methods used to estimate dietary phosphorus content and intake must also be noted (Table 8.1).

8.6 INTAKE AND MORTALITY/CARDIOVASCULAR OUTCOMES

Utilizing in-person 24-hour dietary recall, one prospective study from the NHANES III cohort (9686 participants, median follow-up of 14.7 years) reported that higher phosphorus intake was associated with all-cause mortality, where absolute phosphorus intake ≥1400 mg/d conferred an adjusted HR of 1.89 (95% CI 1.03–3.46) for every 1-unit increase in natural-logarithm (phosphorus intake). Phosphorus intakes below 1400 mg/d were not associated with mortality [13]. Evaluation of the data using phosphorus density demonstrated an association with reduced mortality below the fifth percentile (<0.35 mg/kcal), with an adjusted HR of 0.46 (95% CI 0.24–0.89) per 0.1 mg/kcal increase in phosphorus density, but no association between mortality and phosphorus density ≥0.35 mg/kcal [13]. Similarly, a significant association was seen with lower phosphorus density with reduced CV mortality, although there was no association between CV mortality and absolute phosphorus intake [13]. The addition of serum phosphorus values to these analyses did not change the associations.

Subanalysis of NHANES III, which included only subjects with impaired renal function with an estimated glomerular filtration rate (eGFR) below 60 mL/min/1.73 m^2 (1105 participants), interestingly displayed a lower risk of death associated with higher phosphorus intake, although the association was attenuated after adjusting for demographics, eGFR, other comorbidities, and potential confounders [39]. This study also reported that high dietary phosphorus levels were associated with a very modest increase in serum phosphorus levels.

More recently a post hoc analysis of the Modification of Diet in Renal Disease (MDRD) study, which investigated the relationship between dietary phosphorus intake and hard clinical endpoints in patients with CKD stages 3 to 5, also reported no significant association between baseline dietary phosphorus intake and incidence of end-stage kidney disease, CVD, or mortality [41]. In this study, Cox proportional hazards models were used to assess 24-hour UPE with various outcomes in the MDRD cohort: 795 participants with mean GFR 33 ± 12 mL/min/1.73 m^2. Of note, dietary phosphorus in this study was not associated with serum phosphorus, but serum levels were associated with all-cause mortality (HR 1.15 [95% CI 1.01–1.30] per 0.7 mg/dL higher level).

TABLE 8.1
Observational Studies Reporting Associations between Dietary Phosphorus Intake and Clinical Outcomes and Surrogate Markers of Cardiovascular Disease

Study	Population	Study Design	Outcome	Findings
Chang et al. [13]	NHANES III ($n = 9,686$)	Prospective, median 14.7 yr FU	Mortality	Higher phosphorus intake (>1400 mg/d) associated with all-cause mortality (HR 1.89 [95% CI 1.03–3.46]) for every 1-unit increase in natural log phosphorus intake)
Murtaugh et al. [39]	Sub-analysis of NHANES III (eGFR <60 mL/min) ($n = 1,105$)	Prospective	Mortality	Higher phosphorus intake (>1400 mg/d) associated with all-cause mortality (HR 1.89 [95% CI 1.03–3.46]) for every 1-unit increase in natural log phosphorus intake)
Noori et al. [40]	Dialysis patients ($n = 224$)	Prospective, 5 yr FU	Mortality	All-cause mortality associated with higher dietary intake (HR 2.37 [95% CI 1.01–6.32]) and higher phosphorus-to-protein ratio
Selamet et al. [41]	MDRD study, CKD stages 3–4 ($n = 795$)	Prospective (RCT), mean 16 yr FU	Mortality	No association between mortality and dietary phosphorus (assessed by UPE)
Alonso et al. [42]	ARIC and MESA cohorts ($n = 13,444$)	Prospective, mean 6.2 yr FU	BP	Higher phosphorus intake associated with lower incidence of hypertension, after adjustment for non-dietary factors (no significant association when adjusted for dietary factors)
Kwak et al. [43]	Korean participants, normal kidney function ($n = 23,652$)	Cross-sectional	CAC	No association between CAC and dietary phosphorus intake
Yamamoto et al. [44]	MESA study ($n = 4,494$)	Cross-sectional	LVH	20% increase in dietary phosphorus intake associated with 1.1 g greater LVH (measured by MRI)
Gutierrez et al. [45]	Health Professionals Follow-up study ($n = 1,261$)	Cross-sectional	FGF23	Every 500 mg increase in dietary phosphorus associated with 3.4 RU/mL increase in FGF23
Isakova et al. [46]	CRIC ($n = 3,879$)	Cross-sectional	FGF23	No association between FGF23 and dietary phosphorus

Note: BP, blood pressure; CAC, coronary artery calcification; eGFR, estimated glomerular filtration rate; FGF23, fibroblast growth factor-23; FU, follow-up; LVH, left ventricular hypertrophy; MRI, magnetic resonance imaging; RCT, randomized controlled trial; UPE, urinary phosphorus excretion.

On the contrary, in a smaller cohort study involving 224 prevalent CKD patients undergoing maintenance hemodialysis and followed for up to five years, all-cause mortality was elevated with both higher dietary phosphorus intake and higher phosphorus-to-protein ratio [40]. An HR of 2.37 (95% CI 1.01–6.32) was reported between the highest tertile of dietary phosphorus intake compared to a reference group with the lowest tertile of dietary phosphorus intake. Nutrient intake was estimated from the unmodified 152 multiple-choice Block FFQ. Notably, the FFQ had not previously been validated for use in hemodialysis patients [40].

In the Multi-Ethnic Study of Atherosclerosis (MESA), a large cross-sectional study of 4494 participants, dietary phosphorus intake was estimated using the 120-item modified Block FFQ and was associated with left ventricular mass in a population of community-based individuals. After multivariable adjustment, each 20% increase in dietary phosphorus intake was associated with 1.1 g greater LVH on magnetic resonance imaging (Figure 8.1) [44]. The mean estimated dietary phosphorus intake in this study was 1167 mg/d in men and 1017 mg/d in women. Interestingly, higher dietary phosphorus intake was associated with greater odds of LVH among women, but not men, and the highest gender-specific dietary phosphorus quintile was associated with an estimated 6.1 g greater left ventricular mass compared with the lowest quintile.

The association between dietary phosphorus intake and blood pressure was assessed by Alonso et al. in a cross-sectional study of 13,444 participants combined from the MESA cohort and the Atherosclerosis Risk in Communities (ARIC) cohort [42]. Associations with baseline blood pressure, as well as the incidence of hypertension, were evaluated in this study, and the investigators found that, compared with individuals in the lowest quintile of phosphorus intake, those in the highest quintile had lower systolic and diastolic blood pressure after adjustment for potential confounders. Higher dietary phosphorus intake was also associated with a lower risk of development of future hypertension after adjustment for nondietary factors, although this association was no longer significant after adjustment for dietary factors. Therefore, this study suggested there was no significant relationship between dietary phosphorus and hypertension, with a possible signal for a protective effect of higher phosphorus intake against developing hypertension.

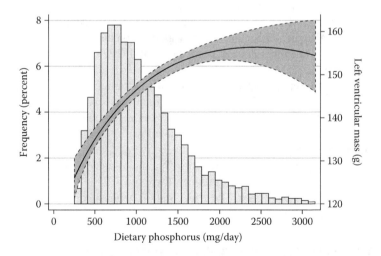

FIGURE 8.1 Functional association of left ventricular mass with estimated dietary phosphorus. In the upper panel, solid and dashed lines depict mean and 95% confidence intervals for left ventricular mass, respectively, by the amount of dietary phosphorus intake. Values were obtained from an unadjusted fractional polynomial linear regression model that included 99% of the study data (dietary phosphorus values <3162 mg/day). In the lower panel, the frequency histogram depicts the distribution of dietary phosphorus consumption across the MESA study population. (From Yamamoto, K.T. et al., *Kidney Int.*, 83, 707–14, 2013. With permission.)

The relationship between dietary phosphorus intake and CAC was assessed in a cross-sectional study of 23,652 Korean participants with normal kidney function and no previous CVD [43]. Self-administered FFQs (assessing eating habits over the previous year) and cardiac computed tomography were performed as part of a health check-up in participating individuals, and there was no significant association between dietary phosphorus (or calcium intake) and CAC in this study. There was also no association between dietary phosphorus and serum phosphorus levels; however, elevated serum phosphorus levels were associated with increasing CAC scores. Lack of a relationship between dietary data and CAC was thought by the authors to result from dietary information collected at one time point not reflecting the long-standing pathological process contributing to vascular disease or because the mean consumption of daily phosphorus intake in this study (810 mg/d for men and 848 mg/d for women) was relatively low compared to Western diets [43].

8.7 INTAKE WITH FIBROBLAST GROWTH FACTOR-23

FGF23 has emerged over the last decade, described not only as a phosphotonin-increasing urinary phosphorus excretion and reducing absorption of phosphorus absorption (through reduction in vitamin D activity), but also as a potential pathogenic factor with significant independent associations with all-cause mortality and CV outcomes [47,48]. These associations were stronger than previously reported with serum phosphorus and suggested that FGF23 was indicative of phosphorus dysregulation and perhaps a better biomarker. Further, in vitro studies have implicated FGF23 as a potential pathogenic factor contributing to cardiac toxicity and suggest a causal role beyond being a biomarker of phosphorus dysregulation [49,50]. Hence, the association between dietary phosphorus intake and FGF23 levels should also be considered.

Numerous observational and interventional studies in the last decade have explored associations between dietary phosphorus intake and FGF23 levels, although with conflicting results. In one cross-sectional study, 1261 male participants of the Health Professionals Follow-Up Study were evaluated for dietary intake, recorded with a self-administered FFQ (of more than 130 food items), and for every 500 mg increase in dietary phosphorus there was an associated 3.4 RU/mL increase in FGF23 levels [45]. In contrast, a study by Isakova et al. showed no association between FGF23 and estimated phosphorus intake in nearly 4000 participants of the Chronic Renal Insufficiency Cohort (CRIC) Study [46]. Another study involving 74 patients with CKD, using four-day dietary records for dietary assessment, also did not demonstrate any association between dietary phosphorus intake and FGF23 [51]. Of note, all three studies used the same FGF23 assay (Immutopics c-terminal FGF23 ELISA) [49,51].

One reason for the discrepancy in these studies of associations between FGF23 and dietary phosphorus could be that phosphorus intake is more strongly associated with FGF23 levels in individuals with normal kidney function than with CKD. Other metabolic disturbances, such as higher serum phosphorus levels and higher PTH, are associated with FGF23 in CKD, and this may limit the ability to detect more modest associations between dietary phosphorus intake and FGF23 in CKD. Klotho, the coreceptor for FGF23, may also be an associated factor and may provide an alternative measure of phosphorus excess, although there are relatively few data on the impact of dietary phosphorus on klotho expression. The effect of dietary phosphorus on FGF23 levels in interventional studies is discussed in Section 8.11.

8.8 SHORT-TERM DIETARY PHOSPHORUS INTERVENTIONS

To determine the potential significance of observational studies reporting associations between serum and urinary phosphorus or FGF23 levels in relation to outcomes, the effect of dietary phosphorus on these markers in interventional studies needs to be reviewed. Recent dietary intervention studies have included measurements of all serum and urinary markers [22,23,38,52–54]. Most of these studies have evaluated a combination of diets, often in cross-over study designs, including

Dietary Phosphorus Intake and Cardiotoxicity

low-phosphorus diets (with either dietary restriction and/or in combination with phosphorus binders) or high-phosphorus diets with supplementation. Studies have also been performed in both healthy volunteers and participants with CKD. Interventional studies evaluating the effect of single meals are not reviewed here.

8.9 EFFECT ON URINARY PHOSPHORUS EXCRETION

A concomitant rise or fall in urinary phosphorus excretion after administration of high- or low-phosphorus diets, respectively, was demonstrated in all except two interventional studies [22,23,38,52–54]. Excretion was measured using 24-hour urinary collections either reported as total UPE or FePi in all studies except one, where phosphorus reabsorption was determined [22,23,38,52–54]. In the latter study, Larsson et al. reported no increase in phosphorus reabsorption in six healthy men subjected to dietary restriction, calculated as approximately 870 mg/d phosphorus intake accompanied by phosphorus binders [55]. Similarly, Isakova et al. did not report any significant reduction in excretion of phosphorus with a prescribed 900 mg/d phosphorus diet, either with or without additional phosphorus binders (in this case, lanthanum carbonate), in a 2×2 factorial study of 39 participants with impaired renal function [56]. These two studies suggest that diets of 870 mg/d or 900 mg/d of phosphorus intake may not involve adequately restricted interventions [55,56]. These studies also did not include a substantially high-phosphorus diet within the cross-over designs, involving either a "normal" diet supplemented with 600 mg inorganic phosphorus or an "*ad libitum*" diet, respectively [55,56].

In other studies where dietary effects on phosphorus excretion were evident, prescribed daily dietary phosphorus restrictions ranged from 500 to 850 mg/d and phosphorus loading ranged from 2000 to 2880 mg/d [22,23,38,52–54]. Interestingly, although phosphorus intake of 850 mg/d decreased urinary excretion, this was not significant compared to baseline levels but provided a large enough separation from the high phosphorus intake values [22]. Collectively, these data imply a reduction in urinary phosphorus excretion may only be evident consistently in phosphorus diets ≤750 mg/d, whereas phosphorus loading ≥2000 mg/d could result in a significantly greater phosphaturic response.

8.10 EFFECT ON SERUM PHOSPHORUS VALUES

Inconsistent results have been reported in studies assessing the effects of dietary phosphorus on serum phosphorus levels. Not surprisingly, in both studies that did not show any effect on urinary phosphorus excretion, no effect was seen on serum phosphorus either [55,56]. There was also no associated rise or fall of serum phosphorus in any of the cross-over designed studies with respective phosphorus interventions.

Two larger studies in healthy volunteers report reduction in serum phosphorus levels with dietary restriction (both less than 600 mg/d), whereas no change was seen in serum levels with dietary phosphorus loading (≥2500 mg/d). Although there were differences in study design and dietary guidance and preparation, both studies also achieved the lowest dietary phosphorus intake values of all studies discussed [23,52]. Dietary phosphorus restrictions in other studies, ranging between 625 and 850 mg/d, showed no effect on serum phosphorus levels [22,38,53,54].

Only one study of healthy volunteers reports an elevation in serum phosphorus levels with dietary phosphorus intake of 2880 mg/day, the largest intake studied to date [22]. Ferrari et al. investigated a similar cohort with a mean daily phosphorus intake of 2860 mg, achieved using a combination of ambulatory dietary intervention with qualified dietitian guidance and 1000 mg phosphorus supplementation, but showed no difference in serum phosphorus values [23]. Interestingly, the differences between these two studies were the food preparation and source of dietary phosphorus despite similar phosphorus intake levels in the loading period [22,23]. Therefore, from these studies one may conclude that serum phosphorus is tightly regulated by normal healthy homeostatic mechanisms,

102   Dietary Phosphorus: Health, Nutrition, and Regulatory Aspects

and such pathways would only be affected at the extremes of dietary phosphorus restriction and supplementation, intakes of <600 mg/d and ≥ 2880 mg/d, respectively.

8.11 EFFECT ON FGF23 LEVELS

A few ELISA kits to measure FGF23 levels are commercially available. The two most common ones have been used in the studies discussed earlier: Immutopics c-terminal FGF23 and Kainos intact FGF23 ELISA kits. Although there are differences between these assays, with readouts that are not interchangeable, both measurements have been used in studies reporting FGF23 associations between mortality and outcomes [57,58]. In this instance, the dietary effects noted by either measure are fairly consistent.

Studies where dietary phosphorus was restricted ≤625 mg/day in healthy participants resulted in a reduction in FGF23 levels, both intact and c-terminal levels [23,52,53]. In a study of 30 CKD patients, phosphorus restriction of 750 mg/d, with or without phosphorus binders, led to decreased intact FGF23 levels; however, in healthy volunteers the same dietary restriction did not affect FGF23 levels to the same extent, and only the addition of phosphorus binders resulted in a small decrease in levels [54]. Of note, another study of four CKD patients reported no difference in c-terminal FGF23 levels with the same phosphorus restriction of 750 mg/d, with or without a phosphorus binder, although the sample size was quite small [38]. Vervloet et al. reported a small decrease in c-terminal FGF23 and no change in intact FGF23 levels with dietary phosphorus restriction of 850 mg/d in healthy individuals [22].

Dietary phosphorus loading ranging from 2000 to 2880 mg/d resulted in elevated FGF23 levels in most studies in both healthy volunteers and CKD participants [22,23,52,54]. Antoniucci et al. did not report any significant elevation of intact FGF23 levels in healthy participants who were normalized with a 1500 mg/d phosphorus diet at baseline prior to the loading phase of 2300 mg/d [53]. In another pilot study, one arm involving patients with CKD treated with a 1500 mg/d phosphorus diet showed an elevation of c-terminal FGF23 levels compared to baseline [38], suggesting that a dietary phosphorus intake of 1500 mg/d may already increase the FGF23 signal and may be inappropriate as a comparator group.

Studies with no or minimal change in FGF23 levels from dietary interventions included the two studies that did not demonstrate any effects on either urinary phosphorus excretion or serum phosphorus levels in either direction with phosphorus loading and restriction [55,56], although with the aforementioned limitations to both studies. Notably, Isakova et al. reported a mild reduction in c-terminal FGF23 levels in one group of four CKD patients treated with a 900 mg/d phosphorus diet in conjunction with a phosphorus binder.

In summary, FGF23 seems to respond more readily, compared with serum phosphorus, to dietary phosphorus intakes at ≤625 mg/d and ≥2000 mg/d. However, urinary phosphorus measurements may better reflect dietary absorption. It is important to remember that these studies are of short duration and the impact of chronic high or low phosphorus consumption beyond three months on serum and urinary parameters is unknown.

8.12 EFFECT ON ENDOTHELIAL FUNCTION AND ARTERIAL STIFFNESS

Higher serum phosphorus may impair endothelial function by increasing oxidative stress and decreasing nitric oxide production. Experimental studies report that changes in dietary phosphorus intake may also lead to endothelial dysfunction. Watari et al. demonstrated varying dietary phosphorus intake in rats impaired endothelial function via increased oxidative stress and inflammatory response [59].

In humans, one small study investigated the effects of postprandial hyperphosphatemia on endothelial function in 11 healthy men served alternate meals of 400 mg or 1200 mg phosphorus in a double-blind cross-over design [60]. Assessment of flow-mediated dilation of the brachial artery

Dietary Phosphorus Intake and Cardiotoxicity

before and two hours after each meal revealed that high dietary phosphorus increased serum phosphorus levels and was associated with decreased flow-mediated dilation. Another study of 74 CKD patients did not report any association between daily dietary phosphorus and augmentation index as a surrogate measure of arterial stiffness [51]. There was also no relationship between augmentation index and other measures of phosphorus (serum levels and 24-hour urinary excretion) in this study.

8.13 EFFECT ON VASCULAR CALCIFICATION

There are experimental studies demonstrating that greater dietary phosphorus intake contributes to worsening of vascular calcification, and dietary phosphorus restriction has the opposite effect in animal models. However, there is limited clinical evidence in humans. In a randomized controlled trial of 90 phosphorus binder-naive patients with CKD stages 3 to 5 not on dialysis, Russo et al. indirectly assessed the effect of dietary phosphorous restriction on vascular calcification [61]. Although this study was not designed to show superiority or an equivalence of dietary phosphorus modification compared with phosphorus binders, CAC scores were increased in the group receiving phosphorus-restricted diet alone and in the group receiving diet in combination with calcium carbonate as a phosphorus binder, whereas there was no progression of calcification in the diet-plus-sevelamer-treated group.

8.14 PHOSPHORUS AND PROTEIN CONSUMPTION

Dietary protein contributes significantly to the total dietary phosphorus intake; thus dietary phosphorus restriction is quite often associated with a concomitant dietary protein restriction, raising concerns that long-term phosphorus restriction may be harmful. One large study of 30,075 prevalent hemodialysis patients was conducted measuring serum phosphorus and normalized protein nitrogen appearance (nPNA) as a surrogate for protein intake assessment [62]. Although this study lacks direct assessment of dietary phosphorus or protein, given the observational nature of the large database analysis, the size of the study population suggested a potential harm of protein/phosphorus restriction using surrogate markers in a cohort that often is prescribed dietary restrictions. Over a three-year period, higher baseline nPNA was associated with lower mortality, and baseline serum phosphorus displayed a J-shaped association, with values lower than 3.5 mg/dL and higher than 4.5 mg/dL related to increased mortality [62]. When assessed together, patients with high nPNA and low serum phosphorus had a better outcome, whereas those with reduced nPNA and concurrent high phosphorus had the worst outcomes. The findings of this study suggest that potential harms of protein restriction may outweigh potential benefits in phosphorus restriction, and further investigation is needed to improve dietary advice in dialysis, as well as to address this issue in the general population.

Two smaller studies have evaluated biochemical changes in relation to changes in protein intake [63,64]. In a short-term study of 19 healthy volunteers provided with low-protein, isocaloric high-protein and *ad libitum* high-protein diets sequentially, no significant changes were seen in PTH or vitamin D metabolites, although a small decrease in intact FGF23 was seen at the end of the two-week isocaloric high-protein diet compared to the end of the two-week low-protein diet. The respective mean dietary phosphorus intakes for the three different dietary interventions within this study were 1556, 2071, and 1622 mg/d. No serum or urine phosphorus measurements were performed in this study [63]. In contrast, a prospective short-term study in 32 non-dialysis-dependent CKD patients evaluated a low-protein diet and a very-low-protein diet, with each undertaken for one week. Patients received considerable education over a three-month run-in period on food preparation, food choices, and salt reduction. The phosphorus compositions in these two diets were 600 to 700 mg/d and 350 to 420 mg/d in the low-protein and very-low-protein diets, respectively. In keeping with the separation of phosphorus consumption, urinary phosphorus excretion, serum phosphorus values, and FGF23 levels were lower at the end of the very-low-protein diet period [64].

104 Dietary Phosphorus: Health, Nutrition, and Regulatory Aspects

One important study by Moe et al. evaluated the differences between meat-based and vegetarian-based diets, suggesting that vegetarian sources may be more beneficial than meat-based sources of protein [65]. Nine CKD patients (mean eGFR 32 mL/min) were provided with the two different diets for one week, each with an intervening 2- to 4-week washout period. Both diets provided similar dietary phosphorus content (~800 mg/d). Serum phosphorus values were marginally lower, FGF23 levels were significantly lower, and PTH was higher with the vegetarian diet when compared to the meat-based diet. Both diets resulted in a lower urinary phosphorus excretion compared to preintervention values; urinary phosphorus values with the vegetarian diet were not significantly lower than the meat-based values. It is likely both diets provided lower phosphorus content than the expected phosphorus content in the average diet, resulting in the lower values seen after either intervention [65]. The higher PTH value may have reflected the marginally higher calcium content in the vegetarian diet (1310 mg/d) compared with the meat-based diet (1176 mg/d) or may have reflected the phytate content of the vegetarian diet possibly affecting calcium absorption.

No clear conclusion is possible from published literature to date with reference to low- or high-protein diets, although a vegetarian diet may provide benefits beyond a predominantly meat-based diet. Larger, longer-term studies assessing different-quantity protein diets from different sources, meat or vegetarian, to determine long-term outcomes are required before any changes to clinical practice and dietary advice are made, not just for subjects at risk such as those with CKD but also for the general population.

8.15 CAN MODIFYING DIETARY PHOSPHORUS AFFECT OUTCOMES?

Although there are robust data linking elevated serum phosphorus with mortality and CV outcomes, causality has not been determined. And although dietary phosphorus loading has been reported in some studies to weakly affect serum phosphorus levels, the reverse—that dietary phosphorus restriction can lower serum phosphorus levels—is not as convincing. The potential independent effect of dietary phosphorus restriction on mortality or CV outcomes needs to be considered; however, there are limited data, apart from observational studies described earlier, addressing associations. There are no prospective studies examining the effect of dietary phosphorus interventions on hard clinical endpoints. It may be unlikely that a study would be conducted to address this issue, as long-term (> 12 month) dietary interventions can be practically difficult. Any study in healthy volunteers would also be difficult to conduct, as the probability of CV events or changes in CV endpoints, such as LVH, within a short time frame is low, necessitating larger study populations and long duration of follow-up.

Studies examining the effects of phosphorus binder therapy on mortality and CV outcomes in the CKD population may be more readily achieved. Phosphorus binders, together with regular dietitian review, are part of routine care in patients with end-stage kidney disease, where phosphate dysregulation occurs resulting in elevated serum phosphorus levels. Currently available binders bind dietary phosphorus within the gastrointestinal tract, either forming an insoluble compound or binding to a resin, thus allowing less phosphorus to be available for absorption and resulting in lower overall dietary phosphorus intake.

A recent large systematic review involving 4622 patients from 11 randomized studies observed a 22% reduction in mortality in dialysis patients assigned non-calcium-based binders compared to calcium-based binders [66]. The effect on mortality was similar in nonrandomized studies analyzed in this systematic review, as well as between dialysis and nondialysis patients separately. CAC was also reduced in patients prescribed non–calcium-based binders compared to calcium-based binders, but CV events were not reported in most studies analyzed. No prospective study in dialysis patients, however, has assessed the effect of phosphorus binders in a placebo-controlled design on hard outcomes.

In nondialysis CKD patients, only three placebo-controlled randomized clinical trials have been published to date assessing the use of phosphorus binders to reduce absorption of dietary phosphorus and evaluating surrogate CV endpoints [36,67,68]. Block et al. reported in 148 CKD subjects

Dietary Phosphorus Intake and Cardiotoxicity

that use of phosphorus binders over nine months lowered serum and urinary phosphorus and attenuated progression of secondary hyperparathyroidism, although with no change in FGF23 levels [36]. The main concerning finding in this study was a significant increase in calcification of the coronary arteries and abdominal aorta with the use of binders compared to placebo, although this was predominantly in the group administered calcium-based binders. Chue et al. found no significant differences between sevelamer and placebo with regard to LV mass, systolic and diastolic function, or pulse wave velocity in 109 CKD subjects after 40 weeks; however, only 56% of subjects took ≥80% of the prescribed therapy [67]. In the compliant subgroup, treatment with sevelamer was associated with lower urinary excretion of phosphorus and serum FGF23, although again binder use was not associated with CV outcomes of interest such as LVH or arterial compliance. In a smaller study of 38 CKD patients, Seifert et al. reported no differences between lanthanum and placebo over 12 months with respect to serum or urinary phosphorus or surrogate CV markers of pulse wave velocity, carotid artery intima-media thickness, or vascular calcification [68].

A newer approach to lower phosphorus absorption may be by inhibition of the electroneutral sodium/hydrogen exchangers (NHE), in particular NHE3. The NHE3 inhibitor tenapanor has been shown to reduce enteric phosphorus absorption in rats and prevent vascular calcification [69], although clinical studies evaluating benefits on CV outcomes in humans are pending.

In summary, despite the epidemiological data linking serum phosphorus and dietary phosphorus and CV outcomes, clinical trials are lacking to support the effect of either reduction in dietary phosphorus intake or the use of phosphorus binders on CV endpoints.

8.16 CONCLUSIONS

There is a plethora of emerging observational evidence showing a strong association between serum phosphorous and FGF23 with increased all-cause mortality and CV burden. However, it is not known whether elevated levels of phosphorus and FGF23 are mere biomarkers of CVD and mortality or play a causative role in the pathogenesis. The epidemiological data are bolstered by many laboratory studies that show a role of phosphorus to induce vascular calcification and endothelial dysfunction. Increasingly, experimental studies report that dietary phosphorus intake in excess may significantly disrupt hormonal regulation of phosphorus, calcium, and vitamin D, contributing to disordered mineral metabolism, vascular calcification, endothelial dysfunction, and the potential for increased CVD and mortality. Few population studies, however, link dietary phosphorus intake to changes in serum phosphorus levels, which may reflect inherent circadian fluctuation in serum phosphorus or the inaccuracies in determining dietary phosphorus intake accurately.

A lack of reliable biomarkers of the effects of dietary phosphorus on CV health may also explain the inconclusive link between dietary phosphorus and cardiotoxicity, although disordered regulation of PTH, FGF23, and klotho by high dietary phosphorus may represent key factors contributing to atherosclerosis and increased CVD. There is a lack of evidence, however, evaluating the potential benefits of modification of dietary phosphorus, either through reduced intake with dietary restriction or with reduced absorption with the use of phosphorus binders. On the contrary, an extremely low phosphorus intake in conjunction with low protein intake may be associated with worse outcome. Large randomized controlled trials are needed to prove or disprove the benefits, risks, and potential economic impact of introducing dietary phosphorus-lowering therapy on CVD.

REFERENCES

1. Berndt, T. and R. Kumar. Phosphatonins and the regulation of phosphate homeostasis. *Annu Rev Physiol.* 2007; 69:341–59.
2. Bergwitz, C. and H. Juppner. Phosphate sensing. *Adv Chronic Kidney Dis.* 2011; 18(2):132–44.
3. Tan, S.J., E.R. Smith, T.D. Hewitson, S.G. Holt, and N.D. Toussaint. The importance of klotho in phosphate metabolism and kidney disease. *Nephrology (Carlton).* 2014; 19(8):439–49.

4. Block, G.A., T.E. Hulbert-Shearon, N.W. Levin, and F.K. Port. Association of serum phosphorus and calcium x phosphate product with mortality risk in chronic hemodialysis patients: A national study. *Am J Kidney Dis.* 1998; 31(4):607–17.

5. Block, G.A., P.S. Klassen, J.M. Lazarus, N. Ofsthun, E.G. Lowrie, and G.M. Chertow. Mineral metabolism, mortality, and morbidity in maintenance hemodialysis. *J Am Soc Nephrol.* 2004; 15(8):2208–18.

6. Dhingra, R., L.M. Sullivan, C.S. Fox, T.J. Wang, R.B. D'Agostino, Sr., J.M. Gaziano, and R.S. Vasan. Relations of serum phosphorus and calcium levels to the incidence of cardiovascular disease in the community. *Arch Intern Med.* 2007; 167(9):879–85.

7. Dhingra, R., P. Gona, E.J. Benjamin, T.J. Wang, J. Aragam, R.B. D'Agostino, Sr., W.B. Kannel, and R.S. Vasan. Relations of serum phosphorus levels to echocardiographic left ventricular mass and incidence of heart failure in the community. *Eur J Heart Fail.* 2010; 12(8):812–8.

8. Foley, R.N., A.J. Collins, C.A. Herzog, A. Ishani, and P.A. Kalra. Serum phosphate and left ventricular hypertrophy in young adults: The coronary artery risk development in young adults study. *Kidney Blood Press Res.* 2009; 32(1):37–44.

9. Foley, R.N., A.J. Collins, C.A. Herzog, A. Ishani, and P.A. Kalra. Serum phosphorus levels associate with coronary atherosclerosis in young adults. *J Am Soc Nephrol.* 2009; 20(2):397–404.

10. O'Seaghdha, C.M., S.J. Hwang, P. Muntner, M.L. Melamed, and C.S. Fox. Serum phosphorus predicts incident chronic kidney disease and end-stage renal disease. *Nephrol Dial Transplant.* 2011; 26(9):2885–90.

11. Calvo, M.S. and Y.K. Park. Changing phosphorus content of the U.S. diet: Potential for adverse effects on bone. *J Nutr.* 1996; 126(4 Suppl):1168S–80S.

12. Uribarri, J. Phosphorus homeostasis in normal health and in chronic kidney disease patients with special emphasis on dietary phosphorus intake. *Semin Dial.* 2007; 20(4):295–301.

13. Chang, A.R., M. Lazo, L.J. Appel, O.M. Gutierrez, and M.E. Grams. High dietary phosphorus intake is associated with all-cause mortality: Results from NHANES III. *Am J Clin Nutr.* 2014; 99(2):320–7. "(erratum Am J Clin Nutr 105:1021-2.)"

14. Block, G., A.M. Hartman, C.M. Dresser, M.D. Carroll, J. Gannon, and L. Gardner. A data-based approach to diet questionnaire design and testing. *Am J Epidemiol.* 1986; 124(3):453–69.

15. Block, G., F.E. Thompson, A.M. Hartman, F.A. Larkin, and K.E. Guire. Comparison of two dietary questionnaires validated against multiple dietary records collected during a 1-year period. *J Am Diet Assoc.* 1992; 92(6):686–93.

16. Block, G., M. Woods, A. Potosky, and C. Clifford. Validation of a self-administered diet history questionnaire using multiple diet records. *J Clin Epidemiol.* 1990; 43(12):1327–35.

17. Day, N., N. McKeown, M. Wong, A. Welch, and S. Bingham. Epidemiological assessment of diet: A comparison of a 7-day diary with a food frequency questionnaire using urinary markers of nitrogen, potassium and sodium. *Int J Epidemiol.* 2001; 30(2):309–17.

18. de Boer, I.H., T.C. Rue, and B. Kestenbaum. Serum phosphorus concentrations in the third National Health and Nutrition Examination Survey (NHANES III). *Am J Kidney Dis.* 2009; 53(3):399–407.

19. Ix, J.H., C.A. Anderson, G. Smits, M.S. Persky, and G.A. Block. Effect of dietary phosphate intake on the circadian rhythm of serum phosphate concentrations in chronic kidney disease: A crossover study. *Am J Clin Nutr.* 2014; 100(5):1392–7.

20. Portale, A.A., B.P. Halloran, and R.C. Morris, Jr. Dietary intake of phosphorus modulates the circadian rhythm in serum concentration of phosphorus. Implications for the renal production of 1,25-dihydroxyvitamin D. *J Clin Invest.* 1987; 80(4):1147–54.

21. Calvo, M.S., R. Kumar, and H. Heath, 3rd. Elevated secretion and action of serum parathyroid hormone in young adults consuming high phosphorus, low calcium diets assembled from common foods. *J Clin Endocrinol Metab.* 1988; 66(4):823–9.

22. Vervloet, M.G., F.J. van Ittersum, R.M. Buttler, A.C. Heijboer, M.A. Blankenstein, and P.M. ter Wee. Effects of dietary phosphate and calcium intake on fibroblast growth factor-23. *Clin J Am Soc Nephrol.* 2011; 6(2):383–9.

23. Ferrari, S.L., J.P. Bonjour, and R. Rizzoli. Fibroblast growth factor-23 relationship to dietary phosphate and renal phosphate handling in healthy young men. *J Clin Endocrinol Metab.* 2005; 90(3):1519–24.

24. Palomino, H.L., D.E. Rifkin, C. Anderson, M.H. Criqui, M.A. Whooley, and J.H. Ix. 24-hour urine phosphorus excretion and mortality and cardiovascular events. *Clin J Am Soc Nephrol.* 2013; 8(7):1202–10.

25. Dominguez, J.R., B. Kestenbaum, M. Chonchol, G. Block, G.A. Laughlin, C.E. Lewis, R. Katz, E. Barrett-Connor, S. Cummings, E.S. Orwoll, J.H. Ix, and Osteoporotic Fractures in Men Study Research. Relationships between serum and urine phosphorus with all-cause and cardiovascular mortality: The Osteoporotic Fractures in Men (MrOS) Study. *Am J Kidney Dis.* 2013; 61(4):555–63.

26. Oliveira, R.B., A.L. Cancela, F.G. Graciolli, L.M. Dos Reis, S.A. Draibe, L. Cuppari, A.B. Carvalho, V. Jorgetti, M.E. Canziani, and R.M. Moyses. Early control of PTH and FGF23 in normophosphatemic CKD patients: A new target in CKD-MBD therapy? *Clin J Am Soc Nephrol*. 2010; 5(2):286–91.

27. Block, G.A., M.S. Persky, M. Ketteler, B. Kestenbaum, R. Thadhani, L. Kooienga, D. Spiegel, J. Asplin, J. Ehrlich, V. Dennis, A. Nissenson, G.M. Chertow, and D.C. Wheeler. A randomized double-blind pilot study of serum phosphorus normalization in chronic kidney disease: A new paradigm for clinical outcomes studies in nephrology. *Hemodial Int*. 2009; 13(3):360–2.

28. Toussaint, N.D., E. Pedagogos, S.J. Tan, S.V. Badve, C.M. Hawley, V. Perkovic, and G.J. Elder. Phosphate in early chronic kidney disease: Associations with clinical outcomes and a target to reduce cardiovascular risk. *Nephrology (Carlton)*. 2012; 17(5):433–44.

29. Tonelli, M., F. Sacks, M. Pfeffer, Z. Gao, G. Curhan, Cholesterol, and Recurrent Events Trial. Relation between serum phosphate level and cardiovascular event rate in people with coronary disease. *Circulation*. 2005; 112(17):2627–33.

30. Kestenbaum, B., J.N. Sampson, K.D. Rudser, D.J. Patterson, S.L. Seliger, B. Young, D.J. Sherrard, and D.L. Andress. Serum phosphate levels and mortality risk among people with chronic kidney disease. *J Am Soc Nephrol*. 2005; 16(2):520–8.

31. Eddington, H., R. Hoefield, S. Sinha, C. Chrysochou, B. Lane, R.N. Foley, J. Hegarty, J. New, D.J. O'Donoghue, R.J. Middleton, and P.A. Kalra. Serum phosphate and mortality in patients with chronic kidney disease. *Clin J Am Soc Nephrol*. 2010; 5(12):2251–7.

32. Moore, J., C.R. Tomson, M. Tessa Savage, R. Borrows, and C.J. Ferro. Serum phosphate and calcium concentrations are associated with reduced patient survival following kidney transplantation. *Clin Transplant*. 2011; 25(3):406–16.

33. Palmer, S.C., A. Hayen, P. Macaskill, F. Pellegrini, J.C. Craig, G.J. Elder, and G.F. Strippoli. Serum levels of phosphorus, parathyroid hormone, and calcium and risks of death and cardiovascular disease in individuals with chronic kidney disease: A systematic review and meta-analysis. *JAMA*. 2011; 305(11):1119–27.

34. Chue, C.D., N.C. Edwards, W.E. Moody, R.P. Steeds, J.N. Townend, and C.J. Ferro. Serum phosphate is associated with left ventricular mass in patients with chronic kidney disease: A cardiac magnetic resonance study. *Heart*. 2012; 98(3):219–24.

35. Adeney, K.L., D.S. Siscovick, J.H. Ix, S.L. Seliger, M.G. Shlipak, N.S. Jenny, and B.R. Kestenbaum. Association of serum phosphate with vascular and valvular calcification in moderate CKD. *J Am Soc Nephrol*. 2009; 20(2):381–7.

36. Block, G.A., D.C. Wheeler, M.S. Persky, B. Kestenbaum, M. Ketteler, D.M. Spiegel, M.A. Allison, J. Asplin, G. Smits, A.N. Hoofnagle, L. Kooienga, R. Thadhani, M. Mannstadt, M. Wolf, and G.M. Chertow. Effects of phosphate binders in moderate CKD. *J Am Soc Nephrol*. 2012; 23(8):1407–15.

37. Gonzalez-Parra, E., M.L. Gonzalez-Casaus, A. Galan, A. Martinez-Calero, V. Navas, M. Rodriguez, and A. Ortiz. Lanthanum carbonate reduces FGF23 in chronic kidney disease Stage 3 patients. *Nephrol Dial Transplant*. 2011; 26(8):2567–71.

38. Isakova, T., O.M. Gutierrez, K. Smith, M. Epstein, L.K. Keating, H. Juppner, and M. Wolf. Pilot study of dietary phosphorus restriction and phosphorus binders to target fibroblast growth factor 23 in patients with chronic kidney disease. *Nephrol Dial Transplant*. 2011; 26(2):584–91.

39. Murtaugh, M.A., R. Filipowicz, B.C. Baird, G. Wei, T. Greene, and S. Beddhu. Dietary phosphorus intake and mortality in moderate chronic kidney disease: NHANES III. *Nephrol Dial Transplant*. 2012; 27(3):990–6.

40. Noori, N., K. Kalantar-Zadeh, C.P. Kovesdy, R. Bross, D. Benner, and J.D. Kopple. Association of dietary phosphorus intake and phosphorus to protein ratio with mortality in hemodialysis patients. *Clin J Am Soc Nephrol*. 2010; 5(4):683–92.

41. Selamet, U., H. Tighiouart, M.J. Sarnak, G. Beck, A.S. Levey, G. Block, and J.H. Ix. Relationship of dietary phosphate intake with risk of end-stage renal disease and mortality in chronic kidney disease stages 3-5: The Modification of Diet in Renal Disease Study. *Kidney Int*. 2016; 89(1):176–84.

42. Alonso, A., J.A. Nettleton, J.H. Ix, I.H. de Boer, A.R. Folsom, A. Bidulescu, B.R. Kestenbaum, L.E. Chambless, and D.R. Jacobs, Jr. Dietary phosphorus, blood pressure, and incidence of hypertension in the atherosclerosis risk in communities study and the multi-ethnic study of atherosclerosis. *Hypertension*. 2010; 55(3):776–84.

43. Kwak, S.M., J.S. Kim, Y. Choi, Y. Chang, M.J. Kwon, J.G. Jung, C. Jeong, J. Ahn, H.S. Kim, H. Shin, and S. Ryu. Dietary intake of calcium and phosphorus and serum concentration in relation to the risk of coronary artery calcification in asymptomatic adults. *Arterioscler Thromb Vasc Biol*. 2014; 34(8):1763–9.

44. Yamamoto, K.T., C. Robinson-Cohen, M.C. de Oliveira, A. Kostina, J.A. Nettleton, J.H. Ix, H. Nguyen, J. Eng, J.A. Lima, D.S. Siscovick, N.S. Weiss, and B. Kestenbaum. Dietary phosphorus is associated with greater left ventricular mass. *Kidney Int*. 2013; 83(4):707–14.

45. Gutierrez, O.M., M. Wolf, and E.N. Taylor. Fibroblast growth factor 23, cardiovascular disease risk factors, and phosphorus intake in the health professionals follow-up study. *Clin J Am Soc Nephrol*. 2011; 6(12):2871–8.

46. Isakova, T., P. Wahl, G.S. Vargas, O.M. Gutierrez, J. Scialla, H. Xie, D. Appleby, L. Nessel, K. Bellovich, J. Chen, L. Hamm, C. Gadegbeku, E. Horwitz, R.R. Townsend, C.A. Anderson, J.P. Lash, C.Y. Hsu, M.B. Leonard, and M. Wolf. Fibroblast growth factor 23 is elevated before parathyroid hormone and phosphate in chronic kidney disease. *Kidney Int*. 2011; 79(12):1370–8.

47. Gutierrez, O.M., M. Mannstadt, T. Isakova, J.A. Rauh-Hain, H. Tamez, A. Shah, K. Smith, H. Lee, R. Thadhani, H. Juppner, and M. Wolf. Fibroblast growth factor 23 and mortality among patients undergoing hemodialysis. *N Engl J Med*. 2008; 359(6):584–92.

48. Xiao, Y., X. Luo, W. Huang, J. Zhang, and C. Peng. Fibroblast growth factor 23 and risk of all-cause mortality and cardiovascular events: A meta-analysis of prospective cohort studies. *Int J Cardiol*. 2014; 174(3):824–8.

49. Faul, C., A.P. Amaral, B. Oskouei, M.C. Hu, A. Sloan, T. Isakova, O.M. Gutierrez, R. Aguillon-Prada, J. Lincoln, J.M. Hare, P. Mundel, A. Morales, J. Scialla, M. Fischer, E.Z. Soliman, J. Chen, A.S. Go, S.E. Rosas, L. Nessel, R.R. Townsend, H.I. Feldman, M. St John Sutton, A. Ojo, C. Gadegbeku, G.S. Di Marco, S. Reuter, D. Kentrup, K. Tiemann, M. Brand, J.A. Hill, O.W. Moe, O.M. Kuro, J.W. Kusek, M.G. Keane, and M. Wolf. FGF23 induces left ventricular hypertrophy. *J Clin Invest*. 2011; 121(11):4393–408.

50. Touchberry, C.D., T.M. Green, V. Tchikrizov, J.E. Mannix, T.F. Mao, B.W. Carney, M. Girgis, R.J. Vincent, L.A. Wetmore, B. Dawn, L.F. Bonewald, J.R. Stubbs, and M.J. Wacker. FGF23 is a novel regulator of intracellular calcium and cardiac contractility in addition to cardiac hypertrophy. *Am J Physiol Endocrinol Metab*. 2013; 304(8):E863–73.

51. Houston, J., K. Smith, T. Isakova, N. Sowden, M. Wolf, and O.M. Gutierrez. Associations of dietary phosphorus intake, urinary phosphate excretion, and fibroblast growth factor 23 with vascular stiffness in chronic kidney disease. *J Ren Nutr*. 2013; 23(1):12–20.

52. Burnett, S.M., S.C. Gunawardene, F.R. Bringhurst, H. Juppner, H. Lee, and J.S. Finkelstein. Regulation of C-terminal and intact FGF-23 by dietary phosphate in men and women. *J Bone Miner Res*. 2006; 21(8):1187–96.

53. Antoniucci, D.M., T. Yamashita, and A.A. Portale. Dietary phosphorus regulates serum fibroblast growth factor-23 concentrations in healthy men. *J Clin Endocrinol Metab*. 2006; 91(8):3144–9.

54. Sigrist, M., M. Tang, M. Beaulieu, G. Espino-Hernandez, L. Er, O. Djurdjev, and A. Levin. Responsiveness of FGF-23 and mineral metabolism to altered dietary phosphate intake in chronic kidney disease (CKD): Results of a randomized trial. *Nephrol Dial Transplant*. 2013; 28(1):161–9.

55. Larsson, T., U. Nisbeth, O. Ljunggren, H. Juppner, and K.B. Jonsson. Circulating concentration of FGF-23 increases as renal function declines in patients with chronic kidney disease, but does not change in response to variation in phosphate intake in healthy volunteers. *Kidney Int*. 2003; 64(6):2272–9.

56. Isakova, T., A. Barchi-Chung, G. Enfield, K. Smith, G. Vargas, J. Houston, H. Xie, P. Wahl, E. Schiavenato, A. Dosch, O.M. Gutierrez, J. Diego, O. Lenz, G. Contreras, A. Mendez, R.B. Weiner, and M. Wolf. Effects of dietary phosphate restriction and phosphate binders on FGF23 levels in CKD. *Clin J Am Soc Nephrol*. 2013; 8(6):1009–18.

57. Smith, E.R., M.M. Cai, L.P. McMahon, and S.G. Holt. Biological variability of plasma intact and C-terminal FGF23 measurements. *J Clin Endocrinol Metab*. 2012; 97(9):3357–65.

58. Smith, E.R., L.P. McMahon, and S.G. Holt. Method-specific differences in plasma fibroblast growth factor 23 measurement using four commercial ELISAs. *Clin Chem Lab Med*. 2013; 51(10):1971–81.

59. Watari, E., Y. Taketani, T. Kitamura, T. Tanaka, H. Ohminami, M. Abuduli, N. Harada, H. Yamanaka-Okumura, H. Yamamoto, and E. Takeda. Fluctuating plasma phosphorus level by changes in dietary phosphorus intake induces endothelial dysfunction. *J Clin Biochem Nutr*. 2015; 56(1):35–42.

60. Russo, D., I. Miranda, C. Ruocco, Y. Battaglia, E. Buonanno, S. Manzi, L. Russo, A. Scafarto, and V.E. Andreucci. The progression of coronary artery calcification in predialysis patients on calcium carbonate or sevelamer. *Kidney Int*. 2007; 72(10):1255–61.

61. Shuto, E., Y. Taketani, R. Tanaka, N. Harada, M. Isshiki, M. Sato, K. Nashiki, K. Amo, H. Yamamoto, Y. Higashi, Y. Nakaya, and E. Takeda. Dietary phosphorus acutely impairs endothelial function. *J Am Soc Nephrol*. 2009; 20(7):1504–12.

62. Shinaberger, C.S., S. Greenland, J.D. Kopple, D. Van Wyck, R. Mehrotra, C.P. Kovesdy, and K. Kalantar-Zadeh. Is controlling phosphorus by decreasing dietary protein intake beneficial or harmful in persons with chronic kidney disease? *Am J Clin Nutr.* 2008; 88(6):1511–8.
63. Kremsdorf, R.A., A.N. Hoofnagle, M. Kratz, D.S. Weigle, H.S. Callahan, J.Q. Purnell, A.M. Horgan, I.H. de Boer, and B.R. Kestenbaum. Effects of a high-protein diet on regulation of phosphorus homeostasis. *J Clin Endocrinol Metab.* 2013; 98(3):1207–13.
64. Di Iorio, B., L. Di Micco, S. Torraca, M.L. Sirico, L. Russo, A. Pota, F. Mirenghi, and D. Russo. Acute effects of very-low-protein diet on FGF23 levels: A randomized study. *Clin J Am Soc Nephrol.* 2012; 7(4):581–7.
65. Moe, S.M., M.P. Zidehsarai, M.A. Chambers, L.A. Jackman, J.S. Radcliffe, L.L. Trevino, S.E. Donahue, and J.R. Asplin. Vegetarian compared with meat dietary protein source and phosphorus homeostasis in chronic kidney disease. *Clin J Am Soc Nephrol.* 2011; 6(2):257–64.
66. Jamal, S.A., B. Vandermeer, P. Raggi, D.C. Mendelssohn, T. Chatterley, M. Dorgan, C.E. Lok, D. Fitchett, and R.T. Tsuyuki. Effect of calcium-based versus non-calcium-based phosphate binders on mortality in patients with chronic kidney disease: An updated systematic review and meta-analysis. *Lancet.* 2013; 382(9900):1268–77.
67. Chue, C.D., J.N. Townend, W.E. Moody, D. Zehnder, N.A. Wall, L. Harper, N.C. Edwards, R.P. Steeds, and C.J. Ferro. Cardiovascular effects of sevelamer in stage 3 CKD. *J Am Soc Nephrol.* 2013; 24(5):842–52.
68. Seifert, M.E., L. de las Fuentes, M. Rothstein, D.J. Dietzen, A.J. Bierhals, S.C. Cheng, W. Ross, D. Windus, V.G. Davila-Roman, and K.A. Hruska. Effects of phosphate binder therapy on vascular stiffness in early-stage chronic kidney disease. *Am J Nephrol.* 2013; 38(2):158–67.
69. Labonte, E.D., C.W. Carreras, M.R. Leadbetter, K. Kozuka, J. Kohler, S. Koo-McCoy, L. He, E. Dy, D. Black, Z. Zhong, I. Langsetmo, A.G. Spencer, N. Bell, D. Deshpande, M. Navre, J.G. Lewis, J.W. Jacobs, and D. Charmot. Gastrointestinal inhibition of sodium-hydrogen exchanger 3 reduces phosphorus absorption and protects against vascular calcification in CKD. *J Am Soc Nephrol.* 2015; 26(5):1138–49.

9 The Relationship between Phosphorus Intake and Blood Pressure

Melissa M. Melough and Alex R. Chang

CONTENTS

Abstract 111
Bullet Points 112
9.1 Introduction 112
9.2 Impact of Dietary Factors on Blood Pressure 112
9.3 Observational Cross-Sectional Studies Examining
       the Relationship between Phosphorus Intake and Blood Pressure 113
9.4 Observational Longitudinal Studies Examining
       the Relationship between Phosphorus Intake and Blood Pressure 115
9.5 Limitations of Nutritional Epidemiology Studies 115
9.6 Observational Studies Examining Relationships between Serum Phosphorus and
       Intact PTH with Blood Pressure 116
9.7 Trials of Different Dietary Levels of Phosphorus Intake on Blood Pressure 116
9.8 Observational and Interventional Studies on Protein Intake and Blood Pressure 117
9.9 Potential Mechanisms Explaining a Phosphorus–Blood Pressure Link 118
9.10 Conclusions 120
References 120

ABSTRACT

Although diet plays a profound role in influencing blood pressure and hypertension, the effects of dietary phosphorus on blood pressure have not been well studied. Other studies of diet and blood pressure have focused more on minerals such as sodium, potassium, magnesium, and calcium. Cross-sectional epidemiologic studies show an inverse relationship between dietary phosphorus intake and blood pressure. However, a longitudinal study of two cohorts suggests that a relationship between phosphorus intake and incident hypertension only exists for dairy-derived phosphorus, which puts into question a direct causal effect of phosphorus. Animal models have not consistently shown a positive or negative effect of phosphorus on blood pressure. One animal study found that a high-phosphate diet could cause parathyroid hormone (PTH)-mediated rises in renin levels, and prospective observational studies suggest that PTH may increase the risk for incident hypertension. Unfortunately, no human experimental study has rigorously examined the effect of phosphorus intake in isolation on blood pressure. Studies of varying protein intake suggest that increasing dietary protein by replacing carbohydrates may result in modestly lower blood pressure, although it is impossible to identify which nutritional factors associated with protein intake drive this benefit. Well-designed interventional trials testing different levels of phosphorus intake while keeping other correlated nutrients constant are needed to determine whether phosphorus affects blood pressure.

BULLET POINTS

- Diet has been shown to influence blood pressure, but little is known about the role that phosphorus plays in this relationship.
- Phosphorus intake is associated with lower blood pressure and incident hypertension, but the association between phosphorus intake and incident hypertension only exists with dairy-derived phosphorus, suggesting that this association may not be driven by phosphorus itself.
- PTH has been shown to be associated with incident hypertension.
- Animal models have been inconclusive, with some showing a direct and others showing an inverse or no relationship between phosphorus intake and blood pressure.
- No large randomized trial has examined the effect of phosphorus intake specifically on blood pressure; future trials are needed to address this question.

9.1 INTRODUCTION

Serum phosphorus concentrations are tightly regulated by parathyroid hormone (PTH), fibroblast growth factor-23 (FGF23), and other factors. There is increasing evidence that high phosphorus intake could have adverse effects on cardiovascular and bone health [1–3]. High phosphorus intake can raise 24-hour mean serum phosphorus concentrations [4], and serum phosphorus has been linked in a number of studies to increased risk of cardiovascular disease, vascular calcification, and death [5–7]. Phosphorus intake can also stimulate PTH and FGF23 [4,8–10], both of which have been associated with increased risk for cardiovascular disease and death [11–16]. Most studies examining phosphorus have thus focused on its effects on PTH, FGF23, and cardiovascular outcomes. However, the majority of observational studies have shown an association between phosphorus intake and reduced blood pressure, raising the question of whether there may be an effect of phosphorus on blood pressure [17–24]. Given the high prevalence of phosphorus-based ingredients used by the food industry, this is an important question [4,25]. In this chapter, we will review the available evidence on this topic, including observational studies, animal studies, and human trials.

9.2 IMPACT OF DIETARY FACTORS ON BLOOD PRESSURE

Dietary factors have long been recognized as having a significant impact on blood pressure and hypertension. Dr. Walter Kempner was one of the first to demonstrate the important effects of diet on blood pressure. He famously treated patients with malignant hypertension with a rice and fruit diet. This diet is notably quite low in phosphorus, although also extremely different from the typical American diet, consisting of about 2000 calories/d, mainly from complex carbohydrates, <20 g of protein, and 150 mg/d of sodium [26]. At a time when the median life expectancy of someone with malignant hypertension was six months, Kempner reported that 107 of the patients treated in his original cohort of 192 showed improvements in blood pressure from a mean of 200/112 to 149/46, although 60 patients had no improvement in blood pressure, and 25 died [27]. He was criticized for not studying his diet in a randomized controlled study, but he successfully treated many patients with conditions ranging from nephrotic syndrome to diabetes and obesity and revolutionized the approach to the management of heart and kidney disease [28].

Other researchers have long noted that vegetarians have lower blood pressure than omnivores, prompting some researchers to speculate a relationship between animal protein and blood pressure [29–32]. Dietary patterns such as the Dietary Approaches to Stop Hypertension (DASH) and the Mediterranean diet that emphasize intake of fresh fruits, vegetables, and legumes while moderating intake of meat, have been shown to have major blood pressure–lowering effects [33]. Recently, a randomized trial of dietary advice to follow a Mediterranean-style diet supplemented with extra-virgin olive oil or nuts decreased the incidence of cardiovascular events [34]. Understanding what elements of these various dietary patterns decrease blood pressure and cardiovascular risk is

The Relationship between Phosphorus Intake and Blood Pressure

challenging, as diet is complex and many nutrients could play a role either in concert or individually. Beyond sodium, several other minerals have been purported to influence blood pressure, including potassium, calcium, magnesium, and phosphorus [23,35–40]. Phosphorus has been the least studied of these minerals in terms of its relationship with blood pressure, although a large body of literature exists on protein, the main source of phosphorus, and blood pressure. Examination of different sources of protein/phosphorus may also be helpful in understanding the relationship between phosphorus and blood pressure, as bioavailability of phytate phosphorus in many vegetable-based products is lower compared to animal or dairy sources [41–43]. Given the dearth of research examining the isolated impact of phosphorus on blood pressure, we consider studies of both phosphorus and protein in this chapter.

9.3 OBSERVATIONAL CROSS-SECTIONAL STUDIES EXAMINING THE RELATIONSHIP BETWEEN PHOSPHORUS INTAKE AND BLOOD PRESSURE

The earliest study examining the relationship between phosphorus intake and blood pressure was done using cross-sectional data from a nationally representative sample of U.S. adults in the National Health and Nutrition Examination Survey I (NHANES I). In this study, a single 24-hour dietary recall was used to determine intakes of sodium, potassium, calcium, phosphorus, iron, and alcohol and examine the relationship between these dietary factors and systolic blood pressure. After adjustment for age, race, and body mass index (BMI), a direct relationship between phosphorus intake and systolic blood pressure was observed [17]. Around the same time, another cross-sectional study was conducted using data from 615 healthy Hawaiian men of Japanese ancestry in the Honolulu Heart Study, who completed a single 24-hour dietary recall [18]. In this study, the relationship between 61 dietary variables (including phosphorus) and blood pressure was examined. Phosphorus intake from food sources was inversely associated with systolic and diastolic blood pressure, whereas phosphorus intake from supplement sources had no relationship with blood pressure after adjustment for age and BMI [18]. Neither of these studies adjusted for multiple comparisons.

The International Study of Macro- and Micro-Nutrients and Blood Pressure (INTERMAP) was a cross-sectional epidemiologic study examining the role of dietary factors on blood pressure in China, Japan, the United Kingdom, and the United States [20]. The study enrolled 4680 men and women aged 40 to 59, and participants presented for four separate visits during which blood pressure measurements, 24-hour urine collections, and 24-hour dietary recalls were obtained. Nutrient totals of the diet as well as food group composition were determined using Nutrition Data System software. In this study, dietary phosphorus intake was inversely associated with blood pressure. Every 232 mg/1000 kcal [2 standard deviation (SD)] increase in phosphorus intake was associated with a reduction in systolic blood pressure between 1.13 and 2.31 mmHg and a reduction in diastolic blood pressure between 0.59 and 1.47 mmHg, depending on how many variables were included in the model. The authors carefully and sequentially adjusted for potential confounders, including age, gender, BMI, physical activity, family history of hypertension, urinary sodium and potassium, intakes of alcohol, cholesterol, fat, vegetable protein, calcium, and magnesium. Findings were similar by country, where sources of phosphorus varied quite substantially.

The same research group used methods similar to genome-wide association studies to examine relationships between nutrients associated with blood pressure in INTERMAP with appropriate adjustment for multiple comparisons and then validate their findings in a separate cohort [22]. Again, dietary phosphorus intake was significantly inversely associated with systolic blood pressure both in INTERMAP and in the NHANES 1999–2006 cohort. Despite these rigorous cross-sectional analyses, there remain the difficulties of interpreting associations between individual nutrients and outcomes, given the high intercorrelation between phosphorus, calcium, and magnesium—all of which were associated with lower blood pressure in INTERMAP [20].

TABLE 9.1

Observational Studies Examining Phosphorus and Blood Pressure

Author	Study Type	Population	Exposure	Outcome	Results	Limitations
Gruchow [17]	Cohort (NHANES I)	9,553 adults from general U.S. population	Phosphorus intake and four other dietary factors (24 hour recall)	Blood pressure	Phosphorus intake directly associated with systolic blood pressure	Minimal adjustment for confounders, multiple comparisons, likely residual confounding
Joffres [18]	Cohort (Honolulu Heart Study)	615 healthy men of Japanese ancestry in Hawaii	Phosphorus intake and 60 other dietary factors (24-hour recall)	Blood pressure	Phosphorus intake from food inversely associated with blood pressure; supplemental phosphorus not associated with blood pressure	Minimal adjustment for confounders, multiple comparisons, likely residual confounding
Zhao [19]	Cohort (INTERMAP)	839 middle-aged Chinese participants from North and South China	Phosphorus intake and 15 other dietary factors (four 24-hour recalls)	Blood pressure	Phosphorus intake inversely associated with blood pressure	Minimal adjustment for confounders, multiple comparisons, likely residual confounding
Elliott [20]	Cohort (INTERMAP)	4,680 adults aged 40–59 from Japan, China, the United Kingdom, and the United States	Phosphorus intake (four 24-hour recalls)	Blood pressure	Phosphorus intake inversely associated with blood pressure	Likely residual confounding
Alonso [21]	Cohort (Atherosclerosis Risk in Communities and Multi-Ethnic Study of Atherosclerosis)	13,444 middle-aged participants from the ARIC and MESA studies	Phosphorus intake (66-item FFQ used in ARIC and 120-item FFQ used in MESA)	Blood pressure and risk of incident hypertension	Phosphorus intake associated with lower cross-sectional blood pressure and risk of incident hypertension; dairy vs. nondairy sources, only dairy sources of phosphorus associated with lower BP and risk of hypertension	Different FFQs used in each cohort, likely residual confounding
Tzoulaki [22]	Cohort (INTERMAP and NHANES 1999–2006)	4,680 adults aged 40–59 from Japan, China, the United Kingdom, and the United States	Phosphorus intake in addition to 81 other nutrients and 3 urine electrolytes (four 24-hour recalls)	Blood pressure	Phosphorus intake inversely associated with systolic blood pressure	Likely residual confounding
Kim [23]	Cross-sectional observational	258 healthy Korean adults	Phosphorus intake and six other dietary factors (three 24-hr recalls)	Blood pressure and blood lipids	Phosphorus intake not significantly correlated with blood pressure	Small sample, likely residual confounding

The Relationship between Phosphorus Intake and Blood Pressure   115

Table 9.1 summarizes published observational studies examining relationships between phosphorus intake and blood pressure. Although the majority of these studies found an inverse relationship between dietary phosphorus and blood pressure, cause and effect cannot be ascribed. These studies also cannot account for changes in dietary behavior that may have occurred as blood pressure increased.

9.4 OBSERVATIONAL LONGITUDINAL STUDIES EXAMINING THE RELATIONSHIP BETWEEN PHOSPHORUS INTAKE AND BLOOD PRESSURE

To our knowledge, only one longitudinal observational study (using data from two well-characterized study cohorts) has been done examining the relationship between phosphorus intake and blood pressure [21]. In this study, researchers used food frequency questionnaire (FFQ) data from the Atherosclerosis Risk in Communities (ARIC) study and the Multi-ethnic Study of Atherosclerosis (MESA) to examine the risk of incident hypertension as well as the cross-sectional relationship between phosphorus intake and blood pressure. Because a number of studies have found a relationship between dairy intake and lower blood pressure [44], these investigators also conducted separate analyses examining the association between phosphorus from dairy sources (31% of total phosphorus intake in ARIC and 29% in MESA) and phosphorus from nondairy sources. Similar to other studies, there was an inverse cross-sectional relationship between total phosphorus intake and blood pressure in both ARIC and MESA. In their longitudinal analysis, there was a 10% decreased risk of incident hypertension among those in the highest quintile of phosphorus intake compared to those in the lowest quintile after adjustment for demographics and other potential confounders (not including other nutrients).

After separating phosphorus intake into dairy and nondairy categories, there was only an association between phosphorus intake from dairy products and incident hypertension; no association existed between phosphorus from nondairy sources and incident hypertension. Further adjustment for other nutrients abolished any relationship between phosphorus intake and incident hypertension. Given these findings, the authors suggested that dairy products, rather than phosphorus specifically, may be responsible for this observed inverse relationship with blood pressure. It is unclear the mechanism by which dairy products may confer lower risk of hypertension, but this study suggests that phosphorus is unlikely to explain this. Other studies have demonstrated the same relationship between dairy intake and blood pressure, including a study of 5880 healthy young adults in Spain in which low-fat dairy consumption was associated with lower risk of incident hypertension even after adjustment for phosphorus and other nutrients [45].

9.5 LIMITATIONS OF NUTRITIONAL EPIDEMIOLOGY STUDIES

All of these nutritional epidemiologic studies have several limitations. First, they rely on dietary self-report. Second, phosphorus intake often correlates highly with other dietary factors such as protein, calcium, magnesium, and potassium. All of these dietary factors have been reported to also correlate inversely with blood pressure [36,38,39,46]. This results in multicollinearity, making it very difficult to determine the individual effect of one nutrient from the effect of others. Third, phosphorus intake related to consumption of inorganic phosphorus additives may not be captured well with current (or past) nutritional databases. As we and several others have shown, there are major limitations in current nutritional databases in capturing phosphorus intake in processed foods that contain phosphorus additives [47,48]. Diets high in processed foods may contain as much as 60% more phosphorus than a similar diet low in processed foods [25,49]. This could cause differential misclassification of phosphorus intake, meaning that individuals eating phosphorus derived from whole foods would have more reported phosphorus than individuals eating phosphorus derived

116 Dietary Phosphorus: Health, Nutrition, and Regulatory Aspects

from processed foods, who may be eating a much unhealthier diet. These studies also suffer from potential residual confounding, as it is unlikely that all nondietary and dietary factors that correlate with phosphorus are measured completely and accounted for in an observational study.

9.6 OBSERVATIONAL STUDIES EXAMINING RELATIONSHIPS BETWEEN SERUM PHOSPHORUS AND INTACT PTH WITH BLOOD PRESSURE

Because high phosphorus intake may increase serum phosphorus concentrations, intact PTH, and/or FGF23, it may be helpful to examine associations between these markers and blood pressure. Data from NHANES I suggested an inverse relationship between serum phosphorus and blood pressure [50]. This was confirmed in a study by Kesteloot in a Belgian population sample [37]. Both of these studies were cross-sectional in nature, and neither had information about parathyroid hormone.

The relationship between serum phosphorus and blood pressure may differ in end-stage renal disease (ESRD) patients, who may be more prone to developing complications from hyperphosphatemia such as vascular calcification and arterial stiffness [51–53]. In a study of 707 incident hemodialysis patients followed prospectively, serum phosphorus was associated with higher systolic blood pressure both in cross-sectional and longitudinal analyses [51]. Every 1 mg/dL increase in serum phosphorus was associated with a 2.5 mmHg higher systolic blood pressure at 27 months.

Other investigators have examined a significant relationship between PTH and incident hypertension and documented an increased risk [54–56]. In a study of 3002 men and women in the MESA study, relationships between PTH and 25-hydroxyvitamin D with incident hypertension were investigated. Compared with PTH <33 pg/mL, PTH ≥65 pg/mL was associated with a higher risk of hypertension (HR 1.27, 95% CI: 1.01–1.59). Adjustment for 25-hydroxyvitamin D, calcium, and phosphorus levels had little effect on findings. Although these findings are intriguing, the elevations in PTH could be driven by low calcium intake or phosphorus intake [57].

9.7 TRIALS OF DIFFERENT DIETARY LEVELS OF PHOSPHORUS INTAKE ON BLOOD PRESSURE

The best way to determine whether a true relationship exists between phosphorus and blood pressure is through interventional studies. Unfortunately, interventional studies that have manipulated dietary phosphorus through feeding studies, prescribed diets, or phosphorus-binding medications have not typically included blood pressure as an outcome. Outcomes have focused on serum phosphorus given the strong relationship between serum phosphorus and risk of cardiovascular disease and mortality [11–16]. Because a clear mechanism has not been identified by which phosphorus might induce hypertension, this may not have been a focus in previous intervention studies. Of published studies where dietary phosphorus is manipulated either by diet or phosphorus-binding medication [43,58–63], only two studies to our knowledge reported effects on blood pressure. In the study by Seifert, 38 patients with stage 3 CKD were randomized to lanthanum carbonate, a phosphorus-binding medication, or placebo. The primary outcome was change in serum phosphorus, and secondary outcomes included measures of phosphorus homeostasis and vascular stiffness after 12 months. Blood pressure, measured at baseline and 12 months, was not an outcome but was reported. There were no differences in blood pressure between the two groups, nor were there differences in serum phosphorus or vascular stiffness outcomes [63].

We recently conducted a randomized, cross-over study examining the effects of phosphorus additives on urinary albumin excretion in 31 patients with eGFR ≥45 mL/min/1.73 m^2 and albuminuria (≥30 mg/d) [64]. Blood pressure was a secondary outcome and was measured using a standardized protocol with an Omron HEM-907 device at three weekly visits during three-week higher and lower phosphorus periods. A contrast of 998 mg/d of dietary phosphorus intake was achieved by supplementing participants' background diet with unaltered, commercially available diet beverages and

The Relationship between Phosphorus Intake and Blood Pressure

breakfast bars, with and without phosphorus additives. Higher phosphorus additive consumption increased 24-hour urine phosphorus excretion by 505 mg/d ($p < 0.001$) and tended to increase albuminuria (higher vs. lower phosphorus period: 14.3%, 95% CI: −2.5%, 34.0%; $p = 0.1$), although this result was not statistically significant. Higher phosphorus additive consumption had no significant effect on systolic blood pressure (higher vs. lower phosphorus period: −1.1 mmHg, 95% CI: −4.1, 1.9; $p = 0.5$) or diastolic blood pressure (higher vs. lower phosphorus period: −0.8 mmHg, 95% CI: −2.7, 1.0; $p = 0.4$). However, this study was likely underpowered for the blood pressure outcome as the minimal detectable difference was estimated to be ~5 to 6 mmHg for systolic blood pressure and ~4 to 5 mmHg for diastolic blood pressure.

9.8 OBSERVATIONAL AND INTERVENTIONAL STUDIES ON PROTEIN INTAKE AND BLOOD PRESSURE

It bears mention that many epidemiologic studies have investigated the effects of protein intake on blood pressure because the majority of phosphorus is derived from protein. A systematic review done in 2010 summarizes available evidence of an effect of protein intake on blood pressure [65]. Cross-sectional studies generally show an inverse relationship between reported protein intake and blood pressure. However, when broken down by source of protein, studies investigating vegetable sources of protein more consistently reported significant inverse associations with blood pressure, whereas studies of animal protein intake have been less consistent in showing an association with blood pressure. Prospective studies also show an inverse relationship between plant protein and blood pressure [66–69], whereas one prospective study found a direct relationship and two studies found no relationship between animal protein intake and blood pressure [66–68].

An important randomized feeding trial that manipulated dietary protein intake is the OmniHeart trial, which included 164 participants with prehypertension or stage 1 hypertension [70]. Healthy DASH-style diets were compared with different macronutrient profiles (higher carbohydrate, higher fat, and higher protein). Participants received each diet for six weeks, and the main outcomes were systolic blood pressure and low-density lipoprotein cholesterol. Phosphorus content of each diet was not reported, although 24-hour urine collections were completed; mean 24-hour urine phosphorus on the higher protein diet was 916 mg/d compared to 845 mg/d on the higher carbohydrate diet and 813 mg on the higher fat diet. Compared to the higher carbohydrate diet, the higher protein diet reduced blood pressure by 1.4 mmHg and by 3.5 mmHg in those with hypertension [70]. However, there was no difference when the higher protein diet was compared to the higher fat diet. Thus, it is possible that both higher protein and higher fat intake could lower blood pressure, or alternatively, that lower carbohydrate intake could have lowered blood pressure.

A pair of studies conducted in Australia produced similar results. The 36 subjects who completed the first of these studies were randomized to receive either a soy protein supplement or an isocaloric maltodextrin supplement for eight weeks. Dietary assignments were further divided so that half received a psyllium fiber supplement [71]. Compared to controls (low fiber and low protein), mean systolic blood pressure fell by 10.5 mmHg and 2.9 mmHg in those on the high-protein diets, with and without added fiber, respectively. Thus, dietary protein and soluble fiber supplements lowered blood pressure additively in hypertensive patients. In another trial conducted in Australia, lean red meat was substituted for carbohydrate-rich foods in the usual diet of participants [72]. Compared to controls who maintained their usual diet, the 24-hour systolic blood pressure was 4 mmHg lower in those consuming higher protein from lean red meat [72]. In another cross-over trial of adults with prehypertension or early hypertension, participants were assigned to take 40 g/day soy protein, milk protein, or carbohydrate supplements [73]. Even though the phosphorus content of each supplement was roughly equal (120 mg/day in soy, 90 mg/day in milk, and 90 mg/day in carbohydrate supplements), compared to carbohydrate, milk protein reduced systolic blood pressure 2.3 mmHg and soy protein reduced it 2.0 mmHg. Based on these findings, it seems that there may be a small beneficial

118   Dietary Phosphorus: Health, Nutrition, and Regulatory Aspects

effect of protein on blood pressure, although further research is needed, particularly on specific sources of protein. Again, these studies are unable to discern whether these effects were due to protein itself, reduced carbohydrate intake, or other specific micronutrients such as phosphorus. They also illustrate the difficulties in designing a study to test the effects of a specific macronutrient or micronutrient on blood pressure.

9.9 POTENTIAL MECHANISMS EXPLAINING A PHOSPHORUS–BLOOD PRESSURE LINK

A handful of animal studies have examined the effect of phosphorus intake on blood pressure (Table 9.2). Unfortunately, these studies have demonstrated no relationship [74,75], a direct relationship [76–78], and an inverse relationship between phosphorus intake and blood pressure [79]. Bindels et al. compared a control diet to a diet supplemented with 2% K2HPO4*KH2PO4 drinking water and a diet supplemented with 1.41% KCl drinking water in spontaneously hypertensive rats (SHR) and age-matched normotensive Wistar-Kyoto rats. SHR rats have been noted to have hypophosphatemia and hypophosphaturia, although it is unclear if this is due to intestinal phosphate absorption and/or more positive phosphorus balance [79,80]. Supplementation with potassium phosphate normalized plasma phosphate levels in the SHR group and systolic blood pressure declined at 20 weeks (mean 25 mmHg) and persisted. Control normotensive Wistar-Kyoto rats had no change in phosphate level but experienced systolic blood pressure decreases at 24 weeks that also persisted. The potassium chloride diet had no effect on blood pressure, and the authors noted that the potassium given was not as much as in other studies showing an effect of potassium on blood pressure. In another study of SHR rats, a high-calcium (4.3%) diet reduced blood pressure, and SHR rats were noted to have marked hypophosphatemia and hypophosphaturia and decreased intestinal phosphate absorption compared to SHR rats fed a lower calcium (1.2%) diet [81]. Interestingly, intravenous phosphate administration abrogated the antihypertensive effect of high calcium intake, contrary to Bindels' study.

In studies that specifically examined CKD animal models, results were null in two studies [74,75], and a third suggested a direct effect of phosphorus on blood pressure [76]. A study by Yamada used adenine-induced CKD rats, which were given diets of different phosphate concentrations ranging from 0.3% to 1.2% for eight weeks. These rats then received lanthanum carbonate. No changes in blood pressure were observed compared to control rats at all time points, although there were increases in markers of oxidative stress, vascular calcification, and premature death. Findings were similar to another study that used uninephrectomized, partially nephrectomized, and intact rats fed diets ranging from 0.5% to 2% phosphate for 18 weeks. No significant difference in blood pressure was noted at 18 weeks despite increasing histologic findings (calcium phosphate deposits, interstitial fibrosis, tubular dilatation, inflammatory cell infiltration) with lower renal functional mass. In the third study, a high-phosphate diet (1.5%) was shown to increase blood pressure at week 27 in male Sprague-Dawley rats who underwent 5/6 nephrectomy [76].

Bozic compared the effects of a high-phosphate diet (1.2%) to a moderate-phosphate diet (0.6%) in Sprague-Dawley rats and conducted a series of experiments to elucidate potential mechanisms for an effect of phosphorus on blood pressure [77]. In this study, significant increases in systolic and diastolic blood pressure occurred, and addition of lanthanum carbonate restored blood pressure levels to previous values. This study found no changes in endothelium-dependent or independent relaxation. There were increases in renin, angiotensin, and PTH that occurred with the high-phosphorus diet that were attenuated by addition of lanthanum. When parathyroidectomy was done in animals fed a high-phosphate diet that were then given a constant PTH infusion, there was no increase in blood pressure even though phosphate levels were high, suggesting that PTH was responsible for a renin-mediated increase in blood pressure, although the investigators did not report changes in renin after parathyroidectomy. This relationship between PTH and renin has been

TABLE 9.2

Animal Studies Examining Phosphorus and Blood Pressure

Author	Population	Exposure	Main Outcome(s)	BP Results	Other Results
Bindels [79]	Spontaneously hypertensive, hypophosphatemic rats (SHR) and normotensive Wistar-Kyoto rats (WKY)	Drinking water with 2% potassium phosphorus	Blood pressure	High-phosphorus diet lowered blood pressure after 15 weeks in SHR rats and after 24 weeks in WKY rats	
Lau [81]	Spontaneously hypertensive rats (SHR) and normotensive Wistar-Kyoto rats (WKY)	Low (0.22%), normal (1.2%), or high (4.3%) calcium diets	Blood pressure	High-calcium (4.3%) diet caused decrease in blood pressure, which was negated when IV phosphorus was administered	
Eraranta [76]	5/6 nephrectomy rat model (5/6 NX) and sham-operated rats	High phosphorus (1.5%) diet	Renal angiotensin-converting enzyme (ACE) expression	High-phosphorus diet had no effect on blood pressure, blood pressure lowered when given phosphorus binder (3% calcium carbonate)	High-phosphorus diet increased renal ACE expression and tissue damage in the 5/6 NX rats
Bozic [77]	Sprague-Dawley rats	High phosphorus (1.2%) diet	Blood pressure	High-phosphorus diet increased blood pressure, phosphorus binder normalized blood pressure	High-phosphorus diet also increased renin, which appeared to be mediated by PTH
Suzuki [78]	Spontaneously hypertensive rats/NDmcr-cp (SHR/cp) and normotensive Wistar-Kyoto rats (WKY)	High-phosphorus (1.2%) and zinc-free diet	Blood pressure and cardiac function	High-phosphorus/zinc-free diet increased blood pressure	High-phosphorus/zinc-free diet reduced left ventricular systolic and diastolic function and myocardial fibrosis
Haut [75]	Sprague Dawley rats; 1/3 with intact kidneys, 1/3 with partial nephrectomy, 1/3 with uninephrectomy	0.5% phosphorus, 1.0% phosphorus, and 2% phosphorus diets	Renal histology	High-phosphorus diet had no effect on blood pressure	Increasing calcium–phosphate deposition with increasing phosphate excreted per nephron
Yamada [74]	Sprague-Dawley rats fed synthetic diet to model CKD with robust arterial medial calcification	0.3% phosphorus, 0.6% phosphorus, 0.9% phosphorus, and 1.2% phosphorus diets	Inflammation, malnutrition, and vascular calcification	Higher phosphorus diet had no effect on blood pressure	Higher phosphorus diet increased TNF-alpha, urinary, and tissue levels of oxidative stress markers and malnutrition

shown experimentally and in hypertensive patients with primary hyperparathyroidism undergoing parathyroidectomy [82–84]. Further, a recent study found that PTH was an independent risk factor for incident hypertension [54].

9.10 CONCLUSIONS

Current data examining the relationship between phosphorus intake and blood pressure are limited and inconclusive. Cross-sectional observational studies suggest an inverse association between phosphorus intake and blood pressure, whereas one prospective study suggests this is limited to phosphorus from dairy sources. No randomized trial has compared the effects of differences in phosphorus intake on blood pressure as an outcome without manipulating other aspects of diet. Studies that have increased protein intake (at the expense of carbohydrate intake) tend to show a modest, beneficial effect of lowering blood pressure, although this cannot be ascribed to phosphorus intake. More research is needed in this area, given the high prevalence of phosphorus-based ingredients in the food supply.

REFERENCES

1. Calvo MS, Park YK. Changing phosphorus content of the U.S. diet: Potential for adverse effects on bone. *J Nutr.* 1996;126(4 Suppl):1168S–1180S.
2. Uribarri J, Calvo MS. Dietary phosphorus intake and health. *Am J Clin Nutr.* 201499:247–248. doi:10.3945/ajcn.113.080259.
3. Chang AR, Lazo M, Appel LJ, Gutiérrez OM, Grams ME. High dietary phosphorus intake is associated with all-cause mortality: Results from NHANES III. *Am J Clin Nutr.* 2014;99(2):320–327. doi:10.3945/ajcn.113.073148. "(erratum *Am J Clin Nutr* 105:1021-2.)"
4. Portale AA, Halloran BP, Morris RC. Dietary intake of phosphorus modulates the circadian rhythm in serum concentration of phosphorus. Implications for the renal production of 1,25-dihydroxyvitamin D. *J Clin Invest.* 1987;80(4):1147–1154.
5. Tonelli M, Sacks F, Pfeffer M, Gao Z, Curhan G. Relation between serum phosphate level and cardiovascular event rate in people with coronary disease. *Circulation.* 2005;112(17):2627–2633. doi:10.1161/CIRCULATIONAHA.105.553198.
6. Dhingra R, Sullivan LM, Fox CS et al. Relations of serum phosphorus and calcium levels to the incidence of cardiovascular disease in the community. *Arch Intern Med.* 2007;167(9):879–885. doi:10.3201/eid1206.060292.
7. Palmer SC, Hayen A, Macaskill P et al. Serum levels of phosphorus, parathyroid hormone, and calcium and risks of death. *JAMA.* 2011;305(11):1119–1127.
8. Burnett S-AM, Gunawardene SC, Bringhurst FR, Jüppner H, Lee H, Finkelstein JS. Regulation of C-terminal and intact FGF-23 by dietary phosphate in men and women. *J Bone Miner Res.* 2006;21(8):1187–1196. doi:10.1359/jbmr.060507.
9. Antoniucci DM, Yamashita T, Portale AA. Dietary phosphorus regulates serum fibroblast growth factor-23 concentrations in healthy men. *J Clin Endocrinol Metab.* 2006;91(8):3144–3149. doi:10.1210/jc.2006-0021.
10. Jubiz W, Canterbury JM, Reiss E, Tyler FH. Circadian rhythm in serum parathyroid hormone concentration in human subjects: Correlation with serum calcium, phosphate, albumin, and growth hormone levels. *J Clin Invest.* 1972;51(8):2040–2046.
11. Ärnlöv J, Carlsson AC, Sundstrom J et al. Serum FGF23 and risk of cardiovascular events in relation to mineral metabolism and cardiovascular pathology. *Clin J Am Soc Nephrol.* 2013;8(5):781–786. doi:10.2215/CJN.09570912.
12. Gutiérrez OM, Januzzi JL, Isakova T et al. Fibroblast growth factor-23 and left ventricular hypertrophy in chronic kidney disease. *Circulation.* 2009;119(19):2545–2552. doi:10.1161/CIRCULATIONAHA.108.844506.
13. Gutiérrez OM, Wolf M, Taylor EN. Fibroblast growth factor 23, cardiovascular disease risk factors, and phosphorus intake in the health professionals follow-up study. *Clin J Am Soc Nephrol.* 2011;6(12):2871–2878. doi:10.2215/CJN.02740311.
14. Isakova T, Xie H, Yang W et al. Fibroblast growth factor 23 and risks of mortality and end-stage renal disease in patients with chronic kidney disease. *JAMA.* 2011;305(23):2432–2439. doi:10.1001/jama.2011.826.

15. Ix JH, Katz R, Kestenbaum BR et al. Fibroblast growth factor-23 and death, heart failure, and cardiovascular events in community-living individuals: CHS (Cardiovascular Health Study). *J Am Coll Cardiol.* 2012;60(3):200–207. doi:10.1016/j.jacc.2012.03.040.

16. Parker BD, Schurgers LJ, Brandenburg VM, Christenson RH, Vermeer C. The associations of fibroblast growth factor 23 and uncarboxylated matrix Gla protein with mortality in coronary artery disease: The Heart and Soul Study. *Ann Intern Med.* 2010;152(10):640–648.

17. Gruchow HW, Sobocinski KA, Barboriak JJ. Alcohol, nutrient intake, and hypertension in US adults. *J Am Med Assoc.* 1985;253(11):1567–1570.

18. Joffres MR, Reed DM, Yano K. Relationship of magnesium intake and other dietary factors to blood pressure: The Honolulu heart study. *Am J Clin Nutr.* 198745:469–475.

19. Zhao L, Stamler J, Yan LL et al. Blood pressure differences between northern and southern chinese: Role of dietary factors the international study on macronutrients and blood pressure. *Hypertension.* 200443:1332–1337. doi:10.1161/01.HYP.0000128243.06502.bc.

20. Elliott P, Kesteloot H, Appel LJ et al. Dietary phosphorus and blood pressure: International study of macro- and micro-nutrients and blood pressure. *Hypertension.* 200851:669–675. doi:10.1161/HYPERTENSIONAHA.107.103747.

21. Alonso A, Nettleton JA, Ix JH et al. Dietary phosphorus, blood pressure, and incidence of hypertension in the atherosclerosis risk in communities study and the multi-ethnic study of atherosclerosis. *Hypertension.* 201055:776–784. doi:10.1161/HYPERTENSIONAHA.109.143461.

22. Tzoulaki I, Patel CJ, Okamura T et al. A nutrient-wide association study on blood pressure. *Circulation.* 2012;126(21):2456–2464. doi:10.1161/CIRCULATIONAHA.112.114058.

23. Kim MH, Choi MK. Seven dietary minerals (Ca, P, Mg, Fe, Zn, Cu, and Mn) and their relationship with blood pressure and blood lipids in healthy adults with self-selected diet. *Biol Trace Elem Res.* 2013;153 (1–3):69–75. doi:10.1007/s12011-013-9656-1.

24. Calvo MS, Uribarri J. Public health impact of dietary phosphorus excess on bone and cardiovascular health in the general population. *Am J Clin Nutr.* 2013;98(1):6–15. doi:10.3945/ajcn.112.053934.

25. Leon JB, Sullivan CM, Sehgal AR. The prevalence of phosphorus containing food additives in top selling foods in grocery stores. *J Ren Nutr.* 2013;23(4):265–270. doi:10.1053/j.jrn.2012.12.003 Secreted

26. Klemmer P, Grim CE, Luft FC. Who and what drove Walter Kempner?: The rice diet revisited. *Hypertension.* 2014;64(4):684–688. doi:10.1161/HYPERTENSIONAHA.114.03946.

27. Kempner W. Some effects of the rice diet treatment of kidney disease and hypertension. *Bull N Y Acad Med.* 1946;22(7):358–370.

28. Kempner W. Treatment of heart and kidney disease and of hypertensive and arteriosclerotic vascular disease with the rice diet. *Ann Intern Med.* 1949;31(5):821–856.

29. Sacks FM, Wood PG, Kass EH. Stability of blood pressure in vegetarians receiving dietary protein supplements. *Hypertension.* 2015;6(2 Pt 1):199–201. doi:10.1161/01.HYP.6.2_Pt_1.199.

30. Sacks FM, Rosner B, Kass EH. Blood pressure in vegetarians. *Am J Epidemiol.* 1974;100(5):390–398.

31. Pettersen BJ, Anousheh R, Fan J, Jaceldo-Siegl K, Fraser GE. Vegetarian diets and blood pressure among white subjects: Results from the Adventist Health Study-2 (AHS-2). *Public Health Nutr.* 2012;15(10):1909–1916. doi:10.1017/S1368980011003454.

32. Armstrong B, Van Merwyk AJ, Coates H. Blood pressure in Seventh-day Adventist vegetarians. *Am J Epidemiol.* 1977;105(5):444–449.

33. Sacks FM, Svetkey LP, Vollmer WM et al. Effects on blood pressure of reduced dietary sodium and the Dietary Approaches to Stop Hypertension (DASH) diet. *N Engl J Med.* 2001;344(1):3–10.

34. Estruch R, Ros E, Salas-Salvado J et al. Primary prevention of cardiovascular disease with a Mediterranean diet. *N Engl J Med.* 2013;368(14):1279–1290. doi:10.1056/NEJMoa1200303.

35. Whelton PK, He J, Cutler JA et al. Effects of oral potassium on blood pressure; Meta-analysis of randomized controlled clinical trials. *J Am Med Assoc.* 1997;277(20):1624–1632. doi:10.1001/jama.1997.03540440058033.

36. Geleijnse JM, Kok FJ, Grobbee DE. Blood pressure response to changes in sodium and potassium intake: A metaregression analysis of randomised trials. *J Hum Hypertens.* 2003;17(7):471–480. doi:10.1038/sj.jhh.1001575.

37. Kesteloot H, Joossens JV. Relationship of serum sodium, potassium, calcium, and phosphorus with blood pressure. *Hypertension.* 198812:589–593. doi:10.1161/01.HYP.12.6.589.

38. Cappuccio FP, Elliot P, Allender PS, Pryer J, Follman DA, Cutler J. Epidemiologic association between dietary calcium intake and blood pressure: A meta-analysis of published data. *Am J Epidemiol.* 1995;142(9):935–945.

39. Pörsti I, Fan M, Kööbi P et al. High calcium diet down-regulates kidney angiotensin-converting enzyme in experimental renal failure. *Kidney Int.* 2004;66(6):2155–2166. doi:10.1111/j.1523-1755.2004.66006.x.
40. Song Y, Sesso HD, Manson JE, Cook NR, Buring JE, Liu S. Dietary magnesium intake and risk of incident hypertension among middle-aged and older US women in a 10-year follow-up study. *Am J Cardiol.* 2006;98(12):1616–1621. doi:10.1016/j.amjcard.2006.07.040.
41. Karp HJ, Vaihia KP, Kärkkäinen MUM, Niemistö MJ, Lamberg-Allardt CJE. Acute effects of different phosphorus sources on calcium and bone metabolism in young women: A whole-foods approach. *Calcif Tissue Int.* 2007;80(4):251–258. doi:10.1007/s00223-007-9011-7.
42. Iqbal TH, Lewis KO, Cooper BT. Phytase activity in the human and rat small intestine. *Gut.* 1994;35(9):1233–1236. doi:10.1136/gut.35.9.1233.
43. Moe SM, Zidehsarai MP, Chambers MA et al. Vegetarian compared with meat dietary protein source and phosphorus homeostasis in chronic kidney disease. *Clin J Am Soc Nephrol.* 2011;6(2):257–264. doi:10.2215/CJN.05040610.
44. Ralston RA, Lee JH, Truby H, Palermo CE, Walker KZ. A systematic review and meta-analysis of elevated blood pressure and consumption of dairy foods. *J Hum Hypertens.* 2012;26(1):3–13. doi:10.1038/jhh.2011.3.
45. Alonso A, Beunza JJ, Delgado-Rodríguez M, Martínez JA, Martínez-González MA. Low-fat dairy consumption and reduced risk of hypertension: The Seguimiento Universidad de Navarra (SUN) cohort. *Am J Clin Nutr.* 2005;82(5):972–979.
46. Jee SH, Miller ER, Guallar E, Singh VK, Appel LJ, Klag MJ. The effect of magnesium supplementation on blood pressure: A meta-analysis of randomized clinical trials. *Am J Hypertens.* 2002;15(8):691–696. doi:10.1016/S0895-7061(02)02964-3.
47. Moser M, White K, Henry B et al. Phosphorus content of popular beverages. *Am J Kidney Dis.* 2015;65(6):969–971. doi:10.1053/j.ajkd.2015.02.330.
48. Sullivan CM, Leon JB, Sehgal AR. Phosphorus containing food additives and the accuracy of nutrient databases: Implications for renal patients. *J Ren Nutr.* 2007;17(5):350–354.
49. Carrigan A, Klinger A, Choquette SS et al. Contribution of food additives to sodium and phosphorus content of diets rich in processed foods. *J Ren Nutr.* 2014;24(1):13–19. doi:10.1097/WAD.0b013e3181aba588. MRI.
50. Harlan WR, Hull AL, Schmouder RL, Landis JR, Thompson FE, Larkin FA. Blood pressure and nutrition in adults. The National Health and Nutrition Examination Survey. *Am J Epidemiol.* 1984;120(1):17–28.
51. Huang CX, Plantinga LC, Fink NE, Melamed ML, Coresh J, Powe NR. Phosphate levels and blood pressure in incident hemodialysis patients: A longitudinal study. *Adv Chronic Kidney Dis.* 2008;15(3):321–331. doi:10.1053/j.ackd.2008.04.012.
52. Raggi P, Boulay A, Chasan-Taber S et al. Cardiac calcification in adult hemodialysis patients. *J Am Coll Cardiol.* 2002;39(4):695–701. doi:10.1016/S0735-1097(01)01781-8.
53. Ashkar ZM. Association of calcium-phosphorus product with blood pressure in dialysis. *J Clin Hypertens.* 2010;12(2):96–103. doi:10.1111/j.1751-7176.2009.00220.x.
54. Van Ballegooijen AJ, Kestenbaum B, Sachs MC et al. Association of 25-hydroxyvitamin D and parathyroid hormone with incident hypertension: MESA (Multi-Ethnic Study of Atherosclerosis). *J Am Coll Cardiol.* 2014;63(12):1214–1222. doi:10.1016/j.jacc.2014.01.012.
55. Taylor EN, Curhan GC, Forman JP. Parathyroid hormone and the risk of incident hypertension. *J Hypertens.* 2008;26(7):1390–1394. doi:10.1097/HJH.0b013e3282ffb43b.
56. Anderson JL, Vanwoerkom RC, Horne BD et al. Parathyroid hormone, vitamin D, renal dysfunction, and cardiovascular disease: Dependent or independent risk factors? *Am Heart J.* 2011;162(2):331–339.e2. doi:10.1016/j.ahj.2011.05.005.
57. Jorde R, Sundsfjord J, Haug E, Bonaa KH. Relation between low calcium intake, parathyroid hormone, and blood pressure. *Hypertension.* 2000;35(5):1154–1159. doi:10.1161/01.HYP.35.5.1154.
58. Oliveira RB, Cancela ALE, Graciolli FG et al. Early control of PTH and FGF23 in normophosphatemic CKD patients: A new target in CKD-MBD therapy? *Clin J Am Soc Nephrol.* 2010;5(2):286–291. doi:10.2215/CJN.05420709.
59. Isakova T, Barchi-Chung A, Enfield G et al. Effects of dietary phosphate restriction and phosphate binders on FGF23 levels in CKD. *Clin J Am Soc Nephrol.* 2013;8(6):1009–1018. doi:10.2215/CJN.09250912.
60. Block GA, Wheeler DC, Persky MS et al. Effects of phosphate binders in moderate CKD. *J Am Soc Nephrol.* 2012;23(8):1407–1415. doi:10.1681/ASN.2012030223.
61. Block GA, Fishbane S, Rodriguez M et al. A 12-week, double-blind, placebo-controlled trial of ferric citrate for the treatment of iron deficiency anemia and reduction of serum phosphate in patients with CKD stages 3-5. *Am J Kidney Dis.* 2014;65(5):728–736. doi:10.1053/j.ajkd.2014.10.014.

62. Chue CD, Townend JN, Moody WE et al. Cardiovascular effects of sevelamer in stage 3 CKD. *J AmSocNephrol*. 2013;24(5):842–852. doi:10.1681/ASN.2012070719.

63. Seifert ME, de las Fuentes L, Rothstein M et al. Effects of phosphate binder therapy on vascular stiffness in early stage chronic kidney disease. *Am J Nephrol*. 2013;38(2):358–366. doi:10.1016/j.jsbmb.2011.07.002. Identification.

64. Chang AR, Miller ER 3rd, Anderson CA et al. Phosphorus additives and albuminuria in early stages of CKD: A randomized controlled trial. *Am J Kidney Dis*. 2017 Feb;69(2):200-209. doi: 10.1053/j.ajkd.2016.08.029. Epub 2016 Nov 16. PubMed PMID: 27865566; PubMed Central PMCID: PMC5263092.

65. Altorf-van der Kuil W, Engberink MF, Brink EJ et al. Dietary protein and blood pressure: A systematic review. *PLOS ONE*. 2010;5(8):e12102. doi:10.1371/journal.pone.0012102.

66. Alonso A, Beunza JJ, Bes-Rastrollo M, Pajares RM, Martínez-González MÁ. Vegetable protein and fiber from cereal are inversely associated with the risk of hypertension in a Spanish cohort. *Arch Med Res*. 2006;37(6):778–786. doi:10.1016/j.arcmed.2006.01.007.

67. Stamler J, Liu K, Ruth KJ, Pryer J, Greenland P. Eight-year blood pressure change in middle-aged men relationship to multiple nutrients. *Hypertension*. 2002;39(5):1000–1006. doi:10.1161/01.HYP.0000016178.80811.D9.

68. Liu K, Ruth KJ, Flack JM et al. Blood pressure in young blacks and whites: Relevance of obesity and lifestyle factors in determining differences: The CARDIA Study. *Circulation*. 1996;93(1):60–66. doi:10.1161/01.CIR.93.1.60.

69. Wang YF, Yancy WS, Yu D, Champagne C, Appel LJ, Lin PH. The relationship between dietary protein intake and blood pressure: Results from the PREMIER study. *J Hum Hypertens*. 2008;22(11):745–754. doi:10.1038/jhh.2008.64.

70. Appel LJ, Sacks FM, Carey VJ et al. Effects of protein, monounsaturated fat, and carbohydrate intake on blood pressure and serum lipids: Results of the OmniHeart randomized trial. *JAMA*. 2005;294(19):2455–2464. doi:10.1001/jama.294.19.2455.

71. Burke V, Hodgson JM, Beilin LJ, Giangiulioi N, Rogers P, Puddey IB. Dietary protein and soluble fiber reduce ambulatory blood pressure in treated hypertensives. *Hypertension*. 2001;38(4):821–826. doi:10.1161/hy1001.092614.

72. Hodgson JM, Burke V, Beilin LJ, Puddey IB. Partial substitution of carbohydrate intake with protein intake from lean red meat lowers blood pressure in hypertensive persons. *Am J Clin Nutr*. 2006;83(4):780–787.

73. He J, Wofford MR, Reynolds K et al. Effect of dietary protein supplementation on blood pressure a randomized, controlled trial. *Circulation*. 2011124:589–595. doi:10.1161/CIRCULATIONAHA.110.009159.

74. Yamada S, Tokumoto M, Tatsumoto N et al. Phosphate overload directly induces systemic inflammation and malnutrition as well as vascular calcification in uremia. *Am J Physiol Renal Physiol*. 2014;306(12):F1418–F1428. doi:10.1152/ajprenal.00633.2013.

75. Haut LL, Alfrey AC, Guggenheim S, Buddington B, Schrier N. Renal toxicity of phosphate in rats. *Kidney Int*. 1980;17(6):722–731. doi:10.1038/ki.1980.85.

76. Eräranta A, Riutta A, Fan M et al. Dietary phosphate binding and loading alter kidney angiotensin-converting enzyme mRNA and protein content in 5/6 nephrectomized rats. *Am J Nephrol*. 201235:401–408. doi:10.1159/000337942.

77. Bozic M, Panizo S, Sevilla MA et al. High phosphate diet increases arterial blood pressure via a parathyroid hormone mediated increase of renin. *J Hypertens*. 201432:1822–1832. doi:10.1097/HJH.0000000000000261.

78. Suzuki Y, Mitsushima S, Kato A, Yamaguchi T, Ichihara S. High-phosphorus/zinc-free diet aggravates hypertension and cardiac dysfunction in a rat model of the metabolic syndrome. *Cardiovasc Pathol*. 2014;23(1):43–49. doi:10.1016/j.carpath.2013.06.004.

79. Bindels RJ, van den Broek LA, Hillebrand SJ, Wokke JM. A high phosphate diet lowers blood pressure in spontaneously hypertensive rats. *Hypertension*. 19879:96–102. doi:10.1161/01.HYP.9.1.96.

80. Bourgoin P, Lucas P, Roullet C et al. Developmental changes of Ca2+, P04, and calcitriol metabolism in spontaneously hypertensive rats. *Am J Physiol*. 1990;259(1 Pt 2):F104–F110.

81. Lau K, Chen S, Eby B. Evidence for the role of PO4 deficiency in antihypertensive action of a high-Ca diet. *Am J Physiol*. 1984;246(3 Pt 2):H324–H331.

82. Gennari, C, Nami, R, Gonnelli S. Hypertension and primary hyperparathyroidism: The role of adrenergic and renin-angiotensin-aldosterone systems. *Miner Electrolyte Metab*. 1995;21(1–3):77–81.

83. Bernini G, Moretti A, Lonzi S, Bendinelli C, Miccoli P, Salvetti A. Renin-angiotensin-aldosterone system in primary hyperparathyroidism before and after surgery. *Metabolism*. 1999;48(3):298–300.

84. Smith JM, Mouw DR, Vander AJ. Effect of parathyroid hormone on renin secretion. *Exp Biol Med*. 1983;172(4):482–487. doi:10.3181/00379727-172-41591.

10 Phosphorus Intake Contribution to Dietary Acid–Base Balance and Bone Health

Tanis R. Fenton and David A. Hanley

CONTENTS

Abstract 125
Bullet Points 126
10.1 Introduction 126
10.2 Methods 128
    10.2.1 Literature Search 128
    10.2.2 Urine and Blood pH Changes from Alkaline Salt Supplementation
         or Diet Changes 128
    10.2.3 The Role of Phosphorus in Calcium and Bone Metabolism 128
    10.2.4 Revised Potential Renal Acid Load Food Lists 129
10.3 Results 129
    10.3.1 Literature Search 129
    10.3.2 Urine and Blood pH Changes from Alkaline Salt Supplementation
         or Diet Changes 129
    10.3.3 The Role of Phosphorus in Calcium and Bone Metabolism 129
    10.3.4 Revised Potential Renal Acid Load Food Lists 136
10.4 Discussion 136
10.5 Conclusions 137
References 137

ABSTRACT

Phosphorus deficiency is associated with defective bone mineralization, but dietary phosphate has been considered an acidic antinutrient for bone maintenance under the acid-ash hypothesis.

We undertook a systematic review to (1) conduct meta-analyses of the urine and blood pH changes from alkaline or acid load changes; (2) assess the role of phosphorus in calcium (urine calcium, calcium balance); and (3) revise the Potential Renal Acid Load (PRAL) food lists.

The literature search identified 13 dietary phosphate intervention studies that met the inclusion criteria. Alkaline versus acidogenic treatments altered blood pH by only 0.01 or 0.02 pH units and urine by 7 to 177 times greater, by 0.2 to 1.2 pH units. No study participants had blood within the acidosis range. Phosphate supplements decreased urine calcium (0.6 mmol/day [95% confidence interval, CI] −0.6 to −0.9) and increased calcium balance by 0.9 mmol/day (95% CI 0.6–1.1) for every 32 mmol (1000 mg) of phosphorus, whether or not the supplement was acidic or alkaline. Because phosphate is anabolic to calcium balance, we revised the PRAL tables with phosphorus

126 Dietary Phosphorus: Health, Nutrition, and Regulatory Aspects

omitted. Several foods that changed PRAL from a positive "acidic load" to an estimated negative "alkaline load" include milk, yogurt, breads (white and whole-wheat), rice, oats, and lentils.

Contrary to the acid-ash hypothesis, urine pH changes markedly from alkaline versus acidogenic treatments, whereas blood pH does not change appreciably. Also contrary to the hypothesis, phosphate supplements decrease urine calcium and increase calcium balance.

BULLET POINTS

- Although dietary phosphate has been considered an acidic antinutrient for bone maintenance, the evidence of the effect of phosphate on bone metabolism does not support the acid-ash hypothesis.
- Phosphate supplements decrease urine calcium and increase calcium balance, whether or not the supplement is acidic or alkaline.
- Alkaline versus acidogenic treatments altered blood pH by only 0.01 or 0.02 pH units and urine by 0.2 to 1.2 pH units, 7 to 177 times greater.
- The revised Potential Renal Acid Load tables with phosphorus omitted changed the estimated acid load from a positive "acidic load" to an estimated negative "alkaline load" for milk, yogurt, breads (white and whole-wheat), rice, oats, and lentils.
- The promoter of the alkaline diet has been convicted in a court of law to be practicing medicine without a license.

10.1 INTRODUCTION

Phosphorus as phosphate plays a vital role in metabolism, energy production, growth, and cell repair; it is included in compounds such as ATP, DNA, RNA, and phospholipids, the main constituent of cell membranes. Phosphate is an essential component of bone mineral, incorporated in hydroxyapatite in a 3:5 ratio with calcium. The importance of calcium as a mineral nutrient required for the development and maintenance of bone strength is widely recognized. In comparison to calcium, phosphorus has almost been ignored.

Phosphate deficiency and hypophosphatemia are associated with defective mineralization and serious bone disorders (osteomalacia and rickets), but dietary phosphate has also been considered an acidic antinutrient for bone maintenance, under the concept of the acid-ash hypothesis. Although this hypothesis has been discounted in systematic reviews [1,2], it has had a significant influence on the scientific study of phosphate over the past century.

The alkaline diet, which is based on the acid-ash hypothesis, is currently being actively promoted through the lay literature and web pages as the cure for almost any situation of ill health in modern society [1,3]. The ideas behind both the alkaline diet and the acid-ash hypothesis were originally developed between 1907 and 1920 [4,5], based on early food chemical analysis and early nutrition studies. Researchers observed that when foods were burned, the remnants, the ash, were the nonorganic minerals' constituents. Some early nutrition researchers fed the food ash to research subjects and assessed their urine composition and reported that urine pH changed based on the ash composition. The acid-ash hypothesis was based on these early studies.

Some investigators observed that calcium excretion was higher in more acidic urine than alkaline urine. From these observations, some proposed the acid-ash hypothesis as a possible mechanism for the development of osteoporosis. Over the intervening century, these theories have been continued, mostly based on observational studies, small short-term clinical trials, and narrative review papers. Many other diseases have been added to the list proposed to be caused by the acid-generating modern diet, based on associations between diet composition and disease occurrence, using the acid-ash hypothesis as an explanation [3]. Associations do not mean causation, and the data from well-conducted randomized clinical trials provide much stronger evidence [6].

One of the most-cited papers of the acid-ash hypothesis is a calculation paper that estimated the acid load (referred to as Potential Renal Acid Load, or PRAL) of foods based on the hypothesis published by Remer and Manz in 1995 [7]. Although often cited, the food categorization by Remer and Manz remains theoretical. Apart from their secondary analysis of urine pH and acid excretion from six subjects who consumed four mixed diets for five days, this food categorization has not been confirmed [8]. The explained variance of the urine pH by the estimates of their food intakes was 0.69 (R^2), a moderate correlation. Bland and Altman describe the weaknesses of correlations as a statistic [9]. Although a correlation reflects the strength of a relationship, it does not assess agreement between two variables. The results from this study do not prove that the individual foods' PRALs are correctly estimated.

In the scientific literature, narrative reviews continue to support the concepts of the acid-ash hypothesis and the alkaline diet [10,11]; however, higher level evidence (randomized studies and systematic reviews) do not support these ideas [1,3]. In contrast with the acid-ash hypothesis and the alkaline diet, higher-level evidence from systematic reviews has revealed that protein may be protective and not detrimental to bone health [12,13]. Further several recent well-designed randomized controlled medium-term feeding trials (4–7 weeks) have further supported that, contrary to the acid-ash hypothesis and the alkaline diet, protein is not detrimental and rather is likely supportive of bone mineralization [14–16]. Diet-induced acid excretion is not associated with whole-body loss of calcium [13]. Evidence is lacking that fruit and vegetables are important for bone health [17,18]. Information about the acid-generating potential of grains has been lacking since the contradictory study published in 1914 [19]. These many lines of evidence all indicate that the acid-ash hypothesis is not well founded.

Under the concepts of the acid-ash hypothesis and the alkaline diet, protein and grain-based foods are considered to contribute to bone mineral loss, whereas fruit and vegetables are protective. Consumption of dairy products, which are high in phosphate and protein, are discouraged in the alkaline diet. Under Remer's PRAL food estimates, milk is considered slightly detrimental for bone health because it has a slightly positive PRAL (0.7) and cheese is considered highly detrimental to bone health (PRAL = 11.1–34.2). These theories have not been validated in experimental studies. In contrast to the acid load expected of milk, a study revealed that milk raises urine pH slightly, making it more alkaline [20]. Additionally, studies have not assessed the effects of individual foods on acid excretion; therefore the values in the Remer tables have not been validated.

The 1995 food lists that classified foods as acid or alkaline producing [7] relied on the 1912 acid-ash hypothesis that assumed that phosphorus is harmful to bone health because it was considered to reflect part of the detrimental acid content of foods [4]. However, a systematic review of the randomized controlled trials of 269 human subjects' phosphorus intakes found that phosphorus contributes to higher calcium retention, regardless of whether calcium intakes were high or moderate and whether the phosphorus source was acidic or alkaline [2]. More recent phosphorus supplementation studies have supported these findings and found that diets low in phosphorus are detrimental to bone health [21] and phosphorus with moderate calcium intakes contribute to calcium retention [22]. These findings that phosphorus contributes to higher calcium retention, when calcium intakes are at least moderate, casts further doubt upon the acid-ash hypothesis and whether it provides useful dietary recommendations to preserve bone health.

Concern has been expressed that the body becomes acidic from ingestion of the modern diet [8,10,11]. As far as we are aware, the effect of phosphate salts on systemic and urinary pH has not been systematically reviewed. A systematic review is a systematic search for and summary of all studies conducted, using strategies to limit bias in the gathering, critical appraisal, and synthesis of all relevant studies on a topic [23]. The Cochrane Collaboration recommends that systematic reviews should be kept up to date and updated every two to three years with new literature.

The purpose of this chapter is to address the question of what role phosphorus has in bone health. The primary and secondary objectives were to (1) conduct meta-analyses of the urine and blood pH changes from alkaline salt supplementation or diet changes; (2) assess the role of phosphorus

10.2 METHODS

10.2.1 Literature Search

The literature search was conducted (Ovid MEDLINE, CINAHL, PubMed, EMBASE, and the Cochrane Central Register of Controlled Trials were searched) in January 2016. We searched the studies for analyses of differences of urine and/or blood pH in response to food and/or nutrient supplementation and for studies on the effect of phosphate supplementation on bone health, as calcium balance and bone markers.

We combined four comprehensive themes using both keywords and text words: phosphorus, phosphate, and phosphates; acid excretion (net acid excretion, acid excretion, acid–base equilibrium, pH); and the following outcomes: bone health (bone, bones, bone density, bone mineral density, fractures, biopsy, bone resorption markers) or calcium metabolism and excretion (calcium, calcium, calciuria, excretion, urine, urinary, balance, retention). The search was limited to adult humans older than 18 years of age. Our search was not limited by language. Reference lists were also reviewed for relevant studies.

10.2.2 Urine and Blood pH Changes from Alkaline Salt Supplementation or Diet Changes

We identified studies that measured urine pH through diet changes and supplements and compared the differences of urine pH to blood pH. Additionally, we examined the data to determine if any of the participants' blood pH was within the acidotic range (i.e., below 7.35).

10.2.3 The Role of Phosphorus in Calcium and Bone Metabolism

We conducted multiple linear regression analyses to examine the effect of dietary phosphate on urinary calcium excretion, calcium balance, and markers of bone resorption or turnover. Interaction terms were included in the regression models to test the hypotheses that the estimated effects of the phosphate supplements were the same whether the subjects were on high or low calcium intakes or whether the phosphate supplement was acidic or not. One study did not report the age of their subjects, who they described as "young women," and the median age of 22 was assumed to keep this study in the analysis. The analyses were weighted for study sample size.

The cutoff point used to stratify the analysis by calcium intake was a value greater than or equal to versus less than the value considered adequate by the Institute of Medicine of 1000 mg/day (25 mmol/day) for adults aged 19 through 50 years and 1200 mg/day (30 mmol/day) for those aged 51 or older [24].

We interpreted our regression results in terms of differences in calcium metabolism with differences of 1 gram/day of phosphate intake because this amount is similar to a difference of approximately 2 standard deviations of phosphate intake among populations in Western societies [25–27].

Phosphorus Intake Contribution to Dietary Acid–Base Balance and Bone Health 129

10.2.4 REVISED POTENTIAL RENAL ACID LOAD FOOD LISTS

Because the phosphorus and bone health analysis revealed that phosphorus is anabolic and not detrimental to calcium retention [2], we revised the Remer/Manz PRAL tables [7] to omit phosphorus from the calculation.

10.3 RESULTS

10.3.1 LITERATURE SEARCH

The literature search identified 13 dietary phosphate intervention studies that met the inclusion criteria [22,28–39] (Tables 10.1 and 10.2). These studies comprised 32 intervention arms and 317 participant intakes. No non-English language papers met the criteria for acceptance.

Relative to the 2009 systematic review [2], this search located one additional study that fit the inclusion criteria [22], and the numerical results on urinary calcium were obtained directly from the authors to include these data in a revised systematic review. An additional paper [40] was originally reviewed and considered. However, this study did not collect 24-hour urine samples or calcium balance data; it reported the bone resorption markers as a change from baseline, which did not permit calculation of differences between groups [41]. Therefore, the study was not included in the analyses.

10.3.2 URINE AND BLOOD pH CHANGES FROM ALKALINE SALT SUPPLEMENTATION OR DIET CHANGES

One of the randomized trials that measured both urine and blood pH differences after phosphorus supplements observed that phosphorus supplements raised urine pH (a difference of 0.21 pH units: 6.58–6.79), whereas the change in blood pH was not clinically meaningful (a difference of 0.023 pH units within the normal range: 7.388–7.411) [36]. Two additional studies were identified that altered urine pH through dietary changes [42] and bicarbonate supplements [43] (Table 10.3). Each of these studies had the participants consume diets designed to be acid producing and tested interventions expected to alter the acid load, as well as the blood and urine pH. The studies each revealed differences in urine pH of 0.2 to 1.2 pH units, whereas blood pH did not change appreciably: 0.01 [42,43] or 0.02 [36] pH units. Comparing the urine pH differences to the blood pH differences, the urine pH changes were 7.5 [36] to 177 [43] times larger than those of the blood pH differences. As estimated from the mean less 2 standard deviations, none of the participants during the "acidogenic" interventions had acidemia (blood pH < 7.35).

It is important to note that the person who actively promoted the alkaline diet to "alkalinize" the body has been found guilty in a court of law to be practicing medicine without a license [44]. He was treating cancer patients with intravenous bicarbonate, and the patients had adverse outcomes [44]. The alkaline diet for cancer prevention and/or treatment was found to lack evidence to support it in a systematic review of the published and gray literature [3].

10.3.3 THE ROLE OF PHOSPHORUS IN CALCIUM AND BONE METABOLISM

In the meta-analysis of the effect of phosphate supplements on urine calcium, phosphate supplements decreased urine calcium by 0.6 mmol/day (95% confidence interval [CI] −0.6 to −0.9) (26 mg, 95% CI 18–34 mg) for every 32 mmol (1000 mg) of phosphate. In the calcium balance analysis, phosphate supplements increased calcium balance by 0.9 mmol/day (95% CI 0.6–1.1) (36 mg, 95% CI 25–46 mg) for every 32 mmol (1000 mg) of phosphate.

TABLE 10.1
Phosphate Study Arm Calcium Intakes, Phosphate Doses, Urine Calcium, and Calcium Balance

Study	n	Phosphate Dose (mmol/ day)	Phosphate Source	Calcium Intake (mmol/ day)	Days on Calcium Intake[a]	Days on Each Balance Study after Adaption[b]	Change uCalcium (mmol/ day)	Change Calcium Balance (mmol/ day)
Patton	18	10	Na_2, HPO_4, and Na glycerophosphate	9	7	7	−0.4	−0.2
Patton	18	19	"	9	7	7	−1.0	0.6
Patton	18	10	"	24	7	7	−0.4	−0.6
Patton	18	19	"	24	7	7	−1.5	0.3
Patton	18	10	"	39	7	7	−1.0	0.03
Patton	18	19	"	39	7	7	−0.4	1.1
Malm	4	24	H_3PO_4	-	98	7	−0.9	n/a
Malm	2	32	H_3PO_4	11	98	28	−0.7	0.7
Malm	4	26	H_3PO_4	20	98	28	−0.9	0.1
Malm	2	19	H_3PO_4	13	56	56	−1	0.03
Goldsmith	7(4))	32	K_2H and KH_2	21	7	4	−0.9	0.45
Bell	5	37	Na PolyP	18	6	22	−1.7	n/a
Spencer	10	37	Naglycerophosphate	5	0	22	−0.8	0.03
Spencer	8	37	Naglycerophosphate	21	0	40	−1.7	0.70
Spencer	3	39	Naglycerophosphate	36	0	34	−2.3	−0.35
Spencer	6	36	Naglycerophosphate	50	0	31	−2.1	0.10
Hegsted	8	49	KH+PO+	13	0	12	−2.5	0.94
Zemel	8	32	KH_2PO_4	10	2	11	−2.0	2.7
Zemel	8	32	$(NaPO_3)_6$	10	2	11	−2.0	1.3
Schuette	8	25	KH_2PO_4	15	2	6	−0.9	0.03
Spencer	1	35	Naglycerophosphate	6	0	w	−3.2	0.5
Spencer	4	34	Naglycerophosphate	20	0	42	−3.0	1.3
Spencer	2	41	Naglycerophosphate	34	0	33	−3.6	0.00
Spencer	3	40	Naglycerophosphate	51	0	40	−3.5	0.2
Whybro	9	32	NaH_2PO_4	25	5	2	−1.1	n/a
Whybro	11	48	Not stated	25	5	9	−2.4	n/a
Kemi	14	8	Na_2 Na_3 HPO_4	6	0	1	−0.2	n/a
Kemi	14	24	Na_2 Na_3 HPO_4	6	0	1	−0.5	n/a
Kemi	14	48	Na_2 Na_3 HPO_4	6	0	1	−0.5	n/a
Krapf	6	9.6	IV PO4 vs. Cl	35	4	3	−3.5	n/a
Karp	14	48	NaH2PO42H2O	9	0	n/a	−0.5	n/a
Karp	14	48	Na5P3O10	9	0	n/a	−1.2	n/a

[a] Days on calcium intake prior to the measurement of outcomes.

[b] The shortest number of days on the balance study is reported if it varied within the comparison interventions.

In the stratified analyses of the effect of phosphate supplements, the results differed depending on calcium intakes (Figure 10.1a and b), and there was a lack evidence of differences depending on whether or not the supplement was acidic or basic (Figure 10.2a and b, Table 10.4).

The effect of phosphate supplements was greater when calcium intakes were higher than the Dietary Reference Intakes (DRI) adequate intakes [24] compared to lower calcium intakes, $p = 0.001$ (Table 10.4). Phosphate supplements had a greater effect on both urine calcium and

Phosphorus Intake Contribution to Dietary Acid–Base Balance and Bone Health   131

TABLE 10.2

Included Studies in the Meta-Analysis of Calcium Balance from a Change of Phosphate Intake

Study	Year	Subjects	Age Range (years)	% Female	Study Design	Baseline PO_4 Intake (mmol/day)	Ethics Approval	Food Weighted	Food lab Analysis	Usual Calcium Intake
Patton	1953	Young women	N/A	0	RCO	25	N/A	Yes	Yes	No
Malm	1953	Male prisoners	20–56	0	CO	Unclear	N/A	Yes	Yes	Yes
Goldsmith	1976	Postmenopausal women with osteoporosis	63–75	100%	CO	40	N/A	No	No	Yes
Bell	1977	Young adults	24–36	38%	CO	32	Yes	Yes	Yes	No
Spencer	1978	Adult men	38–65	0	CO	25	N/A	Yes	yes	No
Hegsted	1981	v	19–25	0	CO	33	Yes	Yes	Yes	No
Zemel	1981	Young men	18–24	0	CO	27	Yes	Yes	Yes	No
Schuette	1982	Young men	19–26	0	CO	29	Yes	Yes	Yes	No
Spencer	1986	Adult males	48–71	0	CO	26	Yes	Yes	Yes	no
Whybro	1998	Healthy men	19–38	0	RCO	26/32	Yes	No	no	No
Kemi	2006	Young women	20–28	100%	RCO	16	Yes	No	No	No
Krapf	1995	Young men	22	0	CO	49	Yes	No	No	No
Karp	2013	Young women	19–31	100%	RCO	16	Yes	No	No	No

TABLE 10.3
Meta-Analysis of the Urine and Blood pH Changes from Alkaline Salt or Diet Supplementation

	Intervention	Difference in Urine pH	Difference in Blood pH	Multiple Urine vs. Blood	Study Design
Krapf (1995)	IV neutral Na phosphate vs. NaCl	0.21	0.028	7.5	Before and after study
Buclin (2001)	Alkaline diet vs. Western diet	1.02	0.014	73	Random cross-over
Maurer (2003)	Na and K bicarbonates vs. NaCl and KCl	1.24	0.007	177	Before and after study

TABLE 10.4
Meta-Analysis of the Difference in Urine Calcium and Calcium Balance from 32 mmol (1000 mg) of Phosphate Intake

	Urine calcium				Calcium balance			
Analysis	B_1 mmol (mg)	p-Value for Slope	p-Value for Interaction	R^2	B_1 mmol (mg)	p-Value for Slope	p-Value for Interaction	R^2
Low calcium intakes	−0.59 (24)	< 0.001	0.001	0.248	1.32 (53)	< 0.001	0.046	0.216
High calcium intakes	−1.32 (53)				0.41 (17)			
Neutral or alkaline phosphate supplement	−0.84 (34)	< 0.001	0.18	0.118	0.74 (30)	< 0.001	0.48	0.224
Acidic phosphate supplement	−0.84 (34)				0.74 (30)			

calcium balance when calcium intakes were higher than the DRI adequate intakes compared to lower calcium intakes (Table 10.4, Figure 10.1a and b). For urine calcium, when calcium intakes were lower than the DRI, phosphate supplements decreased urine calcium by 0.6 (95% CI −0.3 to −0.8) mmol/day for every 32 mmol (1000 mg) of phosphate; when calcium intakes were higher than the DRI, phosphate supplements decreased urine calcium by 1.3 mmol/day for every 32 mmol (1000 mg) of phosphate (Table 10.4, Figure 10.1a). For calcium balance, when calcium intakes were lower than the DRI, phosphate supplements increased calcium balance by 0.3 (95% CI 0.2–0.4) mmol/day for every 32 mmol (1000 mg) of phosphate, whereas when calcium intakes were higher than the DRI, phosphate supplements increased the calcium balance by 0.1 mmol/day for every 32 mmol (1000 mg) of phosphate (Table 10.4, Figure 10.1b).

Phosphorus Intake Contribution to Dietary Acid–Base Balance and Bone Health

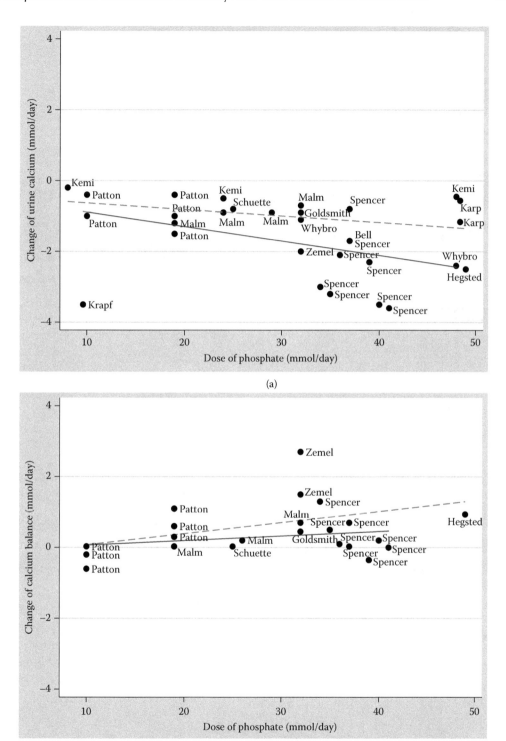

FIGURE 10.1 (a) Effect of PO_4 dose on urine calcium: stratified by calcium intake: low calcium intakes; slope = −0.018 mmol/day; high calcium intakes: slope = −0.041 mmol/day, p-value for slope: $p < 0.001$, p-value for interaction: $p = 0.001$. (b) Effect of PO_4 dose on calcium balance: stratified by calcium intake: low calcium intakes: slope = 0.031 mmol/day; high calcium intakes:slope = 0.013 mmol/day, p-value for slope: $p < 0.001$, p-value for interaction: $p = 0.046$. Dashed line = low calcium intake; Solid line = high calcium intake.

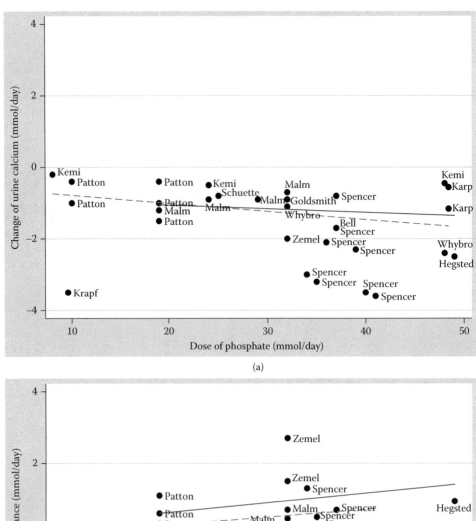

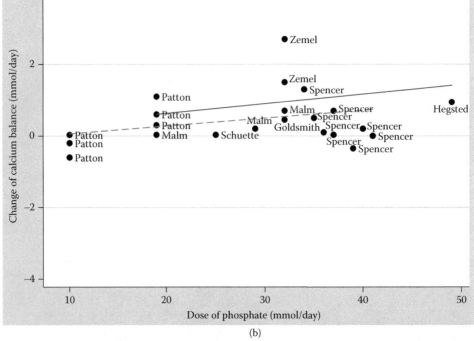

FIGURE 10.2 (a) Effect of PO$_4$ dose on urine calcium: stratified by "acidity" of PO$_4$ supplement: slope = 0.023 $p < 0.001$. Acidic supplement vs. neutral or basic supplement: p-value for interaction: $p = 0.18$. (b) Effect of PO$_4$ dose on calcium balance: stratified by "acidity" of PO$_4$ supplement: slope = 0.021 $p < 0.001$. Acidic supplement vs neutral or basic supplement: p-value for interaction: $p = 0.48$. Dashed line = acidic supplement; Solid line = neutral or basic supplement.

TABLE 10.5
Revised Estimates of Potential Renal Acid Load with Phosphorus Omitted Because It Supports Bone Mineralization

Food group and foods	Protein g	Na mg	K	Ca	Mg	P	Cl	SO$_4$ mEq	Old PRAL[a]	Revised PRAL-P[b]
Dairy products										
Cheddar-type, reduced fat	31.5	670	110	840	39	620	1110	15.4	**26.4**	**3.7**
Cheese, Gouda	24	910	91	740	38	490	1440	11.7	**18.6**	**0.6**
Milk, whole	3.2	55	140	115	11	92	100	1.6	**0.7**	**−2.6**[c]
Processed cheese	20.8	1320	130	600	22	800	2033	10.2	**28.7**	**−0.6**[c]
Yogurt, fruit	5.1	82	210	160	16	130	150	2.5	**1.2**	**−3.6**[c]
Yogurt	5.7	80	280	200	19	170	170	2.8	**1.5**	**−4.7**[c]
Grain products										
Bread, white wheat flour	6.2	553	177	17	0	127	852	3	**3.8**	**−0.8c**
Bread, whole wheat	7	380	270	63	92	196	585	3.4	**1.8**	**−5.3**[c]
Rice, easy cook white, boiled	2.6	1	54	18	11	54	4	1.3	**1.7**	**−0.3**[c]
Rolled oats	12.5	5	335	54	139	391	61	6.1	**10.7**	**−3.7**[c]
Spaghetti, white	12	3	250	25	56	190	25	5.9	**6.5**	**−0.5**[c]
Spaghetti, whole meal	13.4	130	390	31	120	330	210	6.5	**7.3**	**−4.7**[c]
White flour, whole meal	12.7	3	340	38	120	320	38	6.2	**8.2**	**−3.5**[c]
Meat and alternates										
Beef, lean only	20.3	61	350	7	20	180	59	9.9	**7.8**	**1.2**
Chicken, meat only	20.5	81	320	10	25	200	78	10	**8.7**	**1.4**
Cod, fillets	17.4	77	320	16	23	170	110	8.5	**7.1**	**0.9**
Haddock	16.8	120	300	18	23	170	160	8.2	**6.8**	**0.6**
Herring	16.8	67	340	33	29	210	76	8.2	**7**	**−0.7**[c]
Lentils, whole, dried	24.3	12	940	71	110	350	87	11.9	**3.5**	**−9.3**[c]
Trout, brown, steamed	23.5	88	370	36	31	270	70	11.5	**10.8**	**0.9**
Veal, fillet	21.1	110	360	8	25	260	68	10.3	**9**	**−0.5**[c]
Vegetables										
Asparagus	2.9	1	260	27	13	72	60	1.4	**−0.4**	**−3.0**
Beans, green	1.9	0	230	36	17	38	9	0.9	**−3.1**	**−4.4**
Broccoli	4.4	8	370	56	22	87	100	2.2	**−1.2**	**−4.4**
Carrots	0.7	40	240	34	9	25	39	0.3	**−4.9**	**−5.8**
Cauliflower	3.6	9	380	21	17	64	28	1.8	**−4**	**−6.4**
Lettuce	0.8	3	220	28	6	28	47	0.4	**−2.5**	**−3.5**
Onions	1.2	3	160	25	4	30	25	0.6	**−1.5**	**−2.6**
Peppers, green	0.8	4	120	8	10	19	19	0.4	**−1.4**	**−2.1**
Potatoes	2.1	7	360	5	17	37	66	1	**−4**	**−5.4**
Tomatoes	0.7	9	250	7	7	24	55	0.3	**−3.1**	**−4.0**
Zucchini	1.8	1	360	25	22	45	45	0.9	**−4.6**	

[a] Old PRAL = Remer and Manz's original calculated PRAL.

[b] "Revised PRAL-P" = the revised estimates.

[c] Foods that changed PRAL category from positive "acidic" to negative "alkaline."

10.3.4 Revised Potential Renal Acid Load Food Lists

The findings from this systematic review indicate that phosphate is anabolic to calcium balance, contrary to the acid-ash hypothesis. We therefore revised the well-quoted tables of Potential Renal Acid Load (PRAL) [7,8], with phosphorus omitted (Table 10.5). Table 10.5 includes Remer and Manz's original calculated PRAL as column "R.PRAL" and the revised estimates as column "PRAL-P." Several foods that changed PRAL from a positive "acidic load" to an estimated negative "alkaline load" include milk, yogurt, processed cheese, breads (white and whole-wheat), pasta, rice, rolled oats, lentils, herring, trout, and veal.

10.4 DISCUSSION

This is a systematic review of randomized control trials, which were combined in a meta-regression analysis. The primary findings indicate that increased phosphate intake consistently decreased urine calcium and consistently increased calcium balance, whether calcium intakes were high or low, whether the supplements were acidic versus neutral or basic. Of importance, these findings are all in contradiction to the acid-ash hypothesis, which suggests that phosphate is detrimental to calcium balance and bone health on the basis that it represents "acid," and early studies of dietary acid have been associated with higher urine calcium. There are several limits to this theory, because urine calcium is a poor surrogate of calcium nutritional status or calcium balance given that it ignores calcium absorption. The simple categorization of foods as acidic and alkaline based on the acid-ash hypothesis ignores the complexity and the evolution of nutrition science that has occurred in the 100 years since this hypothesis was developed [4].

The other identified phosphate study that did not have data in the format to include in these meta-analyses supports the findings of this systematic review [40]. These researchers tested whether providing both calcium and phosphorus is more supportive of bone health than calcium alone in a year-long randomized controlled trial among women with osteoporosis taking teriparatide and vitamin D. The acid-ash hypothesis would predict that providing phosphate and calcium would lead to poorer bone mineralization, because phosphate is considered acid-producing. In contrast with the acid-ash hypothesis, there were no differences between the groups for bone mineralization, urine calcium, or bone resorption biomarkers [40].

Indeed, the findings of these meta-analyses attack the basis of the acid-ash hypothesis. Under the hypothesis, the cations (calcium, sodium, potassium, and magnesium) are supportive of bone health and do not contribute to bone demineralization to stabilize systemic pH. Under the hypothesis, the anions (phosphate, chloride, sulfate) lead to acidosis and bone demineralization to stabilize the acid–base balance. This meta-analysis found that phosphate contributes to higher calcium balance (regardless of whether the calcium intakes were high or low or whether the supplements were acidic versus neutral or basic) and supports the position that phosphate intake is anabolic for bone mineral and not deleterious to bone health.

In agreement with our revised estimates that milk is not an acidogenic food, other investigators estimated that milk would supply an alkaline load [4,45], and a recent study revealed that milk actually increases urine pH and decreases net acid excretion [20]. Grains were considered in Remer's 1995 food lists as acid generating [7], but as far as we are aware, grains have not been evaluated for their hypothesized acidogenic and calciuric responses or effect on bone health. The study that found milk increases urine pH and decreases net acid excretion provided bread and butter with the milk [20], which suggests that grains do not produce acid when metabolized. Our revised estimates (Table 10.5) reveal that grain foods are not acid generating.

We found only three studies of acid load interventions that measured both urine and blood pH differences as a result of the interventions. Because the urine pH differences ranged from 7.5 [36] to 177 [43] times greater than those of the blood pH differences and none of the subjects provided the "acidogenic" diet and supplements were acidemic, research does not support the claim that diet

Phosphorus Intake Contribution to Dietary Acid–Base Balance and Bone Health   **137**

can acidify the body or that changes in urine pH provides any information about blood pH. In fact, an acidic urine just indicates that the kidneys are effectively excreting acid.

The acid-ash hypothesis predicts that phosphorus would lower urine pH because phosphate is an anion. In contrast to this notion, the identified study that provided phosphate supplements and measured urine pH observed an increase of urine pH (by 0.21 pH units) [36].

10.5   CONCLUSIONS

This systematic review of randomized trial interventions revealed that dietary supplemental phosphorus supports calcium retention, and these findings are consistent whether the participants' calcium intakes are high or low and whether the phosphate supplements are acidic or basic. These findings are contradictory to the acid-ash hypothesis that theorizes that phosphate is detrimental to bone mineralization.

This systematic review also found that even diets designed to be acid generating did not produce acidosis among the study participants, who were healthy individuals [36,42,43]. The phosphate supplement, which was expected to lower urine and blood pH under the hypothesis, actually raised the urine pH and blood pH remained unchanged [36]. All three studies designed to alter the acid–base status of the participants changed urine pH but not blood pH [36,42,43].

Given the lack of support of the acid-ash hypothesis with respect to the entire body of literature [1,3] and the strong evidence that phosphorus is protective of calcium retention, we suggest the acid-ash hypothesis should be abandoned.

REFERENCES

1. Fenton TR, Tough SC, Lyon AW, Eliasziw M, Hanley DA. Causal assessment of dietary acid load and bone disease: A systematic review & meta-analysis applying Hill's epidemiologic criteria for causality. *Nutrition Journal* 2011; 10: 41.
2. Fenton TR, Lyon AW, Eliasziw M, Tough SC, Hanley DA. Phosphate decreases urine calcium and increases calcium balance: A meta-analysis of the osteoporosis acid-ash diet hypothesis. *Nutrition Journal* 2009; 8: 41.
3. Fenton TR, Huang T. Systematic review of the association between dietary acid load, alkaline water and cancer. *BMJ Open* 2016; 6: e010438.
4. Sherman H, Gettler A. The balance of acid-forming and base-forming elements in foods, and its relation to ammonia metabolism. *Journal of Biological Chemistry* 1912; 11: 323–338.
5. Goto K. Mineral metabolism in experimental acidosis. *Journal of Biological Chemistry* 1918; 17: 355–376.
6. Guyatt GH, Oxman AD, Sultan S et al. GRADE guidelines: 9. Rating up the quality of evidence. *Journal of Clinical Epidemiology* 2011; 64: 1311–1316.
7. Remer T, Manz F. Potential renal acid load of foods and its influence on urine pH. *Journal of the American Dietetic Association* 1995; 95: 791–797.
8. Remer T, Manz F. Estimation of the renal net acid excretion by adults consuming diets containing variable amounts of protein. *The American Journal of Clinical Nutrition* 1994; 59: 1356–1361.
9. Bland JM, Altman DG. Statistical methods for assessing agreement between two methods of clinical measurement. *Lancet (London, England)* 1986; 1: 307–310.
10. Remer T, Krupp D, Shi L. Dietary protein's and dietary acid load's influence on bone health. *Critical Reviews in Food Science and Nutrition* 2014; 54: 1140–1150.
11. Nicoll R, McLaren Howard J. The acid-ash hypothesis revisited: A reassessment of the impact of dietary acidity on bone. *Journal of Bone and Mineral Metabolism* 2014; 32: 469–475.
12. Darling AL, Millward DJ, Torgerson DJ, Hewitt CE, Lanham-New SA. Dietary protein and bone health: A systematic review and meta-analysis. *The American Journal of Clinical Nutrition* 2009; 90: 1674–1692.
13. Fenton TR, Lyon AW, Eliasziw M, Tough SC, Hanley DA. Meta-analysis of the effect of the acid-ash hypothesis of osteoporosis on calcium balance. *Journal of Bone and Mineral Research* 2009; 24: 1835–1840.
14. Hunt JR, Johnson LK, Fariba Roughead ZK. Dietary protein and calcium interact to influence calcium retention: A controlled feeding study. *The American Journal of Clinical Nutrition* 2009; 89: 1357–1365.

15. Cao JJ, Johnson LK, Hunt JR. A diet high in meat protein and potential renal acid load increases fractional calcium absorption and urinary calcium excretion without affecting markers of bone resorption or formation in postmenopausal women. *The Journal of Nutrition* 2011; 141: 391–397.
16. Cao JJ, Pasiakos SM, Margolis LM et al. Calcium homeostasis and bone metabolic responses to high-protein diets during energy deficit in healthy young adults: A randomized controlled trial. *The American Journal of Clinical Nutrition* 2014; 99: 400–407.
17. Hamidi M, Boucher BA, Cheung AM, Beyene J, Shah PS. Fruit and vegetable intake and bone health in women aged 45 years and over: A systematic review. *Osteoporosis International* 2011; 22: 1681–1693.
18. Macdonald HM, Black AJ, Aucott L et al. Effect of potassium citrate supplementation or increased fruit and vegetable intake on bone metabolism in healthy postmenopausal women: A randomized controlled trial. *The American Journal of Clinical Nutrition* 2008; 88: 465–474.
19. Blatherwick N. The specific role of food in relation to the composition of the urine. *Archives of Internal Medicine* 1914; 14: 409–450.
20. Heaney RP, Rafferty K. Carbonated beverages and urinary calcium excretion. *The American Journal of Clinical Nutrition* 2001; 74: 343–347.
21. Heaney RP. Phosphorus nutrition and the treatment of osteoporosis. *Mayo Clinic Proceedings* 2004; 79: 91–97.
22. Karp HJ, Kemi VE, Lamberg-Allardt CJE, Kärkkäinen MUM. Mono- and polyphosphates have similar effects on calcium and phosphorus metabolism in healthy young women. *European Journal of Nutrition* 2013; 52: 991–996.
23. Moher D, Shamseer L, Clarke M et al. Preferred reporting items for systematic review and meta-analysis protocols (PRISMA-P) 2015 statement. *Systematic Reviews* 2015; 4: 1.
24. Institute of Medicine. *Dietary Reference Intakes for Calcium and Vitamin D*. Washington, DC: The National Academies Press, 2011.
25. Rosilene WVR, Cumming R, Travison T et al. Relative validity of a diet history questionnaire against a four-day weighed food record among older men in Australia: The Concord Health and Ageing in Men Project (CHAMP). *The Journal of Nutrition, Health & Aging* 2015; 19: 603–610.
26. Adatorwovor R, Roggenkamp K, Anderson JJB. Intakes of calcium and phosphorus and calculated calcium-to-phosphorus ratios of older adults: NHANES 2005-2006 data. *Nutrients* 2015; 7: 9633–9639.
27. Zhang R, Wang Z, Fei Y et al. The difference in nutrient intakes between Chinese and Mediterranean, Japanese and American diets. *Nutrients* 2015; 7: 4661–4688.
28. Malm OJ. On phosphates and phosphoric acid as dietary factors in the calcium balance of man. *Scandinavian Journal of Clinical and Laboratory Investigation* 1953; 5: 75–84.
29. Patton MB, Wilson ED, Leichsenring JM, Norris LM, Dienhart CM. The relation of calcium-to-phosphorus ratio to the utilization of these minerals by 18 young college women. *The Journal of Nutrition* 1953; 50: 373–382.
30. Goldsmith RS, Jowsey J, Dubé WJ, Riggs BL, Arnaud CD, Kelly PJ. Effects of phosphorus supplementation on serum parathyroid hormone and bone morphology in osteoporosis. *The Journal of Clinical Endocrinology and Metabolism* 1976; 43: 523–532.
31. Spencer H, Kramer L, Osis D, Norris C. Effect of phosphorus on the absorption of calcium and on the calcium balance in man. *The Journal of Nutrition* 1978; 108: 447–457.
32. Zemel MB, Linkswiler HM. Calcium metabolism in the young adult male as affected by level and form of phosphorus intake and level of calcium intake. *The Journal of Nutrition* 1981; 111: 315–324.
33. Hegsted M, Schuette SA, Zemel MB, Linkswiler HM. Urinary calcium and calcium balance in young men as affected by level of protein and phosphorus intake. *The Journal of Nutrition* 1981; 111: 553–562.
34. Schuette SA, Linkswiler HM. Effects on Ca and P metabolism in humans by adding meat, meat plus milk, or purified proteins plus Ca and P to a low protein diet. *The Journal of Nutrition* 1982; 112: 338–349.
35. Spencer H, Kramer L, Rubio N, Osis D. The effect of phosphorus on endogenous fecal calcium excretion in man. *The American Journal of Clinical Nutrition* 1986; 43: 844–851.
36. Krapf R, Glatz M, Hulter HN. Neutral phosphate administration generates and maintains renal metabolic alkalosis and hyperparathyroidism. *The American Journal of Physiology* 1995; 268: F802–F807.
37. Whybro A, Jagger H, Barker M, Eastell R. Phosphate supplementation in young men: Lack of effect on calcium homeostasis and bone turnover. *European Journal of Clinical Nutrition* 1998; 52: 29–33.
38. Kemi VE, Kärkkäinen MUM, Lamberg-Allardt CJE. High phosphorus intakes acutely and negatively affect Ca and bone metabolism in a dose-dependent manner in healthy young females. *The British Journal of Nutrition* 2006; 96: 545–552.

39. Karp HJ, Vaihia KP, Kärkkäinen MUM, Niemistö MJ, Lamberg-Allardt CJE. Acute effects of different phosphorus sources on calcium and bone metabolism in young women: A whole-foods approach. *Calcified Tissue International* 2007; 80: 251–258.
40. Heaney RP, Recker RR, Watson P, Lappe JM. Phosphate and carbonate salts of calcium support robust bone building in osteoporosis. *The American Journal of Clinical Nutrition* 2010; 92: 101–105.
41. Bland JM, Altman DG. Best (but oft forgotten) practices: Testing for treatment effects in randomized trials by separate analyses of changes from baseline in each group is a misleading approach. *The American Journal of Clinical Nutrition* 2015; 102: 991–994.
42. Buclin T, Cosma M, Appenzeller M et al. Diet acids and alkalis influence calcium retention in bone. *Osteoporosis International* 2001; 12: 493–499.
43. Maurer M, Riesen W, Muser J, Hulter HN, Krapf R. Neutralization of Western diet inhibits bone resorption independently of K intake and reduces cortisol secretion in humans. *American Journal of Physiology. Renal Physiology* 2003; 284: F32–F40.
44. Dodgson L. Creator of a bogus diet faces 3 years in prison [Internet]. [cited 2017 Jan 25] Available from: http://uk.businessinsider.com/alkaline-ph-diet-founder-arrested-2017-1
45. Gonick HC, Goldberg G, Mulcare D. Reexamination of the acid-ash content of several diets. *The American Journal of Clinical Nutrition* 1968; 21: 898–903.

11 Dietary Phosphorus Regulation of Vitamin D Metabolism in the Kidneys

Adriana S. Dusso, M. Vittoria Arcidiacono,
Natalia Carrillo-López, and Jorge B. Cannata-Andía

CONTENTS

Abstract 141
Bullet Points 142
11.1 Background and Significance 142
11.2 High Dietary Phosphorus Downregulation of Renal Calcitriol Production 143
11.3 Low Dietary Phosphorus Upregulation of Renal Calcitriol Production 144
11.4 Calcitriol Maintenance of the Phosphorus/Calcitriol/FGF23-α-Klotho
     Axis for Healthy Aging and Enhanced Survival 145
     11.4.1 Calcitriol Induction of Renal α-Klotho 145
     11.4.2 Calcitriol Induction of FGF23 Synthesis in Bone 145
     11.4.3 Calcitriol's Tight Control of Its Own Renal Production 146
11.5 Potential Survival Benefits of the Local Bioactivation of Vitamin D to
     25-Hydroxyvitamin D for VDR Induction of FGF23 and α-Klotho Expression 146
References 148

ABSTRACT

Phosphorus, abundant in most diets, is a key structural component of DNA, RNA, phosphoproteins, and phospholipids, all essential biomolecules to ensure cell viability and function. Consequently, normal phosphorus maintains the functional integrity of all tissues. However, high dietary phosphorus induces proinflammatory, pro-aging features that markedly reduce survival in the general population and in chronic kidney disease (CKD) patients. High phosphorus downregulation of the renal content of the longevity molecule α-klotho is a main determinant of the severe mineral, renal, and cardiovascular disturbances increasing mortality rates.

High phosphorus inhibition of renal calcitriol production, an inducer of α-Klotho gene expression, further aggravates the high mortality rates associated with hyperphosphatemia. Indeed, dietary phosphorus restriction, an inducer of renal calcitriol production, effectively counteracts hyperphosphatemia adverse effects on survival.

Calcitriol efficacy to induce both renal α-Klotho and bone synthesis of the phosphaturic hormone fibroblast growth factor-23 (FGF23), while tightly suppressing its own renal production to reduce intestinal calcium and phosphorus absorption and, consequently, the risk of hypercalcemia and hyperphosphatemia, is essential to improve survival.

This chapter updates the molecular mechanisms mediating (1) the opposing regulation of renal calcitriol production by high and low dietary phosphorus; (2) the antagonistic interactions between high phosphorus and the vitamin D system that maintain the phosphorus/calcitriol/FGF23-α-Klotho axis essential for survival; (3) the abnormalities in this critical axis induced by CKD;

142 Dietary Phosphorus: Health, Nutrition, and Regulatory Aspects

and (4) the synergistic interactions between 25-hydroxyvitamin D [25(OH)D] and calcitriol to enhance renal α-Klotho and bone FGF23 expression, which could explain the survival benefits associated with a normal vitamin D status.

BULLET POINTS

- The suppression of renal calcitriol production by high dietary P involves the induction of FGF23, which suppresses renal 1α-hydroxylase mRNA and enzymatic activity.
- FGF23 induction, rather than repression of parathyroid 1α-hydroxylase, demonstrates a tissue-specific modulation of local calcitriol synthesis in response to hyperphosphatemia.
- The induction of renal calcitriol synthesis by low dietary phosphorus requires growth hormone and insulin-like growth factor-1 (IGF-1) signals.
- High-phosphorus–induced reductions in α-klotho in normal individuals contribute to its pro-aging actions.
- Calcitriol fails to induce bone FGF23 synthesis in the absence of hyperphosphatemia.
- Calcitriol induction of renal α-Klotho is essential to maintain FGF23 phosphaturic actions and prevent hyperphosphatemia.

11.1 BACKGROUND AND SIGNIFICANCE

Phosphorus is an abundant component of a regular diet and essential in human health. Normal serum phosphorus not only helps to maintain skeletal integrity and muscle function, but also maintains all cells in a viable and functional state. In fact, phosphorus is an essential structural component of DNA, RNA, phospholipids, phosphoproteins, and adenosine triphosphate (ATP)—all critical biomolecules to ensure normal growth rates and cell differentiation through the regulation of the structural integrity and function of the cell membrane, intracellular cell signalling, enzymatic activities, energy metabolism, etc. However, high dietary phosphorus is sufficient to predispose to systemic inflammation and accelerated aging, two features that markedly increase the risk of cardiovascular mortality (Ellam and Chico 2012).

Part of the pro-aging actions of high dietary phosphorus results from its downregulation of the renal expression of the longevity molecule α-klotho (Kuro-o et al. 1997). In mice, ablation of the α-klotho gene is sufficient to closely resemble human aging, including shortened lifespan, osteopenia, severe hyperphosphatemia, vascular and soft tissue calcification, muscle and skin atrophy, pulmonary emphysema, and infertility (Kuro-o et al. 1997). In contrast, α-klotho overexpression suffices to reduce multiple organ damage and extend the lifespan (Kurosu et al. 2005). The critical contribution of hyperphosphatemia to the severe pro-aging features of the α-klotho knock-out mouse has been conclusively demonstrated by the survival benefits achieved simply through dietary phosphorus restriction (Kurosu and Kuro-o 2008; Razzaque and Lanske 2007; Yoshida et al. 2002).

High phosphorus downregulation of renal calcitriol production (Portale et al. 1989), a transcriptional inducer of α-Klotho expression (Forster et al. 2011), is an additional contributor to the accelerated aging and poor survival rates associated with hyperphosphatemia. Indeed, in chronic kidney disease (CKD), a disorder characterized by renal klotho deficiency and impaired calcitriol production, renal phosphate retention aggravates the severity of renal and cardiovascular damage, as well as the degree of vascular calcification (Kestenbaum et al. 2005). These adverse consequences of hyperphosphatemia in CKD patients can be efficaciously counteracted with either dietary phosphate restriction or the administration of phosphate-binding agents (Isakova et al. 2009).

Undoubtedly, high serum phosphorus does not suppress renal calcitriol synthesis to blunt calcitriol induction of renal α-klotho, but to prevent further worsening of hyperphosphatemia by reducing calcitriol-induced intestinal calcium and phosphorus absorption. Interestingly, whereas phosphorus antagonizes renal calcitriol production, calcitriol antagonizes the development of hyperphosphatemia through dual mechanisms: inhibition of its own renal production

Dietary Phosphorus Regulation of Vitamin D Metabolism in the Kidneys   **143**

(suppressing its synthesis and stimulating its degradation), which attenuates intestinal phosphorus and calcium absorption, and stimulation of bone synthesis and secretion of FGF23 (reviewed in Dusso et al. 2005; Haussler et al. 2013). This potent phosphaturic hormone not only attenuates renal phosphate retention but also further suppresses renal calcitriol production.

The following sections present the progress in our understanding of the molecular mechanisms underlying (1) high phosphorus suppression and low phosphorus stimulation of renal calcitriol production; (2) calcitriol maintenance of the phosphorus/calcitriol/FGF23-α-klotho axis for healthy aging and enhanced survival; (3) abnormalities in the phosphorus/calcitriol/FGF23-α-klotho axis induced by CKD; and (4) potential benefits of local bioactivation of vitamin D to 25-hydroxivitaminD [25(OH)D] to induce FGF23 in bone and α-klotho in the kidney in attenuating hyperphosphatemia and excessive circulating calcitriol.

11.2 HIGH DIETARY PHOSPHORUS DOWNREGULATION OF RENAL CALCITRIOL PRODUCTION

Oral phosphate supplementation reduces serum calcitriol concentrations in healthy individuals (Portale et al.1989, 1987; Portale et al. 1986). In fact, serum phosphorus correlates inversely with circulating calcitriol levels, an association totally accounted for by changes in renal calcitriol production rates, as calcitriol metabolic clearance remains unchanged. Oral phosphorus supplementation also reduces serum calcitriol in patients with idiopathic hypercalciuria or in children with moderate renal insufficiency (Portale et al. 1984). It is important to emphasize that both the duration of dietary patterns and additional dietary factors, including the short-term use of phosphorus-based food additives, could influence the renal response to a high phosphorus intake in regulating calcitriol production. In fact, despite persistently high serum parathyroid hormone (PTH) and reduced ionized calcium, after a four-week ingestion of a high-phosphorus diet, there were no increases in serum calcitriol levels, which suggests that high dietary phosphorus is impairing the renal response to the most potent inducers of CYP27b1 activity in individuals with normal kidney function (Calvo et al 1990). Furthermore, the intake for one week of similar food items differing exclusively in a low versus high amount of phosphorus-containing food additives markedly increases serum levels of the potent phosphaturic hormone FGF23, a primary downregulator of renal calcitriol synthesis (Gutierrez et al. 2015). High phosphorus induction of FGF23 through mechanisms that remain not completely understood has emerged as a main determinant of decreases in renal 1α-hydroxylase mRNA levels and activity. In fact, a transgenic mouse that constitutively expresses FGF23 has reduced calcitriol levels in spite of low plasma phosphate (Shimada et al. 2004b). FGF23 suppresses 1α-hydroxylase mRNA levels dose dependently (Perwad et al. 2005) and also induces post-transcriptional modifications that impair its enzymatic activity (Bai et al. 2004). Although FGF23 also suppresses monocyte 1α-hydroxylase (Bacchetta et al. 2013), it induces, rather than suppress, parathyroid 1α-hydroxylase (Krajisnik et al. 2007), which suggests a tissue-specific modulation of calcitriol production in response to hyperphosphatemia.

High serum phosphorus also induces the expression of frizzled-related protein 4 (FRP-4) and matrix extracellular phosphoglycoprotein (MEPE), two additional contributors to the suppressive effects of high phosphorus (reviewed in Schiavi and Kumar 2004) on renal calcitriol production. Similar to high levels of FGF23, FRP-4 (Berndt et al. 2003) and MEPE overexpression in vivo results in reduced calcitriol levels despite hypophosphatemia (Rowe et al. 2005).

Proximal tubular cells express α-Klotho (Hu et al. 2010a), a protein essential for FGF receptor activation by FGF23 (Tsujikawa et al. 2003). The gene product is a potent negative regulator of 1α-hydroxylase per se. Indeed, the α-klotho-null mouse has elevated renal 1α-hydroxylase mRNA levels and serum calcitriol levels despite high serum calcium and phosphate levels (Yoshida et al 2002), low PTH (Tsujikawa et al.2003), and high FGF23, which is the same phenotype for calcitriol production as that of the FGF23 null mouse (Nakatani et al.2009).

Furthermore, although FGF23 significantly reduces renal mRNA levels for 1α-hydroxylase (CYP27B1), in hemodialysis patients with very high FGF23, 25(OH)D supplementation can normalize serum calcitriol (Dusso et al. 1988). FGF23 also induces calcitriol degradation by increasing the expression of 24-hydroxylase (CYP24A1). Similar to FGF23 control of CYP27b1, despite the increased CYP24A1 mRNA levels, serum 24,25-dihydroxyvitaminD concentrations were persistently lower than normal in CKD patients nonsupplemented or supplemented with 25(OH)D and/or calcitriol (Dai et al. 2012; Bosworth et al. 2012). Clearly, in advanced CKD, the activity of either of these enzymes fails to reflect FGF23 control of the expression in their respective genes. This suggests that the damaged kidney fails to respond to high FGF23 tight downregulation of renal calcitriol production.

Interestingly, high dietary phosphorus also induces elevations in serum PTH (Slatopolsky et al. 2001). Different from FGF23, PTH is the most potent stimulus for renal calcitriol production in the presence of hypocalcemia (Garabedian et al. 1972). In CKD, however, several abnormalities prevent high PTH induction of renal calcitriol synthesis, even at early stages of renal disease (glomerular filtration rate [GFR] between 50 and 80 mL/min). In fact, different from individuals with normal kidney function, patients with a GFR of 70 mL/min and normal calcitriol levels fail to increase serum calcitriol in response to pharmacological doses of PTH (Ritz et al. 1991). Acidosis, a common feature in CKD patients, may contribute to this impaired response to high PTH.

In dogs, acidosis blunts PTH induction of renal 1α-hydroyxlase of the proximal convoluted tubules through an altered coupling of the PTH receptor with adenylate cyclase (Bellorin-Font et al. 1985), as this inhibition can be overcome by cyclic adenosine monophosphate (cAMP).

Acidosis also blunts the phosphaturic response to PTH (Beck et al.1975), and consequently, phosphate retention may also contribute to impair PTH induction of calcitriol synthesis.

CKD also blunts the increases in serum calcitriol induced by calcium restriction (Prince et al. 1988), possibly through the combination of all of the mechanisms listed earlier that impair the response to high PTH, because hypocalcemia and a low dietary calcium intake are the most potent stimulators of PTH secretion (Slatopolsky et al.1999).

In addition, accumulation of N-terminally truncated or C-terminal PTH fragments or of uremic toxins, all of which directly inhibit renal 1α-hydroxylase (Perwad et al. 2005; Usatii et al. 2007; Hsu and Patel 1992), may account for the blunted response to PTH induction of calcitriol synthesis in CKD.

11.3 LOW DIETARY PHOSPHORUS UPREGULATION OF RENAL CALCITRIOL PRODUCTION

Dietary phosphate restriction in individuals with normal kidney function increases serum calcitriol levels in spite of decreases in serum PTH. The mechanism involves increased renal calcitriol production, as suggested by unchanged calcitriol metabolic clearance rate (Portale et al.1989). Characterization of the underlying mechanisms, using normal mice and rat models, has demonstrated that dietary phosphate restriction not only enhances the activity but also the mRNA levels of renal 1α-hydroxylase (Zhang et al. 2002; Yoshida et al. 2001). Growth hormone plays a critical role in low phosphorus induction of renal-1α-hydroxylase mRNA levels. Indeed, whereas hypophysectomy blocks the stimulation of 1α-hydroxylase activity by dietary phosphate restriction, injection of either growth hormone or IGF-I to hypophysectomized rats restores the induction of renal calcitriol production in response to a low dietary phosphate intake (Gray 1981). The induction of 1α-hydroxylase expression by IGF-1 also suggests that, at least in part, α-klotho inhibition of renal calcitriol synthesis could be accounted for by α-klotho inhibition of IGF-1 signals (Bartke 2006).

An additional mechanism postulated to mediate low phosphate induction of renal 1α-hydroxylase was transepithelial inorganic phosphate transport by the renal tubule. However, in a mouse lacking the phosphate-regulated renal sodium Na/P cotransporter 2a (NaPT2a), the response to low phosphate in inducing 1α-hydroxylase mRNA levels and activity remained intact (Tenenhouse et al. 2001). The lower serum FGF23 levels in the NaPT2a-null mice may partially contribute to augment calcitriol synthesis (Perwad et al. 2005).

Dietary Phosphorus Regulation of Vitamin D Metabolism in the Kidneys

Importantly, phosphate restriction fails to induce measurable increases in serum calcitriol levels in patients with end-stage renal disease (Lucas et al. 1986) or in severely uremic dogs (Lopez-Hilker et al. 1990), an effect possibly attributable to very low amounts of remnant renal 1α-hydroxylase.

11.4 CALCITRIOL MAINTENANCE OF THE PHOSPHORUS/CALCITRIOL/FGF23-α-KLOTHO AXIS FOR HEALTHY AGING AND ENHANCED SURVIVAL

Calcitriol exerts three critical actions that contribute to the enhanced survival associated with the maintenance of a normal phosphorus/calcitriol/FGF23-α-Klotho axis, namely, the induction of the longevity molecule α-klotho in the kidney, the induction of the phosphatonin FGF23 in bone, and the tight control of its own circulating levels to avoid hypercalcemia and hyperphosphatemia.

11.4.1 CALCITRIOL INDUCTION OF RENAL α-Klotho

At present, calcitriol/vitamin D receptor (VDR) induction of the mRNA levels of the longevity gene α-Klotho and the identification of a vitamin D responsive elements (VDRE) in the human α-Klotho promoter (Forster et al. 2011) provide a potential causal link for the epidemiological association between vitamin D deficiency and higher risk of all-cause mortality in the general population (Chowdhury et al. 2014), a risk markedly aggravated in CKD patients. Indeed, whereas α-Klotho disruption confers a premature aging-like syndrome (Kuro-o et al. 1997), its overexpression is sufficient to extend the lifespan in mice (Kurosu et al. 2005).

α-Klotho is expressed in the kidney, the parathyroid gland, and the choroid plexus (Li et al. 2004), where it acts as a high-affinity receptor for circulating FGF23. In fact, appropriate levels of renal and parathyroid α-Klotho are required for FGF23 phosphaturic and PTH suppressive actions, respectively. Therefore, calcitriol induction of renal α-Klotho should attenuate the pro-aging features of hyperphosphatemia. Accordingly, progressive reductions of renal klotho in CKD patients stages 3 to 4 were associated with an impaired response to FGF23, reduced fractional excretion of phosphate, and a four-fold higher propensity for abdominal aortic calcification, measured by the Kaupilla index (Craver et al. 2013), thus supporting the potentiation of FGF23 protective actions in cells harboring α-Klotho .

Importantly, α-klotho can be found as a soluble form in blood, urine, and cerebrospinal fluid. Soluble α-klotho (s-klotho) is generated by proteolytic cleavage of the transmembrane α-klotho (Imura et al. 2004; Hu et al. 2010a) and exerts FGF23-independent endocrine actions, including the modulation of the activity of membrane channels, cotransporters, and multiple signalling pathways not fully characterized, all of which contribute to s-klotho's potent survival benefits. Indeed, the systemic administration of recombinant s-klotho is sufficient to rescue the phenotype of the α-klotho–null mice (Mitani et al. 2002) and, more significantly, the renal and cardiovascular damage associated with acute or chronic renal injury (Hu et al. 2010b, 2011, 2015). Therefore, maintenance of renal and/or circulating klotho has become a priority in nephrology. However, the inaccuracy of current assays prevents the use of measurements of s-klotho as a biomarker of the severity of CKD and of the risk for cardiovascular mortality.

11.4.2 CALCITRIOL INDUCTION OF FGF23 SYNTHESIS IN BONE

Calcitriol transactivation of the FGF23 gene in osteocytes and osteoblasts is an essential pro-survival action, as the dominant role of FGF23 is the renal elimination of phosphorus to prevent hyperphosphatemia and its pro-aging consequences. Indeed, as mentioned earlier, the main features of the FGF23-null mouse are hyperphosphatemia, high circulating calcitriol, ectopic calcifications, premature aging, arteriosclerosis, and osteoporosis (Shimada et al. 2004a), a phenotype that resembles that of the α-Klotho-null mouse and that can also be rescued by dietary phosphorus restriction (Kurosu and Kuro-o 2008; Razzaque and Lanske 2007; Yoshida et al.2002).

Furthermore, double knockouts of FGF23 and either the VDR (Hesse et al. 2007) or CYP27B1 (Renkema et al. 2008) also rescue the adverse pro-aging features of the FGF23-null mice by preventing hyperphosphatemia. As described previously, FGF23 suppresses CYP27B1 and induces CYP24A1 in the kidney (Perwad et al. 2005; Shimada et al. 2004a). Therefore, it is clear that the capability of FGF23 to get rid of excessive phosphorus while tightly preventing elevations in serum calcitriol is essential for its pro-survival effects.

There are several putative VDREs for VDR/RXR binding in the FGF23 promoter. Interestingly, FGF23 gene transactivation by calcitriol decreases from 80-fold to 4-fold in the presence of inhibitors of new protein synthesis, indicating that osteoblasts' full response to calcitriol induction of the FGF23 gene is indirect (Haussler et al. 2012). The low levels of FGF23 in the VDR-null mice and CYP27B1 mice (Yu et al. 2005) also suggest that impaired induction of FGF23 during vitamin D deficiency could contribute to accelerate pro-aging features and mortality. Importantly, calcitriol fails to transactivate the FGF23 gene if high calcitriol and hypophosphatemia occur simultaneously, as demonstrated using a transgenic mouse with an ablation in the gene for the phosphorus transporter NaPi2a (Miedlich et al. 2010). This supports the prevalent role of phosphorus over calcitriol in the upregulation of FGF23.

Because FGF23 requires membrane α-Klotho as a coreceptor for its phosphaturic actions (Urakawa et al. 2006), which protect from hypercalcemia, and calcitriol also induces the α-Klotho gene (Forster et al. 2011), it is clear that the maintenance of a normal bone–kidney FGF23/calcitriol/α-Klotho axis is crucial for survival.

11.4.3 CALCITRIOL'S TIGHT CONTROL OF ITS OWN RENAL PRODUCTION

Several indirect mechanisms are responsible for calcitriol inhibition of 1α-hydroxylase in vivo, including calcitriol-mediated increases in serum calcium and phosphorus levels, decreases in serum PTH, and the recently identified induction of bone synthesis of FGF23 (Barthel et al. 2007; Kolek et al. 2005) and of renal klotho expression (Tsujikawa et al. 2003).

Calcitriol feedback inhibition of 1α-hydroxylase minimizes the potential for vitamin D intoxication. Calcitriol directly suppresses 1α-hydroxylase activity in kidney cell culture (Henry 1979; Trechsel et al.1979) and reduces 1α-hydroxylase mRNA (Monkawa et al. 1997; Shinki et al.1997; St Arnaud et al. 1997; Takeyama et al. 1997). However, there is no conclusive evidence of a direct suppression of the 1α-hydroxylase gene promoter by the calcitriol/VDR complex. Instead, calcitriol appears to inhibit PTH/cAMP-mediated induction of 1α-hydroxylase gene expression (Brenza et al. 1998).

For decades, the most critical action of the calcitriol/VDR complex in the kidney has been the induction of CYP24A1 to maintain serum calcitriol within normal limits which, by degrading excessive circulating calcitriol and/or 25(OH)D, prevents hypercalcemia and hyperphosphatemia. Accordingly, CYP24A1 has a 25-fold higher affinity for calcitriol than for 25(OH)D. Induction of CYP24A1 is a classical genomic action of the calcitriol/VDR complex mainly on two proximal VDREs on this gene promoter (Haussler et al. 2013). The pathophysiological relevance of calcitriol induction of CYP24A1 in almost every vitamin D–responsive tissue was conclusively demonstrated by the severe hypercalcemia and nephrocalcinosis of the CYP24A1-null mouse (St-Arnaud et al. 2000) and in children and adults with a loss of function mutation of this gene (Jacobs et al. 2014; Schlingmann et al. 2011).

11.5 POTENTIAL SURVIVAL BENEFITS OF THE LOCAL BIOACTIVATION OF VITAMIN D TO 25-HYDROXYVITAMIN D FOR VDR INDUCTION OF FGF23 AND α-KLOTHO EXPRESSION

Figure 11.1 presents a previously unrecognized synergy between 25(OH)D and calcitriol for VDR activation, which can be achieved simply by ensuring normal serum 25(OH)D levels through nutritional vitamin D supplementation (Arcidiacono et al. 2015). This synergy could safely improve the

Dietary Phosphorus Regulation of Vitamin D Metabolism in the Kidneys

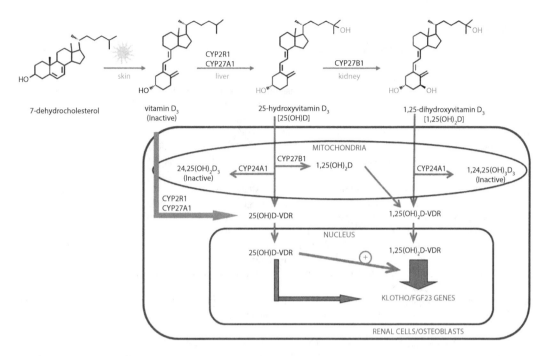

FIGURE 11.1 (see color insert) Vitamin D metabolism and VDR activation. Systemic vitamin D bioactivation to calcitriol [1,25(OH)$_2$D] and subcellular vitamin D bioactivation and degradation processes affecting the degree of transcriptional regulation by liganded VDR. Synergistic interactions between 25-hydroxy vitamin D [25(OH)D] and calcitriol that enhance α-klotho and FGF23 gene transcription (From Bergada, L., J. Pallares, A. Maria Vittoria, A. Cardus, M. Santacana, J. Valls, G. Cao, E. Fernandez, X. Dolcet, A. S. Dusso, and X. Matias-Guiu, *Lab Invest.*, 94, 608–22, 2014. With permission.)

degree of induction of renal α-klotho and bone FGF23 in response to a certain circulating and/or local calcitriol levels for a given local VDR expression in both normal individuals and, more significantly, in CKD patients receiving active vitamin D therapy without increasing active vitamin D dosage. The latter is critical in CKD patients, as Kidney Disease: Improving Global Outcomes (KDIGO) guidelines recommend reducing or stopping any active vitamin dosage during hyperphosphatemia.

Mechanistically, 25(OH)D not only activates the VDR directly, but also synergizes with calcitriol for VDR activation. This clinically relevant synergy has been conclusively demonstrated in the CYP27B1-null mouse (Hoenderop et al. 2004), which lacks the enzyme that converts 25(OH)D to calcitriol, and also in vitro, using 25(OH)D analogs chemically modified to prevent hydroxylation at carbon 1 (Lou et al. 2010; Munetsuna et al. 2011). Furthermore, in advanced experimental CKD, this synergy was proven sufficient in overcoming the parathyroid resistance to low doses of calcitriol (or its analogs) caused by VDR reductions and accumulation of uremic toxins (Arcidiacono et al. 2015).

In contrast to the tight regulation of the constitutive renal CYP27B1 and CYP24A1 hydroxylases by calcium, phosphorus, calcitriol, PTH, and FGF23, the ubiquitously distributed 25-hydroxylases (CYP27A1, CYP2R1) that convert vitamin D to 25(OH)D are loosely regulated. Therefore, vitamin D supplementation, through local 25(OH)D synthesis and the 25(OH)D/calcitriol synergy, could provide a safer alternative compared to increases in calcitriol dosage to counteract the reductions in intracellular levels of the calcitriol/VDR complex induced in the course of CKD. Undoubtedly, an improved VDR activation will be more effective in attenuating progressive reductions of renal α-Klotho content or the resistance of bone cells to produce FGF23 in response to incipient hyperphosphatemia. In fact, in a double-blinded trial in healthy volunteers treated with daily oral cholecalciferol or placebo, FGF23 increased significantly in the cholecalciferol-treated group but not in the placebo group (Nygaard et al. 2014).

REFERENCES

Arcidiacono, M. V., Yang, J. Fernandez, E. and Dusso. A. 2015. The induction of C/EBPbeta contributes to vitamin D inhibition of ADAM17 expression and parathyroid hyperplasia in kidney disease. *Nephrol Dial Transplant* 30 3:423–33. doi:10.1093/ndt/gfu311.

Bacchetta, J., Sea, J. L. Chun, R. F. Lisse, T. S. Wesseling-Perry, K. Gales, B. Adams, J. S. Salusky, I. B. and Hewison. M. 2013. Fibroblast growth factor 23 inhibits extrarenal synthesis of 1,25-dihydroxyvitamin D in human monocytes. *J Bone Miner Res* 28 1:46–55. doi:10.1002/jbmr.1740.

Bai, X., Miao, D. Li, J. Goltzman, D. and Karaplis. A. C. 2004. Transgenic mice overexpressing human fibroblast growth factor 23 (R176Q) delineate a putative role for parathyroid hormone in renal phosphate wasting disorders. *Endocrinology* 145 11:5269–79. doi:10.1210/en.2004-0233.

Barthel, T. K., D. R. Mathern, G. K. Whitfield, C. A. Haussler, H. A. th Hopper, J. C. Hsieh, S. A. Slater, G. Hsieh, M. Kaczmarska, P. W. Jurutka, O. I. Kolek, F. K. Ghishan, and M. R. Haussler. 2007. 1,25-dihydroxyvitamin D3/VDR-mediated induction of FGF23 as well as transcriptional control of other bone anabolic and catabolic genes that orchestrate the regulation of phosphate and calcium mineral metabolism. *J Steroid Biochem Mol Biol* 103 (3-5):381–8. doi: 10.1016/j.jsbmb.2006.12.054.

Bartke, A. 2006. Long-lived Klotho mice: New insights into the roles of IGF-1 and insulin in aging. *Trends Endocrinol Metab* 17 2:33–5. doi:10.1016/j.tem.2006.01.002.

Beck, N., Kim, H. P. and Kim. K. S. 1975. Effect of metabolic acidosis on renal action of parathyroid hormone. *Am J Physiol* 228 5:1483–8.

Bellorin-Font, E., Humpierres, J. Weisinger, J. R. Milanes, C. L. Sylva, V. and Paz-Martinez. V. 1985. Effect of metabolic acidosis on the PTH receptor-adenylate cyclase system of canine kidney. *Am J Physiol* 249 (4 Pt 2):F566–72.

Bergada, L., J. Pallares, A. Maria Vittoria, A. Cardus, M. Santacana, J. Valls, G. Cao, E. Fernandez, X. Dolcet, A. S. Dusso, and X. Matias-Guiu. X. 2014. Role of local bioactivation of vitamin D by CYP27A1 and CYP2R1 in the control of cell growth in normal endometrium and endometrial carcinoma. *Lab Invest* 94 6:608–22.doi: 10.1038/labinvest.2014.57.

Berndt, T., Craig, T. A. Bowe, A. E. Vassiliadis, J. Reczek, D. Finnegan, R. Jan De Beur, S. M. Schiavi, S. C. and Kumar. R. 2003. Secreted frizzled-related protein 4 is a potent tumor-derived phosphaturic agent. *J Clin Invest* 112 5:785–94.

Bosworth, C. R., Levin, G. Robinson-Cohen, C. Hoofnagle, A. N. Ruzinski, J. Young, B. Schwartz, S. M. Himmelfarb, J. Kestenbaum, B. and de Boer. I. H. 2012. The serum 24,25-dihydroxyvitamin D concentration, a marker of vitamin D catabolism, is reduced in chronic kidney disease. *Kidney Int* 82 6:693–700. doi:10.1038/ki.2012.193.

Brenza, H. L., Kimmel-Jehan, C. Jehan, F. Shinki, T. Wakino, S. Anazawa, H. Suda, T. and DeLuca. H. F. 1998. Parathyroid hormone activation of the 25-hydroxyvitamin D3-1alpha-hydroxylase gene promoter. *Proc Natl Acad Sci U S A* 95 4:1387–91.

Calvo, M. S., Kumar, R. and Heath. H. 1990. Persistently elevated parathyroid hormone secretion and action in young women after four weeks of ingesting high phosphorus, low calcium diets. *J Clin Endocrinol Metab* 70 5:1334–40. doi:10.1210/jcem-70-5-1334.

Chowdhury, R., Kunutsor, S. Vitezova, A. Oliver-Williams, C. Chowdhury, S. Kiefte-de-Jong, J. C. Khan, H. Baena, C. P. Prabhakaran, D. Hoshen, M. B. Feldman, B. S. Pan, A. Johnson, L. Crowe, F. Hu, F. B. and Franco. O. H. 2014. Vitamin D and risk of cause specific death: Systematic review and meta-analysis of observational cohort and randomised intervention studies. *BMJ* 348:g1903. doi:10.1136/bmj.g1903.

Craver, L., Dusso, A. Martinez-Alonso, M. Sarro, F. Valdivielso, J. M. and Fernandez. E. 2013. A low fractional excretion of Phosphate/Fgf23 ratio is associated with severe abdominal Aortic calcification in stage 3 and 4 kidney disease patients. *BMC Nephrol* 14:221. doi:10.1186/1471-2369-14-221.

Dai, B., David, V. Alshayeb, H. M. Showkat, A. Gyamlani, G. Horst, R. L. Wall, B. M. and Quarles. L. D. 2012. Assessment of 24,25(OH)2D levels does not support FGF23-mediated catabolism of vitamin D metabolites. *Kidney Int* 82 10:1061–70. doi:10.1038/ki.2012.222.

Dusso, A. S., Brown, A. J. and Slatopolsky. E. 2005. Vitamin D. *Am J Physiol Renal Physiol* 289 (1):F8–28.

Dusso, A., S. Lopez-Hilker, Rapp, N. and Slatopolsky. E. 1988. Extra-renal production of calcitriol in chronic renal failure. *Kidney Int* 34 3:368–75.

Ellam, T. J. and Chico. T. J. 2012. Phosphate: The new cholesterol? The role of the phosphate axis in non-uremic vascular disease. *Atherosclerosis* 220 2:310–8. doi:10.1016/j.atherosclerosis.2011.09.002.

Forster, R. E., Jurutka, P. W. Hsieh, J. C. Haussler, C. A. Lowmiller, C. L. Kaneko, I. Haussler, M. R. and Kerr Whitfield. G. 2011. Vitamin D receptor controls expression of the anti-aging klotho gene in mouse and human renal cells. *Biochem Biophys Res Commun* 414 3:557–62. doi:10.1016/j.bbrc.2011.09.117.

Garabedian, M., Holick, M. F. Deluca, H. F. and Boyle. I. T. 1972. Control of 25-hydroxycholecalciferol metabolism by parathyroid glands. *Proc Natl Acad Sci U S A* 69 7:1673–6.

Gray, R. W. 1981. Control of plasma 1,25-(OH)2-vitamin D concentrations by calcium and phosphorus in the rat: Effects of hypophysectomy. *Calcif Tissue Int* 33 5:485–8.

Gutierrez, O. M., Luzuriaga-McPherson, A. Lin, Y. Gilbert, L. C. Ha, S. W. and Beck, G. R. Jr. 2015. Impact of phosphorus-based food additives on bone and mineral metabolism. *J Clin Endocrinol Metab* 100 11:4264–71. doi:10.1210/jc.2015-2279.

Haussler, M. R., Whitfield, G. K. Kaneko, I. Forster, R. Saini, R. Hsieh, J. C. Haussler, C. A. and Jurutka. P. W. 2012. The role of vitamin D in the FGF23, klotho, and phosphate bone-kidney endocrine axis. *Rev Endocr Metab Disord* 13 1:57–69. doi:10.1007/s11154-011-9199-8.

Haussler, M. R., Whitfield, G. K. Kaneko, I. Haussler, C. A. Hsieh, D. Hsieh, J. C. and Jurutka. P. W. 2013. Molecular mechanisms of vitamin D action. *Calcif Tissue Int* 92 2:77–98. doi:10.1007/s00223-012-9619-0.

Henry, H. L. 1979. Regulation of the hydroxylation of 25-hydroxyvitamin D3 in vivo and in primary cultures of chick kidney cells. *J Biol Chem* 254 8:2722–9.

Hesse, M., Frohlich, L. F. Zeitz, U. Lanske, B. and Erben. R. G. 2007. Ablation of vitamin D signaling rescues bone, mineral, and glucose homeostasis in Fgf-23 deficient mice. *Matrix Biol* 26 2:75–84. doi:10.1016/j.matbio.2006.10.003.

Hoenderop, J. G., Chon, H. Gkika, D. Bluyssen, H. A. Holstege, F. C. R. St-Arnaud, Braam, B. and Bindels. R. J. 2004. Regulation of gene expression by dietary Ca2+ in kidneys of 25-hydroxyvitamin D3-1 alpha-hydroxylase knockout mice. *Kidney Int* 65 2:531–9. doi:10.1111/j.1523-1755.2004.00402.x.

Hsu, C. H. and Patel. S. 1992. Uremic plasma contains factors inhibiting 1 alpha-hydroxylase activity. *J Am Soc Nephrol* 3 4:947–52.

Hu, M. C., Shi, M. Cho, H. J. B. Adams-Huet, Paek, J. Hill, K. Shelton, J. Amaral, A. P. Faul, C. Taniguchi, M. Wolf, M. Brand, M. Takahashi, M. Kuro, O. M. Hill, J. A. and Moe. O. W. 2015. Klotho and phosphate are modulators of pathologic uremic cardiac remodeling. *J Am Soc Nephrol* 26 6:1290–302. doi:10.1681/ASN.2014050465.

Hu, M. C., Shi, M. Zhang, J. Pastor, J. Nakatani, T. Lanske, B. Razzaque, M. S. K. P. Rosenblatt, Baum, M. G. Kuro-o, M. and Moe. O. W. 2010a. Klotho: A novel phosphaturic substance acting as an autocrine enzyme in the renal proximal tubule. *FASEB J* 24 9:3438–50. doi:10.1096/fj.10-154765.

Hu, M. C., Shi, M. Zhang, J. Quinones, H. Griffith, C. Kuro-o, M. and Moe. O. W. 2011. Klotho deficiency causes vascular calcification in chronic kidney disease. *J Am Soc Nephrol* 22 1:124–36. doi:10.1681/ASN.2009121311.

Hu, M. C., Shi, M. Zhang, J. Quinones, H. Kuro-o, M. and Moe. O. W. 2010b. Klotho deficiency is an early bio-marker of renal ischemia-reperfusion injury and its replacement is protective. *Kidney Int* 78 12:1240–51. doi:10.1038/ki.2010.328.

Imura, A., Iwano, A. Tohyama, O. Tsuji, Y. Nozaki, K. Hashimoto, N. Fujimori, T. and Nabeshima. Y. 2004. Secreted Klotho protein in sera and CSF: Implication for post-translational cleavage in release of Klotho protein from cell membrane. *FEBS Lett* 565 (1–3):143–7. doi:10.1016/j.febslet.2004.03.090.

Isakova, T., Gutierrez, O. M. Chang, Y. Shah, A. Tamez, H. Smith, K. Thadhani, R. and Wolf. M. 2009. Phosphorus binders and survival on hemodialysis. *J Am Soc Nephrol* 20 2:388–96. doi:10.1681/ASN.2008060609.

Jacobs, T. P., Kaufman, M. Jones, G. Kumar, R. Schlingmann, K. P. Shapses, S. and Bilezikian. J. P. 2014. A lifetime of hypercalcemia and hypercalciuria, finally explained. *J Clin Endocrinol Metab* 99 3:708–12. doi:10.1210/jc.2013-3802.

Kestenbaum, B., Sampson, J. N. Rudser, K. D. Patterson, D. J. Seliger, S. L. Young, B. Sherrard, D. J. and Andress. D. L. 2005. Serum phosphate levels and mortality risk among people with chronic kidney disease.

Kolek, O. I., E. R. Hines, M. D. Jones, L. K. LeSueur, M. A. Lipko, P. R. Kiela, J. F. Collins, M. R. Haussler, and F. K. Ghishan. 2005. 1alpha,25-dihydroxyvitamin D3 upregulates FGF23 gene expression in bone: The final link in a renal-gastrointestinal-skeletal axis that controls phosphate transport. *Am J Physiol Gastrointest Liver Physiol* 289 (6):G1036-42. doi: 10.1152/ajpgi.00243.2005.

Krajisnik, T., Bjorklund, P. Marsell, R. Ljunggren, O. Akerstrom, G. Jonsson, K. B. Westin, G. and Larsson. T. E. 2007. Fibroblast growth factor-23 regulates parathyroid hormone and 1alpha-hydroxylase expression in cultured bovine parathyroid cells. *J Endocrinol* 195 1:125–31. doi:10.1677/JOE-07-0267.

Kuro-o, M., Matsumura, Y. Aizawa, H. Kawaguchi, H. Suga, T. Utsugi, T. Ohyama, Y. Kurabayashi, M. Kaname, T. Kume, E. Iwasaki, H. Iida, A. Shiraki-Iida, T. Nishikawa, S. Nagai, R. and Nabeshima. Y. I. 1997. Mutation of the mouse klotho gene leads to a syndrome resembling ageing. *Nature* 390 6655:45–51.

Kurosu, H. and Kuro-o. M. 2008. The Klotho gene family and the endocrine fibroblast growth factors. *Curr Opin Nephrol Hypertens* 17 4:368–72. doi:10.1097/MNH.0b013e3282ffd994.

Kurosu, H., Yamamoto, M. Clark, J. D. Pastor, J. V. Nandi, A. Gurnani, P. McGuinness, O. P. Chikuda, H. Yamaguchi, M. Kawaguchi, H. Shimomura, I. Takayama, Y. Herz, J. Kahn, C. R. Rosenblatt, K. P. and Kuro-o. M. 2005. Suppression of aging in mice by the hormone Klotho. *Science* 309 5742:1829–33. doi: 10.1126/science.1112766.

Li, S. A., Watanabe, M. Yamada, H. Nagai, A. Kinuta, M. and Takei. K. 2004. Immunohistochemical localization of Klotho protein in brain, kidney, and reproductive organs of mice. *Cell Struct Funct* 29 4:91–9.

Lopez-Hilker, S., Dusso, A. S. Rapp, N. S. Martin, K. J. and Slatopolsky. E. 1990. Phosphorus restriction reverses hyperparathyroidism in uremia independent of changes in calcium and calcitriol. *Am J Physiol* 259 (3 Pt 2):F432–7.

Lou, Y. R., Molnar, F. Perakyla, M. Qiao, S. Kalueff, A. V. R. St-Arnaud, Carlberg, C. and Tuohimaa. P. 2010. 25-Hydroxyvitamin D(3) is an agonistic vitamin D receptor ligand. *J Steroid Biochem Mol Biol* 118 3:162–70. doi:10.1016/j.jsbmb.2009.11.011.

Lucas, P. A., Brown, R. C. Woodhead, J. S. and Coles. G. A. 1986. 1,25-dihydroxycholecalciferol and parathyroid hormone in advanced chronic renal failure: Effects of simultaneous protein and phosphorus restriction. *Clin Nephrol* 25 1:7–10.

Miedlich, S. U., Zhu, E. D. Sabbagh, Y. and Demay. M. B. 2010. The receptor-dependent actions of 1,25-dihydroxyvitamin D are required for normal growth plate maturation in NPt2a knockout mice. *Endocrinology* 151 10:4607–12. doi:10.1210/en.2010-0354.

Mitani, H., Ishizaka, N. Aizawa, T. Ohno, M. Usui, S. Suzuki, T. Amaki, T. Mori, I. Nakamura, Y. Sato, M. Nangaku, M. Hirata, Y. and Nagai. R. 2002. In vivo klotho gene transfer ameliorates angiotensin II-induced renal damage. *Hypertension* 39 4:838–43.

Monkawa, T., T. Yoshida, S. Wakino, T. Shinki, H. Anazawa, H. F. Deluca, T. Suda, M. Hayashi, and T. Saruta. 1997. Molecular cloning of cDNA and genomic DNA for human 25-hydroxyvitamin D3 1 alpha-hydroxylase. *Biochem Biophys Res Commun* 239 (2):527-33. doi: 10.1006/bbrc.1997.7508.

Munetsuna, E., Nakabayashi, S. Kawanami, R. Yasuda, K. Ohta, M. Arai, M. A. Kittaka, A. Chen, T. C. Kamakura, M. Ikushiro, S. and Sakaki. T. 2011. Mechanism of the anti-proliferative action of 25-hydroxy-19-nor-vitamin D(3) in human prostate cells. *J Mol Endocrinol* 47 2:209–18. doi:10.1530/JME-11-0008.

Nakatani, T., Ohnishi, M. and Razzaque. M. S. 2009. Inactivation of klotho function induces hyperphosphatemia even in presence of high serum fibroblast growth factor 23 levels in a genetically engineered hypophosphatemic (Hyp) mouse model. *FASEB J* 23 11:3702–11. doi:10.1096/fj.08-123992.

Nygaard, B., Frandsen, N. E. Brandi, L. Rasmussen, K. Oestergaard, O. V. Oedum, L. Hoeck, H. C. and Hansen. D. 2014. Effects of high doses of cholecalciferol in normal subjects: A randomized double-blinded, placebo-controlled trial. *PLOS ONE* 9 (8):e102965. doi:10.1371/journal.pone.0102965.

Perwad, F., Azam, N. Zhang, M. Y. Yamashita, T. Tenenhouse, H. S. and Portale. A. A. 2005. Dietary and serum phosphorus regulate fibroblast growth factor 23 expression and 1,25-dihydroxyvitamin D metabolism in mice. *Endocrinology* 146 12:5358–64.

Portale, A. A., Booth, B. E. Halloran, B. P. and Morris, R. C. Jr. 1984. Effect of dietary phosphorus on circulating concentrations of 1,25-dihydroxyvitamin D and immunoreactive parathyroid hormone in children with moderate renal insufficiency. *J Clin Invest* 73 6:1580–9.

Portale, A. A., Halloran, B. P. and Morris, R. C. Jr. 1987. Dietary intake of phosphorus modulates the circadian rhythm in serum concentration of phosphorus. Implications for the renal production of 1,25-dihydroxyvitamin D. *J Clin Invest* 80 4:1147–54. doi:10.1172/JCI113172.

Portale, A. A., Halloran, B. P. and Morris, R. C. Jr. 1989. Physiologic regulation of the serum concentration of 1,25-dihydroxyvitamin D by phosphorus in normal men. *J Clin Invest* 83 5:1494–9.

Portale, A. A., Halloran, B. P. Murphy, M. M. and Morris, R. C. Jr. 1986. Oral intake of phosphorus can determine the serum concentration of 1,25-dihydroxyvitamin D by determining its production rate in humans. *J Clin Invest* 77 1:7–12. doi:10.1172/JCI112304.

Prince, R. L., Hutchison, B. G. Kent, J. C. Kent, G. N. and Retallack. R. W. 1988. Calcitriol deficiency with retained synthetic reserve in chronic renal failure. *Kidney Int* 33 3:722–8.

Razzaque, M. S. and Lanske. B. 2007. The emerging role of the fibroblast growth factor-23-klotho axis in renal regulation of phosphate homeostasis. *J Endocrinol* 194 1:1–10. doi:10.1677/JOE-07-0095.

Renkema, K. Y., Alexander, R. T. Bindels, R. J. and Hoenderop. J. G. 2008. Calcium and phosphate homeostasis: Concerted interplay of new regulators. *Ann Med* 40 2:82–91. doi:10.1080/07853890701689645.

Ritz, E., Seidel, A. Ramisch, H. Szabo, A. and Bouillon. R. 1991. Attenuated rise of 1,25 (OH)2 vitamin D3 in response to parathyroid hormone in patients with incipient renal failure. *Nephron* 57 3:314–8.

Rowe, P. S., Garrett, I. R. Schwarz, P. M. Carnes, D. L. Lafer, E. M. Mundy, G. R. and Gutierrez. G. E. 2005. Surface plasmon resonance (SPR) confirms that MEPE binds to PHEX via the MEPE-ASARM motif: A model for impaired mineralization in X-linked rickets (HYP). *Bone* 36 1:33–46. doi:10.1016/j. bone.2004.09.015.

Schiavi, S. C. and Kumar. R. 2004. The phosphatonin pathway: New insights in phosphate homeostasis. *Kidney Int* 65 1:1–14.

Schlingmann, K. P., Kaufmann, M. Weber, S. Irwin, A. Goos, C. John, U. Misselwitz, J. Klaus, G. Kuwertz-Broking, E. Fehrenbach, H. Wingen, A. M. Guran, T. Hoenderop, J. G. Bindels, R. J. Prosser, D. E. Jones, G. and Konrad. M. 2011. Mutations in CYP24A1 and idiopathic infantile hypercalcemia. *N Engl J Med* 365 5:410–21. doi:10.1056/NEJMoa1103864.

Shimada, T., Kakitani, M. Yamazaki, Y. Hasegawa, H. Takeuchi, Y. Fujita, T. Fukumoto, S. Tomizuka, K. and Yamashita. T. 2004a. Targeted ablation of Fgf23 demonstrates an essential physiological role of FGF23 in phosphate and vitamin D metabolism. *J Clin Invest* 113 4:561–8. doi:10.1172/JCI19081.

Shimada, T., Urakawa, I. Yamazaki, Y. Hasegawa, H. Hino, R. Yoneya, T. Takeuchi, Y. Fujita, T. Fukumoto, S. and Yamashita. T. 2004b. FGF-23 transgenic mice demonstrate hypophosphatemic rickets with reduced expression of sodium phosphate cotransporter type IIa. *Biochem Biophys Res Commun* 314 2:409–14.

Shinki, T., H. Shimada, S. Wakino, H. Anazawa, M. Hayashi, T. Saruta, H. F. DeLuca, and T. Suda. 1997. Cloning and expression of rat 25-hydroxyvitamin D3-1alpha-hydroxylase cDNA. *Proc Natl Acad Sci U S A* 94 (24):12920-5.

Slatopolsky, E., Brown, A. and Dusso. A. 1999. Pathogenesis of secondary hyperparathyroidism. *Kidney Int Suppl* 73:S14–9.

Slatopolsky, E., Brown, A. and Dusso. A. 2001. Role of phosphorus in the pathogenesis of secondary hyper-parathyroidism. *Am J Kidney Dis* 37 (1 Suppl 2):S54–7.

St-Arnaud, R., Arabian, A. Travers, R. Barletta, F. Raval-Pandya, M. Chapin, K. Depovere, J. Mathieu, C. Christakos, S. Demay, M. B. and Glorieux. F. H. 2000. Deficient mineralization of intramembranous bone in vitamin D-24-hydroxylase-ablated mice is due to elevated 1,25-dihydroxyvitamin D and not to the absence of 24,25-dihydroxyvitamin D. *Endocrinology* 141 7:2658–66.

St-Arnaud, R., S. Messerlian, J. M. Moir, J. L. Omdahl, and F. H. Glorieux. 1997. The 25-hydroxyvitamin D 1-alpha-hydroxylase gene maps to the pseudovitamin D-deficiency rickets (PDDR) disease locus. *J Bone Miner Res* 12 (10):1552-9. doi: 10.1359/jbmr.1997.12.10.1552.

Takeyama, K., S. Kitanaka, T. Sato, M. Kobori, J. Yanagisawa, and S. Kato. 1997. 25-hydroxyvitamin D3 1alpha-hydroxylase and vitamin D synthesis. *Science* 277 (5333):1827-30.

Tenenhouse, H. S., Martel, J. Gauthier, C. Zhang, M. Y. and Portale. A. A. 2001. Renal expression of the sodium/phosphate cotransporter gene, Npt2, is not required for regulation of renal 1 alpha-hydroxylase by phosphate. *Endocrinology* 142 3:1124–9.

Trechsel, U., Bonjour, J. P. and Fleisch. H. 1979. Regulation of the metabolism of 25-hydroxyvitamin D3 in primary cultures of chick kidney cells. *J Clin Invest* 64 1:206–17. doi:10.1172/JCI109441.

Tsujikawa, H., Kurotaki, Y. Fujimori, T. Fukuda, K. and Nabeshima. Y. 2003. Klotho, a gene related to a syndrome resembling human premature aging, functions in a negative regulatory circuit of vitamin D endocrine system. *Mol Endocrinol* 17 12:2393–403. doi:10.1210/me.2003-0048.

Urakawa, I., Yamazaki, Y. Shimada, T. Iijima, K. Hasegawa, H. Okawa, K. Fujita, T. Fukumoto, S. and Yamashita. T. 2006. Klotho converts canonical FGF receptor into a specific receptor for FGF23. *Nature* 444 7120:770–4. doi:10.1038/nature05315.

Usatii, M., Rousseau, L. Demers, C. Petit, J. L. Brossard, J. H. Gascon-Barre, M. Lavigne, J. R. Zahradnik, R. J. Nemeth, E. F. and D'Amour. P. 2007. Parathyroid hormone fragments inhibit active hormone and hypocalcemia-induced 1,25(OH)2D synthesis. *Kidney Int* 72 11:1330–5.

Yoshida, T., Fujimori, T. and Nabeshima. Y. 2002. Mediation of unusually high concentrations of 1,25-dihydroxyvitamin D in homozygous klotho mutant mice by increased expression of renal 1alpha-hydroxylase gene. *Endocrinology* 143 2:683–9. doi:10.1210/endo.143.2.8657.

Yoshida, T., Yoshida, N. Monkawa, T. Hayashi, M. and Saruta. T. 2001. Dietary phosphorus deprivation induces 25-hydroxyvitamin D(3) 1alpha-hydroxylase gene expression. *Endocrinology* 142 5:1720–6.

Yu, X., Sabbagh, Y. Davis, S. I. Demay, M. B. and White. K. E. 2005. Genetic dissection of phosphate- and vitamin D-mediated regulation of circulating Fgf23 concentrations. *Bone* 36 6:971–7. doi:10.1016/j. bone.2005.03.002.

Zhang, M. Y., Wang, X. Wang, J. T. Compagnone, N. A. Mellon, S. H. Olson, J. L. Tenenhouse, H. S. Miller, W. L. and Portale. A. A. 2002. Dietary phosphorus transcriptionally regulates 25-hydroxyvitamin D-1alpha-hydroxylase gene expression in the proximal renal tubule. *Endocrinology* 143 2:587–95.

Section II

Dietary Phosphorus Intake and Nutritional Needs

12 Phosphorus
An Essential Nutrient for Bone Health Throughout Life

Jean-Philippe Bonjour

CONTENTS

Abstract 155
Bullet Points 156
12.1 Introduction 156
12.2 Physiology of Phosphorus in Relation to Bone Health and Risk of Fragility Fracture 157
12.3 Direct Activity of Phosphorus Ion on Bone Cell Functions 157
    12.3.1 Phosphorus and Osteogenic Cells 157
    12.3.2 Osteocyte Distribution and Functions 158
    12.3.3 Phosphorus and Osteoclast Lineage Cells 159
    12.3.4 Use of Ca-Phosphorus Biomaterials in Tissue Engineering 159
12.4 Extraskeletal Phosphorus Fluxes in Relation to Bone Metabolism 159
    12.4.1 Intestinal Phosphorus Absorption 160
    12.4.2 Renal Phosphorus Reabsorption 160
    12.4.3 The Bone–Kidney Link in Phosphorus Homeostasis: The Adaptation Concept 160
12.5 Is There a Relationship between Insufficient Phosphorus Intake and Bone Mass and Strength in Postmenopausal Women and Older Men in the Absence of Severe Renal Impairment? 161
    12.5.1 Recommended Phosphorus Intake 161
    12.5.2 Conditions with Insufficient Phosphorus Intake and Bone Structure Impairment 161
    12.5.3 Phosphorus Depletion and Skeletal Muscle Integrity and Function 161
    12.5.4 Vitamin D Deficiency and Skeletal Muscle Weakness: Role of Hypophosphatemia 162
    12.5.5 Inadequate Phosphorus Supply in Relation to Osteoporosis Treatment 162
    12.5.6 Preventing the Risk of Phosphorus Depletion in Osteoporosis Treatment with Anabolic Agents 162
12.6 Conclusions 163
References 163

ABSTRACT

Throughout life, bone is continuously renewed. In the elderly, adequate supply of vitamin D, calcium (Ca), phosphorus, and protein are nutrients required for renewal of bone mass and function. Low supply of these nutrients can accelerate age-related bone loss. Regarding phosphorus, over the last three decades there has been more concern about the possible deleterious effect on bone metabolism of excessive rather than insufficient intake. In this chapter, we recall some fundamental aspects of phosphorus homeostasis, underscoring the essentiality of this element for maintaining many vital cellular processes during aging. In bone, phosphorus associated with Ca is deposited on the organic matrix by mechanisms involving specific osteogenic cell transporters. This mineral deposition strengthens bone mechanical resistance. The phosphorus economy is tightly controlled. The renal tubular reabsorption is the main controlling system. Genetic defects in this renal regulatory capacity lead to severe impairment in bone mineralization that is clinically expressed as rickets during growth and osteomalacia during adulthood. In absence of such selective renal transport defects, phosphorus depletion with hypophosphatemia is uncommon. Besides the renal controlling system, the wide phosphorus distribution in foods and the large net fractional intestinal absorption contribute to this infrequency of phosphorus depletion. Nevertheless, it can be observed in some pathologic conditions, including severe alcoholism, diabetic ketoacidosis, pulmonary infectious diseases, or myocardial infarction. In elderly patients with severe osteoporosis treated with bone anabolic agents in combination with supplemental Ca salts that reduce the intestinal phosphorus absorption, the dietary supply of phosphorus may not be sufficient to cope with the increased phosphorus needs resulting from the stimulated bone mineralization. In this situation, a mineral supplement provided as Ca-phosphorus salt could avoid the high intestinal Ca/phosphorus ratio that would worsen the imbalance between phosphorus supply and bone requirements. In the elderly, such a Ca/phosphorus supplement was shown to reduce hip and other fragility fractures.

BULLET POINTS

- In bone, phosphorus associated with Ca is deposited on the organic matrix and thereby strengthens the mechanical resistance of the skeleton throughout life.
- Nutritional phosphorus depletion can be observed in elderly subjects.
- Osteoporotic patients with low phosphorus intake may not fully benefit from treatment combining bone anabolic agents with Ca supplements made of salts other than phosphorus. The use of Ca-phosphate salt supplements may assure adequacy of both minerals.
- Ca-phosphorus salt associated with vitamin D_3 is not deleterious to bone health. On the contrary, this treatment was shown in elderly subjects to control secondary hyperparathyroidism, increase bone mineral mass, and significantly reduce the risk of hip fracture.

12.1 INTRODUCTION

Over the last 10 years, several reviews have emphasized the negative impact that high dietary phosphorus supply may exert on bone health. The main contention is based on the plausible but putative long-term mechanism that an increased phosphorus intake would tend to lower serum ionized Ca, which, in turn, would stimulate parathyroid hormone (PTH) secretion and thus result in enhanced bone resorption without commensurate elevation in bone formation. Hence, inappropriately high phosphorus intake, exceeding dietary requirements, would induce negative bone mineral balance and, over years, osteoporosis and fragility fractures. This supposed mechanism would worsen the negative impact on bone health when the Ca intake and, thereby, the Ca/phosphorus ratio is inadequately low. As discussed in another chapter of this book and recently reviewed (Calvo and Tucker 2013), there is still uncertainty whether straightforward clinical evidence would favor the long-term deleterious impact of high dietary phosphorus and/or low Ca/phosphorus intake on bone structure and function in healthy individuals.

However, the view of the beneficial role of phosphorus in bone physiology, particularly that needed by aging bone, has been undermined. The aim of this chapter is to recall some fundamental concepts on this crucial role of phosphorus, not only during growth, but also throughout life, particularly in postmenopausal women and elderly. Clinical conditions in which there is a risk of phosphorus depletion are described. Finally, the beneficial, or at least, the nondeleterious effect of Ca-phosphorus supplements on bone health was brought out by large randomized controlled trials (RCT) showing that, associated with vitamin D_3, long-term administration of this phosphorus salt can reduce the risk of hip and other fragility fractures in the elderly.

12.2 PHYSIOLOGY OF PHOSPHORUS IN RELATION TO BONE HEALTH AND RISK OF FRAGILITY FRACTURE

As stated by Charles Scriver in his William Allan Memorial Award Address (Scriver 1979):

"Our cells respire and our skeleton endures against gravity only because we have access to the chemical element—phosphorus."

In living organisms, the element phosphorus (P) is essentially present as phosphate (PO_4^{-3}) whether bound in organic compounds such as DNA, nucleotides, proteins, sugars, or lipids or as inorganic phosphate (Pi) in bone and in extracellular fluid (Griffith et al. 1977). The mineral phase of bone is an analog of the naturally occurring hydroxyapatite [$Ca_{10}(PO_4)_6(OH)_2$] (Boskey and Robey 2013). The total amount of Ca and phosphorus in a human adult of 70 kg is about 1300 and 700 g, respectively. Bone contains about 99% and 80% of whole-body Ca and phosphorus, respectively. In molar and mass ratios the Ca/phosphorus ratio in bone is about 1.7 and 2.2, respectively (Diem and Lentner 1972). Of note, the bone mass ratio of 2.2 is close to that measured in human milk, which may vary from 1.9 to 2.4 (Diem and Lentner 1972).

Phosphorus is an essential factor in bone modeling, a process mainly occurring during growth, and remodeling during adulthood. These physiologic phenomena imply the *de novo* formation of an organic matrix followed by the deposition of specific bone mineral components. This deposition onto the organic matrix requires the translocation of phosphorus and Ca from the systemic extracellular fluid to the unmineralized bone compartment (for review, see Bonjour 2011). This translocation is ensured by specific phosphorus and Ca molecular structures located within the plasma membrane of osteogenic cells. There is evidence that phosphorus is the driving ion, which is translocated through an identified Na/phosphorus transporter. It is followed by the influx of Ca ions, leading to the formation of hydroxyapatite crystal and its subsequent association with collagen fibrils of the organic matrix (Caverzasio and Bonjour 1996; Montessuit et al. 1991, 1995). The key phosphorus transporter present in the plasma membrane of osteogenic cells has been identified at the molecular level and shown to be regulated by insulin-like growth factor-1 (IGF-1) (Palmer et al. 1999), a major bone skeletal growth factor, and by other anabolic agents.

Other contributing actors in the process of bone and cartilage mineralization are enzymes endowed with phosphatase activity that can elevate the phosphorus concentration within the skeletal compartment where hydroxyapatite is formed. Among them, a phosphoethanolamine/phosphocholine phosphatase (PHOSPHO1) has been shown to be essential for normal mineralization and avoidance of spontaneous fractures in mice (Huesa et al. 2011). Hypophosphatasia (HPP) is due to a loss-of-function mutation of alkaline phosphatase that is associated with clinical signs of rickets and osteomalacia (Whyte 2008). In HPP, three phosphocompounds accumulate: phosphoethanolamine, pyridoxal 5'-phosphate, and inorganic pyrophosphate (PPi) (Whyte 2008), a well-characterized inhibitor of hydroxyapatite crystal formation (Fleisch 1978). In HPP, the impaired skeletal mineralization presumably results from the accumulation of PPi within the extracellular skeletal space that prevents the growth of hydroxyapatite crystal after the rupture of the matrix vesicles (Whyte 2010).

12.3 DIRECT ACTIVITY OF PHOSPHORUS ION ON BONE CELL FUNCTIONS

Besides being an essential constituent of hydroxyapatite crystal, phosphorus can also directly influence bone cell functions that are linked to skeletal modeling and remodeling.

12.3.1 PHOSPHORUS AND OSTEOGENIC CELLS

Early studies using organ culture indicated that increasing phosphorus concentration enhances the rate of the bone matrix production in osteogenic cells (Bingham and Raisz 1974). Later on, several studies aimed at identifying genetic defects responsible for clinical cases of hypophosphatemia revealed fascinating connections between phosphorus and osteogenic cells. Indeed, these cells produce active factors that are implicated in both bone metabolism and systemic phosphorus homeostasis.

Among the three main cells present in the adult skeleton, osteocytes account for more than 90% of all of them, compared to 4% to 6% and 1% to 2% for the osteoblast and osteoclast pools, respectively (Bonewald 2013).

12.3.2 Osteocyte Distribution and Functions

Osteocytes are distributed throughout the bone matrix (Figure 12.1) (Bonewald 2013). They are connected to each other, as well as linked to cells on the bone surface, through radiating canaliculi constituted of cytoplasmic dendritic processes (Bonewald 2013). Osteocytes have the widest interface with the bone matrix. These cells respond to mechanical strain by sending signals to osteoblasts and osteoclasts present on the bone surface, thus modulating the rate of bone formation and resorption. These cells produce promoters of mineralization such as PHEX (phosphate-regulating neutral endopeptidase on chromosome X) and DMP-1 (dentin matrix protein 1), as well as inhibitors of bone mineralization and formation such as SOST/sclerostin and MEPE/OF45 (matrix extracellular phosphoglycoprotein/osteoblast/osteocyte factor-45). It has been shown that osteocytes play a pivotal function in phosphorus homeostasis. Osteocytes have the capacity to deposit and remove bone mineral from their environment. Quantitatively, this is not trivial because the surface area of the osteocyte lacuno-canalicular system, which is embedded in direct contact with the hydroxyapatite mineral, is several orders of magnitude greater than the bone surface area covered by the other bone-forming and resorbing cells (Bonewald 2013). This capability has important implications for sensing the mechanical load exerted on bone structure as well as the mineral homeostasis. The osteocyte network, by controlling the phosphorus

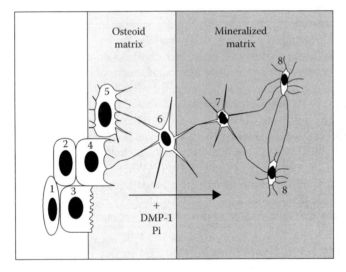

FIGURE 12.1 Transition from osteoblast to osteocyte differentiation and maturation in relation to bone matrix mineralization. Both DMP-1 (dentin matrix protein-1) and Pi (inorganic phosphate) appear to be required for mineralization and maturation of osteoblasts into osteocytes. As described in the text, osteocytes are the main cells producing FGF23 (fibroblast growth factor-23), a factor involved in Pi homeostasis, essentially by inhibiting both the renal Pi reabsorption and the intestinal Pi absorption by reducing the renal production and thereby the circulating level of 1,25(OH)$_2$-vitamin D. (Adapted from Franz-Odendaal et al., Dev Dyn., 235, 176–190, 2006; Dallas and Bonewald, Ann NY Acad Sci., 1192, 437–443, 2010; Zhang et al., J Bone Mineral Res., 26, 1047–1056, 2011.)

Phosphorus: An Essential Nutrient for Bone Health 159

and Ca fluxes, determines the amount of mineral present in its surrounding organic matrix which, inversely, modulates osteocyte maturation (Irie et al. 2008).

In the process of mineralization-induced maturation, osteocytes express factors implicated in osteoblast formation such as sclerostin (van Bezooijen et al. 2005; Irie et al. 2008) and in systemic phosphorus homeostasis such as DMP-1, PHEX, and FGF-23 (fibroblast growth factor-23). DMP-1, which is expressed predominantly in odontoblasts and osteocytes, appears to be a key molecule not only in osteocyte maturation, but also, by controlling FGF23 production, in systemic phosphorus homeostasis. As described later, FGF23 controls the circulating phosphorus concentration and the degree of mineralization, probably by its renal tubular action (Lu et al. 2011). DMP-1 mutation in humans can result in hypophosphatemic rickets during childhood and osteomalacia during adulthood, a condition noted as autosomal-recessive hypophosphatemic rickets (ARHR) (Feng et al. 2006). The skeletal mineralization defect observed in ARHR is associated with an elevation in circulating FGF23 (Feng et al. 2006). An inactivating mutation in PHEX causes X-linked hypophosphatemic rickets (XLH). It is associated with a defect in osteocyte maturation and overproduction of FGF23 that might be the main cause of the low circulating phosphorus level observed in this genetic disease. In favor of such a causal relationship, use of anti-FGF23 antibody in adults with XLH significantly increased TmP/GFR, serum phosphorus, and 1,25D (Carpenter et al. 2014; Imel et al. 2015). Currently, the substrate of PHEX remains to be identified.

Note that the inhibitory effect of FGF23 on the renal tubular phosphorus reabsorption requires the klotho coreceptor protein (Urakawa et al. 2006). Mice defective in the klotho gene have a short lifespan and exhibit a syndrome mimicking human aging, including, hypoactivity, sarcopenia, osteopenia, skin atrophy, vascular calcification, and pulmonary emphysema (Kurosu and Kuro 2009). In contrast, mice overexpressing the klotho gene live longer than congenic controls (Kurosu and Kuro 2009). The klotho gene was named after one of the Greek mythology goddesses who determine the lifespan of every mortal by spinning (Klotho), measuring (Lachesis), and cutting (Atropos) the thread of life.

12.3.3 Phosphorus and Osteoclast Lineage Cells

Exposure of cells of the osteoclast lineage to phosphorus leads to several modifications that favor a reduction in bone-resorbing activity. These changes include both inhibition of preosteoclast differentiation and stimulation of mature osteoclast apoptosis (Kanatani et al. 2003; Mozar et al. 2008). The osteoclastic response to phosphorus exposure could be mediated by an alteration at the molecular level in the local production of osteoprotegerin and RANKL, two essential factors, the balance of which determines the rate of bone resorption (Kanatani et al. 2003; Mozar et al. 2008).

12.3.4 Use of Ca-Phosphorus Biomaterials in Tissue Engineering

The key role of phosphorus as a co-element of Ca is also exemplified in tissue engineering aimed at bone reconstructive surgery after traumatic or pathological injury such as osteoporotic fracture or osteolytic tumor (Verron et al. 2012). Ca-phosphorus materials are considered well-suited alternatives to bone grafting because their chemical properties promote bone remodeling as well as the potential of delivering bone growth factors (Verron et al. 2012; Pastorino et al. 2015).

12.4 EXTRASKELETAL PHOSPHORUS FLUXES IN RELATION TO BONE METABOLISM

At a steady state in young adult humans, the net phosphorus entry into the extracellular compartment, mainly from gut and bone sources, is excreted in the urine. However, as described here, the main physiological process responsible for the regulation of the extracellular phosphorus level is the transport system ensuring its reabsorption along the renal tubules.

12.4.1 Intestinal Phosphorus Absorption

The translocation of phosphorus from the luminal intestinal side to the extracellular compartment uses a specific pathway. The intestinal phosphorus transport system can be stimulated by the hormonal form of vitamin D, namely 1,25-dihydroxy-vitamin-D (1,25D). The renal production of 1,25D is enhanced by IGF-I and PTH, as well as by low phosphorus and Ca exposure. Reduction in phosphorus intake leads to a stimulation of 1,25D and consecutive enhancement of the intestinal capacity to translocate phosphorus across the intestinal epithelium according to the mineral economy requirements (Rizzoli and Bonjour 2006).

12.4.2 Renal Phosphorus Reabsorption

In contrast to their tight association in the processes of formation and resorption of the mineralized organic matrix of skeletal tissues, the renal transport system of phosphorus is independent from that of Ca (Murer and Biber 2010; Prie and Friedlander 2010; Lambers et al. 2006; Bindels 2010). Likewise, the two types of renal transporters are regulated by different homeostatic systems (Rizzoli and Bonjour 2006). PTH is the crucial endocrine factor modulating the tubular reabsorption of Ca in response to fluctuations of its extracellular level. In contrast, although PTH inhibits phosphorus reabsorption, this renal activity can be completely blocked by more specific phosphorus regulators, particularly the intake and demand of phosphorus in relation to bone mineralization needs (Bonjour et al. 1982).

12.4.3 The Bone–Kidney Link in Phosphorus Homeostasis: The Adaptation Concept

Several decades ago, analysis of several well-controlled physiological experiences led us to conceive the existence of a powerful functional link between bone mineralization and the regulation of the tubular phosphorus reabsorption (Bonjour et al. 1977). As recently reviewed (Bonjour 2011), direct blockage of bone mineralization was rapidly followed by a decrease in the maximal capacity to reabsorb phosphorus from the glomerular filtrate (TmP/GFR), as well as a decrease in the 1,25D production and circulating level. The renal adaptation mechanism dominates the regulation of TmP/GFR by responding not only to variation in the dietary phosphorus supply (Trohler et al. 1976a), but also to the phosphorus demand, as influenced by the capacity of bone to incorporate phosphorus in the process of the organic matrix mineralization (Bonjour 2011). Among putative regulatory factors linking bone mineralization to the tubular capacity to reabsorb phosphorus, a serious candidate appears to be FGF23. Its bone production is influenced by phosphorus (Fukumoto 2008). As reported in healthy adults, an increase in the phosphorus supply from foods leads to an increment in the circulating level FGF23 and reduction in the tubular phosphorus reabsorption (Ferrari et al. 2005). Whether FGF23 is the essential renal controlling factor in response to variation in the dietary phosphorus supply is nevertheless not unequivocally established when critically analyzed from human and animal studies with either normal or impaired kidney function (Christov and Juppner 2013).

IGF-I is also an important regulator of the tubular reabsorption of phosphorus (Caverzasio and Bonjour 1991; Caverzasio et al. 1990).

The independent renal regulatory systems of phosphorus vs. Ca may be teleologically explained by their quite distinct influence on nonskeletal cellular functions. Phosphorus exerts key activities in energy storage and delivery, enzyme activity, and acid–base homeostasis, and Ca is essential for intracellular signal transduction, neuronal transmission and excitability, and muscle contraction (for an overview on phosphorus and Ca physiology, see Rizzoli and Bonjour 2006).

Phosphorus: An Essential Nutrient for Bone Health

12.5 IS THERE A RELATIONSHIP BETWEEN INSUFFICIENT PHOSPHORUS INTAKE AND BONE MASS AND STRENGTH IN POSTMENOPAUSAL WOMEN AND OLDER MEN IN THE ABSENCE OF SEVERE RENAL IMPAIRMENT?

12.5.1 RECOMMENDED PHOSPHORUS INTAKE

The Recommended Dietary Allowance (RDA) for phosphorus in the United States is 700 mg/d for most age groups, except in infants and young children (Institute of Medicine Food and Nutrition Board 1997). In the UK, the value for adults is lower (550 mg/d) (Committee on Medical Aspects of Food and Nutrition Policy 1998), whereas in France, the RDA is set at 750 mg/d in adults, with slightly higher value of 800 mg/d in adolescents and the elderly (Guéguen 2001). The main criterion in setting the RDA for phosphorus has been bone, but this has changed recently for the European Union, as discussed in Chapters 19 and 20.

12.5.2 CONDITIONS WITH INSUFFICIENT PHOSPHORUS INTAKE AND BONE STRUCTURE IMPAIRMENT

Counterintuitively, an insufficient phosphorus intake does not necessarily lead to hypophosphatemia (i.e., to a serum level of phosphorus, usually measured in the fasting state) below the adult reference range of 1.5 to 2.0 mmol/L. Two mechanisms explain this phenomenon: the increase in the maximal capacity to reabsorb phosphorus from the glomerular filtrate (TmP/GFR) (Trohler et al. 1976b) as an adaptive response to insufficient phosphorus intake and, concomitantly during the fasting phase, to the net entry of phosphorus into the extracellular compartment (Trohler et al. 1981) from organs and tissues such as liver and skeletal muscle. As described earlier, the renal tubule is equipped with a Na-dependent phosphorus transporter located not only in the brush border membrane of the proximal tubules, but also along the luminal membrane of distal tubules and collecting ducts. This transporter is tightly regulated in response to variation in the phosphorus intake. Reduction in the phosphorus supply leads to a stimulation in TmP/GFR. The extremely tight relationship that exists between TmP/GFR and the level of serum phosphorus reflects the essential role played by the kidney in the regulation of the extracellular phosphorus homeostasis. This close relation and the stimulation of TmP/GFR in response to low phosphorus intake explain why impairment in bone matrix mineralization (i.e., osteomalacia) is not so common in individuals with reduced consumption of this nutrient. Another reason is the fact that even with an elevated phosphorus intake, the fractional intestinal phosphorus absorption remains relatively high (about 55%–80%). Moreover, and as already mentioned, the intestinal Na-dependent phosphorus transporter that responds to 1,25D is stimulated by dietary phosphorus restriction and thus contributes to attenuate or even abrogates any trend toward a decrease in the fasting level of serum phosphorus.

12.5.3 PHOSPHORUS DEPLETION AND SKELETAL MUSCLE INTEGRITY AND FUNCTION

Phosphorus depletion adversely affects skeletal muscle function, as expressed by weakness and, in the most severe cases, damage to the integrity of muscle fibers and rhabdomyolysis (Knochel 1985). In patients with acute respiratory failure, hypophosphatemia can be associated with impairment in the diaphragmatic contractility (Aubier et al. 1985). Parenteral administration of phosphorus as KH_2PO_4 that corrected the severe hypophosphatemia status (serum value < 0.55 mmol/L) restored the contractility of the diaphragm (Aubier et al. 1985). Another prominent consequence of hypophosphatemia is the hypercalcemia-hypercalciuria due to an increase in both the intestinal absorption and the bone release of Ca and a decrease in the tubular reabsorption of Ca (for a review, see Rizzoli and Bonjour 2006).

12.5.4 Vitamin D Deficiency and Skeletal Muscle Weakness: Role of Hypophosphatemia

With aging, the loss of skeletal muscle mass and strength, simply designated by the term sarcopenia, is associated with reduced physical performance (for review, see Mithal et al. 2013). Sarcopenia is an important risk factor for falling and subsequent hip and other fractures of the appendicular skeleton. With advanced age, serum 25OHD decreases, and its level can predict the physical performance score (Wicherts et al. 2007). Vitamin D deficiency is associated with hypophosphatemia. Treatment of vitamin D deficiency increases lower-limb muscle strength in institutionalized elderly (Moreira-Pfrimer et al. 2009). This improvement may be related to the correction of hypophosphatemia per se (Schubert and DeLuca 2010), conceivably through an effect of vitamin D supplementation on muscle energy phosphometabolites (Rana et al. 2014).

12.5.5 Inadequate Phosphorus Supply in Relation to Osteoporosis Treatment

More recently, another situation has occurred where the supply of dietary phosphorus could be inadequate to fulfill an increasing phosphorus body need (Heaney 2004). This could be the case in older women treated for severe osteoporosis with powerful anabolic or bone-forming agents, such as PTH or some of its active fragments (Neer et al. 2001; Greenspan et al. 2007) and, in the future, with sclerostin inhibitors that are currently evaluated in phase III clinical trials (Shah et al. 2015). Use of very active bone-forming agents requires an adequate availability of Ca and phosphorus to keep up with the enhanced laying down of the bone matrix and its commensurate mineral deposition (Heaney 2004). In RCTs testing the antifracture efficacy of anticatabolic or anabolic drugs, vitamin D and Ca have been given to both control and experimental groups. This study design enables us to demonstrate that the tested medication can prevent fragility fracture beyond the antifracture effect of vitamin D and Ca (Boonen et al. 2007). It also implies that (1) in patients not repleted in vitamin D and Ca, the drug might not be as efficacious and (2) in the setting of clinical practice, the prescription of the approved drug concurrently requires the vitamin D and Ca repletion to be secured. In elderly, this requirement is often fulfilled by the administration of vitamin D and Ca supplements, usually taken in the form of carbonate or citrate salts. These Ca preparations may reduce the intestinal phosphorus absorption with the risk of inducing a negative phosphorus balance (Heaney 2004; Heaney and Nordin 2002). Under these circumstances considerations should be given to the use of Ca-phosphate salt supplements to assure adequacy of both minerals.

12.5.6 Preventing the Risk of Phosphorus Depletion in Osteoporosis Treatment with Anabolic Agents

In osteoporotic patients with low phosphorus intake treated by combining a bone anabolic agent and a Ca citrate or carbonate supplement, one may theoretically anticipate that the net intestinal absorption of phosphorus could not be sufficient to secure the increased demand for bone matrix mineralization (Heaney 2004; Heaney and Nordin 2002). Thus, the full potential of the anabolic drug would not be attained unless the Ca supplement is provided in the form of phosphorus salt. Previous reports indicated that tricalcium phosphate, $Ca_3(PO_4)_2$, containing 1200 mg elemental Ca, is not detrimental to bone. In fact, in a large double-blind placebo-controlled study, the Ca-phosphorus salt associated with vitamin D_3 (20 μg/d) resulted in a significant reduced risk of hip fracture and other nonvertebral fractures after 18 months (Chapuy et al. 1992) and 36 months (Chapuy et al. 1994) of intervention. The main results of this large double-blind RCT was further confirmed in another cohort of elderly women (Chapuy et al. 2002). In this second trial, the Ca-phosphorus salt, again combined vitamin D_3 (20 μg/d), was shown to reverse secondary hyperparathyroidism, to prevent the loss in bone mineral density (BMD), and to reduce hip fracture risk in elderly institutionalized women, after 24 months of intervention (Chapuy et al. 2002). Thus, the beneficial effect of vitamin D and Ca for reducing excessive PTH secretion does

Phosphorus: An Essential Nutrient for Bone Health 163

not appear to be mitigated by phosphorus as compared to other Ca salts combined with different anions such as citrate malate (Dawson-Hughes et al. 1997) or carbonate (Heaney 2004; Heaney and Nordin 2002). From a meta-analysis including all RCTs that evaluated the efficacy of supplemental Ca given with vitamin D to prevent hip fracture (Boonen et al. 2007), the most convincing individual study was, as mentioned earlier, the one testing a Ca-phosphorus salt (Chapuy et al. 1992). Whether phosphorus per se would enhance the protective effect of vitamin D and Ca on the risk of hip fracture remains an untested hypothesis.

12.6 CONCLUSIONS

Phosphorus is an essential nutrient for all living organisms. In humans, phosphorus associated with Ca constitutes a key element for the acquisition of bone mineral and its maintenance throughout life. Usual diets provide sufficient phosphorus. Furthermore, the net fractional intestinal absorption is relatively large, thus securing, in most physiological situations, the phosphorus needs of the body, not only for bone mineralization but also for the numerous vital biochemical processes of cells. The powerful adaptation mechanism that responds to dietary phosphorus restriction by markedly enhancing the tubular phosphorus reabsorption reflects the essentiality of phosphorus for human life. Genetic defects that make this adaptation mechanism nonoperational to the dietary phosphorus supply are the cause of severe pathologic disturbances in phosphorus homeostasis, including impairment in bone mineralization. In the context of age-related osteoporosis, patients with relatively low phosphorus intake may not fully benefit from treatment combining strong bone anabolic agents with Ca supplements made of salts other than phosphorus because of inadequate phosphorus supply. In this setting, use of Ca-phosphorus salts can be appropriate. Previous studies have shown that Ca-phosphorus salt associated with vitamin D_3 is not deleterious to bone health. On the contrary, this treatment is associated with a reduction in secondary hyperparathyroidism, increase in bone mineral mass, and reduction in the risk of hip fracture.

REFERENCES

Aubier, M., D. Murciano, Y. Lecocguic, N. Viires, Y. Jacquens, P. Squara, and R. Pariente. 1985. Effect of hypophosphatemia on diaphragmatic contractility in patients with acute respiratory failure. *N Engl J Med* 313 (7):420–424.

Bindels, R. J. 2010. 2009 Homer W. Smith Award: Minerals in motion: From new ion transporters to new concepts. *J Am Soc Nephrol* 21 (8):1263–1269.

Bingham, P. J. and L. G. Raisz. 1974. Bone growth in organ culture: Effects of phosphate and other nutrients on bone and cartilage. *Calcif Tissue Res* 14 (1):31–48.

Bonewald, L. F. 2013. Ostecytes. In *Primer on the Bone Metabolic Diseases and Disorders of Mineral Metabolism*, edited by Rosen,C.J. 34–41. American Society for Bone and Mineral Research, Hoboken, New Jersey: Wiley-Blackwell.

Bonjour, J. P. 2011. Calcium and phosphate: A duet of ions playing for bone health. *J Am Coll Nutr* 30 (5 Suppl 1):438S–448S.

Bonjour, J. P., J, Caverzasio,. H, Fleisch. R, Muhlbauer. and U.Troehler. 1982. The adaptive system of the tubular transport of phosphate. *Adv Exp Med Biol* 151:1–11.

Bonjour, J. P., U. Trohler, R. Muhlbauer, C. Preston, and H. Fleisch 1977. Is there a bone-kidney link in the homeostasis of inorganic phosphate (Pi)? *Adv Exp Med Biol* 81:319–322.

Boonen, S., P. Lips, R. Bouillon, H. A. Bischoff-Ferrari, D. Vanderschueren, and P. Haentjens. 2007. Need for additional calcium to reduce the risk of hip fracture with vitamin d supplementation: Evidence from a comparative metaanalysis of randomized controlled trials. *J Clin Endocrinol Metab* 92 (4):1415–1423.

Boskey, A. L. and P.G.Robey. 2013. The composition of bone. In *Primer on the Metabolic Bone Diseases and Disorders of Mineral Metabolism*, edited by C.J.Rosen, 49–58. Washington, DC: The American Society of Bone and Mineral Research, Wiley-Blackwell.

Calvo, M. S. and K.L.Tucker. 2013. Is phosphorus intake that exceeds dietary requirements a risk factor in bone health? *Ann N Y Acad Sci* 1301:29–35.

Carpenter, T. O., E. A. Imel, M. D. Ruppe, T. J. Weber, M. A. Klausner, M. M. Wooddell, Kawakami, T. Ito, T. Zhang, X. Humphrey, J. K. L. Insogna, and Peacock. M. 2014. Randomized trial of the anti-FGF23 antibody KRN23 in X-linked hypophosphatemia. *J Clin Invest* 124 (4):1587–1597.

Caverzasio, J. and Bonjour. J.P. 1991. IGF-I, a key regulator of renal phosphate transport and 1,25-Dihydroxyvitamine D3 production during growth. *News Physiol Sci* 6:206–210.

Caverzasio, J. and J.P.Bonjour. 1996. Characteristics and regulation of Pi transport in osteogenic cells for bone metabolism. *Kidney Int* 49 (4):975–980.

Caverzasio, J., Montessuit, C. and J.P.Bonjour. 1990. Stimulatory effect of insulin-like growth factor-1 on renal Pi transport and plasma 1,25-dihydroxyvitamin D3. *Endocrinology* 127 (1):453–459.

Chapuy, M. C., M. E. Arlot, P. D. Delmas, and Meunier. P.J. 1994. Effect of calcium and cholecalciferol treatment for three years on hip fractures in elderly women. *BMJ* 308 (6936):1081–1082.

Chapuy, M. C., M. E. Arlot, Duboeuf, F. Brun, J. Crouzet, B. Arnaud, S. P. D. Delmas, and Meunier. P.J. 1992. Vitamin D3 and calcium to prevent hip fractures in the elderly women. *N Engl J Med* 327 (23): 1637–1642.

Chapuy, M. C., Pamphile, R. Paris, E. Kempf, C. Schlichting, M. Arnaud, S. Garnero, P. and Meunier. P.J. 2002. Combined calcium and vitamin D3 supplementation in elderly women: Confirmation of reversal of secondary hyperparathyroidism and hip fracture risk: The Decalyos II study. *Osteoporos Int* 13 (3): 257–264.

Christov, M. and Juppner. H. 2013. Dietary phosphate: The challenges of exploring its role in FGF23 regulation. *Kidney Int* 84 (4): 639–641.

Commitee on Medical Aspects of Food and Nutrition Policy (COMA). 1998. *Nutrition and Bone Health: With Particular Reference to Calcium and Vitamin D*. London, UK: The Stationary Office.

Dallas and Bonewald. 2010. Dynamics of the transition from osteoblast to osteocyte.*Ann NY Acad Sci* 1192:437–443.

Dawson-Hughes, B., S. S. Harris, E. A. Krall, and Dallal. G.E. 1997. Effect of calcium and vitamin D supplementation on bone density in men and women 65 years of age or older. *N Engl J Med* 337 (10): 670–676.

Diem, K. and Lentner. C. 1972. *Tables Scientifiques*. 7th ed. Basel, Switzerland: Ciba-Geigy SA.

Feng, J.Q., L. M. Ward, Liu, S. Lu, Y. Xie, Y. Yuan, B. Yu, X. Rauch, F. S. I. Davis, Zhang, S. Rios, H. M. K. Drezner, L. D. Quarles, L. F. Bonewald, and White. K.E. 2006. Loss of DMP1 causes rickets and osteomalacia and identifies a role for osteocytes in mineral metabolism. *Nat Genet* 38 (11): 1310–1315.

Ferrari, S.L., J. P. Bonjour, and Rizzoli. R. 2005. Fibroblast growth factor-23 relationship to dietary phosphate and renal phosphate handling in healthy young men. *J Clin Endocrinol Metab* 90 (3): 1519–1524.

Fleisch, H. 1978. Inhibitors and promoters of stone formation. *Kidney Int* 13 (5): 361–371.

Franz-Odendaal et al. 2006. Buried alive: How osteoblasts become osteocytes.*Dev Dyn* 235:176–190.

Fukumoto, S. 2008. Physiological regulation and disorders of phosphate metabolism--pivotal role of fibroblast growth factor 23. *Intern Med* 47 (5): 337–343.

Greenspan, S.L., H. G. Bone, M. P. Ettinger, D. A. Hanley, Lindsay, R. J. R. Zanchetta, C. M. Blosch, A. L. Mathisen, S. A. Morris, T. B. Marriott, and Group Treatment of Osteoporosis with Parathyroid Hormone Study. 2007. Effect of recombinant human parathyroid hormone (1-84) on vertebral fracture and bone mineral density in postmenopausal women with osteoporosis: A randomized trial. *Ann Intern Med* 146 (5): 326–339.

Griffith, E.J., Ponnamperuma, C. and Gabel. N.W. 1977. Phosphorus, a key to life on the primitive Earth. *Orig Life* 8 (2): 71–85.

Guéguen, L. 2001. Calcium, phosphore. In *Apports Nutritionnels Conseillés pout la Population Française*, edited by Martin, A. 131–146. Paris, France: Tech & Doc.

Heaney, R.P. 2004. Phosphorus nutrition and the treatment of osteoporosis. *Mayo Clin Proc* 79 (1): 91–97.

Heaney, R.P. and Nordin. B.E. 2002. Calcium effects on phosphorus absorption: Implications for the prevention and co-therapy of osteoporosis. *J Am Coll Nutr* 21 (3): 239–244.

Huesa, C., M. C. Yadav, M. A. Finnila, S. R. Goodyear, S. P. Robins, K. E. Tanner, R. M. Aspden, J. L. Millan, and Farquharson. C. 2011. PHOSPHO1 is essential for mechanically competent mineralization and the avoidance of spontaneous fractures. *Bone* 48 (5): 1066–1074.

Imel, E.A., Zhang, X. M. D. Ruppe, T. J. Weber, M. A. Klausner, Ito, T. Vergeire, M. J. S. Humphrey, F. H. Glorieux, A. A. Portale, Insogna, K. Peacock, M. and Carpenter. T.O. 2015. Prolonged correction of serum phosphorus in adults with X-linked hypophosphatemia using monthly doses of KRN 23. *J Clin Endocrinol Metab* 100 (7): 2565–2573.

Institute of Medicine Food and Nutrition Board. 1997. *Dietary References Intakes for Calcium, Phosphorus, Magnesium, Vitamin D and Fluoride*. Washington, DC: National Academy Press.

Irie, K., Ejiri, S. Sakakura, Y. Shibui, T. and Yajima. T. 2008. Matrix mineralization as a trigger for osteocyte maturation. *J Histochem Cytochem* 56 (6): 561–567.

Phosphorus: An Essential Nutrient for Bone Health

Kanatani, M., Sugimoto, T. Kano, J. Kanzawa, M. and Chihara. K. 2003. Effect of high phosphate concentration on osteoclast differentiation as well as bone-resorbing activity. *J Cell Physiol* 196 (1): 180–189.

Knochel, J.P. 1985. The clinical status of hypophosphatemia: An update. *N Engl J Med* 313 (7): 447–449.

Kurosu, H. and Kuro. O.M. 2009. The Klotho gene family as a regulator of endocrine fibroblast growth factors. *Mol Cell Endocrinol* 299 (1): 72–78.

Lambers, T.T., R. J. Bindels, and Hoenderop. J.G. 2006. Coordinated control of renal Ca2+ handling. *Kidney Int* 69 (4): 650–654.

Lu, Y., Yuan, B. Qin, C. Cao, Z. Xie, Y. S. L. M. M. Dallas, D. Kee, M. K. Drezner, L. F. Bonewald, and Feng. J.Q. 2011. The biological function of DMP-1 in osteocyte maturation is mediated by its 57-kDa C-terminal fragment. *J Bone Miner Res* 26 (2): 331–340.

Mithal, A., J. P. Bonjour, Boonen, S. Burckhardt, P. Degens, H. El Hajj Fuleihan,G. Josse, R. Lips, P. Morales Torres,J. Rizzoli, R. Yoshimura, N. D. A. Wahl, Cooper, C. and Dawson-Hughes.B. 2013. Impact of nutrition on muscle mass, strength, and performance in older adults. *Osteoporos Int* 24 (5): 1555–1566.

Montessuit, C., J. P. Bonjour, and Caverzasio. J. 1995. Expression and regulation of Na-dependent P(i) transport in matrix vesicles produced by osteoblast-like cells. *J Bone Miner Res* 10 (4): 625–631.

Montessuit, C., Caverzasio, J. and Bonjour. J.P. 1991. Characterization of a Pi transport system in cartilage matrix vesicles. Potential role in the calcification process. *J Biol Chem* 266 (27): 17791–17797.

Moreira-Pfrimer, L. D., M. A. Pedrosa, Teixeira, L. and Lazaretti-Castro.M. 2009. Treatment of vitamin D deficiency increases lower limb muscle strength in institutionalized older people independently of regular physical activity: A randomized double-blind controlled trial. *Ann Nutr Metab* 54 (4): 291–300.

Mozar, A., Haren, N. Chasseraud, M. Louvet, L. Maziere, C. Wattel, A. Mentaverri, R. Morliere, P. Kamel, S. Brazier, M. J. C. Maziere, and Massy. Z.A. 2008. High extracellular inorganic phosphate concentration inhibits RANK-RANKL signaling in osteoclast-like cells. *J Cell Physiol* 215 (1): 47–54.

Murer, H. and Biber. J. 2010. Phosphate transport in the kidney. *J Nephrol* 23 (Suppl 16):S145–151.

Neer, R.M., C. D. Arnaud, J. R. Zanchetta, Prince, R. G. A. Gaich, J. Y. Reginster, A. B. Hodsman, E. F. Eriksen, Ish-Shalom,S. H. K. Genant, Wang, O. and Mitlak. B.H. 2001. Effect of parathyroid hormone (1-34) on fractures and bone mineral density in postmenopausal women with osteoporosis. *N Engl J Med* 344 (19): 1434–1441.

Palmer, G., Zhao, J. Bonjour, J. Hofstetter, W. and Caverzasio. J. 1999. In vivo expression of transcripts encoding the Glvr-1 phosphate transporter/retrovirus receptor during bone development. *Bone* 24 (1): 1–7.

Pastorino, D., Canal, C. and Ginebra. M.P. 2015. Drug delivery from injectable calcium phosphate foams by tailoring the macroporosity-drug interaction. *Acta Biomater* 12:250–259.

Prie, D. and Friedlander. G. 2010. Genetic disorders of renal phosphate transport. *N Engl J Med* 362 (25): 2399–2409.

Rana, P., R. K. Marwaha, Kumar, P. Narang, A. M. M. Devi, R. P. Tripathi, and Khushu. S. 2014. Effect of vitamin D supplementation on muscle energy phospho-metabolites: A ^{31}P magnetic resonance spectroscopy-based pilot study. *Endocr Res* 39 (4): 152–156.

Rizzoli, R. and Bonjour. J.P. 2006. Physiology of calcium and phosphate homeostasis. In *Dynamics of Bone and Cartilage Metabolism: Principles and Clinical Applications*, edited by Seibel,M.J. Robins S.P. and Bilezikian,J.P. 345–360. San Diego, CA: Academic Press.

Schubert, L. and DeLuca. H.F. 2010. Hypophosphatemia is responsible for skeletal muscle weakness of vitamin D deficiency. *Arch Biochem Biophys* 500 (2): 157–161.

Scriver, C.R. 1979. The William Allan Memorial Award address: On phosphate transport and genetic screening. "Understanding backward--living forward" in human genetics. *Am J Hum Genet* 31 (3): 243–263.

Shah, A.D., Shoback, D. and Lewiecki. E.M. 2015. Sclerostin inhibition: A novel therapeutic approach in the treatment of osteoporosis. *Int J Womens Health* 7:565–580.

Trohler, U., J. P. Bonjour, and Fleisch. H. 1976a. Inorganic phosphate homeostasis. Renal adaptation to the dietary intake in intact and thyroparathyroidectomized rats. *J Clin Invest* 57 (2): 264–273.

Trohler, U., J. P. Bonjour, and Fleisch. H. 1976b. Renal tubular adaptation to dietary phosphorus. *Nature* 261 (5556): 145–146.

Trohler, U., J. P. Bonjour, and Fleisch. H. 1981. Plasma level and renal handling of Pi: Effect of overnight fasting with and without Pi supply. *Am J Physiol* 241 (5):F509–516.

Urakawa, I., Yamazaki, Y. Shimada, T. Iijima, K. Hasegawa, H. Okawa, K. Fujita, T. Fukumoto, S. and Yamashita. T. 2006. Klotho converts canonical FGF receptor into a specific receptor for FGF 23. *Nature* 444 (7120): 770–774.

van Bezooijen, R.L., ten Dijke,P. S. E. Papapoulos, and Lowik. C.W. 2005. SOST/sclerostin, an osteocyte-derived negative regulator of bone formation. *Cytokine Growth Factor Rev* 16 (3): 319–327.

Verron, E., J. M. Bouler, and Guicheux. J. 2012. Controlling the biological function of calcium phosphate bone substitutes with drugs. *Acta Biomater* 8 (10): 3541–3551.

Zhang et al. 2011. Unique roles of phosphorus in endochondral bone formation and osteocyte maturation. *J Bone Mineral Res* 26:1047–1056.

Whyte, M.P. 2010. Physiological role of alkaline phosphatase explored in hypophosphatasia. *Ann N Y Acad Sci* 1192:190–200.

Whyte, M.-P. 2008. Enzyme defects and the skeleton. In *Primer on the Metabolic Bone Diseases and Disorders of Mineral Metabolism*, edited by Rosen,C.J. Compston J.E. and Lian,J.B. 454–458. Washington, DC: The American Society for Bone and Mineral Research.

Wicherts, I.S., van Schoor,N. M. A. J. Boeke, Visser, M. Deeg, D.J. Smit, J. D. L. Knol, and Lips. P. 2007. Vitamin D status predicts physical performance and its decline in older persons. *J Clin Endocrinol Metab* 92 (6): 2058–2065.

13 Dietary Phosphate Needs in Early Life and Adolescence

Alicia M. Diaz-Thomas, Russell W. Chesney, and Craig B. Langman

CONTENTS

Abstract 167
Bullet Points 167
13.1 Introduction 168
13.2 Phosphorus Economy: An Embarrassment of Wealth 168
    13.2.1 Assessments of Phosphate Homeostasis 169
13.3 Phosphorus Metabolism and Bone 170
13.4 Phosphorus Economy in Fetus and Neonate 171
13.5 Disordered Phosphorus Economy of the Preterm Infant (Metabolic Bone Disease of the Preterm) 176
13.6 Risks to Bone Health in Mid-Childhood and Their Relation to Phosphorus Economy (Childhood Obesity) 177
13.7 Phosphorus Economy in Adolescence (The Effects of Diet and the Road Ahead) 178
13.8 Conclusions 179
Dedication 179
References 179

ABSTRACT

Phosphorus is one of the most abundant minerals in the body, and it is essential for most cellular processes. Only recently, mechanisms governing the regulation of phosphorus have been elucidated. This has provided an opportunity to understand new and emerging roles of phosphorus in the pathophysiology of metabolic bone disease of premature infants. Efforts to understand adequate supplementation of phosphorus in these special populations are underway. Additionally, the role of phosphorus in the genesis of cardiovascular disease is being understood. Adequate dietary evaluation of the growing child and adolescent, with particular attention to phosphorus additives, is needed. Finally, unknown dietary phosphates in foods need to be declared if we are to fully understand the long-term consequences of excess phosphate ingestion in adolescence.

BULLET POINTS

- Phosphate is an integral component of human nutrition that, despite its importance, is regulated exclusively by the kidney.
- Placental transport of this vital mineral is highest in the third trimester of pregnancy.
- Preterm neonates are especially vulnerable to lack of adequate nutritional phosphate intakes.
- In contrast, excess phosphate intake in mid-childhood and adolescence poses additional challenges to healthy bone mineralization.
- Excess phosphate in mid-childhood and adolescence may increase risks for chronic diseases in adulthood.

13.1 INTRODUCTION

Although the history of phosphate itself likely predates the late seventeenth century, Hennig Brand is often credited with the discovery of this element during his alchemical studies into the possibility that the "philosopher's stone" may be hidden in human urine. In the process of heating and purifying urine, he obtained phosphate. Its ability to phosphoresce (basis: Greek "light-bearing") provided its name.

As a nutrient, phosphate is often overlooked due to its ubiquitous presence in most foods. Intake is felt to be adequate unless there is an underlying medical condition, and thus less scrutiny is paid to its daily requirement in contrast to other minerals, such as calcium and magnesium. However, two critical times of ponderal growth, the neonatal and adolescent periods, differ greatly in their need for phosphate when compared to adult life. Preterm infants have significant differences in phosphate metabolism and are at risk for bony demineralization disorders as a consequence. Finally, requirements change through infancy and childhood as a result of growth, changes in the hormonal milieu, and the ensuing mineralization and growth of the human skeleton.

13.2 PHOSPHORUS ECONOMY: AN EMBARRASSMENT OF WEALTH

The role of phosphate in the support of musculoskeletal health is central. The majority of phosphate (85%) in humans is present as hydroxyapatite in the skeleton. The remainder is located in either inorganic or organic form throughout the extracellular and intracellular compartments. Given its widespread distribution, phosphate plays a critical role in many biologic processes, including energy metabolism, membrane composition, nucleotide structure, cellular signaling, and bone mineralization. Excess phosphate is excreted in the urine or stool, but the renal phosphate reclamation or excretion processes appear to be the only ones regulated to any degree.

Intestinal phosphate absorption takes place primarily in the duodenum and jejunum. It occurs by two mechanisms: an active, sodium-dependent transcellular process localized in the mucosal surface by the sodium phosphorous cotransporter IIB (NaPi IIB) and by passive diffusion through a paracellular pathway. Paracellular phosphate movement depends on both the absolute amount of dietary phosphate and the relative concentrations of calcium and phosphate (an excessive amount of either can decrease the absorption of the other). Calcitriol ($1,25(OH)_2D_3$) stimulates NaPi IIB expression and active phosphate absorption. In health, the efficiency of this absorption is high, close to 90% of intake, regardless of the type of feedings provided to the infant or child.

Renal handling of phosphorus occurs through the process of reabsorption. Inorganic serum phosphate is filtered at the glomerulus and reabsorbed in the proximal tubule. Under normal conditions, more than 80% of the filtered load of phosphate is reabsorbed by the proximal tubule. Some additional phosphate (8% to 10%) is reabsorbed in the distal tubule (but not in Henle's loop), leaving about 10% to 12% for excretion in the urine [1]. The transport capacity of the proximal tubule for phosphorus is limited; it cannot exceed a certain number of mmol per unit time. This limit is called the tubular maximum for phosphate (TmP). Renal phosphate transport is primarily regulated by parathyroid hormone (PTH), the FGF23/klotho axis, and the plasma phosphate concentration, each of which alters the Na-phosphate transporter activity, directly or indirectly, thereby affecting the availability or abundance of the high-affinity, low-capacity class of NaPi-II cotransporters. PTH, an 84–amino acid peptide hormone whose release is regulated by the extracellular-calcium sensing receptor in the parathyroid glands, acutely stimulates the translocation of NaPi-II transporters from the brush border membrane though its interaction with sodium–hydrogen exchanger regulatory factor 1 (NHERF1). PTH inhibition of NHERF1 activity results in removal of NaPi-IIa from the brush border, a net decrease in serum phosphate, and an increase in TMP [2,3]. Fibroblast growth factor-23 (FGF23), produced by osteocytes and osteoblasts, is a phosphorus-regulating hormone. Higher levels of FGF23 downregulate the expression of the genes encoding sodium-phosphate cotransporters 2a and 2c (NaPi-IIa and NaPi-IIc) in proximal renal tubules [4]. It also inhibits 25-hydroxy-vitamin

Dietary Phosphate Needs in Early Life and Adolescence

D 1α-hydroxylase (CYP27B1) and increases expression of the 24-hydroyxlase (CYP27A1), both of which lead to a net decrease in both calcitriol levels and intestinal expression of NaPi-IIb [5]. FGF23 hormonal actions are mediated through the klotho/FGFR1 complex[6]. There is some evidence that FGFR4, another fibroblast growth factor receptor, is also important in renal FGF23 actions related to phosphorus metabolism in mice, but its role in humans is directed to off-target actions of FGF23 in the heart [7,8].

Dietary intake of phosphate itself also reciprocally regulates the expression and activity of NaPi II cotransporters and, consequently, the proximal tubular absorption of phosphate, by a mechanism that is independent of PTH. Dietary deprivation of phosphate, for example, leads to a stimulation of phosphate reabsorption that can override the effects of PTH on the proximal tubule. It is likely that this dietary regulation of NaPi II expression may also be mediated by FGF23 [9]. In contrast to calcium, deprivation of phosphate does not appear to improve intestinal phosphorus absorption at low intakes [10]. Intestinal phosphorus absorption appears to continue despite significant hyperphosphatemia [11]. Finally, there is some evidence that in certain clinical conditions, hyperphosphatemia itself can induce hyperparathyroidism and increased release of FGF23 from bone. Here, restoration of blood phosphorus to normal is achieved at the expense of the elevated PTH and FGF23 levels [12,13].

Table 13.1 [14] shows the age-specific normal values of the mineral in blood considering all the previously mentioned regulatory processes for maintenance of phosphate homeostasis.

13.2.1 Assessments of Phosphate Homeostasis

Renal handling of phosphate load can be expressed as either the tubular reabsorption of phosphate (TRP) as a percentage or the Tm renal tubular maximum reabsorption rate of phosphate to

TABLE 13.1
Age-Related Normal Values and Recommended Daily Allowances

Life Stage Group	RDA Phosphorus[b] mg/day	Serum Phosphorus[c] mg/dL	TmP/GFR[d] mmol/L
Term infants	–	–	–
0–3 mo	100[a]	4.8–7.4	1.43–3.43
3–6 mo	100[a]	4.8–7.4	1.48–3.30
6 mo–12 mo	275[a]	4.8–7.4	1.15–2.6
Children	–	–	–
1–3 y	460	4.5–6.5	1.15–2.44
4–8 y	500	3.6–5.8	1.15–2.44
Males	–	–	–
9–13 y	1250	3.6–5.8	1.15–2.44
14–18 y	1250	2.3–4.5	1.15–2.44
19–25 y	700	2.3–4.5	1.0–1.35
Females	–	–	–
9–13 y	1250	3.6–5.8	1.15–2.44
14–18 y	1250	2.3–4.5	1.15–2.44
19–25 y	700	2.3–4.5	0.96–1.44

[a] Denotes adequate intake (AI) rather than RDA

[b] Dietary reference intakes for calcium, phosphorous, magnesium, vitamin D, and fluoride (1997): Food and Nutrition Board, IOM, National Academies.

[c] National Kidney Foundation KDOQI guidelines, 2005.

[d] Payne RB, *Ann Clin Biochem.*, 35, 201–206, 1998.

glomerular filtration rate (TmP/GFR). Reabsorption of phosphate can be calculated using the TRP as follows:

$$\%TRP = 1 - (UPO_4 \times Pcr / PPO_4 \times Ucr) \times 100$$

where UPO_4 = urinary concentration of phosphate, Pcr = plasma creatinine, PPO_4 = plasma concentration of phosphate, and Ucr = urinary concentration of creatinine.

TRP percentage varies with age. It remains quite high until approximately age 15 in girls and age 14 in boys; thereafter it decreases steadily to adult levels. Reference ranges for children between ages 6 and 18 have been published by Kruse et al. [15]. The TmP/GFR was derived as a function of the renal response to a continuous phosphate infusion, initially described by Bijvoet [16]. Some feel that this may be a more useful measurement of renal phosphorus handling in neonates because of their relatively low GFR.

Additional hormonal factors may affect renal handling of phosphate. Modulators of phosphate transport that increase reabsorption include circulating insulin-like growth factor-1, growth hormone acting perhaps through local kidney-produced IGF-1, insulin, thyroid hormone, and calcitriol. PTH-related protein (PTHrP), calcitonin, atrial naturetic factor (ANF), transforming growth factors alpha and beta, and glucocorticoids each inhibit renal reabsorption and promote phosphaturia [17].

13.3 PHOSPHORUS METABOLISM AND BONE

Phosphorus balance is important not only for energy metabolism but also for its role in bone mineralization. Mesenchyme-derived osteoblasts secrete a collagen-rich matrix that is mineralized by apatite crystals, which confer strength and serve as a bio-resource for phosphate release when needed. Bone resorption is carried out by hematopoietically derived osteoclasts. Both of these cells work in concert, linked by several systems but, most importantly, by the RANK-RANKL system that stimulates osteoclastogenesis. Osteoblasts secrete osteoprotegerin (OPG), an inhibitor of RANKL that inhibits osteoclastogenesis. The ratio of RANKL to OPG dictates osteoclast differentiation status and thus release of calcium and phosphate from bone. Bone resorption by osteoclasts releases bone matrix-trapped IGF-1, transforming growth factor-ß (TGF-ß), and bone morphogenic proteins (BMPs), which promote osteoblast migration to the resorption sites and hasten osteoblastogenesis [18,19]. Accordingly, bone mass is a function of the balance between these two processes and is dependent on adequate dietary supply of calcium and phosphorus.

Whereas molar concentrations of Ca:P in the non–bone-forming sites of the body are typically stable and exhibit a ratio of 1:1, those concentrations in the active bone-forming site fluctuate depending on the overriding process: bone resorption or formation. It is here that phosphorus levels seem to influence bone mass and revolve around pyrophosphate (P_2O_7). Typically, pyrophosphate can be produced as a byproduct of cellular processes and can be found both intracellularly and extracellularly [20]. Tissue fluid pyrophosphate found throughout the body inhibits mineral deposition by binding either ionic or crystalline calcium such that mineralization is prevented. Pyrophosphate also induces osteoblast-mediated secretion of osteopontin, an additional inhibitor of mineralization [21]. Tissue-nonspecific alkaline phosphatase (ALPL, TNAP; the bone/kidney/liver isoform of alkaline phosphatase) is an enzyme highly expressed by mineralized tissue cells that degrades pyrophosphate [22]. This hydrolytic process liberates phosphorus, thus elevating local phosphate concentrations and promoting bone mineralization.

In bone, although absolute local phosphate concentrations are important, the phosphate: pyrophosphate ratio (modulated in large measure by the actions of ALPL) provides key molecular regulation in maintaining the equilibrium between promoters and inhibitors necessary for the initiation of normal bone matrix mineralization [23]. Other factors that regulate local phosphate concentrations are also important, such as PHOSPHO1, a phosphatase enzyme that has been proposed to be

Dietary Phosphate Needs in Early Life and Adolescence

present within the matrix vesicle where osteoblast-mediated mineralization begins [24]. Once mineralization is initiated, growth of the hydroxyapatite crystals is regulated by a subcategory of the secreted, calcium-binding phosphoprotein (SCPP) family called the small, integrin-binding ligand, N-linked glycoproteins (SIBLINGs) [25]. This family includes osteopontin (OPN), bone sialoprotein (BSP), dentin matrix protein 1 (DMP1), dentin sialophosphoprotein (DSPP), and matrix extracellular phosphoglycoprotein (MEPE).

13.4 PHOSPHORUS ECONOMY IN FETUS AND NEONATE

The majority of maternal to fetal transfer of phosphate and other minerals occurs during the third trimester. From the analysis of stillbirths and deceased neonates, the rate during this trimester approaches 130 to 250 mg/kg/day of calcium, 60 to 70 mg/kg/day of phosphate, and 3 mg/kg/day of magnesium [26]. The transplacental transport of phosphate is an active process against a concentration gradient and is sodium dependent. Both 1, $25(OH)_2D_3$ and fetal PTH/PTHrP may be involved in the regulation of placental phosphate transfer [27]. Recently, the NaPi IIb cotransporter has been hypothesized to play an important role in placental phosphorus handling [28]. The third-trimester transfer of phosphate to the fetus is vital for achievement of the bone mineral content of term neonates, and its absence due to prematurity is a major risk factor for subsequent inadequate bony demineralization.

After birth, for a term infant, the mean serum phosphate concentration rises rapidly from 2.6 mmol/L (6.2 mg/dL) to reach a typical value of 3.4 mmol/L (8.1 mg/dL) due to both endogenous phosphate release and lower renal excretion when compared to placental clearance. [29,30]. Neonates excrete only 60% of intestinally absorbed phosphate through the kidney and have the highest renal resorption of phosphate at any time in life: they reabsorb 99% of the filtered load of phosphate on the first day of life and 90% by the end of the first week [31]. Reabsorption occurs primarily through the NaPi IIc cotransporter, the expression of which is higher in weaning animals but which has a reduced function in adult animals.

The NaPi IIa cotransporter appears to be involved as well in the high phosphate reabsorption that is present in the term neonate [32]. Renal NaPi II transporter expression is significantly greater in juvenile animals, and a developmental decrease in this specific transporter protein occurs into young adulthood. These patterns in NaPi II expression directly coincide with the increased tubular phosphate reabsorption seen in the juvenile animals [33].

The increase in reabsorption in infants has also been attributed to a blunting of the renal phosphaturic response to PTH [34]. Typically, PTH-induced inhibition of phosphate reabsorption is mediated by several processes: decreased expression of the *SLC34A1* gene responsible for transcription of the NaPi II transporter, endocytosis of NaPi IIa from the brush border, and lysosomal degradation of the endocytosed transporter. This process is likely altered in infants. Immunofluorescent studies in juvenile rats demonstrate that although PTH continues to cause the internalization of the NaPiII cotransporter from the brush border, the cotransporter remained localized in the subapical compartment, rather than being degraded in the lysosomal pathway and thus is more readily available [33]. This may be partly growth hormone dependent, because the endocytic removal and degradation of the PTH-induced NaPi II transporter can occur in juvenile kidneys after growth hormone suppression [35]. Tubular calcium reabsorption in response to PTH seems to remain unaffected, thus increasing both calcium and phosphate retention, allowing for enhanced growth and mineralization at the level of bone [36].

The role of the FGF23/klotho axis in neonates is incompletely described, and FGF23 may have a less critical role in fetal life than in neonates for phosphate homeostasis. For example, *FGF23* null mice have normal length, weight, appearance, and serum calcium and phosphate at birth [37], but disturbed mineral metabolism is evident by 10 days of age. By 2 weeks of age they are smaller in size than their peers [37] and demonstrate both reduced renal phosphorus excretion and an undermineralized skeleton, and limb deformities are present at 3 weeks [38]. Interestingly, at the same time, such mice exhibit increased whole-body mineral content due to excessive pathological mineralization of soft tissues, including heart, lungs, and kidneys. Mortality in such animals is 100% by age 10 to 12 weeks [37, 39–41].

Although FGF23 levels seem to be similar through fetal and neonatal life, there may be differences in c-terminal and intact isoforms. Takaiwa et al. measured FGF23 and c-terminal FGF23 by ELISA in 22 umbilical cord samples (UCS) and in 22 five-day old infants. These levels were also compared to average levels in healthy adults. Overall, the UCS and the infants had c-terminal FGF23 levels that were similar and in both groups higher than the adult FGF23 levels. However, intact FGF23 levels were lower than the adult group and lowest in the fetal group [42]. Finally, in a case series of four infants of parents with hypophosphatemic rickets who were followed from birth, neonatal effects of presumed FGF23 excess resulted in hypophosphatemia between two and six weeks of age and abnormalities in the TRP by six months of age, highlighting the role of FGF23 in early neonatal life in humans too [43].

The growth hormone/somatomedin pathway also contributes to phosphate balance, not only at the level of the bone but also by increasing phosphorus reabsorption. Chronic administration of recombinant IGF-1 increased TMPi/GFR and plasma Pi in hypophesectomized rats as compared to controls. [44] Both GH and IGF-1 mRNA have been localized to apical membranes of proximal tubular epithelial cells, suggesting a role of the GH/IGF-1 axis in phosphate reabsorption [45]. It is not known whether the increase in phosphate retention results directly from GH binding to renal GH receptors or indirectly from GH activation of renal IGF-1, because IGF-1 is also capable of directly increasing phosphate reabsorption in vitro and in vivo [46]. Other suggested mechanisms for GH/IGF-1 effects on renal phosphate handling include well-established, parallel effects of IGF-1 on increases in glomerular filtration and renal plasma flow [47].

Dietary contributions to the phosphate economy in neonates are of utmost importance. Current recommendations for dietary intake of phosphorus in infants are based on the usual dietary intakes of breastfed infants. The concentration of calcium and phosphorus in human breast milk is, on average, significantly lower than in bovine milk or infant formula, but is relatively constant throughout lactation. In mature human milk of term infants, calcium concentrations reported in studies vary from 25 to 35 mg/100 mL and phosphorus from 13 to 16 mg/100 mL [48]. In human milk, minerals are both bound to highly digestible proteins and are present in complexed and ionized states [49]. There is an increase in phosphorus requirements over the first year of life coincident with the addition of solid foods: from 0 to 6 months, infants are recommended to receive 100 mg/d of phosphorus and from 7 to 12 months, the recommendation is 275 mg/day [50] (see Table 13.1).

The mineral intake of an infant's diet is significantly associated with bone mass accretion during the first six months of life. In Specker et al.'s study of term infants, the ones fed human milk during the first six months of life had a greater gain in bone mass during the second six months of life when they were provided a moderate- to high-mineral formula when compared to infants previously fed low- or moderate-mineral formula. These early effects of diet on bone mass accretion resulted in similar total body bone mass at one year of age [51]. Thus although breast milk provides a significantly lower concentration of minerals, bone mass accretion rates appear to be similar over time when compared to formula-fed infants. In a cross-sectional study of infants, 307 healthy participants (63 black), ages 1 to 36 months, had bone mineral content (BMC) and areal bone mineral density (aBMD) of the lumbar spine measured by dual-energy X-ray absorptiometry (DXA). Human milk feeding duration was ascertained by questionnaire. The duration of human milk feeding was associated with lower aBMD among infants <12 months of age. This effect persisted when adjusting for weight, which tends to be lower among infants exclusively receiving human milk compared to those receiving formula. However, this early effect waned in the older infants and toddlers [52]. In infants fed soy-based formulas, the intestinal absorption of phosphate is lower than that of a comparable group of infants fed a similar phosphorus intake from cow milk–based formula [53]. Measurements of BMC have also been found to be lower in soy-fed infants compared with cow milk–based formula-fed infants, consistent with reduced mineral absorption with soy formulas [54].

Dietary Phosphate Needs in Early Life and Adolescence

It is postulated that the phytates in soy formulas can decrease gastrointestinal absorption of calcium and phosphorus [55]. This can be overcome by increasing the amounts of mineral supplements in soy formulas.

Human milk for both term and preterm infants is felt to be an optimal source of nutrition but needs to be fortified to meet the needs for protein and energy of very-low-birth-weight (VLBW <1500 g at delivery) or extremely low-birth-weight (ELBW, 1000 g at delivery) premature infants. Such infants are medically fragile and may have other coincident conditions that would affect mineral metabolism such as poor maternal nutritional status, immature mechanisms of intestinal absorption, ventilator dependence requiring some parenteral nutrition if not all, long-term administration of medications (corticosteroids, methylxanthines, furosemide), and inflammation as a result of infection [56]. Often they receive parenteral feedings initially before being slowly transitioned to oral feedings. Micronutrients such as calcium, phosphorus, sodium, iron, and possibly zinc may also have to be supplemented. In particular, phosphorus levels tend to be quite low, and sufficient supplementation may be impossible parenterally.

Human milk differs in macronutrient, immunological, growth factors, and microbial components both over time (with advancing chronologic age of the infant) and between mothers delivering babies of differing gestational ages. Macronutrient composition differs between preterm and term milk, with preterm milk tending to be higher in protein and fat. Human milk oligosaccharides, sugars that can influence the growth of certain microorganisms, likely influence intestinal colonization and may also influence the bacterial community composition of milk [57]. IGFs and their binding proteins have been found in human milk, with higher quantities present early in lactation. Studies have noted that these growth factors may be delivered in a complexed form, thus giving rise to speculation that they may have a local early role in infant gut maturation [58]. Likely, a combination of all of these factors prime the infant gut to receive individualized nutrition and promote optimal absorption. Thus supplementation of human milk may not be a "one-size-fits-all" endeavor in the youngest and, thus, at highest risk infants for phosphate imbalance.

There are two main types of human milk fortifiers (HMFs): cow's milk–based HMF and human donor milk–based (HDMF). Thomaz et al. [55] compared different ways of processing pooled human milk to manufacture an HMF with a commercial cow's milk–based HMF that is commonly used in Brazil. The human milk was either skimmed, evaporated and lactose free (SEL), and prepared as a liquid, or skimmed, evaporated, lactose free and lyophilized (SELL) and prepared as a powder. They found that overall, human pooled milk fortifiers had lower amounts of minerals and differing calcium/phosphorus ratios from manufactured human milk fortifiers (Table 13.2).

Certainly, direct measurements of micronutrients do not reflect in vivo processes and bioavailability. Chetta et al. followed phosphorus levels in 93 premature infants (25 to 29-wk old and weight <1250 g) receiving breast milk supplemented with HDMF to understand if there were risks related to hyperphosphatemia. There has been some concern that HDMFmay deliver too much phosphorus to these infants. Rates of hyperphosphatemia (>8 mg/dL, 18.3%) were similar to rates of hypophosphatemia (<4.8 mg/dL, 20%) in the 93 infants. The serum phosphate levels reportedly correlated not only with day of life (decreasing with age) and renal function (increasing phosphorus with decreasing renal function) but also apparently with the energy density concentration of HDMF used (phosphorus levels increasing with energy density). Only two instances of hypocalcemia were recorded. The authors concluded that monitoring of serum phosphorus in LBW and ELBW premature infants receiving human milk with HDMF is warranted (Table 13.3).

By contrast, in a prospective study by Kanmaz et al. [59] preterm infants were randomly assigned to receive differing concentrations of fortified human milk, namely standard (1 scoop HMF: 30 mL HM), moderate (1 scoop HMF: 25 mL HM), or aggressive (1 scoop HMF: 20 mL HM). No significant differences in metabolic parameters of calcium, phosphorus, or alkaline phosphatase were noted in any of the three groups. Other parameters were also monitored, and it was felt that higher levels of supplementation than are currently recommended were safe for VLBW infants. This is provided as an alternative to individualized fortification that may not be feasible in all nurseries.

TABLE 13.2
Composition of Pooled Human Donor Milk–Based Fortifiers as Compared to Commercial Cow's Milk–Based Human Milk Fortifiers

	SEL Liquid HM Additive + 100 mL HM	SELL Powdered HM Additive + 100 mL HM	5 g of FM85 (Nestle) + 100 mL HM	P Value
Protein g/dL	1.81	2.38	1.96	< 0.001
Carbs g/dL	6.70	7.25	10.06	0.006
Fat g/dL	3.75	3.75	3.73	0.96
Calcium mg/dL	36.92	44.75	79.37	0.001
Phos mg/dL	20.02	23.28	56.30	0.001
Ca/phos ratio	1.84	1.92	1.41	
Sodium mEq/L	14.32	14.40	20.33	0.143
Osm mOsmol/kgH2O	391.45	412.47	431.00	0.074
Calories kcal in 100 mL	67.78	72.27	81.65	0.001

Source: Thomaz DM et al., *J Pediatr (Rio J).*, 88, 119–124, 2012.

TABLE 13.3
Comparison of Human Donor Milk–Derived Fortifier with Differing Proportions of Human Milk (Commercial HMF Provided as Reference)

	HDMF Prolact + 4	HDMF Prolact + 6	HDMF Prolact + 8	HDMF Prolact + 10	Cow's Milk–Based HMFs
HM:HDMF	80:20	70:30	60:40	50:50	–
Protein g/dL	2.3	2.8	3.2	3.7	–
Carbs g/dL	7.1	7.4	7.6	7.9	–
Fat g/dL	4.9	5.4	5.9	6.5	–
Calcium mg/dL	123	123	123	122	38–138
Phos mg/dL	64	64	64	64	26–67
Ca/Phos ratio	1.91	1.91	1.91	1.91	1.46–2.05
Sodium mEq/L	57	57	57	57	–
Osm mOsmol/kgH2O	< 335[a]	< 360[a]	< 325[a]	< 350[a]	–
Calories kcal 100 mL	82	89	97	104	–

[a] From manufacturer's website: http//www.prolacta.com/human-milk-fortifier, accessed Dec. 15, 2015.

Until recently, most fortifiers were available in powdered form. This raised potential concerns for use in immunocompromised infants after a series of cases of *Cronobacter* sp. infections were reported in infants receiving reconstituted powers (both formula and HMF) [60]. Now liquid preparations of HMF and HDMF have been developed. The composition of these does vary both between manufacturers and among powdered and liquid forms (Table 13.4) [61,62]. There is also concern that the interaction between the components of the particular HMF may have independent and unaccounted for effects on the bioavailability of micronutrients provided in these preparations to preterm infants [63]. Perhaps these recent developments may provide a basis for individualized fortification to promote optimal growth and development of these infants.

Some studies support the concept that ponderal growth in early life, both in utero and during infancy, is a strong predictor of BMC and risk of hip fracture in later adulthood [64,65]. Long-term follow-up of the 5431 children of the Generation R study, conducted in Rotterdam, and enrolled from April 2002 and January 2006, culminated in a DXA at six years of age. Here, growth occurring in the

TABLE 13.4

Comparison of Commercial Cow's Milk–Based HMF Products with Standard Human Milk or Cow's Milk–Based Formula and Comparison of These Products in 100 mL of Standard Human Milk

	Eoprotin (Cow's Milk HMF) 3 g [c]	Similac Powder (Cow's Milk HMF) 0.9 g [a]	5 mL Similac Liquid (Cow's Milk HMF) [a]	5 mL Enfamil Liquid (Cow's Milk HMF) [a]	Breast Milk (HM) in 100 mL [d]	Infant Formula (means) in 100 mL [d]	Cow's Milk in 100 mL [d]	3 g of Eoprotin + 100 mL HM [b]	3.46 g Similac HMF + 100 mL HM [a]	20 mL Similac HMF liquid + 100 mL HM [a]	20 mL Enfamil Liquid HMF + 100 mL of Preterm HM [a]
Protein g/dL	0.6 g	0.25 g	0.349 g	0.55 g	0.9–1.4 [b]	1.45	3.2	2.0	2.28	2.33	3.8
Carbs g/dL	2.1 g	0.45 g	0.807 g	0.3 g	6–7	7.36	4.6	8.74	8.10	8.22	7.9
Fat g/dL	0.02 g	0.09 g	0.266 g	1.45 g	3.9–4.2 [b]	3.51	3.6	3.9	4.02	4.13	5.8
Calcium mg/dL	38 mg	29 mg	35.1 mg	29 mg	24.8–34 mg [b]	51.63	119	62.8	133	137.53	141
Phos mg/dL		16 mg	20.0 mg	15.75 mg		28.65			72.2	77.26	78
Ca/Phos ratio		1.81	1.75			1.80			1.84	1.78	1.8
Sodium mg/dL	20	4	5.39	6.75	24.8 Meq [b]	18.53		44	38	38.63	55
Osm	50 mOsm/L	2.8 mOsm			290 mOsm/kgH2O [b]			340			
Calories kcal	11	3.5	6.85	6	70	67.10	62	78	76	79.92	97

[a] From manufacturer's website: http://abbottnutrition.com/brands/products/similac-human-milk-fortifier-concentrated-liquid, accessed Dec. 17, 2015 and http://www.enfamil.com/products/special-dietary-needs/enfamil-human-milk-fortifier-acidified-liquid, accessed Dec. 17, 2015.

[b] Oval F et al., J Perinatol., 26, 761–763, 2006.

[c] Kanmaz HG et al., J Hum Lact., 29, 400–405, 2012.

[d] Jardi Pinana C et al., An Pediatr (Barc)., 83, 417–429, 2015.

first year of life showed the strongest positive association with bone mass accrual in later childhood [66]. Nevertheless, other studies support a homeostatic set point for individual peak bone mass that is not lastingly affected by interventions in childhood or adolescence [67]. In a group of preterm infants fed supplemented breast milk with increasing caloric density, there was no significant difference in growth parameters, other than the suggestion of a possible trend toward an increase in head circumference in the most heavily supplemented group [53]. Perhaps there may be an effect of patterning early in fetal or neonatal life, and perhaps, this may be affected by early breastfeeding such that bone mineral accrual persists at different rates from infants who are formula fed. Certainly, further understanding of whether breastfeeding has an epigenetic effect, such as changing methylation patterns of genes important for bone mineral accrual and growth, may be of interest in future studies.

13.5 DISORDERED PHOSPHORUS ECONOMY OF THE PRETERM INFANT (METABOLIC BONE DISEASE OF THE PRETERM)

Osteopenia of prematurity, or the metabolic bone disease seen in preterm infants, has become increasingly common with the increasing rates of survival of LBW and VLBW preterm infants. This form of bone disease occurs in up to 23% of newborns weighing <1500 g at birth and in 55% of those weighing <1000 g who have not received fortified breast milk or formula with high Ca and P content. [68]. Overall, the incidence of neonatal osteopenia is inversely correlated with birth weight and gestational age. In a case series, Yeşiltepe Mutlu et al. describe the onset of disease between 6 and 12 weeks in the presence of low serum phosphorus levels [69]. In the acute neonatal phase, this reduction in BMC can lead to fractures in the nursery (described in up to 10% of LBW infants) [70]. Bone mineralization can take a significant time to reach normal levels; in LBW infants at term-age equivalent, BMC is significantly reduced when compared to that of normal term infants and may not approach even median values until after the first year of life [71].

The genesis of the metabolic bone disease of prematurity is felt to be a result of several factors, including a relatively lower bone mineralization at birth given that most bone accrual occurs in the third trimester coincident with placental mineral transfer, dependence on parenteral feeding with a delay in enteral feedings, use of medications such as calciuretic diuretics, and intercurrent illnesses and their therapies. Parenteral routes of nutrition rarely can deliver sufficient phosphorus, due to the risk of precipitation with calcium, although increasing phosphate content can decrease risk of metabolic bone disease of prematurity [26,72]. Additionally, parenteral formulas generally contain trace amounts of aluminum that can be detrimental to bone health [73]. There is some interest in early minimal enteral feeding regimens in preterm infants, but this can be limited by risks for necrotizing enterocolitis and other illnesses [74]. Preterm infants with low serum inorganic phosphate (< 2 mmol/L) are at risk of osteopenia, and levels less than 1.8 mmol/L have been strongly associated with the presence of radiographically evident rickets [75].

Investigating metabolic bone disease in LBW/VLBW infants is performed using both biochemical and radiographic methods. Biochemical assessment of children with osteopenia of prematurity can be problematic as no one single marker has been found to have sufficient sensitivity and specificity early in life to predict children at risk for development of metabolic bone disease. Serum calcium is an unreliable marker for bone disease itself, as it often remains normal due to compensatory elevations in PTH. Urine studies, although technically difficult to perform in infants, can also be difficult to interpret as their normal value may depend on the relative calcium:phosphorus ratio of their formula and the corrected gestational age. Calcium absorption of preterm infants may be limited by transient hypoparathyroidism and an immaturity of the renal hydroxylase enzyme. Formula-fed infants show very low urinary calcium concentrations but a high urinary phosphate, attributable to a low absorption rate of calcium from preterm formulas. In these infants, phosphaturia is noted as a result of the insufficient calcium absorption from the gut. Breast milk contains insufficient phosphate for the needs of preterm infants and therefore infants maximize renal phosphate reabsorption.

Dietary Phosphate Needs in Early Life and Adolescence 177

Hypercalciuria may be noted in the breastfed infant [76,77]. As urinary ratios depend heavily on whether the child is receiving enteral or parenteral feeding and the timing of the sample relative to the feeding, standard reference ranges are less useful. In addition, it has still not been proven that urinary ratios are a reliable substitute for direct measurement of BMC [78].

Combinations of markers may be more promising. In a small study of 43 preterm infants with a median gestational age of 30.3 weeks, Backstrom et al. examined the utility of several biochemical makers (serum Pi, total alkaline phosphatase, and bone-specific alkaline phosphatase) in predicting low bone mineral apparent density (BMAD) at three months of age. BMAD, a calculation used to transform the aBMD measurement to a volumetric measurement, is used to account for bones in smaller individuals. Although bone-specific alkaline phosphatase did not seem to be predictive, in contrast to work done by other investigators, a combination of serum Pi <1.8 mmol/L and total alkaline phosphatase >900 IU/L at three weeks of age gave excellent sensitivity (100%) and reasonable specificity (70%) for low BMAD at three months of the postnatal age in this group. The authors do acknowledge (as have many others) that overall the utility of elevated alkaline phosphatase values in the diagnosis of metabolic bone disease of the preterm infants is low given that some infants will have transient elevations of excessively sialylated liver alkaline phosphatase that is only slowly cleared (transient hyperphosphatasemia) [79]. Other urine and serum markers such as collagen crosslinks are being investigated, but normative data are not fully established.

Radiographic methods for assessment include plain radiograph, DXA measurement, or qualitative ultrasound. On plain radiograph, bone mineralization needs to be markedly decreased by at least 20% to 40% to have changes consistent with osteopenia present, as plain film radiography is much less sensitive than DXA [80]. DXA is increasingly being used as instrument-specific references are developed for neonates [81], but its value may be greater in affording longitudinal measurement and in evaluating body compositional analysis. Some authors have expressed preference for lumbar measurement rather than the total body minus head as it is more easily reproducible. Finally, qualitative ultrasound is available with measurements at the tibia being most common [82]. Research into peripheral quantitative computed tomography (pQCT) and high resolution peripheral quantitative computed tomography (HR-qQCT) for neonatal bone disease are rapidly advancing, as information is obtained about structural strength unavailable by the other methods noted. However, attention to maintenance of low exposures to ionizing radiation will have to be taken into account in this population.

13.6 RISKS TO BONE HEALTH IN MID-CHILDHOOD AND THEIR RELATION TO PHOSPHORUS ECONOMY (CHILDHOOD OBESITY)

Childhood obesity has more than doubled in children and quadrupled in adolescents in the past 30 years. In the United States, the percentage of children aged 6 to 11 years who were obese increased from 7% in 1980 to nearly 18% in 2012. Similar increases were noted in the adolescent population [83]. Currently more than one-third of children in the United States are considered overweight (BMI >85th percentile) with other countries noting similar increases in their pediatric populations. These metabolic changes pose risks not only for increased morbidity from altered glucose metabolism (metabolic syndrome), hypertension, and hyperlipidemia, but also may negatively affect bone metabolism and consequent calcium and phosphorus balance.

Traditionally, obesity has been thought to be associated with increases in bone mineral density, both through increased mechanical forces imposed on the skeleton and estrogen production by adipocyte aromatization. This paradigm, however, is challenged by reports demonstrating increased fracture rates in obese, preadolescent boys compared to their normal-weight counterparts [84,85]. Covariant factors such as location of fat depots and the amount of marrow fat also seem to be important in changes in fracture risk for this population. Obesity may also affect vitamin D metabolism and calcium/phosphorus balance. In leptin-deficient (OB/OB) mice, there is an increase in renal expression of 25-hydroxyvitamin D3-1 alpha hydroxylase and decreases in 24-hydroxylase.

These mice exhibited increases in calcium, phosphorus, and 1,25 dihydroxyvitamin D3. Treatment with leptin normalized these values. The researchers concluded that the low bone mineral density seen in these mice may be explained by the increase in bone resorption effected through stimulation of bone resorption by 1,25 dihydroxyvitamin D3 [86]. Further studies by this group in the same leptin-deficient mice also suggest that these elevations in 25-hydroxyvitamin D3-1 alpha-hydroxylase may be a result of decreases in FGF23 secretion from bone mediated by leptin itself [87]. Thus obesity can affect not only the strength of bone but also its metabolism. Data in obese humans, however, suggest that FGF23 may be elevated rather than decreased and remains a matter of investigation [8].

With the increasing obesity epidemic in mid-childhood years, there seems to be a trend toward earlier pubertal development in females and a relative hypogonadotrophic hypogonadism in obese males. Sex steroids are important for the acquisition of skeletal mass and density, with sexually dimorphic effects present: androgens work directly through the androgen receptor, and estrogens have important effects with respect to an increase in the calcified zone and eventual fusion of the epiphyses. Hypogonadism in both males and females impairs bone size and in males has been shown to reduce volumetric bone mineral density [88]. Some data suggest that estrogens regulate PTH indirectly, possibly through FGF23. For example, estrogen treatment in ovarectomized rats with chronic kidney disease seemed to decrease PTH mRNA and serum PTH levels, serum 1,25(OH) [15] vitamin D_3, and serum phosphorus levels. Notably, increased serum FGF23 and FGF23 mRNA levels were observed after estrogen treatment as well [89]. Thus obesity has both direct and indirect effects on phosphorus metabolism in children.

13.7 PHOSPHORUS ECONOMY IN ADOLESCENCE (THE EFFECTS OF DIET AND THE ROAD AHEAD)

Adolescence is typically a time of rapid growth. With the advent of puberty, females can reach growth rates of 8 cm/yr and male at rates of 10 cm/yr during the peak of the growth spurt. This increased growth is also translated into increased energy and mineral needs. Optimal nutrition is essential to achieving full growth potential. Not only can an inadequate diet result in delayed sexual maturation and slowed or arrested linear growth, but it could also bear on adult diet-related chronic diseases, such as cardiovascular disease, cancer, and osteoporosis. Intakes of phosphorus have been rising in developed countries due to the use of inorganic phosphate-containing food additives and preservatives. This pattern of increased consumption of absorbable phosphates likely affects adolescent populations and/or economically disadvantaged populations disproportionately.

In 2010, the Yale Rudd Center for Food Policy & Obesity issued a report in combination with the Robert Wood Johnson Foundation examining the nutritional quality of fast food menus, marketing, and advertising, called Fast Food FACTS. The report focused on the 12 largest fast food restaurants in the United States and highlighted marketing targeted to children, teens, and black and Hispanic youth in 2009. Findings from the report included targeted marketing to teens, offerings of large-sized soft drinks and French fries, and few choices provided that were considered nutritious. Typical teens in developed countries consume a disproportionately larger intake of processed foods than natural foods, many of which contain phosphoric acid (colas), phosphates, and polyphosphates (processed meats and fish, commercial baked goods) for preservation of shelf life or improvement in flavor.

Excess phosphate ingestion in healthy subjects leads to an increase in circulating FGF23 levels. These changes are accompanied by a decrease in the tubular reabsorption of Pi and a decrease in calcitriol levels. Interestingly these actions have been postulated to be somewhat independent of PTH action [90]. There is some concern that elevations in FGF23 in healthy subjects may be associated with vascular dysfunction [91]. Effects of FGF23 on blood pressure have also been postulated. FGF23- and klotho-deficient mice show renal salt wasting and are hypovolemic, whereas supplementation of normal mice with recombinant FGF23 upregulated the distal tubular sodium-chloride cotransporter and resulted in hypertension [92]. In vitro and in vivo mouse experiments by Faul et al. suggest that there is a direct effect of FGF23 on myocytes that involves specific second-messenger

Dietary Phosphate Needs in Early Life and Adolescence

pathways and results in hypertrophy of the cardiac myocytes [93]. Thus excess phosphorus intake in adolescence may be an independent risk factor for the development of hypertension and cardiovascular dysfunction later in life. In a recent cross-sectional cohort of 130 normotensive African American male adolescents, plasma c-terminal FGF23 levels were associated with abnormal cardiac structure, being higher in the obese adolescents and significantly higher in those showing eccentric or concentric cardiac hypertrophy as assessed by M-mode echocardiography [8]. Further complicating matters are problems with measurement of phosphates in foods, hidden sources of phosphate, lack of prospective studies in healthy populations, and the ubiquity of phosphorus itself.

Measurements of phosphate additives in foods may be difficult: the WHO/FAO (World Health Organization/ Food and Agriculture Organization of the United Nations) acknowledged the need to update specifications and methods for some phosphate additives in foods in their 77th evaluation of food additives and contaminants [94]. Addition of phosphate-rich additives to foods is not typically reported in the food composition tables, and these are easily absorbed and digested [95]. Studies such as the NHANES data set may not be designed to detect excessive phosphate intake in diet due to food additives. Analysis of several questions of the 2005–2010 dataset of dietary recall for 13- to 99-year-old people proposed that increased phosphorus intakes, when combined with equally robust calcium intake, can provide some protective effect in terms of bone health. The concern with using these sources in the future is that perhaps the questionnaires are not powered to effectively detect added phosphate salts in foods [96]. Plant-based diets provide phosphate that is less bioavailable than the inorganic phosphates found in processed diets, proving that one unit of phosphate is not similar between foods themselves [97]. Perhaps with recent attention to obesity in childhood and adolescence and the promotion of plant-based diets, intakes may decrease over time.

13.8 CONCLUSIONS

Phosphate is an integral component of human nutrition that, despite its importance, is regulated exclusively by the kidney. Normal blood values are age related throughout the lifespan. Attention to mineral supplementation in infants has traditionally focused on providing sufficient calcium. However, in certain populations provision of sufficient phosphate can be challenging. In fetal life, placental transport of this vital mineral is maximal in the third trimester. Thus preterm infants are at risk for conditions resulting from lack of adequate phosphorus, namely metabolic bone disease. Careful attention to adequate provision of phosphorus in appropriate ratios in this age group is needed. Furthermore, early identification, optimal treatment regimens, and long-term follow-up are needed to optimize outcomes in relation to phosphorus deficiency in this age group.

In contrast, excess phosphate intakes in mid-childhood and adolescence pose additional challenges to healthy bone mineralization, both through direct (increases in phosphate intake increasing FGF23 levels, changes in local bone microenvironments) and indirect (hormonal changes in obese children) mechanisms. Moreover, there is increasing evidence that FGF23 in excess is a biomarker for cardiovascular disease. Thus, the increasing consumption of hidden phosphates in processed foods may portend further increases in the prevalence of chronic adult diseases such as cardiovascular disease, hypertension, and osteoporosis. Many challenges remain in understanding the long-term implications of excess phosphates in the diets of today's adolescents.

DEDICATION

In memory of Russell Chesney and his brilliant, curious, and insatiable mind.

REFERENCES

1. Bringhurst FR, Demay MB, Kronenberg HM. Hormones and disorders of mineral metabolism. In *Williams Textbook of Endocrinology*, edited by Kronenberg HM, Larsen PR, Melmed S, Polonsky KS. 13th ed., 2016 Chapter 28: pp. 1253–1322.

2. Gisler SM, Stagljar I, Traebert M, Bacic D, Biber J, Murer H. Interaction of the type IIa Na/Pi cotransporter with PDZ proteins. *J Biol Chem* 2001; 276: 9206–9213.
3. Hernando N1, Déliot N, Gisler SM, Lederer E, Weinman EJ, Biber J, Murer HP. DZ domain interactions and apical expression of type IIa Na/P(i) cotransporters. *Proc Natl Acad Sci* 2002; 99: 11957–11962.
4. Silver J, Naveh-Many T. FGF23 and the parathyroid glands. *Pediatr Nephrol* 2010; 25: 2241–2245.
5. Shimada T, Hasegawa H, Yamazaki Y, Muto T, Hino R, Takeuchi Y, Fujita T, Nakahara K, Fukumoto S, Yamashita T. FGF-23 is a potent regulator of vitamin D metabolism and phosphate homeostasis. *J Bone Miner Res* 2004; 19: 429–435.
6. Urakawa I, Yamazaki Y, Shimada T, Iijima K, Hasegawa H, Okawa K, Fujita T, Fukumoto S, Yamashita T. Klotho converts canonical FGF receptor into a specific receptor for FGF23. *Nature* 2006; 444: 770–774.
7. Gattineni J, Alphonse P, Zhang Q, Mathews N, Bates CM, Baum M. Regulation of renal phosphate transport by FGF23 is mediated by FGFR1 and FGFR4. *Am J Physiol Renal Physiol* 2014; 306(3): F351–358.
8. Ali FN, Falkner B, Gidding SS, Price HE, Keith SW, Langman CB. Fibroblast growth factor-23 in obese, normotensive adolescents is associated with adverse cardiac structure. *J Pediatr* 2014 Oct; 1654: 738–743.
9. Saito H, Maeda A, Ohtomo S, Hirata M, Kusano K, Kato S, Ogata E, Segawa H, Miyamoto K, Fukushima N. Circulating FGF-23 is regulated by 1alpha,25-dihydroxyvitamin D3 and phosphate in vivo. *J Biol Chem* 2005; 280: 2543–2549.
10. Lemann J Jr, Worcester EM, Gray RW. Hypercalciuria and stones. *Am J Kidney Dis* 1991; 17: 386–391.
11. Brickman AS, Coburn JW, Massry SG. 1,25 dihydroxy-vitamin D3 in normal man and patients with renal failure. *Ann Intern Med* 1974; 80:161–168.
12. Svenningsen NW, Lindquist B. Postnatal development of renal hydrogen ion excretion capacity in relation to age and protein intake. *Acta Paediatr Scand* 1974; 63(5): 721–731.
13. Segawa H, Kaneko I, Takahashi A, Kuwahata M, Ito M, Ohkido I, Tatsumi S, Miyamoto K. Growth-related renal type II Na/Pi cotransporter. *J Biol Chem* 2002; 277: 19665–19672.
14. Payne RB. Renal Tubular reabsorption of phosphate, (TmP/GFR): Indications and interpretation. *Ann Clin Biochem* 1998; 35: 201–206.
15. Kruse K, Kracht U, Gopfert G. Renal threshold phosphate concentration (TmPO4/GFR). *Arch Dis Child* 1982; 57: 217–223.
16. Walton RJ, Bijvoet OL. Nomogram for derivation of renal threshold phosphate concentration. *Lancet* 1975; 2: 309–310.
17. Tenenhouse HS. Cellular and molecular mechanisms of renal phosphate transport. *J Bone Miner Res* 1997; 12: 159–164.
18. Manolagas SC, Jilka RL. Bone marrow, cytokines, and bone remodeling. Emerging insights into the pathophysiology of osteoporosis. *N Engl J Med* 1995 Feb. 2; 332(5): 305–311.
19. Boyle WJ, Simonet WS, Lacey DL. Osteoclast differentiation and activation. *Nature* 2003; 423(6937): 337–342.
20. Russell RG, Fleisch H. Pyrophosphate and diphosphonates in skeletal metabolism. Physiological, clinical and therapeutic aspects. *Clin Orthop Relat Res* 1975; 108: 241–263.
21. Harmey D, Johnson KA, Zelken J, Camacho NP, Hoylaert MF, Noda M, Terkeltaub R, Millán JL. Elevated osteopontin levels contribute to the hypophosphatasia phenotype in Akp2–/– mice. *J Bone Miner Res* 2006; 21: 1377–1386.
22. Millan JL. Alkaline phosphatases: Structure, substrate specificity and functional relatedness to other members of a large superfamily of enzymes. *Purinergic Signal* 2006; 2: 335–341.
23. Murshed M, McKee MD. Molecular determinants of extracellular matrix mineralization in bone and blood vessels. *Curr Opin Nephrol Hypertens* 2010; 19: 359–365.
24. Roberts S, Narisawa S, Harmey D, Millan JL, Farquharson C. Functional involvement of PHOSPHO1 in matrix vesicle-mediated skeletal mineralization. *J Bone Miner Res* 2007; 22: 617–627.
25. Staines KA, MacRae VE, Farquharson C. The importance of the SIBLING family of proteins on skeletal mineralisation and bone remodelling. *J Endocrinol* 2012; 214(3): 241–255.
26. Rigo J, De Curtis M, Pieltain C, Picaud JC, Salle BL, Senterre J. Bone mineral metabolism in the micro-premie. *Clin Perinatol* 2000; 27(1): 147–170.
27. Weisman J. Maternal, fetal and neonatal vitamin D and calcium metabolism during pregnancy and lactation. In *Vitamin D and Rickets. Endocrine Development*, Hochberg Z (ed.). Basel, Switzerland: Karger, 2003, vol 6:pp. 34-49

Dietary Phosphate Needs in Early Life and Adolescence

28. Shibasaki Y, Etoh N, Hayasaka M, Takahashi MO, Kakitani M, Yamashita T, Tomizuka K, Hanaoka K. Targeted deletion of the tybe IIb Na(+)-dependent Pi-co-transporter, NaPi-IIb, results in early embryonic lethality. *Biochem Biophys Res Commun* 2009; 381: 482–486.

29. Langhendries JP, François A, Chedid F, Battisti O, Bertrand JM, Senterre J. Phosphate intake in preterm babies and variation of tubular reabsorption for phosphate per liter glomerular filtrate. *Biol Neonate* 1992; 61: 345–350.

30. Senterre J, Salle B. Renal aspects of calcium and phosphate metabolism in preterm infants. *Biol Neonate* 1988; 53: 220–229.

31. Hohenauer L, Rosenberg TF, Oh W. Calcium and phosphorus homeostasis on the first day of life. *Biol Neonate* 1970; 15: 49–56.

32. Brodehl J, Gellissen K, Weber HP. Postnatal development of tubular phosphate reabsorption. *Clin Nephrol* 1982; 17(4): 163–171.

33. Woda C, Mulroney SE, Halaihel N, Sun L, Wilson PV, Levi M, Haramati A. Renal tubular sites of increased phosphate transport and NaPi-2 expression in the juvenile rat. *Am J Physiol Regul Integr Comp Physiol* 2001; 280: R1524–R1533.

34. Silverstein DM, Spitzer A, Barac-Nieto M. Parathormone sensitivity and responses to protein kinases in subclones of opossum kidney cells. *Pediatr Nephrol* 2005; 20(6): 721–724.

35. Woda CB, Halaihel N, Wilson PV, Haramati A, Levi M, Mulroney SE. Regulation of renal NaPi-2 expression and tubular phosphate reabsorption by growth hormone in the juvenile rat. *Am J Physiol Renal Physiol* 2004; 287: F117–F123.

36. Tsang RC, Chen IW, Friedman MA, Chen I. Neonatal parathyroid function: Role of gestational age and postnatal age. *J Pediatr* 1973; 83(5): 728–738.

37. Shimada T, Kakitani M, Yamazaki Y, Hasegawa H, Takeuchi Y, Fujita T, Fukumoto S, Tomizuka K, Yamashita T. Targeted ablation of Fgf23 demonstrates an essential physiological role of FGF23 in phosphate and vitamin D metabolism. *J Clin Invest* 2004; 113: 561–568.

38. Sitara D, Kim S, Razzaque MS, Bergwitz C, Taguchi T, Schuler C, Erben RG, Lanske B. Genetic evidence of serum phosphate-independent functions of FGF-23 on bone. *PLoS Genet* 2008; 4: e1000154.

39. Nakatani T, Sarraj B, Ohnishi M, Densmore MJ, Taguchi T, Goetz R, Mohammadi M, Lanske B, Razzaque MS. In vivo genetic evidence for klotho-dependent, fibroblast growth factor 23 (Fgf23)-mediated regulation of systemic phosphate homeostasis. *FASEB J* 2009; 23(2): 433–441.

40. Sitara D, Kim S, Razzaque MS, Bergwitz C, Taguchi T, Schuler C, Erben RG, Lanske B. Genetic evidence of serum phosphate-independent functions of FGF-23 on bone. *PLoS Genet* 2008; 4: e1000154.

41. Sitara D, Razzaque MS, Hesse M, Yoganathan S, Taguchi T, Erben RG, Jüppner H, Lanske B. Homozygous ablation of fibroblast growth factor-23 results in hyperphosphatemia and impaired skeletogenesis, and reverses hypophosphatemia in Phex-deficient mice. *Matrix Biol* 2004; 23: 421–432.

42. Takaiwa M, Aya K, Miyai T, Hasegawa K, Yokoyama M, Kondo Y, Kodani N, Seino Y, Tanaka H, Morishima T. Fibroblast growth factor 23 concentrations in healthy term infants during the early postpartum period. *Bone* 2010; 47: 256–262.

43. Moncrieff MW. Early biochemical findings in familial hypophosphataemic, hyperphosphaturic rickets and response to treatment. *Arch Dis Child* 1982; 57: 70–72.

44. Caverzasio J, Faundez R, Fleisch H, Bonjour JP. Tubular adaptation to Pi restriction in hypophysectomized rats. *Pflugers Arch* 1981 Nov; 3921: 17–21.

45. Hammerman MR, Karl IE, Hruska KA. Regulation of canine renal vesicle Pi transport by growth hormone and parathyroid hormone. *Biochim Biophys Acta* 1980; 603: 322–335.

46. Caverzasio J, Bonjour JP. Growth factors and renal regulation of phosphate transport. *Pediatr Nephrol* 1993; 7: 802–806.

47. Corvilian J, Arnwiow M. Some effects of human growth hormone on renal hemodynamics and on tubular phosphate transport in man. *J Clin Invest* 1962; 41: 1230–1235.

48. Jenness R. The composition of human milk. *Semin Perinatol* 1979 Jul; 33: 225–239.

49. Neville MC. Calcium secretion into milk. *J Mammary Gland Biol Neoplasia* 2005 Apr; 102: 119–128.

50. Klienman RE (ed.). *Pediatric Nutrition Handbook*, 5th ed. Washington, DC: American academy of Pediatrics Committee on Nutrition, 2004, p. 292–293.

51. Specker BL, Beck A, Kalkwarf H, Ho M. Randomized trial of varying mineral intake on total body bone mineral accretion during the first year of life. *Pediatrics* 1997; 99(6): E12.

52. Kalkwarf HJ, Zemel BS, Yolton K, Heubi JE. Bone mineral content and density of the lumbar spine of infants and toddlers: Influence of age, sex, race, growth, and human milk feeding. *J Bone Miner Res* 2013; 28(1): 206–212.

53. Shenai JP, Jhaveri BM, Reynolds JW, Huston RK, Babson SG. Nutritional balance studies in very low-birth-weight infants: Role of soy formula. *Pediatrics* 1981; 67: 631–637.

54. Chan GM, Leeper L, Book LS. Effects of soy formulas on mineral metabolism in term infants. *Am J Dis Child* 1987; 141: 527–530.

55. Thomaz DM, Serafim PO, Palhares DB, Melnikov P, Venhofen L, Vargas MO. Comparison between homologous human milk supplements and a commercial supplement for very low birth weight infants. *J Pediatr (Rio J)* 2012 Mar-Apr; 882: 119–124.

56. Viswanathan S, Khasawneh W, McNelis K, Dykstra C, Amstadt R, Super DM, Groh-Wargo S, Kumar D. Metabolic bone disease: A continued challenge in extremely low birth weight infants. *JPEN J Parenter Enteral Nutr* 2014 Nov; 388: 982–990.

57. Ballard O, Morrow AL. Human milk composition: Nutrients and bioactive factors. *Pediatr Clin North Am* 2013 Feb; 601: 49–74.

58. Milsom SR, Blum WF, Gunn AJ. Temporal changes in insulin-like growth factors I and II and in insulin-like growth factor binding proteins 1, 2, and 3 in human milk. *Horm Res* 2008; 69(5): 307–311.

59. Kanmaz HG, Mutlu B, Canpolat FE, Erdeve O, Oguz SS, Uras N, Dilmen U. Human milk fortification with differing amounts of fortifier and its association with growth and metabolic responses in preterm infants. *J Hum Lact* 2013 Aug; 293: 400–405.

60. Reich F, Konig R, von Wiese W, Klein G. Prevalence of Cronobacter spp. in a powdered infant formula processing environment. *Int J Food Microbiol* 2010 Jun 15; 140(2–3): 214–217.

61. Oval F, Çiftçi H, Çetinkaya Z, Bükülmez A. Effects of human milk fortifier on the antimicrobial properties of human milk. *J Perinatol* 2006; 26: 761–763. doi:10.1038/sj.jp.7211610; published online 5 October 2006.

62. Jardí Pinana C, Aranda Pons N, Bedmar Carretero C, Arija Val V. Composición nutricional de las leches infantiles. Nivel de cumplimiento en su fabricación y adecuación a las necesidades nutricionales. *An Pediatr (Barc)* 2015; 83: 417–429.

63. Thoene M, Hanson C, Lyden E, Dugick L, Ruybal L, Anderson-Berry A. Comparison of the effect of two human milk fortifiers on clinical outcomes in premature infants. *Nutrients* 2014 Jan. 3; 6(1): 261–275.

64. Dennison EM, Syddall HE, Sayer AA, Gilbody HJ, Cooper C. Birth weight and weight at 1 year are independent determinants of bone mass in the seventh decade: The Hertfordshire cohort study. *Pediatr Res* 2005; 57: 582–586.

65. Gale CR, Martyn CN, Kellingray S, Eastell R, Cooper C. Intrauterine programming of adult body composition. *J Clin Endocrinol Metab* 2001; 86: 267–272.

66. Heppe DH, Medina-Gomez C, de Jongste JC, Raat H, Steegers EA, Hofman A, Rivadeneira F, Jaddoe VW. Fetal and childhood growth patterns associated with bone mass in school-age children: The Generation R Study. *J Bone Miner Res* 2014; 29(12): 2584–2593.

67. Gafni RI, Baron J. Childhood bone mass acquisition and peak bone mass may not be important determinants of bone mass in late adulthood. *Pediatrics* 2007; 119(Suppl 2): S131–136.

68. Bozzetti V, Tagliabue P. Metabolic bone disease in preterm newborns: An update on nutritional issues. *Ital J Pediatr* 2009; 35: 20–26.

69. Yeşiltepe Mutlu G, Kırmızıbekmez H, Ozsu E, Er I, Hatun S. Metabolic bone disease of prematurity: Report of four cases. *J Clin Res Pediatr Endocrinol* 2014; 6(2): 111–115.

70. Dabezies EJ, Warren PD. Fractures in very low birth weight infants with rickets. *Clin Orthop Relat Res* 1997; 335: 233–239.

71. Abrams SA, Schanler RJ, Tsang RC, Garza C. Bone mineralization in former very low birthweight infants fed either human milk or commercial formula: One year follow-up observation. *J Pediatr* 1989; 114: 1041–1044.

72. Prestridge LL, Schanler RJ, Shulman RJ, Burns PA, Laine LL. Effect of parenteral calcium and phosphorus therapy on mineral retention and bone mineral content in very low birth weight infants. *J Pediatr* 1993; 122(5 Pt 1): 761–768.

73. Koo WW, Kaplan LA. Aluminum and bone disorders: With specific reference to aluminum contamination of infant nutrients. *J Am Coll Nutr* 1988; 7(3): 199–214.

74. Weiler HA, Fitzpatrick-Wong SC, Schellenberg JM, Fair DE, McCloy UR, Veitch RR, Kovacs HR, Seshia MM. Minimal enteral feeding within 3 d of birth in prematurely born infants with birth weight < or = 1200 g improves bone mass by term age. *Am J Clin Nutr* 2006; 83(1): 155–162.

75. Aiken CGA, Sherwood RA, Lenney W. Role of plasma phosphate measurements in detecting rickets of prematurity and in monitoring treatment. *Ann Clin Biochem* 1993; 30: 469–475.

76. Pohlandt F. Prevention of postnatal bone demineralization in very low-birth-weight infants by individually monitored supplementation with calcium and phosphorus. *Pediatr Res* 1994 Jan; 351: 125–129.

Dietary Phosphate Needs in Early Life and Adolescence

77. Visser F, Sprij AJ, Brus F. The validity of biochemical markers in metabolic bone disease in preterm infants: A systematic review. *Acta Paediatr* 2012 Jun; 1016: 562–568.

78. Harrison CM, Johnson K, McKechnie E. Osteopenia of prematurity: A national survey and review of practice. *Acta Paediatr* 2008; 97(4): 407–413.

79. Backström MC, Kouri T, Kuusela AL, Sievänen H, Koivisto AM, Ikonen RS, Mäki M. Bone isoenzyme of serum alkaline phosphatase and serum inorganic phosphate in metabolic bone disease of prematurity. *Acta Paediatr* 2000; 89: 867–873.

80. Mazess RB, Peppler WW, Chesney RW, Lange TA, Lindgren U, Smith E, Jr. Total body and regional bone mineral by dual-photon absorptiometry in metabolic bone disease. *Calcif Tissue Int* 1984; 36(1): 8–13.

81. Rigo J, Nyamugabo K, Picaud JC. Reference values of body composition obtained by DEXA in preterm and term neonates. *J Pediatr Gastroenterol Nutr* 1998; 27: 184–190.

82. Littner Y, Mandel D, Mimouni FB, Dollberg S. Bone ultrasound velocity curves of newly born term and preterm infants. *J Pediatr Endocrinol Metab* 2003; 16: 43.

83. Ogden CL, Carroll MD, Kit BK, Flegal KM. Prevalence of childhood and adult obesity in the United States, 2011-2012. *JAMA* 2014; 311(8): 806–814.

84. Joeris A, Lutz N, Wicki B, Slongo T, Audigé L. An epidemiological evaluation of pediatric long bone fractures—A retrospective cohort study of 2716 patients from two Swiss tertiary pediatric hospitals. *BMC Pediatr* 2014; 14: 314.

85. Moon RJ, Lim A, Farmer M, Segaran A, Clarke NM, Dennison EM, Harvey NC, Cooper C, Davies JH. Differences in childhood adiposity influence upper limb fracture site. *Bone* 2015; 79: 88–93.

86. Matsunuma A, Kawane T, Maeda T, Hamada S, Horiuchi N. Leptin corrects increased gene expression of renal 25-hydroxyvitamin D3-1 alpha-hydroxylase and -24-hydroxylase in leptin-deficient, ob/ob mice. *Endocrinology* 2004; 145(3): 1367–1375.

87. Tsuji K, Maeda T, Kawane T, Matsunuma A, Horiuchi N. Leptin stimulates fibroblast growth factor 23 expression in bone and suppresses renal 1alpha,25-dihydroxyvitamin D3 synthesis in leptin-deficient mice. *J Bone Miner Res* 2010; 25(8): 1711–1723.

88. Vanderschueren D, Vandenput L, Boonen S. Reversing sex steroid deficiency and optimizing skeletal development in the adolescent with gonadal failure. *Endocr Dev* 2005; 8: 150–165.

89. Carrillo-López N, Román-García P, Rodríguez-Rebollar A, Fernández-Martín JL, Naves-Díaz M, Cannata-Andía JB. Indirect regulation of PTH by estrogens may require FGF23. *J Am Soc Nephrol* 2009 Sep; 209: 2009–2017.

90. Ferrari S, Bonjour J, Rizzoli R. Fibroblast growth factor-23 relationship to dietary phosphate and renal phosphate handling in healthy young men. *J Clin Endocrinol Metab* 2005; 90: 1519–1524.

91. Mirza MA, Larsson A, Lind L, Larsson TE. Circulating fibroblast growth factor-23 is associated with vascular dysfunction in the community. *Atherosclerosis* 2009; 205(2): 385–390.

92. Andrukhova O, Slavic S, Smorodchenko A, Zeitz U, Shalhoub V, Lanske B, Pohl EE, Erben RG. FGF23 regulates renal sodium handling and blood pressure. *EMBO Mol Med* 2014; 6(6): 744–759.

93. Faul C, Amaral AP, Oskouei B, Hu MC, Sloan A, Isakova T. FGF23 induces left ventricular hypertrophy. *J Clin Invest* 2011 Nov. 1; 121: 4393–4408.

94. World Health Organization. Evaluation of certain food additives and contaminants. *World Health Organ Tech Rep Ser* 2013; 983: 1–75.

95. Lou-Arnal LM, Arnaudas-Casanova L, Caverni-Muñoz A, Vercet-Tormo A, Caramelo-Gutiérrez R, Munguía-Navarro P, Campos-Gutiérrez B, García-Mena M, Moragrera B, Moreno-López R, Bielsa-Gracia S, Cuberes-Izquierdo M, Grupo de Investigación ERC Aragón. Hidden sources of phosphorus: Presence of phosphorus-containing additives in processed foods. *Nefrologia* 2014; 34(4): 498–506.

96. Lee AW, Cho SS. Association between phosphorus intake and bone health in the NHANES population. *Nutr J* 2015; 14(1): 28–33.

97. McCarty MF, DiNicolantonio JJ. Bioavailable dietary phosphate, a mediator of cardiovascular disease, may be decreased with plant-based diets, phosphate binders, niacin, and avoidance of phosphate additives. *Nutrition* 2014; 30(7–8): 739–747.

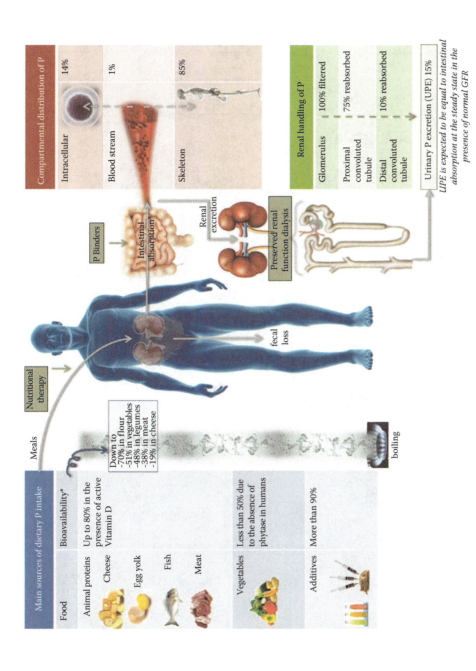

FIGURE 4.1 Phosphate homeostasis. P homeostasis depends on the nutritional intake of P, its intestinal absorption, compartmental distribution, and renal excretion. Nutrition, P binders, and preservation of renal function (and dialysis for ESRD patients) represent the current interventions to affect P balance in humans. Intestinal absorption depends on the bioavailability of nutritional P, presence of P binders in the gut lumen, cooking methods, and levels of active vitamin D.

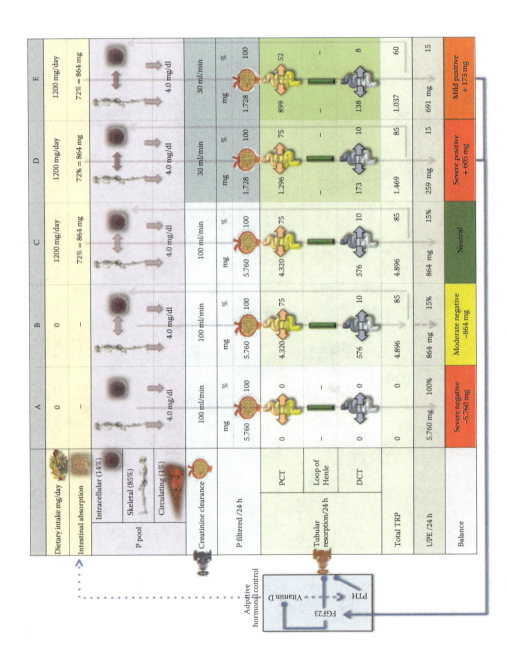

FIGURE 4.2 For description, see Page 48 in text.

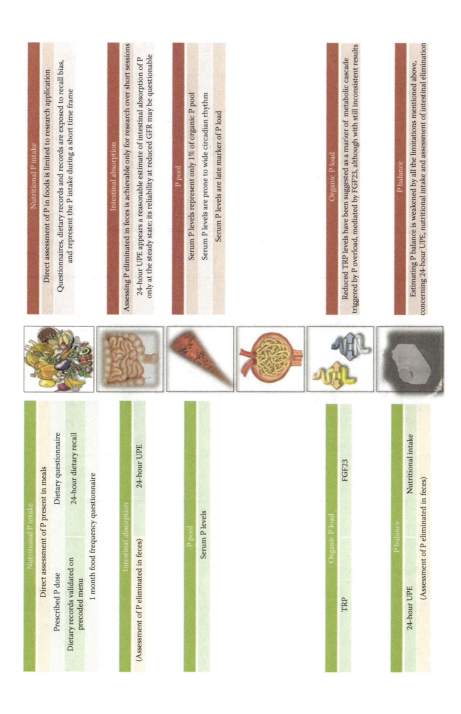

FIGURE 4.3 Assessment of P balance: Methods and weaknesses. Techniques available to assess P balance are reported in green boxes (orange boxes report the methods limited to research application). Weaknesses of techniques are briefly described in red boxes.

ABBREVIATIONS FGF23: fibroblast growth factor 23, P: phosphate, TRP: tubular resorption of P, UPE: urinary P excretion.

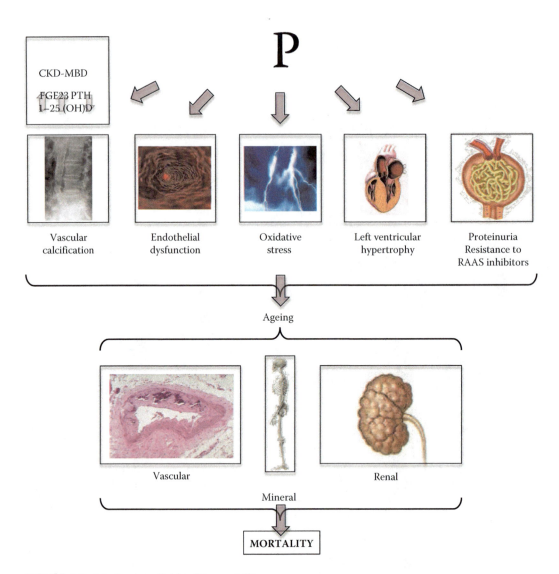

FIGURE 4.4 Mechanisms linking P to mortality.

ABBREVIATIONS CKD-MBD: chronic kidney disease and mineral bone disorder, FGF23: fibroblast growth factor 23, P: phosphate, PTH: parathyroid hormone, RAAS: renin–angiotensin–aldosterone system.

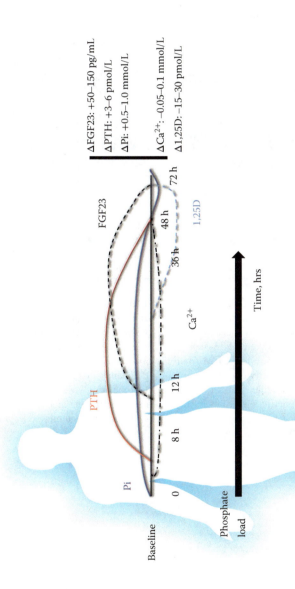

FIGURE 6.2 Response of endocrine regulators to an intravenous or oral phosphate load over time in human volunteers. Graph represents change from baseline (not drawn to scale) illustrating the timing and magnitude of the homeostatic responses that are triggered by a high-dose phosphate challenge. The increase in serum phosphate level is sufficient to induce a small reduction in ionized calcium concentration that results in a robust increase in PTH level. The mild hyperphosphatemia is furthermore associated with an increase in FGF23 concentration that is followed by a decrease in 1,25(OH)2 vitamin D concentration. For further details, see reference. (Adapted from Scanni R et al., *J Am Soc Nephrol.*, 25, 2730–2739, 2014.)

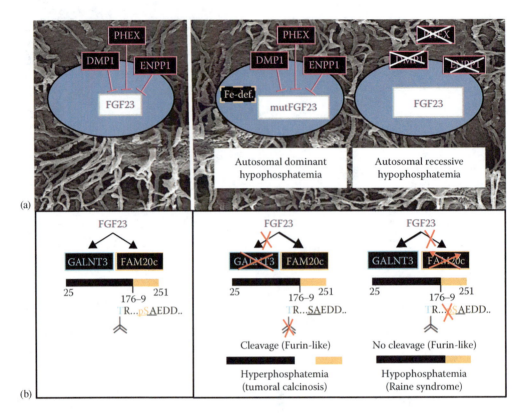

FIGURE 6.3 Factors regulating FGF23 synthesis. FGF23 production in bone by osteocytes (background image in 3) is regulated by a number of other genes through unclear mechanisms. Panel (a): PHEX, DMP1, and ENPP1 appear to reduce FGF23 production (left) because homozygous loss-of-function mutations in PHEX, DMP1, and ENPP1 cause autosomal-recessive FGF23-dependent forms of hypophosphatemia (right). Heterozygous mutations at the RXXR cleavage site in FGF23 (mutFGF23) cause an autosomal-dominant form of hypophosphatemia that becomes particularly apparent when iron deficiency increases FGF23 synthesis through largely unknown mechanisms (middle). Panel (b): FGF23 undergoes O-glycosylation at T178 and phosphorylation at S180 (left). Loss-of-function mutations in the enzymes affecting the amount of post-translational processing of FGF23, namely GALNT3 and FAM20c, lead to hyperphosphatemia and hypophosphatemia, respectively (middle and right).

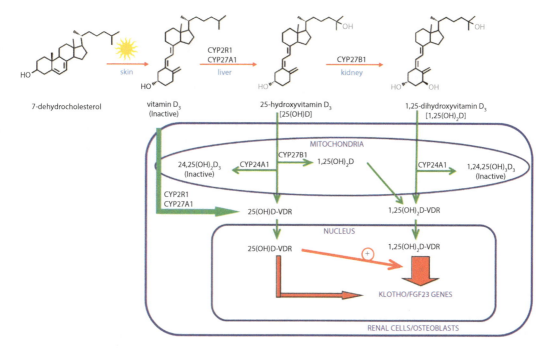

FIGURE 11.1 Vitamin D metabolism and VDR activation. Systemic vitamin D bioactivation to calcitriol [1,25(OH)$_2$D] and subcellular vitamin D bioactivation and degradation processes affecting the degree of transcriptional regulation by liganded VDR. Synergistic interactions between 25-hydroxy vitamin D [25(OH)D)] and calcitriol that enhance α-klotho and FGF23 gene transcription (From Bergada, L., J. Pallares, A. Maria Vittoria, A. Cardus, M. Santacana, J. Valls, G. Cao, E. Fernandez, X. Dolcet, A. S. Dusso, and X. Matias-Guiu, *Lab Invest.*, 94, 608–22, 2014. With permission.)

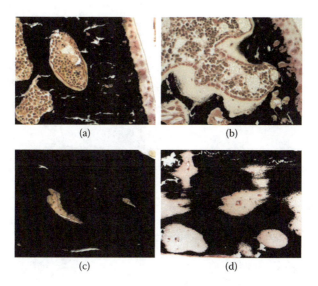

FIGURE 14.2 Von Kossa mineral stain of wild type control mice compared to HYP mice, a murine model of X-linked hypophosphatemia. (a) and (b): Control and HYP tibia, respectively showing articular cartilage and subchondral bone; (b), osteomalacia and defective zone of mineralized articular cartilage are evident. (c) and (d): Control and HYP cortical bone, respectively; (d), osteomalacia and the apparent cortical porosity of unmineralized osteoid.

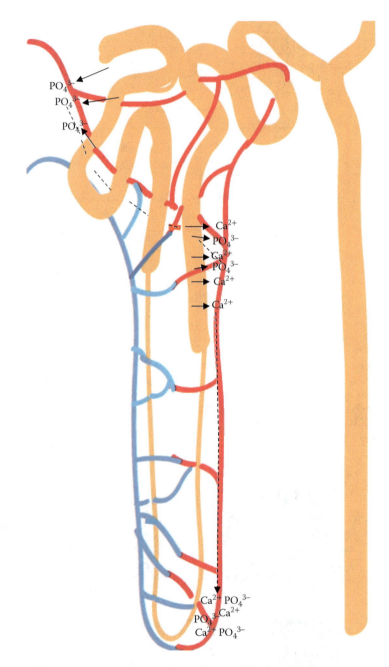

FIGURE 15.3 Reabsorption of calcium and phosphate in the proximal tubules and thick ascending loop of Henle, with possible intravascular transport of both ions to the papillary region. (Interpretation of data from Taylor, ER and ML Stoller, *Urolithiasis*, 43, 41–45, 2015; Blaine, J et al., *Clin J Am Soc Nephrol.*, 10, 1257–1272, 2014.)

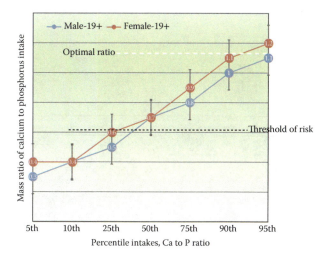

FIGURE 19.4 NHANES, 2009–2010: Distribution of daily individual Ca to P intake ratios across selected percentiles of intake for men and women ≥19 y. Daily individual calcium-to-phosphorus (Ca:P) mass intake ratios for men ($n = 2880$) and women ($n = 3038$) age ≥19 y across selected percentiles of intake from day-1 dietary intake estimates of NHANES 2009–2010. (Reproduced from Calvo MS, Moshfegh AJ, Tucker KL, *Adv Nutr.*, 5, 104–13, 2014. With permission.)

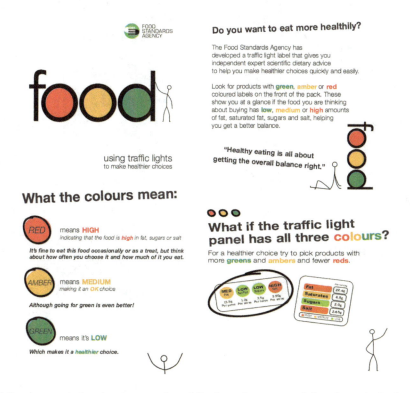

FIGURE 22.2 A suggested system to warn the public about the content of phosphorus in food.

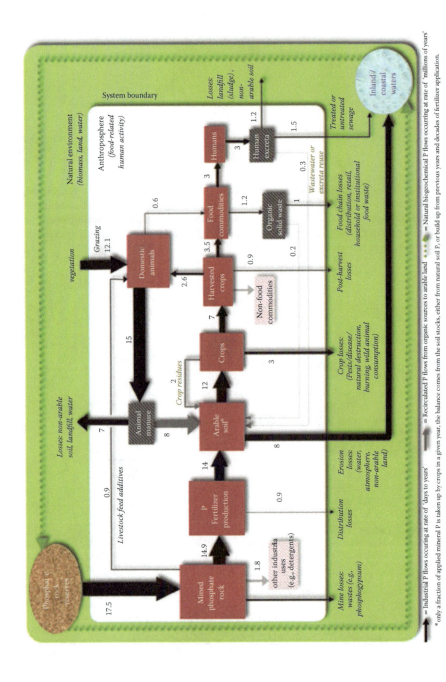

FIGURE 23.1 Global flows of phosphorus (P) among major food system components. Flows are in units of million metric tons (MT) of P and arrows are approximately proportional to the size of the flux. Grey arrows represent recycling fluxes. The dotted arrow represents the natural geological cycle that operates over millions of years. (From Cordell, D et al., *Glob. Environ. Chang.*, 19, 292–305, 2009.)

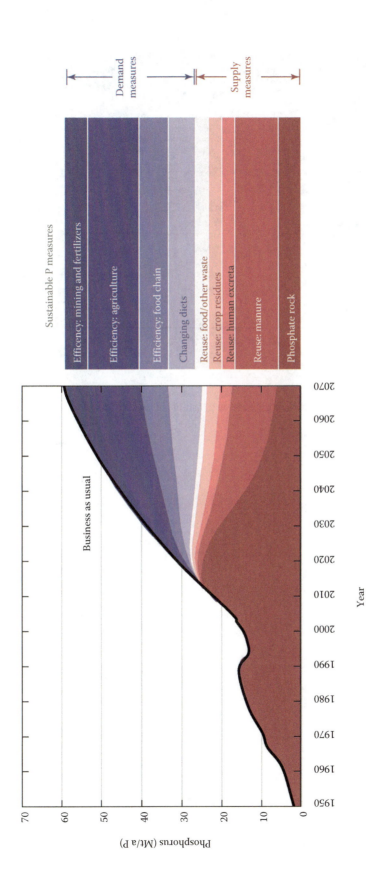

FIGURE 23.2 A scenario from Cordell and White (2014) for achieving long-term P sustainability in which the food system no longer relies on use of "fossil P" (phosphate rock) for fertilizer production. Note that the "business-as-usual" scenario would result in more than a doubling of global P use by ~2100, with enormous implications for water quality and access to P fertilizers. In this scenario, achieving P sustainability requires a combination of demand-side (diet shifts, food chain efficiency, improved farm practices) and supply-side (implementation of large-scale P recycling from organic waste streams) measures.

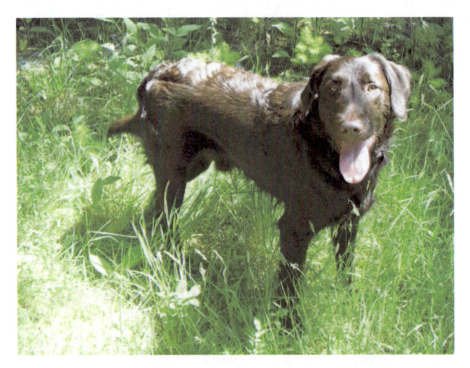

FIGURE 24.3 In the struggle for global phosphate sustainability, even family pets will have to contribute.

14 Overview of Phosphorus-Wasting Diseases and Need for Phosphorus Supplements

Carolyn M. Macica

CONTENTS

Abstract 185
Bullet Points 186
14.1   Introduction 186
14.2   Physiology of Phosphorous 186
14.3   Phosphate Homeostasis 187
14.4   Disturbances in Phosphorous Homeostasis 189
14.5   Hypophosphatemia and Overview of Phosphorus-Wasting Diseases 190
      14.5.1   X-Linked Hypophosphatemia 191
      14.5.2   Autosomal-Dominant Hypophosphatemic Rickets 192
      14.5.3   Tumor-Induced Osteomalacia 192
      14.5.4   Autosomal-Recessive Hypophosphatemia 193
14.6   Phosphate Salts in the Therapy of Persistent Urinary Phosphate Wasting 193
14.7   Adjunct Therapy of Phosphate Salts 193
14.8   Impact of Phosphate Replacement Therapy on Comorbid Features of
      Phosphate-Wasting Disorders 194
14.9   Management of Phosphate-Wasting Diseases During Periods of High Mineral Demand 195
14.10 Limitations of Current Combined Therapies: Calcification of Soft Tissues 196
14.11 Conclusions 196
References 197

ABSTRACT

Total body phosphorus is determined by net intestinal absorption and the amount of phosphate excreted by the kidneys, which are equal under steady-state conditions. A typical Western diet includes high-protein foods such as meat and dairy products that are abundant in elemental phosphorus; thus, dietary hypophosphatemia is rare. An increased consumption of processed foods, especially those including phosphoric acid as an additive, contributes to the daily dietary load of exogenous phosphorus absorbed in the intestine. Despite these variations, in the setting of uncompromised renal function, balance is maintained by excretion of excess phosphate by the kidneys.

However, acute or chronic hypophosphatemia can occur as a consequence of decreased intestinal absorption, redistribution of phosphate from extracellular into intracellular compartments, or renal phosphate-wasting disorders. Metabolic disturbances account for most cases of acute, and potentially severe, hypophosphatemia. Hereditary and acquired diseases of excess renal phosphate wasting and depletion of total phosphorus stores account for the majority of chronic cases of moderate hypophosphatemia. The clinical presentation of familial disorders includes phosphaturia, bone and muscle pain, diminished growth, and defective skeletal and articular mineralization. Oral phosphorus agents are used in the management of these disorders.

BULLET POINTS

- Phosphate homeostasis is regulated over a wide dietary range through an integrated hormonal system, with 85% of total body phosphate stored in bone as hydroxyapatite.
- Phosphatonins represent a relatively recently described class of humoral mediators of phosphorus homeostasis that also include FGF23, a circulating hormone produced in bone that has an overall negative effect on phosphorus homeostasis.
- Alterations in phosphate homeostasis may be related to metabolic disturbances or genetic mutations that affect the handling of phosphate in the kidney or gut.
- Characterization of familial phosphate-wasting disorders has provided valuable insight into phosphate homeostasis and its impact on mineralized tissues over the lifespan.
- Phosphate salts are an essential therapy for acute hypophosphatemia and are used in conjunction with calcitriol in the management of familial phosphate-wasting disorders. Nonetheless, significant deficits in bone integrity as well as debilitating comorbidities may be better managed using newer therapies targeting the actions of phosphatonins.

14.1 INTRODUCTION

The primary focus of this review is an overview of the etiology of hereditary phosphate-wasting disorders and the therapeutic use of high and frequent doses of oral phosphate salts. Generally speaking, disruption of normal phosphate homeostasis arises as a consequence of an intrinsic defect in the renal handling of phosphate, or of factors that regulate renal phosphate excretion. Of the latter, fibroblast growth factor-23 (FGF23), a circulating phosphaturic hormone, has been implicated in several familial disorders. A brief review of phosphate homeostasis and its regulation will be followed by an overview of causes of hypophosphatemia, its impact during periods of high mineral demand, and finally, the efficacy and adverse effects associated with use of phosphate salts as replacement therapy.

14.2 PHYSIOLOGY OF PHOSPHOROUS

At physiological pH, phosphorus exists in the body predominantly as two inorganic phosphate anions, monohydrogenphosphate (HPO_4^{-2}) or its conjugate acid dihydrogenphosphate ($H_2PO_4^{-1}$), collectively abbreviated Pi by convention. In serum, ionizable inorganic phosphate (or in cationic complex with calcium, sodium, or magnesium) makes up a majority of the species with the remaining 10% to 15% bound to serum albumin. The normal range of total inorganic fasting serum phosphate in adults is 3 to 4.5 mg/dL (1.8–2.3 mmol/L) and is subject to endocrine regulation. Serum phosphate is also subject to diurnal variation and is higher in infants and children. Phosphate excretion gradually increases with age, with serum levels ranging from 4.5 to 7.5 mg/dL in infancy (1.45–2.42 mmol/L) to 4 to 6.5 mg/dL (2.3–3.8 mEq/L) in children. This is especially relevant in the diagnosis of familial phosphate-wasting disorders that can be unintentionally missed if age-appropriate serum concentrations are not considered along with elevated alkaline phosphatase activity (Carpenter et al. 2011).

Phosphate is a critical constituent of membrane phospholipids and of several macromolecules including high-energy phosphate bonds of nucleoside triphosphates, phosphodiester bonds of nucleic acids, and erythrocyte 2,3 diphosphoglycerate (2,3-DPG) that facilitates the release of oxygen from hemoglobin. It also plays a role in kinase-dependent modulation of proteins and in cell-signaling pathways involved in growth, differentiation, and the cell cycle. In addition, phosphate plays an important role in maintaining acid–base homeostasis, with the excreted fraction of phosphate serving as a urinary buffer for H^+ in response to a dietary acid load (Koeppen and Stanton 2012).

Although phosphate is the most abundant intracellular anion serum phosphate represents a small fraction of total body phosphorous. A majority is found in physiologically mineralized tissues, including bone, teeth (dentin, enamel, and cementum), articular cartilage, and the fibrocartilaginous

Overview of Phosphorus-Wasting Diseases and Need for Phosphorus Supplements

tendon and ligament insertion sites (entheses), existing as a complex of predominantly calcium and inorganic phosphate that forms crystalline hydroxyapatite with the formula $[(Ca)_5(PO_4)_3(OH)]$. The organic phase of mineralized tissues is dominated by type I collagen in bone and teeth (dentin and cementum) and type II collagen in cartilaginous tissues, which serves as a scaffold for the production of hydroxyapatite. Mineralization of these tissues imparts material properties consistent with their function as providing structural support for the body and serving as transitional tissues subject to high mechanical forces.

Demand for calcium and phosphorus is highest with increasing bone mass during childhood and adolescence. During this period, a positive phosphate balance is established with a majority of bone mass accrued by 18 years in females and 20 years in males. The endochondral growth plate is also sensitive to phosphate levels. Endochondral bone growth occurs at the growth plate in the long bones of the axial and appendicular skeleton. The epiphyseal growth plate can be viewed as a snapshot of type II collagen–producing chondrocytes progressing through a differentiation program regulated by local autocrine factors (Broadus et al. 2007). The cells progress from resting to proliferating chondrocytes that form columns of chondrocytes along the long axis of the bone to prehypertrophic chondrocytes. Finally, terminally differentiated chondrocytes undergo hypertrophy, resulting in a significant increase in cell volume. Hypertrophic chondrocytes secrete matrix vesicles, which serve as a nidus for the first crystals of hydroxyapatite. This supports provisional calcification and serves as a template for osteoblastic ossification. Consistent with this physiological role, hypertrophic chondrocytes now express high alkaline phosphatase activity and type X collagen (Anderson et al. 2005). The epiphyseal growth plate size remains constant as long as cartilage proliferation keeps pace with the rate of bone formation. Disruption of this program in a hypophosphatemic environment manifests itself as a rachitic or expanded growth plate, the result of hypertrophic chondrocyte accumulation. The failure to undergo programmed cell death results in defective long bone growth and short stature. The growth plate is specifically sensitive to levels of phosphate due its role in phosphate-sensitive caspase C that initiates the apoptotic events of the hypertrophic chondrocyte (Sabbagh et al. 2005).

14.3 PHOSPHATE HOMEOSTASIS

The regulation of total body phosphorus involves multiple organs and endocrine feedback loops (Figure 14.1). In the gut, a majority of ingested phosphate following a meal is absorbed in the small intestine by passive paracellular diffusion with the remaining excreted in the feces. The percentage of paracellular diffusion is proportionate to the ingested phosphate load, although the net amount of phosphate absorbed in the gut can be altered by a transport-dependent process via the NaPi-IIb cotransporter or by medications that decrease ionized phosphate such as calcium, aluminum, or magnesium-containing antacids; phosphate binders; or calcium supplements. Adjustment to rising serum phosphate levels occurs at the level of the kidney by altering phosphate excretion. Alternatively, when serum phosphate levels decrease, mitochondrial 1-alpha hydroxylase activity is stimulated in the renal proximal tubule, thereby increasing the synthesis of $1,25(OH)_2D$ (calcitriol). Calcitriol increases intestinal phosphate absorption via the apical membrane NaPi-IIb cotransporter in the small intestine. There is also a reduction in urinary phosphate excretion, so that the fine-tuning of serum phosphate again occurs at the level of the kidney (Bindels et al. 2012).

Ionized, unbound phosphate is freely filtered by the kidney and primarily reabsorbed in the proximal renal tubule via the NaPi-IIa and NaPi-IIc cotransporters using the favorable sodium gradient to drive phosphate reabsorption across the apical membrane. NaPi-IIa transports sodium and phosphate at a ratio of 3:1 and carries positive charge into the cell, and NaPi-IIc transports sodium and phosphate at a ratio of 2:1 and is electrically neutral. The *SLC34A1* and *SCL34A3* genes encode the phosphate cotransporters, respectively. The NaPi-IIa cotransporter is responsive to acute changes in dietary phosphate and is under hormonal control. However, the identification of a heritable form

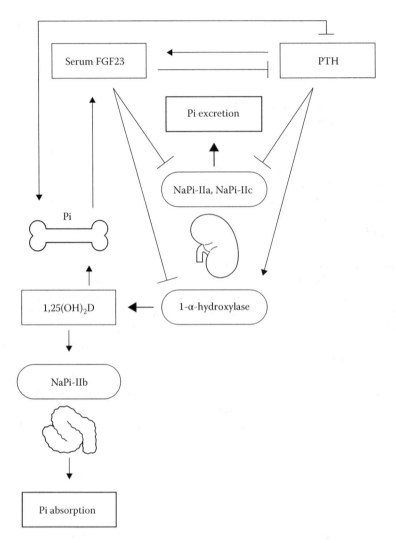

FIGURE 14.1 Phosphorus homeostasis in health.

of hypophosphatemia that arises from a mutation in the *SLC34A3* gene underscores the relative contribution of this transporter in phosphate homeostasis (Bergwitz et al. 2006). Renal tubular Pi cotransporters, like Na-glucose cotransporters, are saturable and exhibit a transfer maximum (T_m) when presented with a high filtered phosphate load.

As the major regulatory organ of phosphate homeostasis, the kidney is responsive to dietary intake and a number of hormones that directly modulate phosphate excretion. Renal NaPi cotransporters are subject to negative regulation primarily by the phosphaturic actions of both PTH and FGF23 in response to changes in phosphate levels, effectively adapting to rises or falls in serum phosphate. Secreted PTH is the major regulator of acute changes in serum calcium, with ionized calcium acting as a rapid-response ligand of the calcium-sensing receptor (CSR) of the parathyroid chief cells to restore calcium levels (Koeppen and Stanton 2012). PTH also acts to mobilize calcium from the skeleton indirectly by regulating RANKL expression to stimulate osteoclast activity. Following a postprandial rapid rise in serum Pi and decrease in serum ionized calcium, PTH is secreted and acts via its adenylyl cyclase-coupled GPCR to stimulate the endocytotic removal and lysosomal degradation of the sodium phosphate transporter to enhance urinary Pi excretion. This mechanism also ensures that phosphate levels, also released during bone resorption, are not disproportionately

Overview of Phosphorus-Wasting Diseases and Need for Phosphorus Supplements **189**

elevated in the restoration of serum calcium levels. In addition to fluxes in ionized calcium, a direct effect of phosphate on PTH secretion has been suggested (Bindels et al. 2012).

PTH-independent phosphaturia is mediated by phosphatonins, including secreted frizzled related protein-4 (sFRP-4), matrix extracellular phosphoglycoprotein (MEPE), and the circulating hormone FGF23, first identified as a phosphatonin responsible for the phosphate wasting of autosomal-dominant hypophosphatemic rickets (Consortium 2000). FGF23 inhibits the renal NaPi cotransporters to decrease phosphate reabsorption and increase phosphate excretion (Gattineni et al. 2009). Response by FGF23 to changes in serum phosphate has a much slower temporal profile than does PTH, and recent evidence suggests that unlike PTH, the action of FGF23 on the kidney occurs indirectly via changes in FGF receptor coupling (Bourgeois et al. 2013).

Although the tyrosine kinase receptors for FGF23 have been identified as FGFR1, FGFR2c, and FGFR3, specificity of the receptor-mediated effects is achieved by the restricted pattern of its coreceptor klotho, including its expression in the renal tubule (Yu et al. 2005; Urakawa et al. 2006). However, klotho expression is restricted to the distal convoluted tubule (DCT), which is spatially distinct from proximal tubular NaPi-IIa and NaPi-IIc expression. A potential feedback mechanism by FGF23 acting via FGFR1/klotho in the DCT and mediated by p-ERK1/2 signaling to the proximal tubule has been proposed to explain the disparity between klotho expression and altered transport in the proximal tubule (Farrow et al. 2009). FGF23 also inhibits 1-α-hydroxylase and the synthesis of 1,25(OH)$_2$D to decrease intestinal phosphate absorption, an important contributor to the enhanced loss of phosphate in FGF23-mediated disorders (Saito et al. 2003).

14.4 DISTURBANCES IN PHOSPHOROUS HOMEOSTASIS

Given the critical role of phosphorus, severe acute hypophosphatemia or moderate chronic hypophosphatemia can affect multiple cellular functions (Smogorzewski et al. 2012). However, most cases of hypophosphatemia are rate limiting once the underlying cause is treated (i.e., the hypophosphatemia resolves). To determine the underlying etiology of hypophosphatemia, urine phosphate is measured and will reflect the origin as being due to (1) limited intestinal absorption or excess gastrointestinal loss, (2) shifts of phosphate into intracellular compartments, or (3) increased urinary phosphate excretion. This is used to discriminate between hypophosphatemia without an increase in urine phosphate and hypophosphatemia with an increase in urine phosphate (phosphaturia).

Compromised intestinal absorption or losses can result in a negative phosphate balance. Limited intestinal absorption of phosphate can arise from overuse of chelating antacids, phosphate binders, or vitamin D deficiency. Increased intestinal loss due to chronic diarrhea or malabsorption syndromes may result in hypophosphatemia. In both cases, normal intestinal phosphate transport can be resolved if the underlying disorder is addressed. Redistribution of phosphate into the intracellular space can occur with insulin therapy, especially in the setting of phosphate depletion associated with diabetic ketoacidosis, and in response to respiratory alkalosis. Respiratory alkalosis results in the rapid redistribution of extracellular phosphate into the intracellular space. Alcohol withdrawal in alcoholic patients can also result in severe hypophosphatemia, with the mechanism likely being multifactorial, involving both intestinal and renal abnormalities. Severe hypophosphatemia (<1 mg/dL, 0.32 mmol/L) is symptomatic and results in decreased intracellular levels of ATP and availability of oxygen to the tissues, secondary to 2,3-DPG depletion. Many of the coincident cardiopulmonary, hematologic, endocrine, neuromuscular, and central nervous system (CNS) effects of hypophosphatemia can be attributed to the latter and requires urgent correction with oral phosphate (intravenous phosphate is used only in cases when the patient is not ambulatory) (Geerse et al. 2010).

Alternatively, increased urinary phosphate excretion and moderate hypophosphatemia (1.0–2.5 mg/dL [0.32–0.80 mmol/L]) can be caused by elevated levels of the phosphaturic hormones or by defects in renal NaPi-II cotransporters. Phosphaturia can also occur with either primary or secondary hyperparathyroidism. As a phosphaturic hormone, elevation of PTH secretion can produce hypophosphatemia by decreasing the abundance of the NaPi cotransporters in the apical membrane of renal proximal tubule cells. This occurs in primary hyperparathyroidism and is generally mild and resolved upon parathyroidectomy. Secondary hyperparathyroidism occurs due to calcium or 1,25(OH)$_2$D deficiency, both of which stimulate PTH and result in NaPi cotransporter-mediated phosphaturia, both directly and indirectly, via increased FGF23. Endocytotic removal of the NaPi-IIc protein in response to PTH treatment has been shown to be delayed relative to NaPi-IIa, suggesting differences in the temporal response by PTH in the regulation of phosphate (Leblanc et al. 2011). A deficiency of 1,25(OH)$_2$D also contributes to hypophosphatemia due to diminished intestinal reabsorption. Administration of vitamin D supplements in the setting of 1,25(OH)$_2$D deficiency can normalize PTH levels and calcium status as well as potentiate intestinal absorption of phosphate.

Increased urinary phosphate excretion may also involve either an effect on tubular transporters or impairment of proximal phosphate transport. Two syndromes include mutations that affect proximal tubular NaPi cotransporters. Hereditary hypophosphatemic rickets with hypercalciuria (HHRH) results from a homozygous loss-of-function mutation in the *SLC34A3* gene encoding the NaPi-IIc protein, and transmission is autosomal recessive. Identification of the mutation also established a role for this renal phosphate transporter that was previously thought to be minimal relative to the NaPi-IIa protein (Tenenhouse et al. 2003; Bergwitz et al. 2006). Calcitriol levels are appropriately elevated in HHRH given the state of hypophosphatemia (Tieder et al. 1985). Consequently, intestinal calcium absorption is high, resulting in hypercalciuria with potential for nephrolithiasis and nephrocalcinosis. Thus, treatment with phosphate salts, but without the activated vitamin D metabolite calcitriol to minimize further hypercalciuria, is a standard therapy.

Disordered NaPi-IIa-mediated phosphate transport can alternatively occur due to a mutation that indirectly affects the regulation of the cotransporter by PTH. The predominant form of Dent disease, a rare X-linked recessive disease with approximately 250 known cases, results from an X-linked recessive mutation in the *CLCN5* gene (chloride channel, voltage-sensitive 5) encoding an endosomal H$^+$/Cl$^-$ exchanger localized to the renal proximal tubule (Fisher et al. 1995). The channel is important in maintaining the acidic endosome environment. The disorder manifests itself with proteinuria, hypophosphatemia, phosphaturia, hypercalciuria and nephrocalcinosis, and nephrolithiasis. Endosomal uptake of proteins, including PTH, is disrupted. Increased delivery of PTH to the late proximal tubule stimulates the PTH receptor to inhibit phosphate reabsorption by the NaPi-IIa transporter, resulting in phosphaturia. Hypercalciuria presumably results from PTH-mediated activation of 1α-hydroxylase and an increase in 1,25(OH)$_2$D and stimulation of intestinal calcium absorption. Therapy of Dent's disease is primarily supportive, and presentation of rickets and osteomalacia can be treated with phosphate salts and calcitriol. Calcitriol should be carefully titrated to minimize exacerbation of the already high risk of hypercalciuria (Carpenter et al. 2011).

14.5 HYPOPHOSPHATEMIA AND OVERVIEW OF PHOSPHORUS-WASTING DISEASES

Unlike the PTH-mediated phosphaturia of primary and secondary hyperparathyroidism, FGF23-mediated hypophosphatemia predominantly occurs due to mutations that alter levels of the circulating hormone. Several acquired and inherited hypophosphatemic disorders have been associated with excess FGF23. X-linked hypophosphatemia (XLH) is the most prevalent form of the familial phosphate-wasting disorders; thus, most clinical data of the etiology and presentation of these disorders as a group have been derived from this patient population (Holm et al. 2003). In addition to XLH, a number of phosphate-wasting disorders involve elevated levels of bioactive FGF23, including tumor-induced osteomalacia (TIO), autosomal-dominant hypophosphatemic rickets (ADHR), and autosomal-recessive hypophosphatemic rickets (ARHR) (Yu and White 2005).

14.5.1 X-Linked Hypophosphatemia

X-Linked hypophosphatemia (XLH) is the most common form of heritable hypophosphatemia, affecting approximately 1 in 20,000 (Carpenter 1997). XLH is transmitted in an X-linked–dominant inheritance pattern, and although penetrance is thought to be 100%, the severity of clinical symptoms can vary considerably (Sabbagh et al. 2015). It is currently unknown if other genetic, environmental, and lifestyle factors affect the patient phenotype. In XLH, hypophosphatemia results from elevation of the bone-derived hormone, FGF23. A murine model of XLH, the HYP (hypophosphatemic) mouse, as well as mice genetically modified to inactivate or overexpress FGF23, have proven invaluable in illuminating the physiological role of FGF23 as an important regulator of phosphate homeostasis and of bone as an endocrine organ (Figure 14.2). FGF23 is expressed in osteocytes and osteoblasts and accesses the plasma as a circulating hormone. It was identified as a phosphatonin that acts via the renal FGFR1/alpha-klotho receptor to regulate phosphate reabsorption and the synthesis of biologically active $1,25(OH)_2D$.

XLH arises as a result of a mutation in the *PHEX* (phosphate-regulating gene with homologies to endopeptidases on the X chromosome) gene sequence and subsequent inactivity of the PHEX protein. The X-linked dominant pattern of inheritance is due to PHEX haploinsufficiency and thus only requires inactivation of one allele for full expression on the disorder (Wang et al. 1999). Consistent with this finding is the similarity in the severity of the disease between males and females and the finding that gene dosage (one or two mutant alleles) has similar abnormalities in mineral homeostasis (Ichikawa et al. 2013). Inactivation of PHEX results in elevated circulating levels of both bioactive FGF23 and an inactive C-terminal FGF23 fragment by a mechanism not yet understood. As a consequence of this mutation, patients with XLH are unable to effectively reabsorb the filtered tubular load of phosphate.

Aberrant regulation of vitamin D production also occurs due to elevated FGF23 levels and leading to impaired intestinal calcium and phosphate absorption. It is this abnormality in the biosynthesis of $1,25(OH)_2D$ that underlies the use of the term "inappropriately low" vitamin D in the context of hereditary hypophosphatemia because the normal physiological response to hypophosphatemia should be induction of $1,25(OH)_2D$ activity to facilitate intestinal phosphate reabsorption to re-establish serum levels.

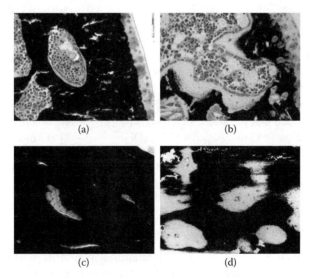

FIGURE 14.2 (See color insert.) Von Kossa mineral stain of wild type control mice compared to HYP mice, a murine model of X-linked hypophosphatemia. (a) and (b): Control and HYP tibia, respectively showing articular cartilage and subchondral bone; (b), osteomalacia and defective zone of mineralized articular cartilage are evident. (c) and (d): Control and HYP cortical bone, respectively; (d), osteomalacia and the apparent cortical porosity of unmineralized osteoid.

The typical clinical presentation of XLH in children includes radiographical evidence of rickets, lower leg deformities (varus or valgus deformity), and internal tibial torsion with in-toeing, dental abscesses without caries, and short stature. Patients may also present with craniosynostosis with craniofacial deformities, including frontal bossing and symptoms of vertigo and hearing impairment. The adult disorder is dominated by persistent osteomalacia and bone and joint pain, degenerative osteoarthritis and osteophytes (bone spurs at the margins of the joint) and a pervasive mineralizing enthesopathy affecting numerous fibrocartilaginous entheses (tendon/ligament insertion sites) (Liang et al. 2009, 2011). There is also a lack of resolution of dental abscess, abscesses or hearing impairment, if involved. Current treatment consists of oral phosphate salts and calcitriol that improve, but do not resolve, the abnormalities in children (Carpenter et al. 2011). The impact of replacement therapy on the clinical management of the childhood versus adult disorder is discussed in Section 14.7 and should be considered separately as the clinical goals are *not* identical.

14.5.2 Autosomal-Dominant Hypophosphatemic Rickets

ADHR has an indistinguishable biochemical and radiographical presentation from XLH, consistent with the identification of a missense mutation at an $_{176}RXXR_{179}/S_{180}$ cleavage site involved in the processing of FGF23 (Consortium 2000). Termination of the phosphaturic activity of FGF23 activity is mediated by proteolytic cleavage of the hormone at this site, and disruption gives rise to ADHR. Variability in the onset and symptoms of the disorder between affected individuals is one of the factors that distinguish ADHR from XLH. Some patients display varying levels of intact FGF23, mirrored in the hypophosphatemia and associated clinical symptoms of these patients that, in some cases, spontaneously resolve. In experiments involving ADHR patients and a mouse model of ADHR, a possible explanation for this variability has been proposed to involve the positive modulation of FGF23 synthesis and secretion as an inverse function of iron status. In unaffected controls without a cleavage defect, low serum iron likewise stimulates FGF23 production but is offset by an increase in the proteolytic cleavage of FGF23 to the inactive C-terminal fragment (Imel et al. 2011; Farrow et al. 2011).

Within the spectrum of the comorbidities of phosphate-wasting disorders, the enthesopathy is particularly challenging to manage given the lack of understanding of the pathophysiology in this setting. The enthesis, or tendon/ligament insertion site, serves to function as a transitional tissue between the tendon and bone and is subject to pathological processes, the most common enthesopathy being mineralization of the insertion site, commonly known as an enthesophyte or bone spur. The enthesis is a structurally continuous tissue that transitions from the tendon to calcified bone. The enthesis exhibits gradients in tissue organization classified into four distinct zones with varying cellular compositions, mechanical properties, and functions in order to facilitate joint movement. As discussed later, patients with ADHR also develop mineralizing enthesophytes (Karaplis et al. 2012). Data showing the same phenotypic changes in the entheses of XLH mice and a mouse model overexpressing FGF23 suggest that FGF23 is a common etiological factor in the progression of this paradoxical bony disorder (Karaplis et al. 2012; Liang et al. 2009).

14.5.3 Tumor-Induced Osteomalacia

Tumor-induced osteomalacia (TIO) is a rare, nonfamilial phosphate-wasting disease, with the causative factor being ectopic tumor–derived FGF23 production (Kumar 2000). Once the tumor is identified and removed, serum chemistries return to normal. However, the origin of the causative tumor is sometimes obscure or may not be amenable to surgical resection, and so it is included in disorders managed with phosphate salts. The tumors are predominantly benign and of mesenchymal origin with a morphologically distinct phenotype described as a phosphaturic mesenchymal tumor, mixed connective tissue variant (Weidner and Santa Cruz 1987). The resultant mineral disorder and

Overview of Phosphorus-Wasting Diseases and Need for Phosphorus Supplements 193

clinical presentation of TIO is similar to XLH and it is managed as such. Pediatric patients present with hypophosphatemia and phosphaturia and inappropriately low $1,25(OH)_2D_3$ levels, rickets, bowing of lower limbs, and diminished growth. Because it is not a common disorder, perhaps the biggest challenge of TIO in adults is its inclusion in the differential diagnosis as it may present with bone symptoms of generalized pain and weakness.

14.5.4 AUTOSOMAL-RECESSIVE HYPOPHOSPHATEMIA

ARHR is a rare phosphate-wasting disorder that has been described in patients with a mutation in the human dentin matrix acidic phosphoprotein 1 gene (*DMP1*) (Lorenz-Depiereux et al. 2006; Feng et al. 2006). Elevated FGF23 levels characterize ARHR, although the mechanism is unknown. The *DMP1* gene product is an extracellular noncollagenous matrix protein with multiple acidic and phosphorylation domains and an integrin-binding RGD sequence. DMP1 belongs to the small, integrin-binding, ligand N-linked glycoprotein (SIBLING) family and is expressed in dentin and bone, where it is localized to osteocytes and osteoblasts. Patients exhibit elevated levels of FGF23, which is responsible for the observed phosphaturia. DMP1 knock-out mice are phenotypically similar to HYP mice. The Dmp1 protein itself may also contribute to the phenotype of ARHR. Dmp1 plays a putative role in mechanical sensing as well as in the development of osteoblasts into terminally differentiated osteocytes. It is also phosphorylated and transported to the extracellular matrix where it regulates mineralization.

14.6 PHOSPHATE SALTS IN THE THERAPY OF PERSISTENT URINARY PHOSPHATE WASTING

Due to a common etiology involving FGF23 in phosphate-wasting disorders, much of the discussion on the use of phosphate salts and adjunct therapies will be presented in the context of XLH. A common feature of these disorders is the use of relatively high doses of inorganic phosphate salts in the management of the disorder, supplied as the sodium or potassium salt of phosphate, in three to five divided doses per day (Carpenter et al. 2011). Hypophosphatemia due to persistent urinary phosphate wasting is more of a therapeutic challenge because the underlying disorder is frequently familial, and raising the serum phosphate concentration with phosphate supplements will result in a further increase in phosphate excretion that minimizes the elevation in serum phosphate. The rachitic growth plate of children with XLH and HYP mice is sensitive to oral phosphate salts, the result of increased Pi absorption in the gut, even in the face of an increase in the fractional excretion of Pi (Glorieux et al. 1978; Marie et al. 1981).

Therapy also improves bone pain and bone turnover, as indicated by an increase in both osteoblast and osteoclast activity and lowering of serum alkaline phosphatase. The impact on bone cells is multifaceted. In the untreated environment, elevated serum alkaline phosphatase activity is a hallmark of these disorders and may be reflective of sustained osteoblast and chondrocyte activity, which continue to synthesize and secrete matrix but fail to adequately mineralize the matrix in the hypophosphatemic environment (Liang et al. 2011; Marie et al. 1981). Osteoclast number and activity are diminished, presumably due to reduced mineralized surfaces available for remodeling. Improved, but not normalized, serum alkaline phosphatase activity suggests new bone formation once replacement therapy is initiated. Nonetheless, despite improved growth, osteomalacia persists throughout adulthood (Marie et al. 1981).

14.7 ADJUNCT THERAPY OF PHOSPHATE SALTS

The concomitant use of calcitriol, or analogs of calcitriol, along with oral phosphate salts is also indicated in the therapy of familial hypophosphatemia and is available in solution, tablet, or capsule forms (Carpenter et al. 2011). Calcitriol facilitates the absorption of intestinal phosphate and calcium, improves bone mineralization, and prevents the hypocalcemia that can result with phosphate therapy. Unopposed supplementation with phosphate salts can precipitate secondary hyperparathyroidism with parathyroid hyperplasia due to a decrease in serum ionized calcium (Portale et al. 1984) and to the suppression of $1,25(OH)_2D$ biosynthesis (Slatopolsky et al. 1996), both negative regulators of PTH secretion. Untreated HYP mice have elevated PTH, and untreated patients are either in the normal or higher range of PTH levels (Carpenter et al. 1996). Thus, the addition of $1,25 (OH)_2D$ serves to suppress the secretion of PTH in an endocrine feedback loop. In addition to offsetting secondary hyperparathyroidism, linear growth has been shown to be more responsive to combined therapy (Glorieux and Scriver 1972). Yet another factor in the precipitation of sustained hyperparathyroidism in the therapeutic use of phosphate is phosphorus itself. In situ hybridization showed that hypophosphatemia decreases PTH mRNA in parathyroid cells, whereas a high-phosphate diet stimulates PTH synthesis (Wu et al. 2000). These and other findings await elucidation of the mechanism(s) by which a putative phosphate sensor can modulate gene expression and protein biosynthesis (Kilav et al. 1995). Recent studies conducted in *Drosophila* have increased the understanding of cellular responses to phosphate by phosphate response elements (PRE) involved in a number of cellular processes (Bergwitz et al. 2013). Identification of a phosphate response element of the murine gene that encodes NaPi-IIa further supports the role of Pi as a primary signaling molecule (Kido et al. 1999).

Calcimimetic agents that act at the Ca^{++}-sensing receptor to reduce PTH secretion secondary to hyperplasia represent a novel therapeutic approach to secondary hyperparathyroidism, and reports of their efficacy in XLH, although sparse, suggest that they may serve as an effective adjunct therapy (Alon et al. 2008; Grove-Laugesen and Rejnmark 2014).

Finally, and of significant importance in the management of these patients, both phosphate supplements and calcitriol stimulate the production of FGF23, setting the stage for a vicious cycle of dysregulated phosphate homeostasis (Imel et al. 2010). This underscores the need for better therapies, including newer biologics like a recombinant FGF23 monoclonal antibody that displays efficacy in a murine model of XLH with normalization of serum phosphate and $1,25(OH)_2D$ levels and improved TmP/GFR in patients in a randomized study (Carpenter et al. 2014; Yamazaki et al. 2008).

14.8 IMPACT OF PHOSPHATE REPLACEMENT THERAPY ON COMORBID FEATURES OF PHOSPHATE-WASTING DISORDERS

Although randomized, controlled studies on patients have not been conducted to assess the impact of the disorder on joints, the combined use of phosphate and calcitriol has been shown to restore the normal architecture of the synovial joint in a murine model of phosphate wasting (Liang et al. 2011). This is important because degenerative osteoarthritis, osteophytes, and joint pain are significant comorbidities of XLH, characterized by thinning of articular joints and subchondral sclerosis (Hardy et al. 1989; Reid et al. 1989).

Histological and EPIC (equilibrium partitioning of an ionic contrast)-microCT analyses to obtain quantitative and high-resolution three-dimensional images from HYP mice reveals an absence of a mineralized zone of articular cartilage as well as significant changes in noncollagenous proteins. In addition, significant thinning of cartilage is evident in adult untreated HYP mice. The zone of mineralized cartilage serves as a transitional tissue that reduces mechanical stress at the interface between cartilage and subchondral bone, having material properties of both cartilage and bone. Loss of this zone in the hypophosphatemic environment affects the entire zonal arrangement of the articular surface as well as its function in resisting compressive forces (Figure 14.2).

A dramatic recovery of mineralization and of noncollagenous proteins following treatment suggests that phosphate is a key regulator of chondrocyte mineralization and that mineralization fails to occur in the hypophosphatemic environment. Because articular chondrocytes are terminally differentiated cells, they are programmed to continually synthesize and secrete matrix proteins for the

Overview of Phosphorus-Wasting Diseases and Need for Phosphorus Supplements 195

life of the cell. Thus, it is possible that discontinuation of therapy, as variably occurs following the epiphyseal closure, removes an important stimulus in the maintenance of the extracellular matrix that may predispose patients to degenerative osteoarthritis (Liang et al. 2011).

An additional benefit to replacement therapy is in the management of the multiple dental abscesses that arise in this patient population. Abscesses without caries ranks as one of the more significant quality-of-life issues, with hypophosphatemia affecting the quality and integrity of the enamel and dentin and cementum (Cremonesi et al. 2014).

14.9 MANAGEMENT OF PHOSPHATE-WASTING DISEASES DURING PERIODS OF HIGH MINERAL DEMAND

Periods of high mineral demand present a unique challenge to patient management in mineral-wasting disorders. One of the most recognized periods of high mineral demand occurs during puberty and long bone growth. Increased intestinal absorption and decreased urinary losses normally establish a positive phosphate balance during this period to support rapid growth. Pediatric patients with phosphate-wasting disorders are unable to achieve these adjustments to ensure normal growth and mineralization. Consequently, the pediatric disorder has received much attention to ensure improved growth, to correct varus or valgus alignment, and to reduce the severity of the bone disease. This includes both pharmacologic and surgical interventions.

Management of the adult disorder is variable and inconsistent (Carpenter et al. 2011). In addition, attention to adult management during periods of high mineral demand has been relatively neglected. Pregnancy and lactation represent unique maternal demands to meet the needs of the developing fetal skeleton, especially during the latter period of pregnancy in which the accretion of mineral is at its highest and during lactation in which the maternal skeleton is the primary contributor of calcium and phosphorus. No studies have evaluated the use of phosphate and calcitriol in pregnant women who have XLH. Generally, therapy is maintained if the patient is already receiving therapy and monitored for hypercalciuria. Alternatively, therapy is not initiated if the patient is not being treated at the time of conception (Ruppe 1993).

There are no current recommendations for women who are considering breastfeeding. During pregnancy, maternal adaptations to high mineral demand include more than doubling intestinal calcium absorption by increasing $1,25 (OH)_2D$ production, normally impaired in states of elevated FGF23. In addition, the greatest loss of mineral during lactation occurs from the trabecular skeleton, especially from the trabecular-rich spine (Hayslip et al. 1989; Kent et al. 1990). However, the mechanism for bone resorption in an already hypophosphatemic skeleton with low trabecular bone volume and diminished osteoclast activity is unclear.

Recent studies were performed in HYP mice in order to examine the endocrine response to pregnancy and lactation in mature cortical bone, which represents the highest density of mineral in HYP mice (Macica et al. 2016). It was hypothesized that mineral demand is met by utilizing intracortical mineral reserves as an alternative mechanism of bone resorption that either creates new mineralized surfaces available for resorption by osteoclasts or frees up matrix mineral independently of osteoclasts. Indeed, using high-resolution micro-CT a significant increase in intracortical porosity during pregnancy and lactation was observed. In addition, a significant increase in a type I collagen proteinase (MMP-13) and in the number of osteoclasts was observed, suggesting that the cortical bone acts as a mineral reserve during this period. There were also surprisingly similar changes in maternal serum biochemistries between HYP and control unaffected mice revealing the same pattern in the upregulation of $1,25(OH)_2D$ production with concomitant increases in serum calcium and phosphate (to a level within the normal range). PTH also fell to the lower end of the normal range (Cross et al. 1995; Dahlman et al. 1994; Gallacher et al. 1994; Rasmussen et al. 1990), potentially protecting the maternal skeleton from excessive bone resorption and indicating that PTH is not the source driving the increase in $1,25(OH)_2D$ (Turner et al. 1988). Instead, other regulators of 1α-hydroxylase must account for most of the circulating 1,25(OH)$_2$D during pregnancy (Singh et al. 1999). The additional finding of increased carbonate ion substitution into the hydroxyapatite mineral in the phosphate-wasting milieu of HYP mice (Macica et al. 2016) has been evaluated by Raman analysis in tooth dentin from individuals with XLH as a proxy for human bone. Dentin likewise shows increased carbonate substitution (unpublished data). Increased ion substitution of phosphate for carbonate has an impact on several parameters, including an increase in solubility of the bioapatite, which facilitates the resorption of bone mineral during normal turnover (Nelson et al. 1982). Further studies are being conducted to better understand the impact of these physiological adaptations to phosphate wasting and may help to model a standard of care during the maternal period.

14.10 LIMITATIONS OF CURRENT COMBINED THERAPIES: CALCIFICATION OF SOFT TISSUES

Perhaps one of the most significant limitations of combined phosphate therapy with calcitriol is the reported documentation of hypercalcemia and soft tissue calcification in both pediatric and adult patients, with nephrocalcinosis being the most commonly reported (Alon et al. 1992; Petersen et al. 1992; Verge et al. 1991). The toxicity of 1,25(OH)$_2$D should not be underestimated and requires both careful titration by the clinician and regular diagnostic imaging to detect deposition of calcium salts in the renal parenchyma, especially in the setting of secondary hyperparathyroidism.

In addition, one of the most common and debilitating comorbidities of XLH is the pervasive mineralizing enthesopathy that occurs at fibrocartilaginous insertion sites throughout the body. Enthesophytes, or bone spurs, cause a considerable amount of pain and contribute significantly to range of motion and mobility issues. Phosphate therapy does not appear to affect the onset or progression of the enthesopathy (Ramonda et al. 2005). In addition, several lines of evidence suggest that the enthesopathy is not unique to XLH but a common feature of FGF23-mediated phosphate-wasting disorders, including a severe mineralizing enthesopathy demonstrated in patients with ARHR. To test this, we examined the Achilles insertion in a mouse model overexpressing FGF23 and demonstrated the development of the same progression on mineralization of the entheses as previously demonstrated in HYP mice, inconsistent with a direct role of the PHEX mutation (Karaplis et al. 2012). Immunological evidence of the FRFR3 receptor and klotho coreceptor in fibrochondrocytes provides evidence of direct FGF23-mediated effects of fibrochondrocyte hyperplasia (Liang et al. 2009).

14.11 CONCLUSIONS

The use of phosphate salts has proven to be effective in the therapy of acute, life-threatening severe hypophosphatemia and in chronic cases of moderate hypophosphatemia. Although oral phosphate salts, in conjunction with calcitriol to improve growth and reduce the severity of bone disease, have been the mainstay of the pediatric disorder, such therapies have proven to be ineffective in minimizing the long-term impact of phosphate-wasting disorders on mineralized tissues. Newer therapies are targeted to neutralizing circulating FGF23 in an attempt to reconstitute endogenous levels of phosphorus (Carpenter et al. 2014; Zhang et al. 2016). Although phosphate levels and bone quality improve, it remains to be seen if immune neutralization will positively affect outcomes of the cartilage disease dental manifestations and the enthesopathy and the enthesopathy, either directly or indirectly, by improving the mineral substrate into which tendons and ligaments insert. Regardless of the tissue mineralization defect in these tissues, a phosphate-deficient environment affects the inorganic anabolic product of mineral apatite formation (Macica et al. 2016). The study of XLH and other rare bone diseases has contributed a great deal to our understanding of mineral homeostasis and the role of minerals like phosphorus in the physiological setting.

REFERENCES

Alon, U., D. L. Donaldson, S. Hellerstein, B. A. Warady, and D. J. Harris. 1992. Metabolic and histologic investigation of the nature of nephrocalcinosis in children with hypophosphatemic rickets and in the Hyp mouse. *J Pediatr* 120 (6):899–905.

Alon, U. S., R. Levy-Olomucki, W. V. Moore, J. Stubbs, S. Liu, and L. D. Quarles. 2008. Calcimimetics as an adjuvant treatment for familial hypophosphatemic rickets. *Clin J Am Soc Nephrol* 3 (3):658–64. doi:10.2215/CJN.04981107.

Anderson, H. C., R. Garimella, and S. E. Tague. 2005. The role of matrix vesicles in growth plate development and biomineralization. *Front Biosci* 10:822–37.

Bergwitz, C., N. M. Roslin, M. Tieder, J. C. Loredo-Osti, M. Bastepe, H. Abu-Zahra, D. Frappier, K. Burkett, T. O. Carpenter, D. Anderson, M. Garabedian, I. Sermet, T. M. Fujiwara, K. Morgan, H. S. Tenenhouse, and H. Juppner. 2006. SLC34A3 mutations in patients with hereditary hypophosphatemic rickets with hypercalciuria predict a key role for the sodium-phosphate cotransporter NaPi-IIc in maintaining phosphate homeostasis. *Am J Hum Genet* 78 (2):179–92. doi:10.1086/499409.

Bergwitz, C., M. J. Wee, S. Sinha, J. Huang, C. DeRobertis, L. B. Mensah, J. Cohen, A. Friedman, M. Kulkarni, Y. Hu, A. Vinayagam, M. Schnall-Levin, B. Berger, L. A. Perkins, S. E. Mohr, and N. Perrimon. 2013. Genetic determinants of phosphate response in Drosophila. *PLOS ONE* 8 (3):e56753. doi:10.1371/journal. pone.0056753.

Bindels, R. J. M., J. G. J. Hoenderop, and J. Biber. 2012. Transport of calcium, magnesium, and phosphate. *In Brenner and Rector's The Kidney*, edited by M. W. Taal, G. M. Chertow, P. A. Marsden, K. Skorecki, A. S. L. Yu and B. M. Brenner, pp. 226–51. Philadelphia, PA: Elsevier Saunders.

Bourgeois, S., P. Capuano, G. Stange, R. Muhlemann, H. Murer, J. Biber, and C. A. Wagner. 2013. The phosphate transporter NaPi-IIa determines the rapid renal adaptation to dietary phosphate intake in mouse irrespective of persistently high FGF23 levels. *Pflugers Arch* 465 (11):1557–72. doi:10.1007/ s00424-013-1298-9.

Broadus, A. E., C. Macica, and X. Chen. 2007. The PTHrP functional domain is at the gates of endochondral bones. *Ann N Y Acad Sci* 1116:65–81.

Carpenter, T. O. 1997. New perspectives on the biology and treatment of X-linked hypophosphatemic rickets. *Pediatr Clin North Am* 44 (2):443–66.

Carpenter, T. O., E. A. Imel, I. A. Holm, S. M. Jan de Beur, and K. L. Insogna. 2011. A clinician's guide to X-linked hypophosphatemia. *J Bone Miner Res* 26 (7):1381–8. doi:10.1002/jbmr.340.

Carpenter, T. O., E. A. Imel, M. D. Ruppe, T. J. Weber, M. A. Klausner, M. M. Wooddell, T. Kawakami, T. Ito, X. Zhang, J. Humphrey, K. L. Insogna, and M. Peacock. 2014. Randomized trial of the anti-FGF23 antibody KRN23 in X-linked hypophosphatemia. *J Clin Invest* 124 (4):1587–97. doi:10.1172/ JCI72829.

Carpenter, T. O., M. Keller, D. Schwartz, M. Mitnick, C. Smith, A. Ellison, D. Carey, F. Comite, R. Horst, R. Travers, F. H. Glorieux, C. M. Gundberg, A. R. Poole, and K. L. Insogna. 1996. 24,25 Dihydroxyvitamin D supplementation corrects hyperparathyroidism and improves skeletal abnormalities in X-linked hypophosphatemic rickets—A clinical research center study. *J Clin Endocrinol Metab* 81 (6):2381–8.

Consortium, A. 2000. Autosomal dominant hypophosphataemic rickets is associated with mutations in FGF23. *Nat Genet* 26 (3):345–8. doi:10.1038/81664.

Cremonesi, I., C. Nucci, G. D'Alessandro, N. Alkhamis, S. Marchionni, and G. Piana. 2014. X-linked hypophosphatemic rickets: Enamel abnormalities and oral clinical findings. *Scanning* 36 (4):456–61. doi:10.1002/sca.21141.

Cross, N. A., L. S. Hillman, S. H. Allen, G. F. Krause, and N. E. Vieira. 1995. Calcium homeostasis and bone metabolism during pregnancy, lactation, and postweaning: A longitudinal study. *Am J Clin Nutr* 61 (3):514–23.

Dahlman, T., H. E. Sjoberg, and E. Bucht. 1994. Calcium homeostasis in normal pregnancy and puerperium. A longitudinal study. *Acta Obstet Gynecol Scand* 73 (5):393–8.

Farrow, E. G., S. I. Davis, L. J. Summers, and K. E. White. 2009. Initial FGF23-mediated signaling occurs in the distal convoluted tubule. *J Am Soc Nephrol* 20 (5):955–60. doi: 10.1681/ASN.2008070783.

Farrow, E. G., X. Yu, L. J. Summers, S. I. Davis, J. C. Fleet, M. R. Allen, A. G. Robling, K. R. Stayrook, V. Jideonwo, M. J. Magers, H. J. Garringer, R. Vidal, R. J. Chan, C. B. Goodwin, S. L. Hui, M. Peacock, and K. E. White. 2011. Iron deficiency drives an autosomal dominant hypophosphatemic rickets (ADHR) phenotype in fibroblast growth factor-23 (Fgf23) knock-in mice. *Proc Natl Acad Sci U S A* 108 (46):E1146–55. doi:10.1073/pnas.1110905108.

Feng, J. Q., L. M. Ward, S. Liu, Y. Lu, Y. Xie, B. Yuan, X. Yu, F. Rauch, S. I. Davis, S. Zhang, H. Rios, M. K. Drezner, L. D. Quarles, L. F. Bonewald, and K. E. White. 2006. Loss of DMP1 causes rickets and osteomalacia and identifies a role for osteocytes in mineral metabolism. *Nat Genet* 38 (11):1310–5.

Fisher, S. E., I. van Bakel, S. E. Lloyd, S. H. Pearce, R. V. Thakker, and I. W. Craig. 1995. Cloning and characterization of CLCN5, the human kidney chloride channel gene implicated in Dent disease (an X-linked hereditary nephrolithiasis). *Genomics* 29 (3):598–606.

Gallacher, S. J., W. D. Fraser, O. J. Owens, F. J. Dryburgh, F. C. Logue, A. Jenkins, J. Kennedy, and I. T. Boyle. 1994. Changes in calciotrophic hormones and biochemical markers of bone turnover in normal human pregnancy. *Eur J Endocrinol* 131 (4):369–74.

Gattineni, J., C. Bates, K. Twombley, V. Dwarakanath, M. L. Robinson, R. Goetz, M. Mohammadi, and M. Baum. 2009. FGF23 decreases renal NaPi-2a and NaPi-2c expression and induces hypophosphatemia in vivo predominantly via FGF receptor 1. *Am J Physiol Renal Physiol* 297 (2):F282–91. doi:10.1152/ajprenal.90742.2008.

Geerse, D. A., A. J. Bindels, M. A. Kuiper, A. N. Roos, P. E. Spronk, and M. J. Schultz. 2010. Treatment of hypophosphatemia in the intensive care unit: A review. *Crit Care* 14 (4):R147. doi:10.1186/cc9215.

Glorieux, F. H., P. J. Bordier, P. Marie, E. E. Delvin, and R. Travers. 1978. Inadequate bone response to phosphate and vitamin D in familial hypophosphatemic rickets (FHR). *Adv Exp Med Biol* 103:227–32.

Glorieux, F. and C. R. Scriver. 1972. Loss of a parathyroid hormone-sensitive component of phosphate transport in X-linked hypophosphatemia. *Science* 175 (25):997–1000.

Grove-Laugesen, D. and L. Rejnmark. 2014. Three-year successful cinacalcet treatment of secondary hyperparathyroidism in a patient with x-linked dominant hypophosphatemic rickets: A case report. *Case Rep Endocrinol* 2014:479641. doi:10.1155/2014/479641.

Hardy, D. C., W. A. Murphy, B. A. Siegel, I. R. Reid, and M. P. Whyte. 1989. X-linked hypophosphatemia in adults: Prevalence of skeletal radiographic and scintigraphic features. *Radiology* 171 (2):403–14.

Hayslip, C. C., T. A. Klein, H. L. Wray, and W. E. Duncan. 1989. The effects of lactation on bone mineral content in healthy postpartum women. *Obstet Gynecol* 73 (4):588–92.

Holm, I. A., M. J. Econs, and T. O. Carpenter. 2003. Familial hypophosphatemia and related disorders. *In Pediatric Bone: Biology & Diseases*, edited by F. Glorieux, H. Juppner and J. M. Pettifor, pp. 603–31. San Diego, CA: Academic Press.

Ichikawa, S., A. K. Gray, E. Bikorimana, and M. J. Econs. 2013. Dosage effect of a Phex mutation in a murine model of X-linked hypophosphatemia. *Calcif Tissue Int* 93 (2):155–62. doi:10.1007/s00223-013-9736-4.

Imel, E. A., L. A. DiMeglio, S. L. Hui, T. O. Carpenter, and M. J. Econs. 2010. Treatment of X-linked hypophosphatemia with calcitriol and phosphate increases circulating fibroblast growth factor 23 concentrations. *J Clin Endocrinol Metab* 95 (4):1846–50. doi:10.1210/jc.2009-1671.

Imel, E. A., M. Peacock, A. K. Gray, L. R. Padgett, S. L. Hui, and M. J. Econs. 2011. Iron modifies plasma FGF23 differently in autosomal dominant hypophosphatemic rickets and healthy humans. *J Clin Endocrinol Metab* 96 (11):3541–9. doi:10.1210/jc.2011-1239.

Karaplis, A. C., X. Bai, J. P. Falet, and C. M. Macica. 2012. Mineralizing enthesopathy is a common feature of renal phosphate-wasting disorders attributed to FGF23 and is exacerbated by standard therapy in hyp mice. *Endocrinology* 153 (12):5906–17. doi:10.1210/en.2012-1551.

Kent, G. N., R. I. Price, D. H. Gutteridge, M. Smith, J. R. Allen, C. I. Bhagat, M. P. Barnes, C. J. Hickling, R. W. Retallack, S. G. Wilson et al. 1990. Human lactation: Forearm trabecular bone loss, increased bone turnover, and renal conservation of calcium and inorganic phosphate with recovery of bone mass following weaning. *J Bone Miner Res* 5 (4):361–9. doi:10.1002/jbmr.5650050409.

Kido, S., K. Miyamoto, H. Mizobuchi, Y. Taketani, I. Ohkido, N. Ogawa, Y. Kaneko, S. Harashima, and E. Takeda. 1999. Identification of regulatory sequences and binding proteins in the type II sodium/phosphate cotransporter NPT2 gene responsive to dietary phosphate. *J Biol Chem* 274 (40):28256–63.

Kilav, R., J. Silver, and T. Naveh-Many. 1995. Parathyroid hormone gene expression in hypophosphatemic rats. *J Clin Invest* 96 (1):327–33. doi:10.1172/JCI118038.

Koeppen, B. M. and B. A. Stanton. 2012. *Renal Physiology,Mosby Physiology Monograph Series (with Student Consult Online Access),5: Renal Physiology*. Philadelphia, PA: Elsevier Mosby.

Kumar, R. 2000. Tumor-induced osteomalacia and the regulation of phosphate homeostasis. *Bone* 27 (3):333–8.

Leblanc, E. S., T. A. Hillier, K. L. Pedula, J. H. Rizzo, P. M. Cawthon, H. A. Fink, J. A. Cauley, D. C. Bauer, D. M. Black, S. R. Cummings, and W. S. Browner. 2011. Hip fracture and increased short-term but not long-term mortality in healthy older women. *Arch Intern Med* 171 (20):1831–7. doi:10.1001/archinternmed.2011.447.

Liang, G., L. D. Katz, K. L. Insogna, T. O. Carpenter, and C. M. Macica. 2009. Survey of the enthesopathy of X-linked hypophosphatemia and its characterization in Hyp mice. *Calcif Tissue Int* 85 (3):235–46. doi:10.1007/s00223-009-9270-6.

Liang, G., J. Vanhouten, and C. M. Macica. 2011. An atypical degenerative osteoarthropathy in Hyp mice is characterized by a loss in the mineralized zone of articular cartilage. *Calcif Tissue Int* 89 (2):151–62. doi:10.1007/s00223-011-9502-4.

Lorenz-Depiereux, B., M. Bastepe, A. Benet-Pages, M. Amyere, J. Wagenstaller, U. Muller-Barth, K. Badenhoop, S. M. Kaiser, R. S. Rittmaster, A. H. Shlossberg, J. L. Olivares, C. Loris, F. J. Ramos, F. Glorieux, M. Vikkula, H. Juppner, and T. M. Strom. 2006. DMP1 mutations in autosomal recessive hypophosphatemia implicate a bone matrix protein in the regulation of phosphate homeostasis. *Nat Genet* 38 (11):1248–50.

Macica, C. M., H. E. King, M. Wang, C. L. McEachon, C. W. Skinner, and S. M. Tommasini. 2016. Novel anatomic adaptation of cortical bone to meet increased mineral demands of reproduction. *Bone* 85:59–69. doi:10.1016/j.bone.2015.12.056.

Marie, P. J., R. Travers, and F. H. Glorieux. 1981. Healing of rickets with phosphate supplementation in the hypophosphatemic male mouse. *J Clin Invest* 67 (3):911–4.

Nelson, D. G., J. D. Featherstone, J. F. Duncan, and T. W. Cutress. 1982. Paracrystalline disorder of biological and synthetic carbonate-substituted apatites. *J Dent Res* 61 (11):1274–81. doi:10.1177/0022034582061 0111301.

Petersen, D. J., A. M. Boniface, F. W. Schranck, R. C. Rupich, and M. P. Whyte. 1992. X-linked hypophosphatemic rickets: A study (with literature review) of linear growth response to calcitriol and phosphate therapy. *J Bone Miner Res* 7 (6):583–97. doi:10.1002/jbmr.5650070602.

Portale, A. A., B. E. Booth, B. P. Halloran, and R. C. Morris, Jr. 1984. Effect of dietary phosphorus on circulating concentrations of 1,25-dihydroxyvitamin D and immunoreactive parathyroid hormone in children with moderate renal insufficiency. *J Clin Invest* 73 (6):1580–9. doi:10.1172/JCI111365.

Ramonda, R., P. Sfriso, M. Podswiadek, F. Oliviero, C. Valvason, and L. Punzi. 2005. The enthesopathy of vitamin D-resistant osteomalacia in adults. *Reumatismo* 57 (1):52–6.

Rasmussen, N., A. Frolich, P. J. Hornnes, and L. Hegedus. 1990. Serum ionized calcium and intact parathyroid hormone levels during pregnancy and postpartum. *Br J Obstet Gynaecol* 97 (9):857–9.

Reid, I. R., D. C. Hardy, W. A. Murphy, S. L. Teitelbaum, M. A. Bergfeld, and M. P. Whyte. 1989. X-linked hypophosphatemia: A clinical, biochemical, and histopathologic assessment of morbidity in adults. *Medicine (Baltimore)* 68 (6):336–52.

Ruppe, M. D. 1993. X-linked hypophosphatemia. *In GeneReviews(R)*, edited by R. A. Pagon, M. P. Adam, H. H. Ardinger, S. E. Wallace, A. Amemiya, L. J. H. Bean, T. D. Bird, C. R. Dolan, C. T. Fong, R. J. H. Smith and K. Stephens. University of Washington, Seattle.

Sabbagh, Y., T. O. Carpenter, and M. B. Demay. 2005. Hypophosphatemia leads to rickets by impairing caspase-mediated apoptosis of hypertrophic chondrocytes. *Proc Natl Acad Sci U S A* 102 (27):9637–42.

Sabbagh, Y., M. Tenenbaum, M. J. Econs, and A. Auricchio. 2015. Mendelian hypophosphatemias. *In The Online Metabolic and Molecular Bases of Inherited Disease (OMMBID)*, edited by D. Valle, A. L. Beaudet, B. Vogelstein, K. W. Kinzler, S. E Antonarakis, A. Ballabio, K. Gibson and G. Mitchell. New York, NY: McGraw-Hill.

Saito, H., K. Kusano, M. Kinosaki, H. Ito, M. Hirata, H. Segawa, K. Miyamoto, and N. Fukushima. 2003. Human fibroblast growth factor-23 mutants suppress Na+-dependent phosphate co-transport activity and 1alpha,25-dihydroxyvitamin D3 production. *J Biol Chem* 278 (4):2206–11.

Singh, H. J., N. H. Mohammad, and A. Nila. 1999. Serum calcium and parathormone during normal pregnancy in Malay women. *J Matern Fetal Med* 8 (3):95–100. doi:10.1002/(SICI)1520-6661(199905/06)8:3<95::AID-MFM5>3.0.CO;2-4.

Slatopolsky, E., J. Finch, M. Denda, C. Ritter, M. Zhong, A. Dusso, P. N. MacDonald, and A. J. Brown. 1996. Phosphorus restriction prevents parathyroid gland growth. High phosphorus directly stimulates PTH secretion in vitro. *J Clin Invest* 97 (11):2534–40. doi:10.1172/JCI118701.

Smogorzewski, M. J., R. K. Rude, and A. S. L. Yu. 2012. Disorders of calcium, magnesium, and phosphate balance. *In Brenner and Rector's The Kidney*, edited by M. W. Taal, G. M. Chertow, P. A. Marsden, K. Skorecki, A. S. L. Yu and B. M. Brenner, pp. 689–725. Philadelphia, PA: Elsevier Saunders.

Tenenhouse, H. S., J. Martel, C. Gauthier, H. Segawa, and K. Miyamoto. 2003. Differential effects of Npt2a gene ablation and X-linked Hyp mutation on renal expression of Npt2c. *Am J Physiol Renal Physiol* 285 (6):F1271–8. doi:10.1152/ajprenal.00252.2003.

Tieder, M., D. Modai, R. Samuel, R. Arie, A. Halabe, I. Bab, D. Gabizon, and U. A. Liberman. 1985. Hereditary hypophosphatemic rickets with hypercalciuria. *N Engl J Med* 312 (10):611–7. doi:10.1056/NEJM198503073121003.

Turner, M., P. E. Barre, A. Benjamin, D. Goltzman, and M. Gascon-Barre. 1988. Does the maternal kidney contribute to the increased circulating 1,25-dihydroxyvitamin D concentrations during pregnancy? *Miner Electrolyte Metab* 14 (4):246–52.

Urakawa, I., Y. Yamazaki, T. Shimada, K. Iijima, H. Hasegawa, K. Okawa, T. Fujita, S. Fukumoto, and T. Yamashita. 2006. Klotho converts canonical FGF receptor into a specific receptor for FGF23. *Nature* 444 (7120):770–4.

Verge, C. F., A. Lam, J. M. Simpson, C. T. Cowell, N. J. Howard, and M. Silink. 1991. Effects of therapy in X-linked hypophosphatemic rickets. *N Engl J Med* 325 (26):1843–8. doi:10.1056/NEJM199112263252604.

Wang, L., L. Du, and B. Ecarot. 1999. Evidence for Phex haploinsufficiency in murine X-linked hypophosphatemia. *Mamm Genome* 10 (4):385–9.

Weidner, N. and D. Santa Cruz. 1987. Phosphaturic mesenchymal tumors. A polymorphous group causing osteomalacia or rickets. *Cancer* 59 (8):1442–54.

Wu, C. J., Y. M. Song, and W. H. Sheu. 2000. Tertiary hyperparathyroidism in X-linked hypophosphatemic rickets. *Intern Med* 39 (6):468–71.

Yamazaki, Y., T. Tamada, N. Kasai, I. Urakawa, Y. Aono, H. Hasegawa, T. Fujita, R. Kuroki, T. Yamashita, S. Fukumoto, and T. Shimada. 2008. Anti-FGF23 neutralizing antibodies show the physiological role and structural features of FGF23. *J Bone Miner Res* 23 (9):1509–18. doi:10.1359/jbmr.080417.

Yu, X., O. A. Ibrahimi, R. Goetz, F. Zhang, S. I. Davis, H. J. Garringer, R. J. Linhardt, D. M. Ornitz, M. Mohammadi, and K. E. White. 2005. Analysis of the biochemical mechanisms for the endocrine actions of fibroblast growth factor-23. *Endocrinology* 146 (11):4647–56.

Yu, X. and K. E. White. 2005. FGF23 and disorders of phosphate homeostasis. *Cytokine Growth Factor Rev* 16 (2):221–32. doi:10.1016/j.cytogfr.2005.01.002.

Zhang, X., E. A. Imel, M. D. Ruppe, T. J. Weber, M. A. Klausner, T. Ito, M. Vergeire, J. Humphrey, F. H. Glorieux, A. A. Portale, K. Insogna, T. O. Carpenter, and M. Peacock. 2016. Pharmacokinetics and pharmacodynamics of a human monoclonal anti-FGF23 antibody (KRN23) in the first multiple ascending-dose trial treating adults with X-linked hypophosphatemia. *J Clin Pharmacol* 56 (2):176–85. doi:10.1002/jcph.570.

15 Phosphate and Calcium Stone Formation

Hans-Göran Tiselius

CONTENTS

Abstract 201
Bullet Points 201
15.1 Epidemiological Aspects of Calcium Stone Formation in the Urinary Tract 202
15.2 Determinants of Supersaturation with CaOx and CaP 203
15.3 Renal Handling of Phosphate 203
15.4 Interaction between CaP and CaOx in Stone Formation 206
15.5 How Can Deposits of CaP Cause Precipitation of CaOx? 206
15.6 How Are Subepithelial CaP Deposits and Intratubular Plugs Formed? 207
15.7 What Is the Role of Phosphate in the Formation of Subepithelial Plaques and
Intratubular Plugs of CaP? 207
15.8 Preventive Considerations against Recurrence 208
References 210

ABSTRACT

According to our current view of calcium oxylate (CaOx) stone formation, subepithelial deposits (plaques) and intratubular plugs of CaP (HAP) are considered to be of great importance. It also is obvious that without a sufficient renal supply of phosphate, no intratubular or interstitial CaP precipitates will form. Despite these conclusions, we need a more complete understanding of how and where the initial CaP precipitation takes place. Such information is necessary to elucidate the exact role of phosphate in patients with calcium oxalate stone disease. Irrespective of our shortcomings so far, there is sufficient evidence that phosphate needs appropriate attention.

In this chapter some mechanisms that might underlie the development of CaP solid phases and their role in subsequent crystallization of CaOx are discussed briefly. Dietary phosphate thus apparently has stone-promoting properties, but intestinal phosphate also forms complexes with calcium and reduces calcium absorption. Moreover, urinary pyrophosphate is a crystallization inhibitor.

Increased research efforts are highly desirable in order to better understand when, where, and how pathological precipitation of CaP occurs and how it possibly can be counteracted.

BULLET POINTS

- Calcium phosphate is of fundamental importance for calcium oxalate stone formation.
- Calcium phosphate can form intratubularly, preferably in the loop of Henle.
- Interstitial subepithelial deposits of calcium phosphate at the papillary tip might serve as a surface for nucleation of calcium oxalate crystals.
- Increased phosphate load to the kidney increases the risk of intratubular and interstitial precipitation of calcium phosphate.
- For prevention of calcium oxalate stone formation, it is apparently necessary to pay attention to periods with high supersaturation levels of both calcium oxalate and calcium phosphate.

15.1 EPIDEMIOLOGICAL ASPECTS OF CALCIUM STONE FORMATION IN THE URINARY TRACT

During the past decades extensive research efforts have been made to reveal the fundamental mechanisms of calcium stone formation. It thereby is well recognized that the vast majority of concrements formed in the kidney are dominated by calcium oxalate (CaOx) (Knoll et al. 2011; Herring 1962; Wood et al. 2013), but also that a considerable fraction of these stones contain calcium phosphate (CaP), although usually only in small quantities (Öhman et al. 1992; Tiselius 2011). This is at least the case for patients from the industrialized parts of the world who develop stones, and moreover, it has been estimated that stone disease afflicts around 10% of the population in Europe and North America. The disease is more commonly encountered in men than in women. The clinical impact of calcium stone formation is, however, related to its high recurrence rate. In a 10-year perspective, approximately 50% of all calcium stone patients will form one or more new stones (Ahlstrand and Tiselius 1990). Understanding the mechanisms of calcium stone formation thus has remained fundamental for the design of rational recurrence prevention programs (Goldfarb and Coe 1999; Tiselius 2015).

As a consequence of findings from the analysis of calcium stones, summarized in Table 15.1, CaOx has been the focus of both laboratory research and clinical management, with the goal of finding rational methods for arresting, or at least reducing, the risk of recurrent stone formation. Despite the common occurrence of CaP in CaOx stones, it is of note that pure CaP stones are formed much less frequently and usually when a high urine pH occurs simultaneously with a low urinary concentration of citrate. This combination is mainly encountered in patients with complete or partial renal tubular acidosis (Goldfarb and Coe 1999; Osther et al. 1993) or during treatment with acetazolamide (Ahlstrand and Tiselius 1987; Welch et al. 2006). Pure CaP stones are occasionally also seen in patients with hyperparathyroidism (Bouzidi et al. 2011). Brushite (calcium hydrogen phosphate) is a specific crystal phase of pure CaP that rarely is formed. The prerequisites for brushite precipitation are not fully understood, but the clinical significance of the latter crystal phase is that patients who have formed such stones suffer a particularly high risk of recurrent stone formation (>70%). Factors considered important for brushite stone formation are a high calcium excretion and a pH that is higher than for patients with CaOx stones but lower than that seen in patients with hydroxyapatite (HAP) or octacalcium phosphate (OCP) (Siener et al. 2013; Krambeck et al. 2010; Mandel et al. 2003).

It is of interest to note that according to several observations during the past decades, there seems to be an increased incidence of CaP stone formation (Mandel et al. 2003). Increased formation of both HAP and brushite has been reported (Knoll et al. 2011). Although the incidence of brushite has increased, the real number of such stones is still very small. The reason for this shift in calcium stone composition, as well as for the conversion of CaOx to CaP stone disease, is not known and might be explained by changed dietary habits, use of pharmacological agents, or altered lifestyle (Mandel et al. 2003). A possible relationship to shockwave lithotripsy (SWL) has been suggested, but this hypothesis remains highly speculative, and it needs to be emphasized that CaP stones have become more common in both children and in patients treated with other stone-removing procedures than SWL (Wood et al. 2013).

TABLE 15.1

Average Frequency of Stone Components in Swedish Patients with Calcium Stone Disease

Stone Component	Percentage
Pure calcium oxalate	24
Calcium oxalate + calcium phosphate	72
Pure calcium phosphate[a]	4

[a] Stones containing carbonate apatite as a result of urinary tract infection are excluded.

Phosphate and Calcium Stone Formation 203

In summary it can be concluded that calcium stones account for approximately 85% of all stones formed, whereby pure CaOx, CaOx+CaP and pure CaP stones occur in 20%, 60%, and 5% of patients, respectively.

15.2 DETERMINANTS OF SUPERSATURATION WITH CaOx AND CaP

The basic prerequisite for formation of a solid phase is a sufficiently high crystallization driving force, determined by the level of supersaturation, conveniently expressed in terms of ion activity products (AP) of the corresponding salts (Tiselius 1996a). The determinants of greatest importance for AP_{CaOx} are concentrations of calcium, oxalate, citrate, and magnesium, whereas those for AP_{CaP} are concentrations of calcium phosphate, pH, and citrate (Tiselius 1996a, 2002). Calculation of AP levels can be made from a large number of urine constituents with iterative approximation in complex computer programs. Simplified estimates of AP_{CaP} can be derived from the determinants mentioned earlier, and for CaP an approximation can be obtained with the following formula (Tiselius 1984):

$$AP(CaP)index = \frac{F \cdot Calcium^{1.07} \cdot Phosphate^{0.70} \cdot \left(pH - 4.5\right)^{6.8}}{Citrate^{0.20} \cdot Volume^{1.31}}$$

In this index the urine variables are expressed in mmols excreted during a defined period of time and the volume in liters. The collection period determines factor F, which for 24 hours is 2.7×10^{-3}. The AP(CaP) index is numerically related to the more accurately calculated AP_{CaP}.

Although CaP does not correspond to a specific crystal phase, the AP(CaP) index can be used to derive approximate estimates of HAP, OCP, and brushite (Tiselius 1984). The relative importance of phosphate in relation to calcium is obvious from the exponents.

In addition to the AP levels (supersaturation) of CaOx and/or CaP, a large number of macromolecular as well as small molecular crystallization modulating substances have been identified in urine (Khan and Kok 2004). In view of the calcium-binding properties of these compounds, they might inhibit crystal growth and crystal aggregation, but they also have the property of inducing crystal nucleation (initial precipitation of a calcium salt). Most experimental and clinical observations on such effects have been made for CaOx, but there is experimental evidence as well as strong logical reasons to believe that what has been shown for CaOx in most cases also is valid for CaP. It is likely that modulating factors for the crystallization of calcium salts are important in both final urine (in the calyces and renal pelvis) and in nephron urine, but at considerably different concentrations and excretion patterns.

The primary precipitation product of calcium phosphate in urine is thought to be amorphous calcium phosphate (ACP), which usually is converted to OCP and HAP. In this regard it is of note that phosphoric acid has three different pKa values: 2.25, 6.8, and 11.6. The first one is without clinical interest, but for the finally precipitated CaP phase, it is important to know that PO_4^{3-} is a prerequisite for the formation of ACP, OCP, and HAP, whereas HPO_4^{2-} is required for calcium hydrogen phosphate (brushite). The pH conditions of urine in the loop of Henle favor PO_4^{3-}, and it has also been demonstrated that HAP is the crystal phase encountered in the interstitial CaP deposits (discussed later). For one mol of calcium, 0.74 mol of PO_4^{3-} is required for the formation of ACP. The corresponding amounts of phosphate for OCP and HAP are 0.75 mol and 0.60 mol, respectively. The urinary excretion of phosphate normally is much higher than that of calcium, which means that in most cases, as soon as the formation product has been exceeded, enough phosphate is usually available.

15.3 RENAL HANDLING OF PHOSPHATE

There is inconsistent information on whether urinary phosphate differs between normal subjects and those who form stones. Robertson found that whereas the average daily phosphate excretion in normal subjects was 28.9 mmol, higher levels were recorded in patients who form stones from the UK and

Saudi Arabia with values of 47.8 mmol and 49.6 mmol, respectively (Robertson 2015). Moreira et al. (2013) reported a mean 24 h phosphorus excretion of 31 mmol in CaOx stone patients and 27 mmol in CaP stone patients. In Chinese stone-forming patients the mean (SD) 24-hour excretion of phosphate was 17 (9) mmol (Wu et al. 2014). Healy and coworkers analyzed the composition of two 24-hour urine samples and found that the mean (SD) phosphate excretion was 31.2 (10.6) and 32.3 (11.0) in properly collected samples (Healy et al. 2013). Siener et al. (2013) analyzed urine composition in brushite stone-forming patients and healthy controls and noted 24-hour urine phosphate excretion of 34.7 (10.0) and 39.7 (14.0) mmol, respectively. The calcium excretion in these patients was, however, significantly different: 8.41 (2.38) and 4.96 (2.55) mmol.

In some reports on urine composition a lower phosphate excretion was recorded in stone patients compared with that in normal subjects. Accordingly mean (SD) 16-hour phosphate excretion in urine from male Swedish stone formers was 22.5(7.1) mmol and in normal men 24.0(8.0) mmol. The corresponding phosphate excretion levels in women were 17.4(6.0) and 19.0(5.0) mmol, respectively (Tiselius 1997). The lower phosphate excretion in some of the stone forming populations is of note, as it might indicate a consumption of phosphate at high nephron levels of importance for development of subepithelial and intratubular CaP deposits (see below). In recent analysis of 16-hour urine samples from 694 patients with stone disease, the average phosphate excretion was 18.2 mmol (approximately corresponding to 27 mmol during 24 hours). The range of 16-hour excretion was, however, large, and values as high as 50.4 mmol were recorded. This level of phosphate excretion was similar to that reported by Nouvenne et al. (2014): mean 27 to 28 mmol in men and 21 to 22 mmol in women (Nouvenne et al. 2014).

A normal range of 24-hour urine phosphate between 10 and 40 mmol is commonly reported, and the problem related to interpretation of urinary phosphate is that the value is strongly dependent on the diet. The acceptable practical limit for 24-hour phosphate excretion in risk evaluation of patients with calcium stone disease has been set to 35 mmol (Hesse et al. 2009), but the relevance of this limit, of course, can be discussed in view of the meager information on urinary phosphate in stone-forming patients and whether a reduced urinary phosphate is of importance for recurrence prevention.

Urinary phosphate originates from dietary sources and to a small extent also from bone turnover (Figure 15.1). The amount of phosphate excreted in urine depends on the intake and the intestinal absorption of phosphate. Dietary phosphate varies considerably from one patient to another and is highly dependent on what food sources are consumed. It is generally considered that the average daily intake of inorganic phosphorous varies between 25 and 50 mmol. Some foodstuffs have a particularly high content of phosphate. In meat, soft and hard cheese, and nuts the phosphate content is in the range of 13 to 30 mmol/100 g. It is of note that the phosphate content of cocoa powder is as high as 24 mmol/100 g.

With urinary phosphate there is a concomitant excretion of small amounts of pyrophosphate, a substance that has crystal growth and aggregation inhibitory properties of both CaOx and CaP (Wilson et al. 1985). This is one of the reasons why orthophosphate has been used as a pharmacological approach for prevention of recurrent stone formation (Caudarella 2012). Moreover, administration of orthophosphate resulted in decreased calcium excretion, an effect that in addition to reabsorption in the nephron has been explained by formation of calcium phosphate in the gut (Caudarella 2012). In view of our current understanding of calcium stone initiation and the contribution of CaP to the risk of CaOx stone formation, treatment with orthophosphate appears less logical. But this is a field that certainly deserves further analysis.

It has been demonstrated that the circadian rhythm of serum phosphate comprises essentially two peaks: one in midafternoon and another one just after midnight. Moreover, the lowest serum phosphate levels were encountered in the morning between 8 and 10 (Prasad and Bhadauria 2013). Measurements of diurnal variation of phosphate in final urine disclosed that the highest levels were encountered during the daytime (Lederer 2014). Whether this observation also is true for phosphate concentrations in the loop of Henle and other distal parts of the nephron is not known,

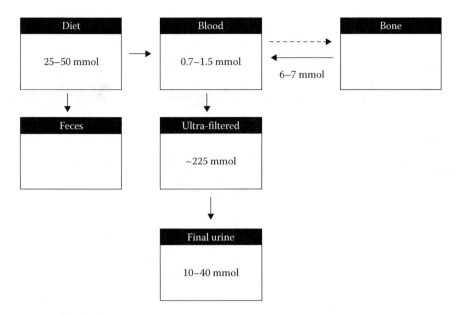

FIGURE 15.1 Approximate daily amounts of phosphate content in diet, blood, and urine.

but it can be assumed that such a relationship exists. It is therefore tempting to speculate that the risk for occasional CaP deposition and formation of intratubular CaP precipitates is particularly high following phosphate-rich meals.

When a standardized AP(CaP) index was calculated, based on 24-hour urine volume of 1.5 L and urine pH of 7, it was theoretically assumed that this value approximately might be extrapolated to conditions in the distal part of the distal tubules (Tiselius 1996b).

Approximately 65% of ingested phosphate is absorbed in duodenum and jejunum, but complex formation with calcium, magnesium, and aluminum reduces phosphate absorption (Prasad and Bhadauria 2013). Complexes between calcium and other intestinal components are facilitated by the alkaline conditions in the gut. In average 225 mmol of phosphate is ultra-filtered by the glomeruli daily. With reabsorption of 80% to 90%, the remaining phosphate that is excreted will be in the approximate range of 25 to 40 mmol. For deposition of interstitial CaP plaques or intratubular CaP plugs, however, what is important is how much of filtered phosphate is present in the loops of Henle. With 80% reabsorbed in the proximal tubules it means that 45 mmol of phosphate passes through the loop of Henle daily.

Following glomerular filtration approximately 80% to 90% of phosphate is reabsorbed in the brush border of proximal tubules. This reabsorption is accomplished by 2a and 2c sodium phosphate cotransporters (Prasad and Bhadauria 2013). Another 5% of filtered phosphate is reabsorbed at nephron levels below the loop of Henle.

With a low phosphate intake most of the filtered phosphate will be reabsorbed in the proximal tubules, and the concentrations of phosphate in the loop of Henle and further down the nephron will be low. Prediction of the role of dietary phosphate on stone formation therefore is complicated.

Reabsorption of filtered phosphate is an important mechanism for phosphate supply to the skeleton. There are a number of factors by which phosphate homeostasis is controlled, and this issue is discussed in detail elsewhere in this book. Here we will just mention that parathyroid hormone, 1,25 vitamin D, and fibroblast growth factor-23, together with its cofactor klotho, are the most important factors for maintaining the plasma level of phosphate between 0.7 and 1.5 mmol/L (Taylor et al. 2015; Lederer 2014; Fukumoto 2014; Prasad and Bhadauria 2013). A complex interaction between these factors determines the fate of ingested phosphate and how much phosphate is present in the nephron and renal interstitial tissues.

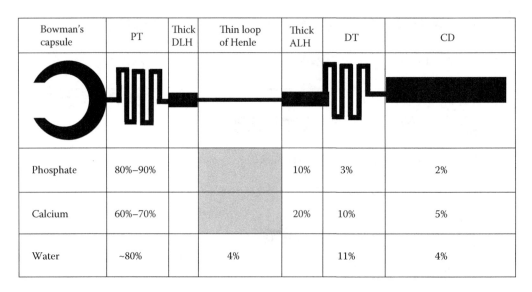

FIGURE 15.2 Approximate reabsorption of phosphate, calcium, and water in different nephron segments. Proximal tubules (PT), thick descending loop of Henle (ThickDLH), thin loop of Henle, thick ascending loop of Henle (ThickALH), distal tubule (DT), and collecting duct (CD). (Based on data from Blaine, J et al., *Clin J Am Soc Nephrol.*, 10, 1257–1272, 2014.)

Approximate fractions of phosphate, calcium, and water reabsorbed in the different nephron segments are shown in Figure 15.2 (Blaine et al.2014).

15.4 INTERACTION BETWEEN CaP AND CaOx IN STONE FORMATION

It is of great interest to note that recent laboratory and clinical observations suggest that accumulations of CaP crystals apparently play an important role in CaOx stone formation.

Inspection of the papillary tips with modern endoscopic optical instruments (Evan 2009; Evan et al. 2008), together with microscopic examinations of tissues and stones, have indicated that CaOx might precipitate and grow on the surface of papillary CaP deposits. This crystallization occurs when CaP is exposed to urine following erosion of the overlying epithelium. A similar process of CaOx crystallization might occur on trapped and fixed plugs of CaP in the distal part of collecting ducts.

Subepithelial deposits and intratubular plugs of CaP were initially described 70 years ago by Randall (1940), and the deposits were termed Randall's plaques 1 and 2. It was also demonstrated that such CaP precipitates were more common in patients with stone disease than in healthy (stone-free) subjects. The clinical relevance of these plaques was, however, initially not understood, and during a considerable period of time it was assumed that Randall's plaques were unrelated to CaOx stone formation. It was not until recently that evidence was obtained for a closer relationship between CaP and CaOx in the CaOx stone formation. Accordingly clinical control of CaOx stone formation might require attention to abnormalities in urinary excretion of phosphate as well as its concentration in the renal tissue in order to counteract subsequent CaP precipitation.

15.5 HOW CAN DEPOSITS OF CaP CAUSE PRECIPITATION OF CaOx?

It is not fully understood how crystallization of CaOx is induced. As stated earlier, it is possible that CaOx at sufficiently high levels of supersaturation deposits on the surface of interstitial CaP deposits following erosion of the covering epithelium or on the surface of plugs in the collecting ducts (Evan 2009; Evan et al. 2008). Arguments against such growth are the surplus supply of

Phosphate and Calcium Stone Formation

growth inhibitors in final urine. Another and possibly more reasonable mechanism is that CaP plaques/plugs are partially dissolved during periods with low urine pH (Tiselius 2011). Theoretical calculations have suggested that even limited dissolution of HAP particles can release substantial amounts of calcium, which subsequently are concentrated to calcium-binding sites on macromolecules (Baumann et al. 2001). Very high local levels of AP_{CaOx} might be obtained when the increased concentration of calcium adds to the ion composition of final urine. The ensuing DG might thus induce nucleation of CaOx rather than growth. The urinary macromolecules that have been suggested as important in the final steps of CaOx crystal formation are osteopontin (OPN) and Tamm Horsfall protein (THP) (Evan et al. 2005). OPN thereby is assumed to provide Ca-binding sites and THP, causing aggregation by self-polymerizing in acid urine with high ion strength (Hess 1994). Crystallization and aggregation of CaOx thus might take place both on denuded plaques of HAP and on intratubular plugs of HAP trapped in collecting ducts. In a recent experimental study it was shown that the presence of phosphate strongly promoted nucleation of calcium oxalate monohydrate. ACP promoted aggregation of amorphous calcium oxalate (Xie et al. 2015).

The interlacing of CaOx and HAP (or any other CaP crystal phase) in the interstitial deposit probably explains why CaP is such a common companion of CaOx in finally dislodged stones.

15.6 HOW ARE SUBEPITHELIAL CaP DEPOSITS AND INTRATUBULAR PLUGS FORMED?

It is important to consider the final steps of CaOx stone formation in order to better understand how the whole process might be initiated. The observations briefly reviewed earlier have undoubtedly brought urinary phosphate and primary CaP precipitation into focus. It has been concluded that for both interstitial deposition of CaP and formation of intratubular plugs of CaP nephron, supersaturation with CaP might be necessary in order to provide sufficient levels of DG. The assumption was made that the highest levels of AP_{CaP} and the greatest risk of CaP precipitation normally are encountered in the ascending loop of Henle (Asplin et al. 1991; DeGanello et al. 1990; Luptak et al. 1994). Calculation of DG for CaP and CaOx disclosed that in most subjects positive values for CaOx might not be encountered until urine reaches the distal part of collecting ducts or the pelvicalyceal system (Luptak et al. 1994). On the other hand, urine at higher levels of the nephron, as a result of its concentrations of calcium, phosphate, and pH, normally has a positive DG only for CaP (Luptak et al. 1994). Positive DG values for CaOx at higher nephron levels than the collecting duct can probably only be expected with particularly high concentrations of oxalate. It was recently shown by Robertson (2015) that CaOx precipitation might occur in the descending loop of Henle in association with high blood levels of oxalate. In the average stone-forming patient the supersaturation at this nephron level usually is in favor of CaP, and it was concluded that precipitation of CaP occasionally might occur already in the descending loop of Henle (Robertson 2015).

15.7 WHAT IS THE ROLE OF PHOSPHATE IN THE FORMATION OF SUBEPITHELIAL PLAQUES AND INTRATUBULAR PLUGS OF CaP?

Formation of intratubular or interstitial CaP precipitates requires sufficiently high concentrations of both calcium and phosphate. There are several theoretical possibilities for the further course of intratubularly formed CaP precipitates in the ascending loop of Henle. Internalization of CaP by the epithelial cells with expulsion into the interstitial tissue is one possibility. Alternatively intracellular dissolution of CaP by lysosomal enzymes might occur. In the latter case, transport of calcium and phosphate ions from dissolved CaP might recrystallize in the basement membrane on the interstitial side of the tubular cells (Khan et al. 2012). Growth and migration of these solids can finally build up the subepithelial deposits referred to as Randall's plaques 1. There is also a possibility that CaP moves from the tubular lumen to the basement membrane between tubular cells.

Intratubularly formed CaP solids might also be transported along the nephron in the direction of the collecting ducts. The vast majority of such CaP particles will certainly be expelled through from the nephron and passed with urine. It needs to be emphasized that CaP is a common constituent of final urine (Herrmann et al. 1991). Under special conditions, with formation of large CaP aggregates, as result of insufficient inhibition of growth/aggregation or increased promotion of crystal aggregation, critically large masses of CaP might form. Such masses will occasionally be trapped in collecting ducts, and these precipitates are referred to as Randall's type 2 plaques. Today these CaP precipitates are termed intratubular CaP plugs (Khan 2014; Khan and Canales 2015). Why the latter pathology does not occur more frequently is not known, but intratubular precipitates of CaP might be completely dissolved during periods with acid urine (Tiselius 2011; Tiselius et al. 2009). For exceptionally large plugs, dissolution of CaP is insufficient, and the precipitate might provide a surface or volume for subsequent CaOx crystallization. But it is of note that precipitation of CaOx on CaP is much more common for the plaques than for the plugs.

Another and perhaps even more interesting hypothesis was presented by Stoller et al. (1996) (Taylor and Stoller 2015). They compared the pathological interstitial deposition of CaP with the pathology of arteriosclerosis. Calcium reabsorption does not occur in the thin ascending loop of Henle, but in the thick part calcium is reabsorbed and subsequently transferred to the vasa recta and transported with the blood alongside the thin loop of Henle to the papilla.

Also phosphate is reabsorbed in the thick ascending part of the loop (Blaine et al. 2014). Accordingly both calcium and phosphate can then reach the basement membrane by a positive gradient. In this process the inflammatory vascular lesion might lead to leakage of cholesterol and lipids that might induce CaP crystal nucleation (Khan and Canales 2015). It is possible that also part of the phosphate that is reabsorbed in the proximal tubules is transported via the vasa recta toward the papilla. Particularly high AP_{CaP} levels can thus be the cause of subepithelial CaP plaques. There are no studies on interstitial concentrations of phosphate, but it can be assumed that reabsorption of large quantities of phosphate result in high interstitial concentrations of phosphate. A hypothetic view of the combined effect of calcium and phosphate transport into the interstitial tissue is shown in Figure 15.3.

Precipitation of CaP might also be associated with an inflammatory response. If such a mechanism can result in elimination of CaP from the interstitium is not known, but the inflammation might cause activation of macrophages and monocytes (Khan and Kok 2004; Khan and Canales 2015), which is an effective tool for the kidney to get rid of interstitial CaP. When the rate of CaP deposition is greater than the crystal-removing capacity, CaP deposits might remain or increase in volume.

15.8 PREVENTIVE CONSIDERATIONS AGAINST RECURRENCE

One of the therapeutic steps that apparently is fundamental to counteract CaOx stone formation is to reduce the supersaturation with CaP. Whereas the risk of crystallization with CaOx might have a peak when low pH coincides with high levels of AP_{CaOx}, the risk of pathological CaP deposition is the result of high AP_{CaP} levels in nephron urine and/or in the interstitial papillary tissue. Under alkaline conditions supersaturation with CaP occurs when high concentrations of calcium and phosphate coincide with a high pH. This risk situation most likely will occur in relation to meals with a rich supply of calcium and phosphate. During the alkaline tide the best prerequisite for CaP precipitation is at hand.

The problem that becomes apparent in terms of preventing calcium stone formation is that whereas reduced intake of calcium and phosphate will have a positive effect on CaP precipitation in the nephron and interstitium, the effect with such a regimen might be negative regarding CaOx precipitation (Robertson et al. 1981; Tiselius 1982). Population studies have shown that with insufficient intake of calcium, the risk of CaOx crystallization and CaOx stone formation increase as a result of increased intestinal absorption and urinary excretion of oxalate (Curhan et al. 2004).

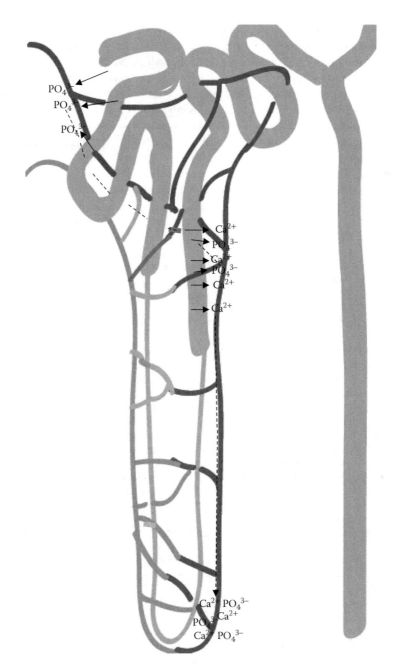

FIGURE 15.3 (See color insert.) Reabsorption of calcium and phosphate in the proximal tubules and thick ascending loop of Henle, with possible intravascular transport of both ions to the papillary region. (Interpretation of data from Taylor, ER and ML Stoller, *Urolithiasis*, 43, 41–45, 2015; Blaine, J et al., *Clin J Am Soc Nephrol.*, 10, 1257–1272, 2014.)

The question that then arises is if we can influence the pathological precipitation of CaP by reducing dietary phosphate. Alternatively, would it be worthwhile to dilute urine in the loop of Henle, distal tubules, or collecting ducts during periods when high levels of AP_{CaP} can be expected? Such therapeutic procedures have, however, not been studied either clinically or experimentally.

REFERENCES

Ahlstrand, C and HG Tiselius. 1987. Urine composition and stone formation during treatment with acetazolamide. *Scand J Urol Nephrol* 21:225–228.

Ahlstrand, C and HG Tiselius. 1990. Recurrences during a 10-year follow-up after first renal stone episode. *Urol Res* 18:397–399.

Asplin, J, S DeGanello, YN Nakgawa, and FL Coe. 1991. Evidence for calcium phosphate supersaturation in the loop of Henle. *Am J Physiol* 270:F604–F613.

Baumann, JM, B Affolter, U Caprez, U Henze, D Lauper, and F Maier. 2001. Hydroxyapatite induction and secondary aggregation, two important processes in calcium stone formation. *Urol Res* 29:417–422.

Blaine, J, M Chonchol, and M. Levi. 2014 Oct 6. Renal control of calcium, phosphate, and magnesium homeostasis. *Clin J Am Soc Nephrol* 10:1257–1272.

Bouzidi, H, D de Brauwere, and M. Daudon. 2011. Does urinary stone composition and morphology help for prediction of primary hyperparathyroidism? *Nephrol Dial Transplant* 26:565–572.

Caudarella, R. 2012. Orthophosphates. *In: Urolithiasis Basic Science and Clinical Practice*. Talati J, Tiselius HG, Albala DM, Ye, Z (Eds.). London: Springer-Verlag London, pp. 751–756.

Curhan, GC, WC Willett, EL Knight, and MJ Stampfer. 2004. Dietary factors and the risk of incident kidney stones in younger women: Nurses' Health Study II. *Arch Intern Med* 164:885–891.

DeGanello, S, J Asplin, and FL Coe. 1990. Evidence that the fluid in the thin segment of the loop of Henle normally is supersaturated and forms poorly crystallized hydroxyapatite that can initiate renal stones. (Abstract). *Kidney Int* 37:472.

Evan, AP. 2009. Physiopathology and etiology of stone formation in the kidney and the urinary tract. *Pediatr Nephrol* 25:831841.

Evan, AP, FL Coe, SR Rittling, SM Bledsoe, Y Shao, JE Lingeman, and EM Worcester. 2005. Apatite plaque particles in inner medulla of kidneys of calcium oxalate stone formers: Osteopontin localization. *Kidney Int* 68:145–154.

Evan, AP, JE Lingeman, FL Coe, and EM Worcester. 2008. Role of interstitial apatite plaque in the pathogenesis of the common calcium oxalate stone. *Semin Nephrol* 28:111–119.

Fukumoto, S. 2014. Phosphate metabolism and vitamin D. *Bonekey Rep* 3:497.

Goldfarb, DS and FL Coe. 1999. Prevention of recurrent nephrolithiasis. *Am Fam Physician* 60:2269–2276.

Healy, KA, SG Hubosky, and DH Bagley. 2013. 24-hour urine collection in the metabolic evaluation of stone formers: Is one study adequate? *J Endourol* 27:374–378.

Herring, LC. 1962. Observations on the analysis of ten thousand urinary calculi. *J Urol* 88:545–562.

Herrmann, U, PO Schwille, and P Kuch. 1991. Crystalluria determined by polarizing microscopy. Technique and results in healthy control subjects and patients with idiopathic recurrent calcium urolithiasis classified in accordance with calciuiria. *Urol Res* 19:151–158.

Hess, B. 1994. Tamm-Horsfall glycoprotein and calcium nephrolithiasis. *Minerl Electrolyte Metab* 20:393–398.

Hesse, A, HG Tiselius, R Siener, and R Hoppe. 2009. Urinary Stones. *Diagnosis, Treatment and Recurrence Prevention*. Basel, Switzerland: Karger.

Khan, SR. 2014. Reactive oxygen species, inflammation and calcium oxalate nephrolithiasis. *Transl Androl Urol* 3:256–276.

Khan, SR and BK Canales. 2015. Unified theory on the pathogenesis of Randall's plaques and plugs. *Urolithiasis* 43:109–123.

Phosphate and Calcium Stone Formation

Khan, SR and DJ Kok. 2004. Modulators of urinary stone formation. *Front Biosci* 9:1450–1482.

Khan, SR, DE Rodriguez, LB Gower, and M Monga. 2012. Association of Randall plaque with collagen fibers and membrane vesicles. *J Urol* 187:1094–1100.

Knoll, T, AB Schuber, D Fahlenkamp, DB Leusmann, G Wendt-Nordahl, and G Schubert. 2011. Urolithiasis through the ages: Data on more than 200,000 urinary stone analyses. *J Urol* 185:1304–1311.

Krambeck, AE, SE Handa, AP Evan, and JE Lingeman. 2010. Profile of the brushite stone former. *J Urol* 184:1367–1371.

Lederer, E. 2014. Regulation of serum phosphate. *J Physiol* 592:3985–3995.

Luptak, J, H Bek-Jensen, AM Fornander, I Hojgaard, MA Nilsson, and HG Tiselius. 1994. Crystallization of calcium oxalate and calcium phosphate at supersaturation levels corresponding to those in different parts of the nephron. *Scanning Microsc* 8:47–62.

Mandel, N, I Mandel, K Fryjoff, T Rejniak, and G Mandel. 2003. Conversion of calcium oxalate to calcium phosphate with recurrent stone episodes. *J Urol* 169:2026–2029.

Moreira, DM, JI Friedlander, C Hartman, SE Elsamra, AD Smith, and Z Okeke. 2013. Differences in 24-hour urine composition between apatite and brushite stone formers. *Urology* 82:768–772.

Nouvenne, A, A Ticinesi, F Allegri, A Guerra, L Guida, I Morelli, L Borghi, and T Meschi. 2014. Twenty-five years of idiopathic calcium nephrolithiasis: Has anything changed? *Clin Chem Lab Med* 52:337–344.

Öhman, S, L Larsson, and HG Tiselius. 1992. Clinical significance of phosphate in calcium oxalate renal stones. *Ann Clin Biochem* 29:59–63.

Osther, PJ, J Bollerslev, AB Hansen, K Engel, and P Kildeberg. 1993. Pathophysiology of incomplete renal tubular acidosis in recurrent renal stone formers: Evidence of disturbed calcium, bone and citrate metabolism. *Urol Res* 21:169–173.

Prasad, N and D Bhadauria. 2013. Renal phosphate handling: Physiology. *Indian J Endocrinol Metab* 17:620–627.

Randall, A. 1940. Papillary pathology as a precursor of primary renal calculus. *J Urol* 44:580.

Robertson, WG. 2015. Potential role of fluctuations in the composition of renal tubular fluid through the nephron in the initiation of Randall's plugs and calcium oxalate crystalluria in a computer model of renal function. *Urolithiasis* 43 (Suppl 1):93–107.

Robertson, WG, DS Scurr, and M Bridge. 1981. Factors influencing the crystallisation of calcium oxalate— Critique. *J Cryst Growth* 53:182–194.

Siener, R, L Netzer, and A Hesse. 2013. Determinants of brushite stone formation: A case-control study. *PLOS ONE* 8:e78996. doi:10.1371/journal.pone.0078996. eCollection 2013.

Stoller, ML, RK Low, GS Shami, VD McCormick, and RL. Kerschmann. 1996. High resolution radiography of cadaveric kidneys: Unraveling the mystery of Randall's plaque formation. *J Urol* 156:1263–1266.

Taylor, EN, AN Hoofnagle, and GC Curhan. 2015. Calcium and phosphorus regulatory hormones and risk of incident symptomatic kidney stones. *Clin J Am Soc Nephrol* 10:667–675.

Taylor, ER and ML Stoller. 2015. Vascular theory of the formation of Randall plaques. *Urolithiasis* 43 (Suppl 1):41–45.

Tiselius, H-G. 1982. An improved method for then routine biochemical evaluation of patients with recurrent calcium oxalate stone disease. *Clin Chim Acta* 122:409–418.

Tiselius, HG. 1984. A simplified estimate of the ion-activity product of calcium phosphate in urine. *Eur Urol* 10:191–195.

Tiselius, HG. 1996b. Estimated levels of superstauration with calcium phosphate and calcium oxalate in the distal tubuli. *Urol Res* 25:153–159.

Tiselius, HG. 1996a. Solution chemistry of supersaturation. *In: Kidney Stones: Medical and Surgical Management.* Coe FL, Favus MJ, Pak CYC, Parks JH, Preminger GM (Eds.). Philadelphia, PA: Lippincott-Raven Publishers, pp. 33–64.

Tiselius, HG. 1997. Metabolic evaluation of patients with stone disease. *Urol Int* 59:131–141.

Tiselius, HG. 2002. Medical evaluation of nephrolithiasis. *Endocrinol Metab Clin North Am* 31:1031–1050.

Tiselius, HG, B Lindbäck, A-M Fornander, and MA Nilsson. 2009. Studies on the role of calcium phosphate in the process of calcium oxalate crystal formation. *Urol Res* 37:181–192.

Tiselius, HG. 2011. A hypothesis of calcium stone formation: An interpretation of stone research during the past decades. *Urol Res* 39:231–243.

Tiselius, HG. 2015. Should we modify the principles of risk evaluation and recurrence preventive treatment of patients with calcium oxalate stone disease in view of the etiologic importance of calcium phosphate? *Urolithiasis* 43:47–57.

Welch, BJ, D Graybea, OW Moe, NM Maalouf, and K Sakhaee. 2006. Biochemical and stone-risk profiles with topiramate treatment. *Am J Kidney Dis* 48:555–563.

Wilson, JW, PG Werness, and LH Smith. 1985. Inhibitors of crystal growth of hydroxyapatite: A constant composition approach. *J Urol* 134:1255–1258.

Wood, KD, IS Stanasel, DS Koslov, PW Mufarrij, GA McLorie, and DG Assimos. 2013. Changing stone composition profile of children with nephrolithiasis. *Urology* 82:210–213.

Wu, W, D Yang, HG Tiselius, L Ou, Y Liang, H Zhu, S Li, and G Zeng. 2014. The characteristics of the stone and urine composition in Chinese stone formers: Primary report of a single-center results. *Urology* 83:732–737.

Xie, B, TJ Halter, BM Borah, and GH Nancollas. 2015. Aggregation of calcium phosphate and oxalate phases in the formation of renal stones. *Cryst Growth Des* 15:204–211.

16 Impact of Socioeconomic Factors on Phosphorus Balance

Orlando M. Gutiérrez

CONTENTS

Abstract 213
Bullet Points 213
16.1 Introduction 214
16.2 Socioeconomic Status and Organic Phosphorus Intake 214
16.3 Socioeconomic Status and Inorganic Phosphorus Intake 216
16.4 Conclusions 218
References 218

ABSTRACT

Total body phosphorus balance is tightly regulated through an intricate system of endocrine feedback loops that coordinate phosphorus trafficking between dietary sources, bone and soft tissue stores, and the kidney. Under normal conditions, excess dietary phosphorus intake is the primary factor leading to disturbances in total body phosphorus balance in free-living adults. Epidemiologic data showing that these disturbances are associated with cardiovascular disease events and death have fueled interest in dietary phosphorus restriction as a potential strategy for improving cardiovascular outcomes, particularly in chronic kidney disease. However, successfully restricting dietary phosphorus intake in free-living adults is challenging because of the wide variety of personal, cultural, and environmental barriers to limiting dietary phosphorus consumption in individuals consuming typical Westernized diets. Among these, low socioeconomic status plays a particularly important role in disturbing systemic phosphorus homeostasis by promoting excess intake of phosphorus with high bioavailability. This occurs not only because of difficulty in affording lower-phosphorus foods, but also because of specific elements of the built environment that can promote excess phosphorus intake via reduced access to low-phosphorus food options. Accordingly, any serious effort to reduce phosphorus intake requires an understanding of both individual and contextual socioeconomic factors that serve as obstacles to reducing total phosphorus intake per day. This chapter focuses on discussing the major socioeconomic factors that affect dietary phosphorus consumption in the interest of increasing the understanding of the most important barriers to maintaining normal phosphorus balance in individuals consuming typical Westernized diets.

BULLET POINTS

- Both individual and contextual socioeconomic factors strongly influence dietary phosphorus intake.
- Dietary phosphorus intake is the primary means of manipulating phosphorus balance in free-living adults.
- Low socioeconomic status promotes the intake of excess dietary phosphorus with high bioavailability; however, phosphate bioavailability cannot be determined in nutrient intake assessment.

- Epidemiological data have demonstrated socioeconomic gradients in the prevalence and severity of disorders of phosphorus balance, supporting the notion that socioeconomic factors strongly affect total phosphorus balance in community-living adults.
- Efforts to reduce phosphorus intake in clinical practice must include an understanding of where and what kinds of foods an individual is able to purchase and the barriers that each individual faces in making healthier food choices.

16.1 INTRODUCTION

Serum phosphorus concentrations are maintained through a tightly coordinated balance between dietary phosphorus absorption; urinary phosphorus excretion; and exchanges with bone, soft tissue, and intracellular stores (Uribarri 2007). The kidneys are the primary organs that regulate this balance by modulating urinary phosphorus excretion in response to changes in dietary intake and bone/soft tissue turnover. Under normal conditions, dietary intake makes up the majority of the obligate phosphorus load that the kidneys must eliminate on a daily basis to maintain total body phosphorus balance (Berndt and Kumar 2007). Because of this, dietary phosphorus intake is the primary means of manipulating phosphorus balance in free-living adults.

Epidemiologic data have shown that disturbances in systemic phosphorus homeostasis are associated with cardiovascular disease events and death independently of traditional risk factors (Block et al. 2004; Dhingra et al. 2007; Kestenbaum et al. 2005; Tonelli et al. 2005). Experimental data have supported the biological plausibility of these findings by demonstrating pathophysiological mechanisms underlying the link between disturbances in phosphorus metabolism and cardiovascular disease (Giachelli et al. 2001; Mathew et al. 2008; Di Marco et al. 2008; Shuto et al. 2009; Lau et al. 2011; El-Abbadi et al. 2009). Because excess dietary phosphorus intake is common in individuals consuming Westernized diets (Uribarri 2007) and can lead to disturbances in phosphorus metabolism, these findings have fueled interest in dietary phosphorus restriction as a potential strategy for improving cardiovascular outcomes, particularly in individuals with chronic kidney disease (CKD).

Successfully restricting dietary phosphorus intake in free-living adults is challenging. A major reason for this is the myriad personal, cultural, and environmental factors that can affect the quantity and quality of dietary phosphorus that individuals consume. For example, both individual-level and contextual socioeconomic factors strongly influence the types of foods that an individual consumes. Individual factors primarily refer to a person's ability to afford foods with higher nutritional quality, whereas contextual factors include those factors related to the specific characteristics of the built environment (e.g., access to grocery stores, density of fast food establishments) that can strongly affect decisions related to food purchase (Diez-Roux et al. 1999; Morland et al. 2002; Morland et al. 2002; Moore and Diez Roux 2006; Moore et al. 2009; Duran et al. 2013; Curl et al. 2013; Dubowitz et al. 2008; Diez Roux 2001) (Figure 16.1). Whereas current clinical practice guidelines primarily focus on modifying individual behavior when it comes to food consumption, less attention is paid to socioeconomic factors that serve as obstacles in making healthier food choices. This is critical to understand as it will strongly affect systemic phosphorus balance via its powerful influence on daily phosphorus consumption. The focus of this chapter will be to review socioeconomic factors that influence dietary phosphorus intake in community-dwelling adults.

16.2 SOCIOECONOMIC STATUS AND ORGANIC PHOSPHORUS INTAKE

Dietary sources of phosphorus can be broadly categorized as organic or inorganic. The distinction between these types of phosphorus is reviewed in detail in Chapter 19. Briefly, organic phosphorus refers to esterified forms of phosphorus found in protein-rich foods such as eggs, fish, meat, dairy products, and vegetables, whereas inorganic forms of phosphorus include those forms commonly added to processed foods and beverages (Sherman and Mehta 2009a, b; Uribarri and Calvo 2003).

Impact of Socioeconomic Factors on Phosphorus Balance

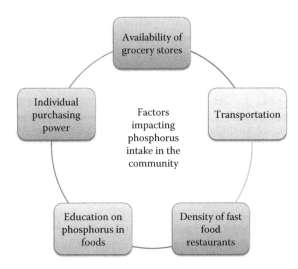

FIGURE 16.1 Factors affecting phosphorus intake in the community.

Epidemiologic data on the association of socioeconomic status with protein intake have been mixed, with some studies showing that lower socioeconomic status is associated with higher protein intake, whereas others show the opposite (Darmon and Drewnowski 2008; Lin et al. 2011). Despite this inconsistency, numerous studies have shown that individuals with lower socioeconomic status tend to purchase cheaper food items such as carbohydrate-rich or fatty foods that are energy dense but nutrient poor (Appelhans et al. 2012; Monsivais and Drewnowski 2009; Drewnowski et al. 2007; Maillot et al. 2007; Aggarwal et al. 2011), in contradistinction to many protein-rich foods. As a result, there is solid indirect evidence supporting the notion that lower socioeconomic status is associated with lower overall intake of organic sources of phosphorus found in protein-rich foods.

More consistent socioeconomic gradients appear to exist when comparing animal to vegetable protein intake. In general, as compared to individuals with higher socioeconomic status, individuals with lower socioeconomic status consume fewer vegetable sources of protein (Darmon and Drewnowski 2008). This has potentially important implications for systemic phosphorus balance in that the bioavailability of phosphorus in animal proteins is higher than in vegetable proteins. This is because phosphorus found in many plant sources, particularly in the form of phytate, is poorly absorbed by humans (see Chapters 17 and 18). Phytate is the most abundant storage form of phosphorus found in grains and seeds (Maga 1982). Because humans lack phytase in the small intestine, they have limited capacity to hydrolyze ingested phytate in order to release phosphorus for absorption (Iqbal et al. 1994). Thus, although current estimates suggest that humans absorb ~60% of dietary phosphorus in the gut, this percentage may be substantially lower among individuals consuming diets rich in plant sources.

The impact of vegetable versus animal protein on phosphorus absorption was highlighted in several feeding studies. The first was a cross-over study of nine patients with mild-to-moderate CKD who were fed diets in which the protein sources were either primarily vegetarian or meat in sequential order (with the order in which the diets were consumed being randomly assigned). This study showed that the diet with primarily vegetarian sources of protein reduced circulating concentrations of phosphorus and fibroblast growth factor-23 (FGF23)—a hormone that regulates phosphorus and vitamin D metabolism—as compared to the diet with meat sources of protein. In the second study, young and elderly Korean females were fed alternating diets containing either high or low phytate content (Joung et al. 2007). Each diet was consumed for 10 days, during which time fecal collections were obtained to estimate gut phosphorus absorption. Despite similar total phosphorus content between the diets, gut phosphorus absorption was significantly lower during the high phytate period than during the low phytate period among the younger volunteers (61 ± 13 vs. 72 ± 9%, $P = 0.02$), although no significant differences were noted in the older volunteers. The third study involved 16 young Finnish females who were fed five experimental diets: a control diet containing 500 mg of phosphorus and four diets containing identical amounts of phosphorus (~1500 mg) but from different sources (meat, cheese, whole grains, or phosphorus supplements) (Karp et al. 2007). Each diet was consumed for one day, during which time serum levels of phosphorus and 24-hour urinary excretion of phosphorus were measured. Whereas the diets containing meat, cheese, and supplements resulted in either stable or higher serum phosphorus concentrations, the grain-based (phytate-rich) diet resulted in a trend toward lower levels. In addition, 24-hour urinary excretion of phosphorus was significantly lower on the grain diet as compared to the meat or supplement diet, suggesting lower gut phosphorus absorption with the grain-based diet. These data indicate that diets containing phosphorus with low bioavailability (i.e., vegetable proteins) can effectively limit dietary phosphorus absorption. Because individuals with low socioeconomic status tend to consume lower amounts of vegetable proteins than individuals with greater affluence, this supports the notion that lower socioeconomic status tends to promote consumption of organic forms of phosphorus with higher phosphorus bioavailability.

There are relatively few data on the role of local food environments in the consumption of animal protein. However, the relationship between access to food stores and consumption of vegetable forms of protein provide important clues. A number of population-based studies have shown that lower access to supermarkets and grocery stores was associated with lower intake of fruits and vegetables (Darmon and Drewnowski 2008). The importance of these findings for phosphorus balance was highlighted in a study in the Chronic Renal Insufficiency Cohort (CRIC) study, which showed that consumption of a higher percentage of protein from plant sources was associated with lower FGF23 concentrations in CKD patients (Scialla et al. 2012). Given that higher animal protein intake is commonly associated with lower fruit and vegetable intake, it is likely that the local food environment plays an important role in contributing to excess animal protein intake and downstream consequences such as higher phosphorus bioavailability.

16.3 SOCIOECONOMIC STATUS AND INORGANIC PHOSPHORUS INTAKE

The complex issues surrounding phosphorus added to processed foods are reviewed in detail in separate chapters of this text (see Chapters 19 and 21 through 23). Socioeconomic status plays an important role in the consumption of inorganic forms of phosphorus in individuals living in developed countries. This is largely due to the nearly ubiquitous presence of phosphorus-based food additives in processed and convenience foods. Phosphorus additives serve a number of critical functions for food manufacturing, including pH stabilization, metal cation sequestration, emulsification, leavening, hydration, and bactericidal actions (Molins 1991). Because of this wide diversity of applications, the use of phosphorus additives in the food manufacturing industry is immense—for example, over 40 million pounds of phosphorus additives were used annually in the United States during the 1970s by the meat industry alone (Molins 1991). The magnitude of the use of phosphorus additives in the meat industry pales in comparison to that of the baking industry, which utilizes the highest quantities of phosphorus additives because of the key role that phosphorus acids play as dough-leavening agents (Stahl and Ellinger 1971). In a report commissioned by the U.S. Department of Commerce, baked goods were estimated to contain nearly 10-fold higher amounts of phosphorus additives than meat products (GRAS [Generally Recognized as Safe] Food Ingredients — Phosphates 1972). Phosphorus additives are also commonly used in dark colas and sodas, principally in the form of phosphoric acid (Murphy-Gutekunst 2005). This is important in that processed meats are often cited as the major source of phosphorus additive consumption in individuals with low socioeconomic status—however, cheap, energy-dense food products such as baked products and dark colas likely represent a more substantial exposure to phosphorus additives among persons with limited financial means.

Phosphorus is naturally abundant in the food supply. Therefore, irrespective of socioeconomic status, most individuals in the United States usually exceed the recommended daily allowance of dietary phosphorus (see Chapter 19). The high levels of phosphorus additives in processed foods augments phosphorus intake even further (Uribarri 2007), with estimates ranging from 250 to 1,000 mg of extra phosphorus per day (Bell et al. 1977; Calvo 2000; Oenning et al. 1988). Several more contemporary studies have shown that the contribution of phosphorus additives to total phosphorus per day remains quite high in diets rich in highly processed foods. León et al. selected the top five best-selling food products containing phosphorus additives within 15 general food categories from a commercially available data set of grocery sales in northeast Ohio and matched them one-to-one to similar products without phosphorus additives (Leon et al. 2013). These investigators then purchased both additive-containing and non-additive-containing products from local food stores and measured the phosphorus content after preparation of the food items according to standard practices. They then developed sample meals using analyzed matched foods to approximate the mean calorie, protein, carbohydrate, and total fat intake of U.S. adults as estimated by recent nutritional databases based on data from the most recent National Health and Nutrition Education Survey. They found that compared to additive-free meals, additive-rich meals had, on average, 736 ± 91 mg more phosphorus. In addition, they found that sample meals consisting of additive-rich foods were, on average, \$2.00 cheaper per day than meals consisting of additive-free foods, an important consideration for individuals living on fixed or limited incomes. Similarly, Carrigan et al. examined the contribution of phosphorus-based food additives to the total phosphorus content of processed foods by developing separate four-day menus for a low-additive and additive-enhanced diet using the most recent Nutrition Data System for Research software (Carrigan et al. 2014). The low-additive diet was designed to conform as close as possible to the 1997 Institute of Medicine's recommended dietary intake guidelines (RDA) for phosphorus of 700 mg per day for adults (IOM 1997). The phosphorus content of the control meals was approximately 900 mg of phosphorus per day and contained minimally processed foods. The additive-enhanced diet contained the same food items as the low-additive diet except that highly processed foods were substituted for minimally processed foods. Food items from both diets were collected, blended, and sent for measurement of energy and nutrient intake. The main findings of this study were that, when averaged over the four menu days, measured phosphorus contents of the additive-enhanced diet were 606 ± 125 higher than the low-additive diet, respectively, representing a 60% increase in total phosphorus content on average.

Given the strong association of neighborhood characteristics with consumption of processed and fast foods reviewed earlier, limited access to healthy food options likely plays an important role in promoting excess phosphorus intake by increasing the consumption of highly processed foods. To date, however, few studies have specifically looked at whether access to food stores or fast food restaurants affects phosphorus intake. Nevertheless, studies looking at the association of individual-level markers of socioeconomic status and biochemical markers of phosphorus homeostasis may provide important clues. Studies have shown that lower annual family income was associated with higher serum phosphorus in participants of the Third National Health and Nutrition Examination Survey and with higher serum phosphorus and FGF23 concentrations in participants of the Chronic Renal Insufficiency Cohort Study (Isakova et al. 2011; Gutierrez et al. 2010, 2011). Similarly, a study of 10,672 participants of the Kidney Early Evaluation Program showed that serum phosphorus was inversely associated with access to medical care and health insurance (Mehrotra et al. 2013), both strong proxies for low socioeconomic status. In contrast, a study using the Multi-Ethnic Study of Atherosclerosis cohort showed no association of annual family income with serum phosphorus concentrations when controlling for other factors, particularly female sex (Gutierrez et al. 2012). Further, this latter study showed that consumption of fast foods was not associated with serum phosphorus concentrations. Possible reasons for the disparate findings in the latter study as compared to the prior studies include differences in sample size, demographics (principally age and sex), and methods of sampling. Nevertheless, in the aggregate, these data suggest that socioeconomic status partly affects biochemical measures of phosphorus homeostasis, although the magnitude and strength of this association were inconsistent and not clearly related to access to food sources. Further studies using more sensitive measures of dietary phosphorus intake such as 24-hour urinary phosphorus excretion are needed to determine the association of neighborhood characteristics with phosphorus intake.

16.4 CONCLUSIONS

Socioeconomic status strongly affects phosphorus balances in several ways. First, individuals with limited purchasing power tend to buy foods that are not only high in total phosphorus content but also have high phosphorus bioavailability. Second, critical aspects of the built environment, such as availability of grocery stores that sell fresh fruits, vegetables, and meats, all of which are unprocessed foods with lower amounts of added phosphorus, can strongly influence the ability of individuals to successfully achieve a low-phosphorus diet. The biological consequences of these factors is supported by epidemiologic data showing economic gradients in markers of bone and mineral metabolism—individuals with lower socioeconomic status have a greater prevalence of disturbances in phosphorus metabolism than individuals with higher socioeconomic status, independent of other potential confounders. Together, these findings have important implications for the approach to dietary phosphorus restriction in free-living adults. Specifically, any serious attempt to limit dietary phosphorus consumption in individuals requires detailed knowledge of not only the general types of foods that an individual consumes but where and what kinds of foods are being purchased, current barriers in terms of accessing healthier food choices, and potential strategies to overcome both individual-level and contextual socioeconomic obstacles to lowering dietary phosphorus intake.

REFERENCES

Aggarwal, A., P. Monsivais, A. J. Cook, and A. Drewnowski. 2011. Does diet cost mediate the relation between socioeconomic position and diet quality? *Eur J Clin Nutr* 65 (9):1059–66.

Appelhans, B. M., B. J. Milliron, K. Woolf, T. J. Johnson, S. L. Pagoto, K. L. Schneider, M. C. Whited, and J. C. Ventrelle. 2012. Socioeconomic status, energy cost, and nutrient content of supermarket food purchases. *Am J Prev Med* 42 (4):398–402.

Bell, R. R., H. H. Draper, D. Y. Tzeng, H. K. Shin, and G. R. Schmidt. 1977. Physiological responses of human adults to foods containing phosphate additives. *J Nutr* 107 (1):42–50.

Berndt, T. and R. Kumar. 2007. Phosphatonins and the regulation of phosphate homeostasis. *Annu Rev Physiol* 69:341–59.

Block, G. A., P. S. Klassen, J. M. Lazarus, N. Ofsthun, E. G. Lowrie, and G. M. Chertow. 2004. Mineral metabolism, mortality, and morbidity in maintenance hemodialysis. *J Am Soc Nephrol* 15 (8):2208–18.

Calvo, M. S. 2000. Dietary considerations to prevent loss of bone and renal function. *Nutrition* 16 (7–8):564–6.

Carrigan, A., A. Klinger, S. S. Choquette, A. Luzuriaga-McPherson, E. K. Bell, B. Darnell, and O. M. Gutierrez. 2014. Contribution of food additives to sodium and phosphorus content of diets rich in processed foods. *J Ren Nutr* 24 (1):13–9, 19e1.

Curl, C. L., S. A. Beresford, A. Hajat, J. D. Kaufman, K. Moore, J. A. Nettleton, and A. V. Diez-Roux. 2013. Associations of organic produce consumption with socioeconomic status and the local food environment: Multi-Ethnic Study of Atherosclerosis (MESA). *PLOS ONE* 8 (7):e69778.

Darmon, N. and A. Drewnowski. 2008. Does social class predict diet quality? *Am J Clin Nutr* 87 (5):1107–17.

Dhingra, R., L. M. Sullivan, C. S. Fox, T. J. Wang, R. B. D'Agostino, Sr., J. M. Gaziano, and R. S. Vasan. 2007. Relations of serum phosphorus and calcium levels to the incidence of cardiovascular disease in the community. *Arch Intern Med* 167 (9):879–85.

Di Marco, G. S., M. Hausberg, U. Hillebrand, P. Rustemeyer, W. Wittkowski, D. Lang, and H. Pavenstadt. 2008. Increased inorganic phosphate induces human endothelial cell apoptosis in vitro. *Am J Physiol Renal Physiol* 294 (6):F1381–7.

Diez Roux, A. V. 2001. Investigating neighborhood and area effects on health. *Am J Public Health* 91 (11):1783–9.

Diez-Roux, A. V., F. J. Nieto, L. Caulfield, H. A. Tyroler, R. L. Watson, and M. Szklo. 1999. Neighbourhood differences in diet: The Atherosclerosis Risk in Communities (ARIC) Study. *J Epidemiol Community Health* 53 (1):55–63.

Drewnowski, A., P. Monsivais, M. Maillot, and N. Darmon. 2007. Low-energy-density diets are associated with higher diet quality and higher diet costs in French adults. *J Am Diet Assoc* 107 (6):1028–32.

Dubowitz, T., M. Heron, C. E. Bird, N. Lurie, B. K. Finch, R. Basurto-Davila, L. Hale, and J. J. Escarce. 2008. Neighborhood socioeconomic status and fruit and vegetable intake among whites, blacks, and Mexican Americans in the United States. *Am J Clin Nutr* 87 (6):1883–91.

Duran, A. C., A. V. Diez Roux, R. Latorre Mdo, and P. C. Jaime. 2013. Neighborhood socioeconomic characteristics and differences in the availability of healthy food stores and restaurants in Sao Paulo, Brazil. *Health Place* 23:39–47.

El-Abbadi, M. M., A. S. Pai, E. M. Leaf, H. Y. Yang, B. A. Bartley, K. K. Quan, C. M. Ingalls, H. W. Liao, and C. M. Giachelli. 2009. Phosphate feeding induces arterial medial calcification in uremic mice: Role of serum phosphorus, fibroblast growth factor-23, and osteopontin. *Kidney Int* 75 (12):1297–307.

Giachelli, C. M., S. Jono, A. Shioi, Y. Nishizawa, K. Mori, and H. Morii. 2001. Vascular calcification and inorganic phosphate. *Am J Kidney Dis* 38 (4 Suppl 1):S34–7.

GRAS (Generally Recognized as Safe) Food Ingredients–Phosphates. 1972. Philadelphia, PA: The Franklin Institute Research Labs.

Gutierrez, O. M., C. Anderson, T. Isakova, J. Scialla, L. Negrea, A. H. Anderson, K. Bellovich, J. Chen, N. Robinson, A. Ojo, J. Lash, H. I. Feldman, and M. Wolf. 2010. Low socioeconomic status associates with higher serum phosphate irrespective of race. *J Am Soc Nephrol* 21 (11):1953–60.

Gutierrez, O. M., T. Isakova, G. Enfield, and M. Wolf. 2011. Impact of poverty on serum phosphate concentrations in the Third National Health and Nutrition Examination Survey. *J Ren Nutr* 21 (2):140–8.

Gutierrez, O. M., R. Katz, C. A. Peralta, I. H. de Boer, D. Siscovick, M. Wolf, A. Diez Roux, B. Kestenbaum, J. A. Nettleton, and J. H. Ix. 2012. Associations of socioeconomic status and processed food intake with serum phosphorus concentration in community-living adults: The Multi-Ethnic Study of Atherosclerosis (MESA). *J Ren Nutr* 22 (5):480–9.

Institute of Medicine. 1997. *Dietary References Intakes for Calcium, Phosphorus, Magnesium, Vitamin D, and Fluoride.* Washington, DC: The National Academics Press. https://doi.org/10.17226/5776

Iqbal, T. H., K. O. Lewis, and B. T. Cooper. 1994. Phytase activity in the human and rat small intestine. *Gut* 35 (9):1233–6.

Isakova, T., P. Wahl, G. S. Vargas, O. M. Gutierrez, J. Scialla, H. Xie, D. Appleby, L. Nessel, K. Bellovich, J. Chen, L. Hamm, C. Gadegbeku, E. Horwitz, R. R. Townsend, C. A. Anderson, J. P. Lash, C. Y. Hsu, M. B. Leonard, and M. Wolf. 2011. Fibroblast growth factor 23 is elevated before parathyroid hormone and phosphate in chronic kidney disease. *Kidney Int* 79 (12):1370–8.

Joung, H., B. Y. Jeun, S. J. Li, J. Kim, L. R. Woodhouse, J. C. King, R. M. Welch, and H. Y. Paik. 2007. Fecal phytate excretion varies with dietary phytate and age in women. *J Am Coll Nutr* 26 (3):295–302.

Karp, H. J., K. P. Vaihia, M. U. Karkkainen, M. J. Niemisto, and C. J. Lamberg-Allardt. 2007. Acute effects of different phosphorus sources on calcium and bone metabolism in young women: A whole-foods approach. *Calcif Tissue Int* 80 (4):251–8.

Kestenbaum, B., J. N. Sampson, K. D. Rudser, D. J. Patterson, S. L. Seliger, B. Young, D. J. Sherrard, and D. L. Andress. 2005. Serum phosphate levels and mortality risk among people with chronic kidney disease. *J Am Soc Nephrol* 16 (2):520–8.

Lau, W. L., A. Pai, S. M. Moe, and C. M. Giachelli. 2011. Direct effects of phosphate on vascular cell function. *Adv Chronic Kidney Dis* 18 (2):105–12.

Leon, J. B., C. M. Sullivan, and A. R. Sehgal. 2013. The prevalence of phosphorus-containing food additives in top-selling foods in grocery stores. *J Ren Nutr* 23 (4):265–70, e2.

Lin, Y., S. Bolca, S. Vandevijvere, H. Van Oyen, J. Van Camp, G. De Backer, L. H. Foo, S. De Henauw, and I. Huybrechts. 2011. Dietary sources of animal and plant protein intake among Flemish preschool children and the association with socio-economic and lifestyle-related factors. *Nutr J* 10:97.

Maga, J. A. 1982. Phytate: Its chemistry, occurrence, food interactions, nutritional significance, and methods of analysis. *J Agric Food Chem* 30:1–9.

Maillot, M., N. Darmon, F. Vieux, and A. Drewnowski. 2007. Low energy density and high nutritional quality are each associated with higher diet costs in French adults. *Am J Clin Nutr* 86 (3):690–6.

Mathew, S., K. S. Tustison, T. Sugatani, L. R. Chaudhary, L. Rifas, and K. A. Hruska. 2008. The mechanism of phosphorus as a cardiovascular risk factor in CKD. *J Am Soc Nephrol* 19 (6):1092–105.

Mehrotra, R., C. A. Peralta, S. C. Chen, S. Li, M. Sachs, A. Shah, K. Norris, G. Saab, A. Whaley-Connell, B. Kestenbaum, and P. A. McCullough. 2013. No independent association of serum phosphorus with risk for death or progression to end-stage renal disease in a large screen for chronic kidney disease. *Kidney Int* 84 (5):989–97.

Molins, R.A. 1991. *Phosphates in Food.* Boca Raton, FL: CRC Press.

Monsivais, P. and A. Drewnowski. 2009. Lower-energy-density diets are associated with higher monetary costs per kilocalorie and are consumed by women of higher socioeconomic status. *J Am Diet Assoc* 109 (5):814–22.

Moore, L. V. and A. V. Diez Roux. 2006. Associations of neighborhood characteristics with the location and type of food stores. *Am J Public Health* 96 (2):325–31.

Moore, L. V., A. V. Diez Roux, J. A. Nettleton, D. R. Jacobs, and M. Franco. 2009. Fast-food consumption, diet quality, and neighborhood exposure to fast food: The multi-ethnic study of atherosclerosis. *Am J Epidemiol* 170 (1):29–36.

Morland, K., S. Wing, and A. Diez Roux. 2002. The contextual effect of the local food environment on residents' diets: The atherosclerosis risk in communities study. *Am J Public Health* 92 (11):1761–7.

Morland, K., S. Wing, A. Diez Roux, and C. Poole. 2002. Neighborhood characteristics associated with the location of food stores and food service places. *Am J Prev Med* 22 (1):23–9.

Murphy-Gutekunst, L. 2005. Hidden phosphorus in popular beverages. *Nephrol Nurs J* 32 (4):443–5.

Oenning, L. L., J. Vogel, and M. S. Calvo. 1988. Accuracy of methods estimating calcium and phosphorus intake in daily diets. *J Am Diet Assoc* 88 (9):1076–80.

Scialla, J. J., L. J. Appel, M. Wolf, W. Yang, X. Zhang, S. M. Sozio, E. R. Miller, 3rd, L. A. Bazzano, M. Cuevas, M. J. Glenn, E. Lustigova, R. R. Kallem, A. C. Porter, R. R. Townsend, M. R. Weir, and C. A. Anderson. 2012. Plant protein intake is associated with fibroblast growth factor 23 and serum bicarbonate levels in patients with chronic kidney disease: The Chronic Renal Insufficiency Cohort study. *J Ren Nutr* 22 (4):379–388, e1.

Sherman, R. A. and O. Mehta. 2009a. Dietary phosphorus restriction in dialysis patients: Potential impact of processed meat, poultry, and fish products as protein sources. *Am J Kidney Dis* 54 (1):18–23.

Sherman, R. A. and O. Mehta. 2009b. Phosphorus and potassium content of enhanced meat and poultry products: Implications for patients who receive dialysis. *Clin J Am Soc Nephrol* 4 (8):1370–3.

Shuto, E., Y. Taketani, R. Tanaka, N. Harada, M. Isshiki, M. Sato, K. Nashiki, K. Amo, H. Yamamoto, Y. Higashi, Y. Nakaya, and E. Takeda. 2009. Dietary phosphorus acutely impairs endothelial function. *J Am Soc Nephrol* 20 (7):1504–12.

Stahl, J. L. and R. H. Ellinger. 1971. The use of phosphate in the cereal and baking industry. *In Symposium: Phosphate in Food Processing*, edited by J. M. Deman and P. Melnychyn. Westport, CT: The Avi Publishing Company.

Tonelli, M., F. Sacks, M. Pfeffer, Z. Gao, and G. Curhan. 2005. Relation between serum phosphate level and cardiovascular event rate in people with coronary disease. *Circulation* 112 (17):2627–33.

Uribarri, J. 2007. Phosphorus homeostasis in normal health and in chronic kidney disease patients with special emphasis on dietary phosphorus intake. *Semin Dial* 20 (4):295–301.

Uribarri, J. and M. S. Calvo. 2003. Hidden sources of phosphorus in the typical American diet: Does it matter in nephrology? *Semin Dial* 16 (3):186–8.

17 Bioavailability of Phosphorus

Suvi T. Itkonen, Heini J. Karp,
and Christel J. E. Lamberg-Allardt

CONTENTS

Abstract 221
Bullet Points 221
17.1 Introduction 222
17.2 *In Vitro* Determinations of Phosphorus Bioavailability 222
    17.2.1 Phosphorus Content and Digestibility of Plant-Based Foods 223
        17.2.1.1 Effects of Processing on Cereal Phosphorus Digestibility 224
    17.2.2 Phosphorus Digestibility and Total Content in Beverages 225
    17.2.3 Phosphorus Digestibility and Total Content in Meat and Meat Products ... 225
    17.2.4 Phosphorus Digestibility and Total Content in Dairy Products 226
17.3 Effects of Different Phosphorus Sources on Phosphorus Metabolism in Humans ... 227
17.4 Future Challenges in Assessing Phosphorus Bioavailability 231
References 231

ABSTRACT

Phosphorus (P) intake in Western countries exceeds the nutritional recommendations two- to three-fold, and the increased use of food additive phosphates by the food industry has augmented total P intake with an estimated 10% to 50% of the total P intake coming from additives. Moreover, in food composition databases, P contents of the recipe-based foodstuffs are calculated based on nutrient content of raw materials and not on chemically analyzed values of the finished food product. Thus, the amount of phosphate from additives may not have been taken into account when estimating the total P content.

    The chemical composition of a foodstuff affects the bioavailability of P. Both human (*in vivo*) and in vitro studies have shown that bioavailability of P differs between the foodstuffs. Bioavailability of P is higher in processed, phosphate additive–containing foods, such as in processed meats, baking powder–containing bakery products, processed cheeses, and cola drinks. In contrast, P bioavailability of plant-based products is low, especially in legumes and seeds. In cereals, P bioavailability increases during processing when, for example, the bread is fermented and P from phytate is released as absorbable, inorganic P through the action of microbial phytase. Phosphorus bioavailability from animal-based products is generally high, with the exception of cottage cheese. Thus, effects of P on health may depend on the source from which it is ingested. However, there is a growing need to develop research methods by which P bioavailability can be taken into account. Data on the use of food additive phosphates by the food industry and updated information on P content in foodstuffs are also needed.

BULLET POINTS

- Phosphorus bioavailability is highest from processed food containing phosphate additives.
- Phosphorus bioavailability from animal-based foods is relatively lower but generally high.
- Phosphorus bioavailability of legumes and seeds is relatively poor.
- Processing (e.g., fermentation) of cereals increases the amount of bioavailable phosphorus.
- Reliable methods to measure phosphorus bioavailability are needed.

17.1 INTRODUCTION

The goal of this chapter is to summarize our findings from a series of studies where we applied two new approaches to determining the bioavailability of phosphorus (P) from a variety of commonly eaten food categories. We developed both an *in vitro* digestion analytical method and an in vivo method, which relies on human consumption of whole foods and changes in serum and urine P as biomarkers of bioavailability. The important practical application of our findings from these studies is relevant to the improvement of the dietary management of chronic kidney disease (CKD) patients through the reduction of dietary P intake. There is a critical gap in our knowledge concerning the actual bioavailability of P from foods, most importantly those foods known to have high total P content, which kidney patients are currently strongly advised to avoid. Accurate knowledge of the poor bioavailability of P from some of these high P foods can help to expand the diet quality and healthy food choices of these patients and hopefully slow the progression of their disease.

P occurs naturally in many foodstuffs; however, bioavailability of P differs depending on the source. To understand the bioavailability of P, one should be aware of the chemical composition of P in each foodstuff. In grains, seeds, and legumes, most of the P is in the form of phytate, which stores inositol and P (Reddy 2002). However, small amounts of P in plant products occur as phospholipids (Molins 1991). Phytate needs to be hydrolyzed to release inorganic P (Pi) in a form available for intestinal absorption. Although phytase activity in the human gut is very low (Iqbal et al. 1994), different food-processing methods can be used to hydrolyze phytic acid (Plaami 1997). Thus, more P is likely to be digestible from processed (i.e., fermented, soaked) plant-derived foodstuffs than from raw or unprocessed foods.

In foodstuffs containing muscle protein (meat, poultry, fish), P is bound to amino acid side chains, which are released during the digestion process as inorganic Pi (Massey 2003). Phosphorus in animals occurs as nucleoproteins, phosphoproteins, phospholipids, and nucleotides and is also present in body fluids and some tissues (Molins 1991) and the high correlation of phosphorus with protein in foods is well established. The most important phosphoproteins found in foods are oval-bumin in eggs and casein in milk (Molins 1991). In milk, P exists in organic and inorganic forms (Gaucheron 2011). One-third occurs as inorganic P, 20% in ester bound casein amino acids, 40% in caseinate micelles, and the rest as water- and fat-soluble esters (Uribarri and Calvo 2003). The organic form is bound to molecules such as casein, phospholipids, DNA, RNA, nucleotides, and sugar Pi (Gaucheron 2011). Pi exists as phosphate ions, and the distribution between different phosphate valences depends on pH (Gaucheron 2011). In the processing of milk, part of the Pi can be transferred to the aqueous phase. Some of the Pi is lost to whey in cheese processing (Gaucheron 2011), which explains the differing Pi contents in various dairy products.

Phosphates can also be added to the foods in the form of inorganic phosphate salts or their derivatives (Uribarri and Calvo 2013). They are used for a number of reasons; they enable food products to achieve, for example, better texture, taste, emulsification, acidification, leavening, anticaking, moisture binding, antimicrobial action, color stability, iron binding, buffering, and freeze–thaw stability (Uribarri and Calvo 2013).

Our studies have revealed how various aspects of processing can increase or decrease the bioavailability of P in a food and how previously avoided, yet known healthy foods such as whole-grain products and nuts, offer very limited digestible P, despite their high total P content. Of further importance to the management of renal disease, we present sound evidence of the greater P bioavailability that occurs when foods are processed with phosphate-containing additives. These findings underscore the need to label the phosphorus content of processed foods.

17.2 *IN VITRO* DETERMINATIONS OF PHOSPHORUS BIOAVAILABILITY

In response to a long-standing gap in our knowledge about P bioavailability in foodstuffs, a new *in vitro* digestion analysis method that mimics the process that the foodstuffs undergo in the intestine was developed by Itkonen et al. (2012). This method utilizes the sample treatment method

Bioavailability of Phosphorus   **223**

described by Asp et al. (1983) for dietary fiber, with some modifications for the determination of digestible phosphorus (DP) (Ekholm et al. 2000). The Itkonen method first digests starch and proteins of the sample enzymatically, in the same manner as in the alimentary tract. The digested samples are subsequently dialyzed, and digestible phosphorus (DP) can be analyzed from the dialysate by inductively coupled plasma mass spectrometry (ICP-MS) or inductively coupled plasma optical emission spectrometry (ICP-OES). The insoluble mineral bound by food components remains in the dialysis residue.

Application of this *in vitro* method determined DP, a surrogate measure for P bioavailability, and was first applied to foods considered to be important P and protein sources. Meat, milk, grains, and legumes are important P and protein sources; thus products from these food groups were analyzed. In addition, foods containing P additives (i.e. cola beverages, processed cheeses, and meats) were analyzed. To clarify P contents of similar products, several labels among processed meats, cola beverages, cheeses, and breads were analyzed. Anticipating differences in composition among various products in a single category due to processing or formulation, several different brands of processed meats, cola beverages, cheeses, and breads were also analyzed. The nationally most popular products in each food category were chosen for analysis to facilitate future determination of specific potentially healthy products for renal patients (Karp et al. 2012a, b). Total phosphorus contents of various foodstuffs were analyzed with routine methods by ICP-MS (Itkonen et al. 2012) and ICP-OES (Karp et al. 2012a, b).

17.2.1 Phosphorus Content and Digestibility of Plant-Based Foods

The results of the total phosphorus (TP) and *in vitro* digestible phosphorus (DP) determinations in plant foods are shown in Table 17.1. Among the studied plant-based foods (Karp et al. 2012a), the highest P content was found in rye crisp (TP 291 mg/100 g), probably due to its low water but high whole-grain content. Apart from the rye crisp, the TP content of all other breads was similar with exception of white wheat bread (Itkonen et al. 2012), which was less than half that of the higher fiber-containing breads analyzed. Greater variation in DP content was observed in these breads. DP content of 89 and 53 mg/100 g was determined for two very similar small rye breads differing only by the potato content. In contrast, high content of both TP (212 mg/100 g) and DP (201 mg/100 g) was also found in commercially made muffins, which contain phosphate additives. The sweet bakery products, sweet buns (leavened with yeast), and cookies (containing no phosphate additives) had a P content similar to that in white wheat bread (Karp et al. 2012a). It is important to note that commercially prepared muffins containing phosphate additives (baking powder) differed from other wheat products; the percentage of DP was almost 100%, indicating greater bioavailability of added phosphate. TP content of muffins was similar to that of rye bread, but DP content was higher than in any cereal products.

In legumes, seeds, and products prepared from legumes, TP content varied between 59 mg/100 g in soaked chickpea and 667 mg/100 g in sesame seed. Legumes contained an average DP content of 83 mg/100 g (38% of TP). The proportion of DP from TP was lowest in legumes and seeds (6%–42% of TP). Earlier results have suggested that bioavailability of P from beans is only 25% (Uribarri 2007). Results of our *in vitro* analyses of phosphorus digestibility indicate that DP contents in legumes are, on average, higher than these earlier estimates. However, similarly to lentils, beans, and peas, sesame seeds with hulls had a low DP content (42 mg/100 g). This is in line with the results of an earlier short-term *in vivo* controlled study, where whole sesame seeds did not affect the concentrations of serum phosphorus (S-Pi), indicating them to be poor sources of bioavailable P (Kärkkäinen et al. 1997). Nevertheless, the cooking time of lentils, green beans, and peas is relatively short, and these products do not require soaking before cooking (except dry peas), which would decrease phytate contents and release inorganic Pi (Sandberg 2002). Thus, it is unlikely that a large proportion of phytate is hydrolyzed during processing, and therefore, DP content in lentils, green beans, and peas would not increase appreciably, if at all, when these products are cooked.

TABLE 17.1
Total Phosphorus (TP) and *In Vitro* Digestible Phosphorus (DP) Content of the Analyzed Plant Foods

Product	TP (mg/100 g)	DP (mg/100 g)
Bakery products		
Rye bread pool	208	123
Rye crisp	291	191
Small rye bread containing potato 1	192	89
Small rye bread containing potato 2	206	54
White wheat bread[*]	83	42
Mixed grain bread with seeds	189	116
Muffin pool[a]	212	201
Sweet bun pool	116	60
Cookie pool	125	43
Legumes and seeds		
Sesame seed (with hull)	667	42
Tofu (firm)	164	51
Green bean	57	24
Green pea (frozen)	118	50
Chickpea (soaked)	149	53
Red lentil	432	167
Green lentil	400	120
Beverages		
Pepsi Max[b]	14	15
Coca-Cola light[b]	13	13
Coca-Cola[b]	19	16
Cola pool[b]	17	16
Freeway Cola light[b]	11	10
Beer	21	22

[a] Contains sodium polyphosphate as an additive.
[b] Contains phosphoric acid as an additive.
[*] Result from Itkonen et al. (2012).

17.2.1.1 Effects of Processing on Cereal Phosphorus Digestibility

The effect of processing at various stages of cereal food production on the DP and TP content of cereals (wheat and rye flours, doughs, home-baked and bakery breads) were analyzed by inductively coupled plasma-mass spectrometry (Itkonen et al. 2012). Different rye breads were found to have similar proportions of DP (68%–78%), whereas in rye dough, the proportion of DP was almost 100%. In earlier studies, the phytic acid content in rye bread was almost reduced to zero during processing (Fretzdorff and Brümmer 1992; Larsson and Sandberg 1991), which probably also occurred in this study, but during the process of baking rye bread some P in the dough may have become insoluble for unknown reasons because the DP content in the baked bread was lower than in dough. The results were similar to those of previous studies in which phytates were mostly degraded in sourdough rye bread (Plaami and Kumpulainen 1995). In support of the finding that microbial action (fermentation) was experienced when making sourdough rye bread, Karp et al. (2007) found that the intake of unfermented cereals did not increase S-Pi concentration compared with other P sources, such as cheese and meat, indicating a lower bioavailability of P in cereals. The bakery breads did not apparently differ in DP or TP contents compared with home-baked bread, even though they most likely were leavened

Bioavailability of Phosphorus

for a shorter time than the home-baked breads. No exact information about fermentation times of the bakery products was available. When compared to other analyzed cereals, the TP content in flour was much higher (about 300 mg/100 g) than in doughs or breads, because doughs and breads also contain ingredients besides flour. TP content in wheat samples was lower than in rye products because the fiber and whole-grain contents were lower. In the analyzed wheat samples, the mean proportion of DP was about 50%, and it increased with processing especially in soured wheat bread. The results showed that the DP content in processed cereals was higher than in unprocessed cereals (Itkonen et al. 2012). This is probably because during processing of foodstuffs, such as bread making, phytate was degraded to lower inositol Pi and the same process formed inorganic Pi, which increased the DP content (Sandberg 2002). The products were processed under circumstances where both enzymatic and nonenzymatic degradation can occur (low pH, high temperature, presence of yeast, hydrothermal processing) (Sandberg 2002; Sandberg and Andlid 2002); some of the doughs were soured and some were leavened with yeast, and baked, which should increase the inorganic Pi contents.

17.2.2 Phosphorus Digestibility and Total Content in Beverages

In beer and cola beverages (Table 17.1), all P was digestible (DP 10–16 mg/100 g in cola drinks; 22 mg/100 g in beer) (Karp et al. 2012a). This result is in line with results on high absorbability of P from food additives such as phosphoric acid in cola drinks, which appears to be absorbed completely in the intestine (Bell et al. 1977; Karp et al. 2007). TP contents in both cola drinks and beer were comparable with values published earlier (Murphy-Gutekunst 2005). In beer, P originates from the grain used in making the product. Based on these results, it seems that during malting and other processing of grain when brewing beer, P is efficiently released from the grain to a highly digestible form, resulting in a high proportion of DP. Processing of beer also includes long-term fermentation of grains with yeast, which are known to contain phytase, and thus, the ability to degrade phytate to bioavailable P (Türk et al. 2006). However, in beer, as in some cola beverages the amount of DP exceeded the amount of TP. This may be explained by the uncertainty of the analysis method under circumstances of low P content.

17.2.3 Phosphorus Digestibility and total Content in Meat and Meat Products

In sausages and cold cuts, the TP content shown in Table 17.2 varied between 175 and 279 mg/100 g (Karp et al. 2012b). The highest values were found in boiled ham that contained phosphate additives.

TABLE 17.2
Total Phosphorus (TP) and *In Vitro* Digestible Phosphorus (DP) Content of the Analyzed Meat and Meat Products

Product	TP (mg/100 g)	DP (mg/100 g)
Processed sausage, 18% fat	210	224
Processed sausage, light, 10% fat[a]	241	242
Frankfurter pool, 20% fat[a]	175	144
Frankfurter pool, light, 13% fat[a]	186	130
Sausage, dry, salami type[a]	244	171
Sausage cold cuts[a]	184	164
Boiled ham[a]	279	255
Raw pork steak	212	161
Raw chicken fillet	229	191
Raw beef	199	147
Raw rainbow trout fillet	232	207

[a] Contains food additive phosphates.

The TP content of a salami-type sausage was similar to that of a low-fat processed sausage, but the DP content of the former was 24% lower than that of the latter. The P content in frankfurters was slightly lower than in other sausages or cold cuts. The TP contents varied between 199 and 232 mg/100 g in raw meats and rainbow trout. Greater variation seemed to exist in the DP content of the meats (147–207 mg/100 g). Among the foods we analyzed, raw meats and meat products did not have very high TP content, but the DP content of some processed meats were among the highest values determined. When raw meats were compared, only small differences were found among chicken, pork, beef, and rainbow trout. TP content of the P-additive–free meats is similar to those of unenhanced meats published earlier (Sullivan et al. 2007; Sherman and Mehta 2009a). The DP content of raw meats varied more than TP content, with the lowest DP content present in beef and the highest in rainbow trout. However, determination of the TP and DP content of cooked meats need more attention in the future, as cooking itself and likely also the cooking method affect the P content of a food (Cupisti et al. 2012; Delgado-Andrade et al. 2011; Cupisti et al. 2006) (Table 17.2).

In sausages and cold cuts, the lowest percentages of DP relative to TP were found in the salami-type sausage and in low-fat frankfurters. The content of P additives in the salami-type sausage was likely lower than that in other sausages, as one of the sausages in the salami-type sausage pool did not contain any P additives. Also, the consistency of salami is different from that of other sausages. Phosphates increase the water content of a product, which is an unwanted quality in a dry salami-type sausage. The results indicate that frankfurters may contain less P than other sausages, but other brands should be analyzed before drawing further conclusions. In addition, some variance between products manufactured in different countries may exist.

17.2.4 Phosphorus Digestibility and Total Content in Dairy Products

As shown in Table 17.3, all processed and hard cheeses had the highest TP and DP contents among all foods analyzed (Karp et al. 2012b). In unprocessed hard cheeses, the TP content varied between 529 and 638 mg/100 g, but the DP content seemed to be lower (53%–76% of TP). These results confirm previous data on cheeses as P-rich foods to be avoided by patients with chronic kidney disease. Notably, an extremely high content of DP was found in processed cheeses, providing evidence in support of earlier

---

TABLE 17.3

Total Phosphorus (TP) and *In Vitro* Digestible Phosphorus (DP) Content of the Analyzed Dairy Foods

Product	TP (mg/100 g)	DP (mg/100 g)
Milk, 1.5% fat	108	85
Skimmed milk	122	75
Processed cheese, individually packed slices, 5% fat[a]	574	589
Processed cheese, individually packed slices, 12% fat[a]	647	720
Processed cheese, individually packed slices, 23% fat[a]	584	576
Cheese spread, 9% fat[a]	92	794
Cheese spread, 22% fat[a]	755	772
Hard cheeses pool, 5%–17% fat	638	484
Hard cheeses pool, 24%–29% fat	529	282
Cottage cheese	146	71

[a] Contains food additive phosphates.

Bioavailability of Phosphorus

warnings to avoid them due to their known higher phosphate additive content. This finding is in accord with earlier study of Karp et al. (2007), in which regular cheese not containing P additives increased the S-Pi concentration more than meat, whole grains, or even a mixture of P additives, suggesting that P from processed cheese is easily and efficiently absorbed. Furthermore, in a cross-sectional study on a randomly selected subgroup of 31- to 43-year-old Finnish women, consumption of processed cheeses was associated with a higher mean serum parathyroid hormone (S-PTH) concentration (Kemi et al. 2009).

Variation in both DP (589–794 mg/100 g) and TP (574–892 mg/100 g) was found among processed cheeses, which also showed very high percentages of total P that is digestible (DP/TP 89%–100%). The P content seems not to depend on the fat or protein content of the processed cheese; the TP and DP contents were higher in cheese spreads than in sliced processed cheese. Possibly, the softer texture of cheese spreads requires more P additives for water retention than the harder texture of sliced, processed cheeses. Contrary to other cheeses, cottage cheese had the lowest absolute DP content and the DP-to-TP proportion among the analyzed dairy products, which may be due to the specific processing method used. In other countries, such as the United States, cottage cheese curd can be set with phosphoric acid or involve other phosphorus containing additives or may not contain them (Joint FAO/WHO Codex Alimentarius Commission 2010). The P contents of fresh cheeses are lower than those of hard cheeses or processed cheeses because of the higher water content of fresh cheeses and possibly because of a different preparation technique from hard cheeses.

To conclude the results of these *in vitro* bioavailability studies, both TP and DP contents varied widely between the different food groups analyzed and also within many food groups. Results of TP can largely be explained by protein content of the food and/or use of P-containing food additives. Proportion of DP to TP content seems to be affected by processing of food in phytic acid–containing plant foods and by the presence of P-containing food additives. Furthermore, the results support previous findings of better P absorbability in foods of animal origin. Variation among similar products, however, seems to exist. This variation often depends not only on the protein or fat content of the food but also on the use of P additives, which can affect the desired texture of the food.

17.3 EFFECTS OF DIFFERENT P SOURCES ON PHOSPHORUS METABOLISM IN HUMANS

Karp et al. (2012a, b) investigated the effects of different phosphorus sources on serum phosphate (S-Pi), urinary phosphate (U-Pi), and serum parathyroid hormone (S-PTH) concentrations in 16 healthy female volunteers who participated in five separate 24-hour sessions (Karp et al. 2007). At the control session, both P and Ca intakes were low (approximately 500 and 250 mg/day, respectively). During the other four sessions, P intake was approximately 1500 mg/day, 1000 mg of which was obtained from meat, cheese, whole grains, or a phosphate supplement, respectively. The S-Pi concentration was elevated during the meat, cheese, whole-grain, and supplement sessions compared with the control session (Figure 17.1a). Cheese increased the S-Pi concentration more than the other Pi sources. The S-Pi concentration also remained higher in the cheese session on the following morning than in all other sessions. U-Pi excretion was higher in all Pi sessions than in the control session and meat as well as the supplement increased U-Pi excretion more than grain or cheese (Figure 17.1b). Compared with the other sessions, cheese decreased S-PTH most (Figure 17.2). By contrast, Pi supplement increased S-PTH concentration compared with the control session, whereas meat or grain had no effect on S-PTH. Differences were observed between study sessions also in S-PTH concentrations of the second-day fasting samples, and the S-PTH concentration was lower in the cheese session on the following morning compared to all other sessions.

In another study, the effects of monophosphates and polyphosphates on S-Pi, U-Pi, and S-PTH in 14 healthy female volunteers were investigated in three separate 24-h sessions (Karp et al. 2013). During each session, the subjects ingested a monophosphate (MP), polyphosphate (PP), or placebo supplement during three meals. The MP supplement contained sodium dihydrogen phosphate, and the PP contained

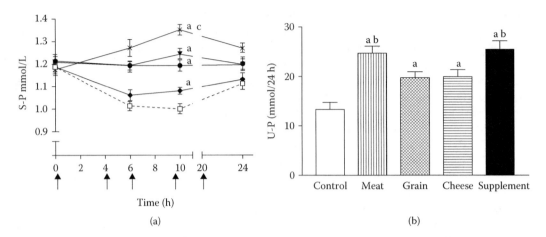

FIGURE 17.1 Changes in serum phosphate (S-P) concentration (a) and 24-hour urinary excretion of phosphate (U-P) (b) during the five study sessions. (a) Control (□), meat (●), supplement (▼), cheese (×), and grain (♦) session. Arrows indicate mealtimes. The different phosphorus sources affected the AUC values of S-P (ANOVA, $P = 0.0001$) and 24-hour U-P (ANOVA, $P = 0.0001$); [a]significantly different from control session, [b]significantly different from grain and cheese sessions, [c]significantly different from all other sessions. (Reproduced from Karp HJ et al., *Calcif Tissue Int.*, 80, 251–258, 2007.)

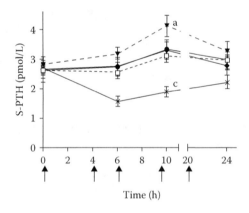

FIGURE 17.2 Changes in serum parathyroid hormone (PTH) concentration during control (□), meat (●), supplement (▼), cheese (x), and grain (♦) session. Arrows indicate mealtimes. The different phosphorus sources affected the AUC values of S-PTH (ANOVA, $p = 0.0001$); [a]significantly different from control session, [c]significantly different from all other sessions. (Reproduced from Karp HJ et al., *Calcif Tissue Int.*, 80, 251–258, 2007).

sodium tripolyphosphate. The Pi supplements contained 1500 mg/d of P, with each dose containing 500 mg of P. The meals served during each study session were identical, containing 500 mg of P and 340 mg of Ca. Both MP and PP increased S-Pi compared with the control session, and the difference between the MP and PP sessions in S-Pi was not statistically significant (Figure 17.3a). Differences were also found in the urinary Pi excretion among the study sessions (Figure 17.3b), whereas both MP and PP increased U-Pi, compared with the control session. However, no differences between the MP and PP sessions in U-Pi excretion were found. S-PTH concentrations differed between the study sessions (Figure 17.4) as both MP and PP increased the S-PTH compared with the control session, the increase in S-PTH being similar with both Pi salts.

As generally known, serum and urinary Pi concentrations are indirect measures of absorbed P, and U-Pi is affected by PTH secretion. Still, in a controlled setting, comparing S- and U-Pi after

Bioavailability of Phosphorus

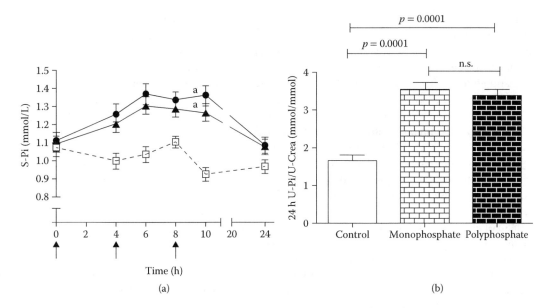

FIGURE 17.3 Changes in serum phosphate (S-Pi) concentration (a) and 24-hour urinary excretion of phosphate (U-Pi/Crea) (b) during the three study sessions. (a): control (□), monophosphate (●), polyphosphate (▲). The supplement administration times are indicated with an arrow. The supplements affected the area under the curve values of S-Pi (ANOVA, $p = 0.0001$) and 24-h U-Pi/Crea (ANOVA, $p = 0.0001$). Significantly different from control session. (Reproduced from Karp HJ et al., *Eur J Nutr.*, 52, 991–996, 2013.)

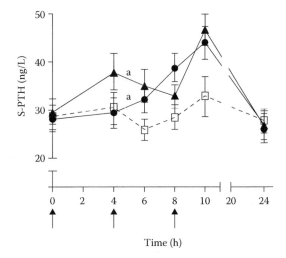

FIGURE 17.4 Changes in serum parathyroid hormone (S-PTH) concentration during the three study sessions. Control (□), monophosphate (●), polyphosphate (▲). The supplement administration times are indicated with an arrow. The supplements affected the AUC values of S-PTH (ANOVA, $p = 0.019$); significantly different from control session. (Reproduced from Karp HJ et al., *Eur J Nutr.*, 52, 991–996, 2013.)

ingesting different P sources provides information on P absorbability. Based on S-Pi and U-Pi results in the Karp et al. (2007) study on healthy young women, P from meat and supplements appears to absorb better than P from whole grains. The whole-grain foods given to the subjects (oatmeal porridge, rye bread) were unfermented. Because fermentation can improve the absorption of minerals in phytate-containing foods, the bioavailability of P may be higher from fermented whole grains and even greater from low-fiber grains. P supplements and meat had similar effects on S-Pi and

U-Pi. As meat did not affect S-PTH, it remains unclear whether this is difference due to variation in absorbability, protein intake, or another factor. The results show that cheese decreases S-PTH, probably due to its high Ca content, meat and grain have no effect on S-PTH, and P additives—both monophosphates and polyphosphates—increase S-PTH relative to control session.

Estimation of the absorbability of P from cheese is more complex than that of whole grains because the high calcium (Ca) content can decrease PTH secretion, which decreases U-Pi excretion. Thus, the low U-Pi excretion in the cheese session was probably due to low S-PTH concentration caused by the high Ca intake. S-Pi increased during the cheese session more than during any other session. Decreased U-Pi caused by low PTH secretion may have caused an increase in S-Pi by increasing the renal P threshold. A decrease in bone resorption in terms of decreased urinary N-terminal telopeptide of type I collagen concentrations was also found (results not shown here), which likely caused a drop in the release of P from bone, which could decrease S-Pi concentration. The effects of these two mechanisms counteract each other's effect on S-Pi. A more likely explanation is that P intake during the cheese session was slightly higher than during other P sessions, which may have increased S-Pi concentration. Probably many of these factors simultaneously affected S-Pi during the cheese ingestion, with the outcome being increased S-Pi. However, based on another short-term controlled study, both milk and cheese increased S-Pi efficiently, which suggests that P from dairy foods is well absorbed and therefore readily bioavailable (Kärkkäinen et al. 1997). Both Pi salts, commonly used in the food industry, affected S-Pi and U-Pi in a similar manner and therefore, were likely to absorb equally well.

The effect on mineral metabolism of P additives apparently differs from that of foods containing natural P. In most interventions, P has been administered as a supplement (Portale et al. 1986; Calvo and Heath 1988; Brixen et al. 1992; Kärkkäinen and Lamberg-Allardt 1996; Kemi et al. 2006; Trautvetter et al. 2016). In all but one of these studies, a rise in PTH secretion as a result of P administration was observed. In addition to our study (Karp et al. 2007), at least two interventions have been conducted using diets assembled from common foods (Calvo et al. 1988, 1990). Also, in these studies a sustained rise in S-PTH concentration with low-Ca, high-P diet was found. In the latter two studies, the intake of P additives was high in the test diet compared to the control diet because the high-P test diet was assembled from grocery foods with P additives, whereas the control was made up of foods largely without P additives. For this reason, the effects of the high-P diets are likely attributed to P additives in these studies. Moreover, Bell et al. (1977) observed enhanced parathyroid activity measured indirectly by biomarkers of PTH action as a response to foods containing P additives compared to the same foods prepared without additives. The PTH-raising effect of P additive intake compared with other sources could be due to their better absorbability.

When investigating different Pi salts in healthy young women (Karp et al. 2013), both MP and PP increased S-PTH, as seen in previous intervention studies conducted with P additives (Kärkkäinen and Lamberg-Allardt 1996; Kemi et al. 2006). Hence, both MP and PP affect PTH secretion similarly, even though previously MP increased urinary cyclic adenosine monophosphate (cAMP) (as a surrogate marker of PTH activity) more than did PP (Zemel and Linkswiler 1981). Because cAMP excretion is an indirect measure of PTH secretion, we consider our results more accurate. The increase in S-PTH may partly have been due to the Ca-binding capacity of Pi, especially PP. In that study, however, it was not possible to detect a difference in S-PTH between the MP and PP sessions. It is possible that more samples would have been required to detect all the differences in the serum measurements. As no samples were taken between 0 and 4 and 10 and 24 hours, we do not know what happened with S-PTH and S-Pi during these periods. With more frequent sampling the diurnal variation of PTH may have been captured in more detail.

One shortcoming in these earlier studies exploring P additive intake is the inability to determine the effects of P on fibroblast growth factor-23 (FGF23) as the assays were not available at that time. A recent German eight-week intervention trial showed a potential adaption to high P intake from supplements when FGF23 was higher after four weeks than at the study endpoint at eight weeks, but the use of P and Ca intakes that do not reflect typical Western dietary patterns make these findings

Bioavailability of Phosphorus

difficult to interpret (Trautvetter et al. 2016). To our present knowledge, no whole-food studies on FGF23 have been carried out.

In conclusion, there are acute differences in metabolic responses to P from different foods and P additives. The effects of high P intake appear to depend on the P sources consumed and other nutrients of the P-containing food. Our study findings provide evidence that P additives commonly used by food industries are absorbed well and likely increase S-PTH, as shown in previous studies; but in contrast, P from meat or whole grains appears not to affect S-PTH.

17.4 FUTURE CHALLENGES IN ASSESSING PHOSPHORUS BIOAVAILABILITY

Chemically analyzed phosphorus contents of foodstuffs often differ from the values of food composition databases, especially among foods containing additive phosphates (Carrigan et al. 2014; León et al. 2013; Benini et al. 2011; Sherman and Mehta 2009a, b; Sullivan et al. 2007). This generally causes inaccuracy and underestimation in the estimates of phosphorus intakes. Due to the lower bioavailability of plant-derived P, the use of a correction factor in P intake for plant-derived P has been proposed (McCarty 2014). However, correction factors may introduce error into results until reliable methods are developed to estimate P bioavailability (Chang et al. 2014). More importantly, the main problems may be the ones that are caused by unknown exposure to food additive phosphates, as well as by food preparation (Chang et al. 2014). For estimating dietary P intake, the 24-h urine Pi excretion measurement has been reported to estimate the amount of dietary phosphorus intake more accurately than estimates from weighed dietary records; however, there was poor agreement between these two measures in a recent study (Morimoto et al. 2014). When adjustment for the phosphorus:protein ratio, a recognized constant, was made for both the diet estimates and urine collections, Morimoto et al. found that the ratios in the 24-hour urine collection were higher than those estimated from the dietary records, indicating that urine P was higher than intake estimates. One explanation offered to explain this difference was the unaccounted phosphate food additives that may have confounded the estimated phosphorus intake in the weighed dietary records and, due to their higher bioavailability, raised urine P concentrations higher than intake estimates. Others have suggested the use of algorithms to better quantify P bioavailability. Algorithms could be developed to adjust for such confounding from these efficiently absorbed P additives and possible interfering interactions with calcium and other nutrients similar to what has been developed for dietary iron or folate bioavailability estimates (Calvo and Tucker 2013). Nonetheless, there is a need to further develop standardized methods to analyze bioavailable P content in foodstuffs (Itkonen 2015) and to better identify and quantify effects of co-consumed foods and nutrients like calcium on phosphorus bioavailability (Kemi et al. 2009).

REFERENCES

Asp NG., Johansson CG., Hallmer H., Siljeström M., Rapid enzymatic assay of insoluble and soluble dietary fiber. *J Agric Food Chem* 1983;31:476–482.

Bell RR., Draper HH., Tzeng DYM., Shin HK., Schmidt GR., Physiological responses of human adults to foods containing phosphate additives. *J Nutr* 1977;107:42–50.

Benini O., D'Alessandro C., Gianfaldoni D., Cupisti A., Extra-phosphate load from food additives in commonly eaten foods: A real and insidious danger for renal patients. *J Ren Nutr* 2011;21:303–308.

Brixen K., Nielsen HK., Charles P., Mosekilde L., Effect of a short course of oral phosphate treatment on serum parathyroid hormone (1-84) and biochemical markers of bone turnover: A dose-response study. *Calcif Tissue Int* 1992;51:276–281.

Calvo MS., Heath H., 3rd. Acute effects of phosphate-salt ingestion on serum phosphorus, serum ionized calcium, and parathyroid hormone in young adults. *Am J Clin Nutr* 1988;47:1025–1029.

Calvo MS., Kumar R., Heath H., 3rd. Elevated secretion and action of serum parathyroid hormone in young adults consuming high phosphorus, low calcium diets assembled from common foods. *J Clin Endocrinol Metab* 1988;66:823–829.

232 Dietary Phosphorus: Health, Nutrition, and Regulatory Aspects

Calvo MS., Kumar R., Heath H., 3rd. Persistently elevated parathyroid hormone secretion and action in young women after four weeks of ingesting high phosphorus, low calcium diets. *J Clin Endocrinol Metab* 1990;70:1334–1340.

Calvo MS., Tucker KL., Is phosphorus intake that exceeds dietary requirements a risk factor in bone health? *Ann NY Acad Sci* 2013;1301:29–35.

Carrigan A., Klinger A., Choquette SS., Luzuriaga-McPherson A., Bell EK., Darnell B., Gutiérrez OM., Contribution of food additives to sodium and phosphorus content of diets rich in processed foods. *J Ren Nutr* 2014;24:13–19.

Chang AR., Lazo M., Appel LJ., Gutiérrez OM., Grams ME., Reply to MF McCarty. *Am J Clin Nutr* 2014;99:966–967.

Cupisti A., Comar F., Benini O., Lupetti S., D'Alessandro C., Barsotti G., Gianfaldoni D., Effect of boiling on dietary phosphate and nitrogen intake. *J Ren Nutr* 2006;16:36–40.

Cupisti A., Benini O., Ferretti V., Gianfaldoni D., Kalantar-Zadeh K., Novel differential measurement of natural and added phosphorus in cooked ham with or without preservatives. *J Ren Nutr* 2012;22:533–540.

Delgado-Andrade C., Seiquer I., Mesías García M., Galdó G., Navarro MP., Increased Maillard reaction products intake reduces phosphorus digestibility in male adolescents. *Nutrition* 2011;27:86–91.

Ekholm P., Virkki L., Ylinen M., Johansson L., Varo P., Effects of natural chelating agents on the solubility of some physiologically important mineral elements in oat bran and oat flakes. *Cereal Chem* 2000;77:562–566.

Fretzdorff B., Brümmer JM., Reduction of phytic acid during breadmaking of whole-meal breads. *Cereal Chem* 1992;69:266–270.

Gaucheron F., Milk and dairy products: A unique micronutrient combination. *J Am Coll Nutr* 2011;30:400S–409S.

Iqbal TH., Lewis KO., Cooper BT., Phytase activity in the human and rat small intestine. *Gut* 1994;35:1233–1236.

Itkonen S., 2015. Dietary Phosphorus—Bioavailability and Associations with Vascular Calcification in a Middle-Aged Finnish Population. Dissertationes Scholae Doctoralis Ad Sanitatem Investigandam Universitatis Helsinkiensis 9, 2015. Academic Dissertation. Hansaprint 2015. E-Thesis. Available at https://helda.helsinki.fi/bitstream/handle/10138/153148/dietaryp.pdf?sequence=1.

Itkonen S., Ekholm P., Kemi V., Lamberg-Allardt C., Analysis of in vitro digestible phosphorus content in selected processed rye, wheat and barley products. *J Food Comp Anal* 2012;25:185–189.

Joint FAO/WHO Codex Alimentarius Commission. Codex Alimentarius: Standard for cottage cheese codex Stan 273-1968. Rome: World Health Organization, Food and Agriculture Organization of the United Nations, 2010.

Kärkkäinen M., Lamberg-Allardt C., An acute intake of phosphate increases parathyroid hormone secretion and inhibits bone formation in young women. *J Bone Miner Res* 1996;11:1905–1912.

Kärkkäinen MUM., Wiersma JW., Lamberg-Allardt CJE., Postprandial parathyroid hormone response to four calcium-rich foodstuffs. *Am J Clin Nutr* 1997;65:1726–1730.

Karp H., Ekholm P., Kemi V., Itkonen S., Hirvonen T., Närkki S., Lamberg-Allardt C., Differences among total and in vitro digestible phosphorus content of plant foods and beverages. *J Ren Nutr* 2012a;22:416–422.

Karp H., Ekholm P., Kemi V., Hirvonen T., Lamberg-Allardt C., Differences among total and in vitro digestible phosphorus content of meat and milk products. *J Ren Nutr* 2012b;22:344–349.

Karp HJ., Kemi VE., Lamberg-Allardt CJE., Kärkkäinen MUM., Mono- and polyphosphates have similar effects on calcium and phosphorus metabolism in healthy young women. *Eur J Nutr* 2013;52:991–996.

Karp HJ., Vaihia KP., Kärkkäinen MU., Niemistö MJ., Lamberg-Allardt CJE., Acute effects of different phosphorus sources on calcium and bone metabolism in young women: A whole foods approach. *Calcif Tissue Int* 2007;80:251–258.

Kemi VE., Kärkkäinen MU., Lamberg-Allardt CJ., High phosphorus intakes acutely and negatively affect Ca and bone metabolism in a dose-dependent manner in healthy young females. *Br J Nutr* 2006;96:545–552.

Kemi VE., Rita HR., Kärkkäinen MUM., Viljakainen HT., Laaksonen MM., Outila TA., Lamberg-Allardt CJE., Habitual high phosphorus intakes and foods with phosphate additives negatively affect serum parathyroid hormone concentrations: A cross-sectional study on healthy premenopausal women. *Public Health Nutr* 2009;12:1885–1892.

Larsson M., Sandberg AS., Phytate reduction in bread containing oat flour, oat bran or rye bran. *J Cereal Sci* 1991;14:141–149.

León JB., Sullivan CM., Sehgal AR., Prevalence of phosphorus-containing food additives in top-selling foods in grocery stores. *J Ren Nutr* 2013;23:265–270.

Massey LK., Dietary animal and plant protein and human bone health: A whole foods approach. *J Nutr* 2003;133:862S–865S.

McCarty MF., Lower bioavailability of plant-derived phosphorus. *Am J Clin Nutr* 2014;99:966.

Molins R., Food Phosphates. Boca Raton, FL: CRC Press, 1991.

Morimoto Y., Sakuma M., Ohta H., Suzuki A., Matsushita A., Umeda M., Ishikawa M., Taketani Y., Takeda E., Arai H., Estimate of dietary phosphorus intake using 24-h urine collection. *J Clin Biochem Nutr* 2014;55:62–66.

Murphy-Gutekunst L., Hidden phosphorus in popular beverages: Part 1. *J Ren Nutr* 2005;15:e1–e6.

Plaami S., Myoinositol phosphates: Analysis, content in foods and effects in nutrition. *LWT Food Sci Technol* 1997;30:633–647.

Plaami S., Kumpulainen J., Inositol phosphate content of some cereal-based foods. *J Food Comp Anal* 1995;8:324–335.

Portale AA., Halloran BP., Murphy MM., Morris RC., Jr. Oral intake of phosphorus can determine the serum concentrations of 1,25-dihydroxyvitamin by determining its production rate in humans. *J Clin Invest* 1986;77:7–12.

Reddy NR., Occurrence, distribution, content, and dietary intake of phytate. In Rukma NR., Sathe SK., (eds.). *Food Phytates.* Boca Raton, FL: CRC Press, 2002.

Sandberg AS., In vitro and in vivo degradation of phytate. In Rukma NR., Sathe SK., (eds.). *Food Phytates.* Boca Raton, FL: CRC Press, 2002.

Sandberg AS., Andlid T., Phytogenic and microbial phytases in human nutrition. *Int J Food Sci Tech* 2002;37:823–833.

Sherman RA., Mehta O., Dietary phosphorus restriction in dialysis patients: Potential impact of processed meat, poultry, and fish products as protein sources. *Am J Kidney Dis* 2009a;54:18–23.

Sherman RA., Mehta O., Phosphorus and potassium content of enhanced meat and poultry products: Implications for renal patients who receive dialysis. *Clin J Am Soc Nephrol* 2009b;4:1370–1373.

Sullivan CM., Leon JB., Sehgal AR., Phosphorus containing food additives and the accuracy of nutrient databases: Implications for renal patients. *J Ren Nutr* 2007;17:350–354.

Trautvetter U., Jahreis G., Kiehntopf M., Glei M., Consequnces of a high phosphorus intake on mineral metabolism and bone remodeling in depence of calcium intake in healthy subjects—A randomized placebo-controlled human intervention study. *Nutr J* 2016;15:7.

Türk M., Carlsson NG., Sandberg AS., Reduction in the levels of phytate during wholemeal bread making: Effect of yeast and wheat phytases. *J Cereal Sci* 1996;23:257–264.

Uribarri J., Phosphorus homeostasis in normal health and in chronic kidney disease patients with special emphasis on dietary phosphorus intake. *Semin Dial* 2007;20:295–301.

Uribarri J., Calvo M., Dietary phosphorus excess: A risk factor in chronic bone, kidney, and cardiovascular disease? *Adv Nutr* 2013;4:542–544.

Uribarri J., Calvo MS., Hidden sources of phosphorus in the typical American diet: Does it matter in nephrology? *Semin Dial* 2003;16:186–188.

Zemel MB., Linkswiler HM., Calcium metabolism in the young adult male as affected by level and form of phosphorus intake. *J Nutr* 1981;111:315–324.

18 Special Nutritional Needs of Chronic Kidney Disease and End-Stage Renal Disease Patients

Rationale for the Use of Plant-Based Diets

Ranjani N. Moorthi and Sharon M. Moe

CONTENTS

Abstract 235
Bullet Points 236
18.1   Introduction 236
18.2   Phytate: The Primary Source of Phosphate from Plants 237
18.3   Comparison of Grain versus Synthetic Feeds on Phosphorus and CKD-MBD in a
          Rodent Model 238
18.4   Effect of a Plant-Based Source of Protein on CKD-MBD in Humans 239
18.5   Other Effects of Plant-Based Diets in CKD 242
18.6   Conclusions 243
References 243

ABSTRACT

As kidney disease progresses, there is a rise in parathyroid hormone (PTH) and fibroblast growth factor-23 (FGF23) to increase urinary phosphate excretion and maintain normal serum phosphate levels until late in the course of kidney disease. At that time, this compensation is inadequate and hyperphosphatemia develops, and this is associated with arterial calcification and mortality in patients with kidney disease. In addition, chronic and persistent elevation in PTH and FGF23 can lead to adverse consequences such as left ventricular hypertrophy and bone loss. Thus, intervening by decreasing intestinal phosphorus absorption may prevent the rise in phosphate, PTH, and FGF23 levels that are observed with progressive kidney disease, leading to beneficial effects over time. One approach to decreasing intestinal phosphorus absorption is to ingest foods with lower bioavailable phosphorus. Grain-based (vegetarian) sources of protein contain phosphorus bound to phytate. Humans lack the enzyme phytase, and thus hydrolysis of phytate to release phosphate is reduced. In a rat model of chronic kidney disease (CKD), a grain-based versus synthetic casein–based protein diet of equivalent total phosphate and protein content led to reduced urinary phosphate excretion, lower PTH and FGF23 levels, and slower progression of kidney disease. In humans with stage 3b to 4 chronic kidney disease, a small cross-over trial found reduced urinary phosphate excretion with 100% vegetarian versus 100% meat-based diet consumed for one week. In a four-week study, a 70% plant-based diet similarly decreased the urinary phosphate excretion in patients with advanced kidney disease. Thus, grain/vegetarian-based diets contain less bioavailable phosphate and can provide an adequate source of protein yet decrease intestinal phosphate absorption. Long-term studies are needed to fully assess safety and efficacy.

BULLET POINTS

- Grain-based foods contain phosphorus bound to phytate, which is less bioavailable than phosphorus additives or meat- and dairy-based organic sources of phosphorus.
- The hydrolysis of phytate to release phosphorus occurs with processing, and thus phosphorus in processed grain foods such as yeast-leavened bread becomes more bioavailable.
- Nutritional databases may be inaccurate in the assessment of bioavailable phosphorus from grain sources.
- Studies in a rat model of CKD demonstrated that grain-based diets slow the progression of CKD and reduce intestinal phosphate absorption.
- A one-week cross-over trial in patients with stage 3b to 4 chronic kidney disease demonstrated decreased urine phosphate excretion and reduced FGF23 levels in a grain-based compared to meat-based diet of equivalent total phosphorus and protein content.
- A four-week study demonstrated persistent decrease in urinary phosphate excretion with a 70% grain-based diet and decreased urinary net acid excretion.

18.1 INTRODUCTION

Higher serum phosphate is associated with an increased risk of mortality in observational studies in patients with normal kidney function (Dhingra et al. 2007; Tonelli et al. 2005), predialysis chronic kidney disease (CKD) (Kestenbaum et al. 2005), and on hemodialysis (Ganesh et al. 2001; Block et al. 1998). As kidney function decreases there is an increase in fibroblast growth factor-23 (FGF23) and parathyroid hormone (PTH) as an appropriate response to maintain serum phosphate within normal ranges until late in the course of disease (Isakova et al. 2011). These adaptive hormone responses, if persistent, may cause bone and cardiac disease, and thus both the K/DOQI (2003) and the KDIGO (KDIGO 2009) guidelines recommended maintaining serum phosphate within "normal" ranges in CKD by decreasing dietary intake and prescribing phosphate binders. Unfortunately, as detailed in Chapters 5 and 7, the serum phosphate level does not reflect intestinal phosphate absorption, especially in patients with CKD, due to the concomitant presence of renal osteodystrophy and altered hormonal regulation. In addition, serum phosphate levels have diurnal variation: they are lower at 8 AM and if subjects are fasting, complicating the interpretation of some clinical studies (Ix et al. 2014; Moe et al. 2011b). However, in steady-state situations, the 24-hour urinary phosphate excretion is a good estimate of dietary phosphorus intake, providing a reasonable endpoint for evaluation of the different intestinal bioavailability of phosphorus sources (Moe et al. 2011b).

Dietary phosphorus restriction indirectly occurs when subjects are placed on a low-protein diet in research studies (Klahr et al. 1994; Zeller et al. 1991; Williams et al. 1991). However, in the low (0.58 g/kg/day) and very low protein (0.28 g/kg/day) arms of the landmark Modification of Diet in Renal Disease study, some nutritional indices worsened, raising concerns for this approach (Kopple et al. 1997; Klahr et al. 1994). Similarly, an observational study in dialysis patients showed increased mortality risk with a decrease in protein consumption (Shinaberger et al. 2008). Therefore, clinical practice guidelines have recommended dietary phosphorus restriction without decreasing the total amount of dietary protein; theoretically this can be achieved with lower phosphorus/protein ratio foods. In the K/DOQI 2003 guidelines, a list of the phosphorus/protein ratio was provided (K/DOQI 2003). Egg whites are an example of a food with a low ratio (2 mg phosphate/g protein), and a study of 13 hemodialysis patients found that eight ounces per day of egg whites for six weeks lowered serum phosphorus by 0.94 mg/dL ($p = 0.003$) (Taylor et al. 2011). Whereas this appears to be a safe and effective dietary intervention to lower phosphorus, this "dose" of egg whites may be difficult to

Special Nutritional Needs of Chronic Kidney Disease

maintain long term. Therefore, we must design diets that are palatable, nutritionally adequate, feasible, and beneficial for patients with CKD and end-stage renal disease (ESRD). Plant-based diets may provide these benefits as described later.

18.2 PHYTATE: THE PRIMARY SOURCE OF PHOSPHATE FROM PLANTS

Organic phosphorus in diets comes from animal-based and plant-based protein sources. Animal based protein is intracellular and is easily hydrolyzed to inorganic phosphate, which is readily absorbed in the intestine of humans; different sources have different phosphate-to-protein ratios, and thus the higher the ratio, the greater the absorption for a given intake of protein (Kalantar-Zadeh et al. 2010). In contrast, grain (organic) sources of protein are largely in the form of phytate-bound phosphate. Phytate, the salt form of phytic acid (myo-inositol 1,2,3,4,5,6 hexakis dihydrogen phosphate), stores phosphate in plants (Schlemmer et al. 2009) (Figure 18.1). The amount of phytate in plants varies and is present in seeds, but less so in tubers and roots (Schlemmer et al. 2009). Phytate-bound phosphate is cleaved with germination of seeds, leading to release of inositol monophosphates and diphosphates for the growing plant. Unprocessed cereals, legumes, oil seeds, and nuts have the highest phytate content. Processing, such as home cooking (pressure cooking or heating to 100°C), will not hydrolyze phytate; however, industrial processing, such as fermenting (as in bread making) and germinating, will release phosphate from phytate (Schlemmer et al. 2009; Troesch et al. 2013). The exact phytate (and thus phosphate) content in plants varies with growing practices such a fertilizer use, soil conditions, water supply, and season (Nitika et al. 2008; Ahmed et al. 2014). From the examples given, it would appear that the traditional American omnivore diet contains approximately half the phytate compared to a lacto-ovo vegetarian diet (average 748 mg vs. 1550 mg in males and 631 vs. 1250 mg in females) (Schlemmer et al. 2009; Ellis et al. 1987). High-dose calcium and magnesium will also enhance phytate hydrolysis (Sandberg et al. 1993), and thus, in theory, high-dose calcium-based phosphate binders may actually lessen the benefits of grain-based diets.

Phytate is naturally cleaved to release phosphorus by phytases (myo-inositol hexaphosphate phosphohydrolase). Phytase is present in the intestinal lumen of most herbivores, but humans lack this enzyme unless exogenously consumed in food. Phytase is present in some animal tissues, bacteria, and fungi, as well as in some whole-grain cereals (Schlemmer et al. 2009). In humans, studies have shown that 37% to 66% of phytate is degraded in the stomach and intestines if the diet is

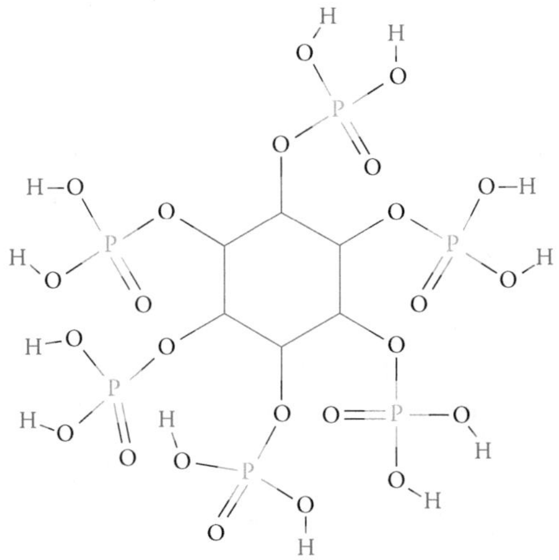

FIGURE 18.1 Structure of phytic acid. (From http://pubchem.ncbi.nlm.nih.gov/compound.)

unprocessed and contains whole-grain cereals and legumes that also contain phytase (McCance and Widdowson 1942). There is also some variable degradation by microbial-produced phytase in the large intestine of humans due to altered microbiome (Schlemmer et al. 2009). The manner of cooking cereals and beans may lead to variable amounts of phosphorus release. Heat cooking to 100°C, pressure cooking, and roasting foods at home may degrade phytase but not phytate, thus limiting phosphorus release. However, the use of added phytases in industrial processing or extended periods of boiling at high temperatures (e.g., 140°C) that occurs in manufacturing of cereals and other products degrades both phytate and phytase and therefore increases phosphorus release and absorption (Schlemmer et al. 2009).

In the past, phytate has thought to be detrimental as it binds essential minerals such as zinc and iron and other minerals are less bioavailable when human subjects are placed on a 100% plant-based diet (Gibson et al. 2010). Absorption of iron in humans is affected by the addition of phytate in a dose-dependent manner (Hallberg et al. 1989). Studies have demonstrated that the addition of phytase to diet increases the bioavailability of dietary iron and zinc (Troesch et al. 2013; Sandberg et al. 1996). The addition of phytase during processing to plant-based foods increases absorption of iron and zinc, as well as that of calcium, phosphorus, and magnesium (Troesch et al. 2013; Hallberg et al. 1989). With limited data available, it appears that a diet balanced in phytate and phytase is important to derive maximum benefit from a plant-based diet.

Despite these potential negative consequences of high-phytate diets, such diets have been shown to be associated with decreased nephrolithiasis (Grases et al. 2007), cardiovascular calcification (Grases et al. 2008), and decreased carcinogenesis (Vucenik and Shamsuddin 2003) in small studies. Additionally high-phytate diets have been associated with favorable blood glucose responses in rodents (Kim et al. 2010) and increased insulin sensitivity of adipocytes in cell culture (Kim et al. 2014). Increasing intake of phytate-rich foods, such as in vegetarian diets, also provides the ability to deliver adequate (0.8–1 mg/kg) protein and thus would be ideal for patients with CKD. The American Dietetic Association defines vegetarian diets as "one that does not include meat (including fowl) or seafood, or products containing those foods" (Craig et al. 2009). Vegetarian diets can be "lacto-ovo vegetarian," which includes eggs and dairy, but excludes meat, including seafood. A lacto-vegetarian consumes dairy products but not eggs, meats, or seafood. A vegan or "total" vegetarian diet is a 100% plant-based diet that excludes dairy products, eggs, meats, and seafood (Craig et al. 2009). Finally, a pesco-vegetarian eating pattern includes fish intake along with eggs and milk products. If planned well, these different vegetarian eating patterns have phytate contents that are higher than an omnivore diet and yet can still provide adequate protein intake (Schlemmer et al. 2009). Thus, vegetarian diets may be a therapy for chronic kidney disease–mineral bone disorder (CKD-MBD).

18.3 COMPARISON OF GRAIN VERSUS SYNTHETIC FEEDS ON PHOSPHORUS AND CKD-MBD IN A RODENT MODEL

In our rat model of progressive CKD, the Cy/+ rat, we have treated animals with both a grain-based diet and a casein/synthetic diet (Moe et al. 2009, 2011a). Three diets were used: (1) the grain diet was made of 20% protein, 0.6% phosphate, 0.8% calcium, and 4.5% fat (Purina 5002 diet with grain source ground corn, whole wheat, dehulled soybean, wheat middling); (2) the casein diet was composed of 18% protein, 0.7% phosphorus, 0.7% calcium, 5% fat (diet from Harlan Teklan TD.04539); and (3) a casein-based diet of only 0.2% phosphorus (Moe et al. 2009, 2011a). The comparison of the two protein sources at an equivalent 0.7% phosphorus (Table 18.1) demonstrated that the progressive rise in blood urea nitrogen (BUN) (a surrogate of kidney dysfunction), phosphorus, and PTH was blunted in the animals fed a grain-based diet compared to a casein-based diet from 20 to 38 weeks. The laboratory results from the 0.7% grain diet were similar to those of the 0.2% phosphate casein diet (not shown in table for clarity) (Moe et al. 2009, 2011a). We also performed metabolic cage studies on

TABLE 18.1

Comparison of 0.7% Phosphorus/20% Protein Diet from Casein/Synthetic Source versus Grain Source

	20 Weeks	34 Weeks	38 Weeks
Phosphorus (mg/dL) Casein diet	5.4 ± 0.2	11.6 ± 0.2	14.8 ± 1.5
Phosphorus (mg/dL) Grain diet	5.4 ± 0.3	5.1 ± 0.3	7.2 ± 0.6
Calcium (mg/dL) Casein diet	9.6 ± 0.4	9.9 ± 0.3	9.8 ± 0.6
Calcium (mg/dL) Grain diet	8.8 ± 0.3	8.9 ± 0.3	8.9 ± 0.3
BUN (mg/dL) Casein diet	38 ± 1	107 ± 13	140 ± 16
BUN (mg/dL) Grain diet	42 ± 2	62 ± 3	86 ± 7
PTH (pg/mL) Casein diet	469 ± 87	3543 ± 648	5151 ± 1067
PTH (pg/mL) Grain diet	347 ± 56	303 ± 116	421 ± 97
FGF23 (pg/mL) Casein diet	1254 (1183–1411)		
FGF23 (pg/mL) Grain diet	869 (799–903)		
Urine phosphorus (mg/24 hr) Casein diet	76.3 (58.3–87.8)		
Urine phosphorus (mg/24 hr) Grain diet	44.3 (39.4–49.0)		

Source: Adapted from Moe, S. M. et al. *J Bone Miner Res.*, 26, 11, 2672–81, 2011; Moe, S. M. et al. *Kidney Int.*, 75, 2, 176–84, 2009.

these diets to confirm that the differences between the casein and grain diets could be attributed to the phytate source of phosphorus in the grain diet. We compared the casein 0.7% total phosphorus diet to casein 0.4% plus phytate phosphorus 0.3% (total phosphorus for both diets = 0.7%) over one week in 20-week-old animals. The 2-hour urine phosphate levels were 4141 ± 1397 in the 7% P casein diet compared to 2161 ± 741 in the 0.4% P casein + 0.3% phosphorus phytate diets ($p < 0.01$; unpublished data). These results confirm that phytate phosphorus is not equivalently absorbed across the intestine as is nonphytate phosphorus. No differences in serum phosphate were found, perhaps because this was an early stage of CKD.

These findings are consistent with reduced bioavailability of P in grain-based diets, which contain much of the phosphate as phytate-phosphate. Thus, the type of animal feed used in research studies in CKD can lead to differences in phosphorus absorption and utility of binders. This is important to account for study designs and critical to report in publications. Cereal or grain-based animal feeds will also vary in phytate and phosphate content from season to season as well as with the use of fertilizers (Nitika et al. 2008; Ahmed et al. 2014). These data provided the rationale for our subsequent studies in humans.

18.4 EFFECT OF A PLANT-BASED SOURCE OF PROTEIN ON CKD-MBD IN HUMANS

To determine if the source of dietary protein/phosphorus could also affect phosphorus homeostasis in humans, we extended our studies to humans with CKD (Moe et al. 2011b). We randomized eight patients with mean eGFR 32.3+/– 6 mL/min to receive prepared grain/soy- (referred to as vegetarian) or meat/dairy- (referred to as meat) based protein diets for seven days (Figure 18.2). Each subject then had a 2- to 4-week washout followed by the other treatment in a cross-over design. Subjects were admitted to a clinical research center for the last 24 hours of each treatment arm (vegetarian and the

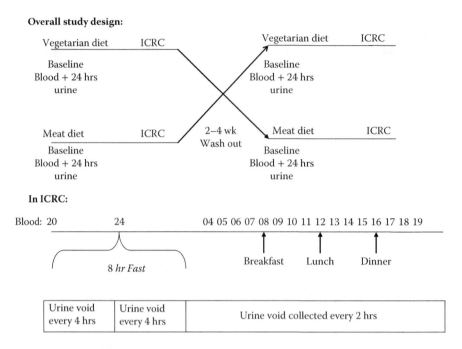

FIGURE 18.2 Overall study design of cross-over pilot study. The top panel demonstrates the overall cross-over design, and the lower panel depicts urine and blood sampling during the 24-hour Indiana Clinical Research Center (ICRC) inpatient stay. (Reprinted with permission from Moe, S. M. et al. Clin J Am Soc Nephrol., 6, 2, 257–64, 2011.)

meat based) and frequent blood and stool urine samples collected. Twenty-four-hour urine collections were also performed at the start of each diet period. The vegetarian and the meat diets were equivalent in calories at 2200 kcals with 20% protein content and 800 mg/day phosphate and no phosphate additives. The daily calcium and sodium were 1000 and 3000 mg per day, respectively. Comparing the change from baseline to end of each arm, the results demonstrated higher serum phosphate, FGF23, and urinary phosphate and a lower PTH in the meat diet compared to the vegetarian diet (Table 18.2). This pilot study demonstrated that adequate protein could be delivered from 100% plant-based sources, with desirable changes in FGF23 and PTH (although the latter may also reflect phytate binding of calcium and changes in serum calcium), indicating a potential that long-term dietary restriction of phosphorus by altering bioavailability might be able to prevent rises in PTH and FGF23. Both of these hormones are associated with bone and cardiac disease (EVOLVE Investigators, 2012; Sprague and Moe 2012; Moe et al. 2015a, 2015b). However, it is unknown if long-term treatment with a 100% plant-based diet would lead to sustained improvements in the biochemical parameters of CKD-MBD.

In people who are not committed to a vegetarian lifestyle, adherence to a complete plant-based diet may be difficult (Lea and Worsley 2003). A diet that allows some daily animal protein intake would likely be considered more palatable and therefore sustainable long term by patients. In another cross-over trial, Azadbakht Esmaillzadeh (2009) studied the effect of seven weeks of a 65% vegetarian diet compared to a 70% animal-based diet in patients with diabetes with baseline serum creatinine of 1 to 2.5 mg/dL and with known macroalbuminuria. They showed that the predominantly vegetarian diet led to decreased albuminuria. Serum phosphate was also lowered by 0.2 ± 0.3 mg/dL in the vegetarian diet compared to 0.03 ± 0.2 mg/dL in the meat diet (Azadbakht and Esmaillzadeh 2009).

We extended these studies and examined a 70% plant-based diet in a cohort of 13 patients with more advanced CKD (median eGFR 26 mL/min). The purpose was to design a more tolerable diet, especially to patients who normally consume a meat diet, by examining the effect of a 70% plant-based protein diet provided to subjects over a four-week period with intensive education (Moorthi et al. 2014).

Special Nutritional Needs of Chronic Kidney Disease

TABLE 18.2

Blood and Urine Measurements after One Week of Diet as Outpatient

	Pre	Post	Pre	Post	
		Meat (Casein) Diet		Vegetarian (Grain) Diet	P Value (Paired t-test)[a]
Average daily phosphorus intake (mg/day)		810 ± 27		795 ± 51	NS
Plasma phosphate (mg/dL)	3.5 ± 0.6	3.7 ± 0.6	3.5 ± 0.6	3.2 ± 0.5	0.02
Plasma intact PTH (pg/mL)	58 ± 31	46 ± 29	58 ± 39	56 ± 30	0.002
Plasma FGF23 (pg/mL)	72 ± 39	101 ± 83	84 ± 65	61 ± 35	0.008
Plasma calcium (mg/dL)	9.2 ± 0.4	9.4 ± 0.7	9.3 ± 0.4	9.1 ± 0.3	NS
Creatinine clearance (mL/min)	47 ± 16	47 ± 16	43 ± 11	44 ± 16	NS
Urine 24-hr calcium excretion (mg/24 hours)	66 ± 69	77 ± 48	60 ± 59	71 ± 43	NS
Urine 24-hr phosphate excretion (mg/24 hours)	836 ± 187	583 ± 216	778 ± 190	416 ± 233	0.07
Urine 24-hr fephosph (%)	38.0 ± 6.2	23.9 ± 5.1	38.2 ± 11.5	20.9 ± 9.9	NS

Source: Moe, S. M. et al. *Clin J Am Soc Nephrol.*, 6, 2, 257–64, 2011. With permission.

[a] By paired t-test comparing results at end (post) each seven-day controlled diet study period drawn at the same time. Results are mean ± SD. The "pre" values are shown to demonstrate what the patients ate on their own during the prestudy and washout periods and to demonstrate no carry-over effect.

The study began after two baseline 24-hour urine collections on subjects' usual home diet and five days of diet records to obtain baseline "usual" phosphorus intake. Subjects were then placed on a study diet for four weeks. Subjects were supplied with a "CKD" diet to deliver 0.8 to 0.9 g/kg protein (mean = 0.84 g/kg), 0.8 to 1.3 g of phosphate, 700 to 1000 mg of calcium, 2 to 4 g sodium (2.2 g mean), and 2 to 3 g of potassium per day. Twenty-four–hour urine collections and blood draws were performed at the two- and four-week time points. The primary endpoint for the study was urinary phosphate excretion, which decreased from 830 ± 244 by 22% at four weeks ($p < 0.001$) (Table 18.3). Serum phosphate levels decreased from 3.7 ± 0.4 to 3.5 ± 0.5 at two weeks to 3.6 ± 0.5 at four weeks, but this was not significant. FGF23 levels decreased by 12% in the study period, but this also did not reach statistical significance, likely due to the variability in levels and small sample size. Importantly, there were no serious adverse consequences observed over the four-week period on the 70% plant-based protein diet in these subjects. There were three isolated incidences of hyperkalemia (all <6 mEq/l), but all controlled with minor diuretic or food choice changes. There was no loss of muscle strength, and there was a trend toward improvement in glucose control. The diet represented a dramatic change from baseline intake: the estimated phytate content of this diet was 1333 ± 215 mg, which was significantly different compared to the prestudy mean phytate of 532 ± 416 mg per day ($p < 0.001$). Therefore a predominantly (70%) plant-based protein diet is well tolerated in CKD stage 4, is safe, and decreases phosphate excretion by a magnitude comparable to high-dose binders (Block et al. 2012).

These studies suggest that lowering dietary phosphorus bioavailability using phytate-bound sources has beneficial effects in short-term studies in CKD-MBD. The traditional CKD diet limits legumes and vegetables due to both potassium and phosphorus content. However, the bioavailable phosphorus/protein ratio is much lower than the measured phosphorus/protein ratio. The results of the studies raises the possibility of expanding the typical CKD diet limitation on phytate-based sources of protein. Unfortunately, there are no measures of phosphorus content on food labels, making it cumbersome, even for motivated CKD patients, to plan their own meals. In the crossover study of a total plant-based diet discussed earlier (Moe et al. 2011b), phosphorus content

TABLE 18.3
Effect of a 70% Plant Protein–Based Diet on Urine Parameters

	Baseline[a]	2 Weeks on Study Diet	4 Weeks on Study Diet	p
		Mean ± SD or Median (25th, 75th percentile)		
Urine P (mg/24 hrs)	830 ± 244	580 ± 215[*]	615+273[*], [**]	0.001
Urine P/Cr	0.48 ± 0.1	0.37 ± 0.1[*]	0.39 ± 0.1[*], [**]	<0.001
Urine Creatinine (mg/24 hrs)	1748 ± 463	1613 ± 508	1543 ± 395[*]	0.038
24-h Creatinine Clearance (mL/min)	51 ± 17	46 ± 13	48 ± 15	0.26
Urine Urea Nitrogen (g/24 hrs)	10.5 ± 4.23	9.08 ± 2.74	9.15 ± 4.04	0.26
24-h Urea Clearance (mL/min)	22 ± 8	19 ± 5	20 ± 9	0.31
Urine Calcium (mg/24 hrs)	19 (10,26)	31 (26,53)[*]	27 (15,33)	0.007
Urine Citrate (mg/24 hrs)	279 ± 147	353 ± 168	317 ± 79	0.107
Urine Sodium (mmol/ 24 hrs)	200 ± 81	142 ± 44[*]	132 ± 51[*]	0.002
Urine Sulfate (meq/24 hrs)	42 ± 17	36 ± 12	36 ± 15	0.162
Urine pH	6.0 ± 0.5	6.2 ± 0.6	6.2 ± 0.5	0.2
Urine Ammonium Excretion (mmol/24 hrs)	18 ± 10	10 ± 6[*]	12 ± 8[*]	0.002
Titratable Acid (meq /24 hrs)	17.9 ± 8.5	10.8 ± 5.6[*]	12.6 ± 9.5[*]	0.003

Source: Moorthi, R. N. et al. *Am J Nephrol.*, 40, 6, 582–91, 2014. With permission.

  Repeated measures testing were used by one-way ANOVA and the Holm-Sidak method for pairwise comparisons for normally distributed data. For non-normally distributed data, repeated measures testing was done using ANOVA on ranks, with Tukey testing for pairwise comparisons.

[a] Average of twobaseline collections done during prestudy period.

[*] Significant when compared to baseline $p < 0.05$.

[**] Significant when compared to two-week value $p < 0.05$.

of prepared meals was measured from frozen, lyophilized food that was ashed, and the measured content was about 33% less than that calculated from the Minnesota Nutrient Database system, but the meat diet matched the database. Thus designing diets with this database may be problematic. In general, plant-based diets appear safe in CKD, but the longest published interventional study of such a diet is seven weeks. As detailed earlier in this chapter, phytate also binds essential minerals such as iron and zinc and other nutrients (Hallberg et al. 1989; Troesch et al. 2013) and this may be important in the long term. Thus, longer studies of plant-based diets in CKD need to be performed to determine compliance and ensure no adverse nutrient deficiencies, especially if plant-based diets are widely recommended for management of CKD-MBD.

18.5 OTHER EFFECTS OF PLANT-BASED DIETS IN CKD

There are additional studies of vegetarian diet studies in CKD with outcomes other that CKD-MBD. An observational study in the NHANES subpopulation with early CKD showed that an increased proportion of plant-based protein to total protein is associated with a decrease in all-cause mortality (Chen et al. 2015). A case control study in Taiwan of vegetarian Buddhist nuns versus omnivores showed that there was no difference in kidney function between these groups, despite lower systolic blood pressures and better fasting glucose in vegetarians (Lin et al. 2010). Increased endogenous acid production based on dietary intake was associated with lower serum bicarbonate levels and CKD progression in a secondary analysis of the African American Study of Kidney Disease and Hypertension trial (Scialla et al. 2011, 2012). Clinical trials have subsequently demonstrated that correction of metabolic acidosis via oral bicarbonate can slow progression of kidney disease (de Brito-Ashurst et al. 2009; Mahajan et al. 2010). More recently, plant-based foods have been tested

Special Nutritional Needs of Chronic Kidney Disease

for this indication in CKD. Patients with CKD stage 1 ($n = 79$) or stage 2 ($n = 120$) were randomized to 30-day treatment with control diet, 0.5 mEq/kg/day of sodium bicarbonate, or "base-producing" fruits and vegetables to reduce their net acid excretion by 50%. The results demonstrated a decrease in biomarkers of kidney injury (urine albumin, N-acetyl β-D-glucosaminidase, and transforming growth factor β) in both the oral bicarbonate and fruits and vegetable arms (Goraya et al. 2012). When a similar fruit and vegetable added diet was compared to sodium bicarbonate prescription in 71 patients with eGFR 15 to 29 mL/min over one year, there was no effect on CKD progression, but there was improvement in markers of kidney injury as well as in metabolic acidosis (Goraya et al. 2013). Of note, these studies did not test the effect of plant-based sources of protein; they tested the effect of correcting metabolic acidosis on kidney disease progression with fruits and vegetables. Study subjects were allowed to eat ad lib, as long as they incorporated prescribed fruits and vegetables to decrease their net acid load by 50%. However, it can be inferred that they likely also decreased the proportion of animal- to plant-based sources of protein. In our four-week study of the 70% vegetarian diet, we also saw a reduction in urine ammonium excretion and titratable acid by two weeks and a reduction in sodium excretion (Table 18.3) (Moorthi et al. 2014). Thus, encouraging patients to consume a more vegetarian diet consisting of fruits and vegetables and less processed foods may also protect against progression of kidney disease.

18.6 CONCLUSIONS

Plant-based sources of protein provide phytate bound phosphorus that is lower in bioavailability than animal protein. In CKD plant-based sources of protein can be used to replace 70% to 100% of animal protein in diets to decrease urine phosphate excretion and limit the use of binders. In short-term studies, these diets reduce urinary excretion of phosphate, sodium, and net acid excretion and appear safe. However, the long-term safety and efficacy in slowing kidney progression and averting the consequences of excess phosphate intake should be evaluated in future long-term studies.

REFERENCES

Ahmed, S. O., A. W. Abdalla, T. Inoue, A. Ping, and E. E. Babiker. 2014. Nutritional quality of grains of sorghum cultivar grown under different levels of micronutrients fertilization. *Food Chem* 159:374–80. doi:10.1016/j.foodchem.2014.03.033.

Azadbakht, L., and A. Esmaillzadeh. 2009. Soy-protein consumption and kidney-related biomarkers among type 2 diabetics: A crossover, randomized clinical trial. *J Ren Nutr* 19 (6):479–86. doi:S1051-2276(09)00153-8.

Block, G. A., T. E. Hulbert-Shearon, N. W. Levin, and F. K. Port. 1998. Association of serum phosphorus and calcium x phosphate product with mortality risk in chronic hemodialysis patients: A national study. *Am J Kidney Dis* 31 (4):607–17.

Block, G. A., D. C. Wheeler, M. S. Persky, B. Kestenbaum, M. Ketteler, D. M. Spiegel, M. A. Allison, J. Asplin, G. Smits, A. N. Hoofnagle, L. Kooienga, R. Thadhani, M. Mannstadt, M. Wolf, and G. M. Chertow. 2012. Effects of phosphate binders in moderate CKD. *J Am Soc Nephrol* 23 (8):1407–15. doi:10.1681/ASN.2012030223.

Chen, X., G. Wei, T. Jalili, J. Metos, A. Giri, M. E. Cho, R. Boucher, T. Greene, and S. Beddhu. 2015. The Associations of Plant Protein intake with all-cause mortality in CKD. *Am J Kidney* Dis 67 (3):423–30. doi:10.1053/j.ajkd.2015.10.018.

Craig, W. J., A. R. Mangels, and Association American Dietetic. 2009. Position of the American Dietetic Association: Vegetarian diets. *J Am Diet Assoc* 109 (7):1266–82.

de Brito-Ashurst, I., M. Varagunam, M. J. Raftery, and M. M. Yaqoob. 2009. Bicarbonate supplementation slows progression of CKD and improves nutritional status. *J Am Soc Nephrol* 20 (9):2075–84. doi:10.1681/ASN.2008111205.

Dhingra, R., L. M. Sullivan, C. S. Fox, T. J. Wang, R. B. D'Agostino, Sr., J. M. Gaziano, and R. S. Vasan. 2007. Relations of serum phosphorus and calcium levels to the incidence of cardiovascular disease in the community. *Arch Intern Med* 167 (9):879–85.

Ellis, R., J. L. Kelsay, R. D. Reynolds, E. R. Morris, P. B. Moser, and C. W. Frazier. 1987. Phytate: Zinc and phytate X calcium: Zinc millimolar ratios in self-selected diets of Americans, Asian Indians, and Nepalese. *J Am Diet Assoc* 87 (8):1043–7.

Ganesh, S. K., A. G. Stack, N. W. Levin, T. Hulbert-Shearon, and F. K. Port. 2001. Association of elevated serum PO(4), Ca x PO(4) product, and parathyroid hormone with cardiac mortality risk in chronic hemodialysis patients. *J Am Soc Nephrol* 12 (10):2131–8.

Gibson, R. S., K. B. Bailey, M. Gibbs, and E. L. Ferguson. 2010. A review of phytate, iron, zinc, and calcium concentrations in plant-based complementary foods used in low-income countries and implications for bioavailability. *Food Nutr Bull* 31 (2 Suppl):S134–46.

Goraya, N., J. Simoni, C. Jo, and D. E. Wesson. 2012. Dietary acid reduction with fruits and vegetables or bicarbonate attenuates kidney injury in patients with a moderately reduced glomerular filtration rate due to hypertensive nephropathy. *Kidney Int* 81 (1):86–93. doi:10.1038/ki.2011.313.

Goraya, N., J. Simoni, C. H. Jo, and D. E. Wesson. 2013. A comparison of treating metabolic acidosis in CKD stage 4 hypertensive kidney disease with fruits and vegetables or sodium bicarbonate. *Clin J Am Soc Nephrol* 8 (3):371–81. doi:10.2215/CJN.02430312.

Grases, F., B. Isern, P. Sanchis, J. Perello, J. J. Torres, and A. Costa-Bauza. 2007. Phytate acts as an inhibitor in formation of renal calculi. *Front Biosci* 12:2580–7.

Grases, F., P. Sanchis, J. Perello, B. Isern, R. M. Prieto, C. Fernandez-Palomeque, and C. Saus. 2008. Phytate reduces age-related cardiovascular calcification. *Front Biosci* 13:7115–22.

Hallberg, L., M. Brune, and L. Rossander. 1989. Iron absorption in man: Ascorbic acid and dose-dependent inhibition by phytate. *Am J Clin Nutr* 49 (1):140–4.

Investigators, Evolve Trial, G. M. Chertow, G. A. Block, R. Correa-Rotter, T. B. Drueke, J. Floege, W. G. Goodman, C. A. Herzog, Y. Kubo, G. M. London, K. W. Mahaffey, T. C. Mix, S. M. Moe, M. L. Trotman, D. C. Wheeler, and P. S. Parfrey. 2012. Effect of cinacalcet on cardiovascular disease in patients undergoing dialysis. *N Engl J Med* 367 (26):2482–94. doi:10.1056/NEJMoa1205624.

Isakova, T., P. Wahl, G. S. Vargas, O. M. Gutierrez, J. Scialla, H. Xie, D. Appleby, L. Nessel, K. Bellovich, J. Chen, L. Hamm, C. Gadegbeku, E. Horwitz, R. R. Townsend, C. A. Anderson, J. P. Lash, C. Y. Hsu, M. B. Leonard, and M. Wolf. 2011. Fibroblast growth factor 23 is elevated before parathyroid hormone and phosphate in chronic kidney disease. *Kidney Int* 79 (12):1370–8. doi: ki201147.

Ix, J. H., C. A. Anderson, G. Smits, M. S. Persky, and G. A. Block. 2014. Effect of dietary phosphate intake on the circadian rhythm of serum phosphate concentrations in chronic kidney disease: A crossover study. *Am J Clin Nutr* 100 (5):1392–7. doi:10.3945/ajcn.114.085498.

K/DOQI, National Kidney Foundation. 2003. Clinical practice guidelines for bone metabolism and disease in chronic kidney disease. *Am J Kidney Dis 42 (Supplement):S1–201.* doi: S0272638603009053 [pii].

Kalantar-Zadeh, K., L. Gutekunst, R. Mehrotra, C. P. Kovesdy, R. Bross, C. S. Shinaberger, N. Noori, R. Hirschberg, D. Benner, A. R. Nissenson, and J. D. Kopple. 2010. Understanding sources of dietary phosphorus in the treatment of patients with chronic kidney disease. *Clin J Am Soc Nephrol* 5 (3):519–30. doi:10.2215/CJN.06080809.

KDIGO. 2009. Clinical practice guidelines for the management of CKD-MBD. *Kidney Int* 76 (S113):S1–130.

Kestenbaum, B., J. N. Sampson, K. D. Rudser, D. J. Patterson, S. L. Seliger, B. Young, D. J. Sherrard, and D. L. Andress. 2005. Serum phosphate levels and mortality risk among people with chronic kidney disease. *J Am Soc Nephrol* 16 (2):520–8.

Kim, J. N., S. N. Han, and H. K. Kim. 2014. Phytic acid and myo-inositol support adipocyte differentiation and improve insulin sensitivity in 3T3-L1 cells. *Nutr Res* 34 (8):723–31. doi:10.1016/j.nutres.2014.07.015.

Kim, S. M., C. W. Rico, S. C. Lee, and M. Y. Kang. 2010. Modulatory effect of rice bran and phytic acid on glucose metabolism in High Fat-Fed C57BL/6N Mice. *J Clin Biochem Nutr* 47 (1):12–7. doi:10.3164/jcbn.09-124.

Klahr, S., A. S. Levey, G. J. Beck, A. W. Caggiula, L. Hunsicker, J. W. Kusek, and G. Striker. 1994. The effects of dietary protein restriction and blood-pressure control on the progression of chronic renal disease. Modification of Diet in Renal Disease Study Group. *N Engl J Med* 330 (13):877–84.

Kopple, J. D., A. S. Levey, T. Greene, W. C. Chumlea, J. J. Gassman, D. L. Hollinger, B. J. Maroni, D. Merrill, L. K. Scherch, G. Schulman, S. R. Wang, and G. S. Zimmer. 1997. Effect of dietary protein restriction on nutritional status in the Modification of Diet in Renal Disease Study. *Kidney Int* 52 (3):778–91.

Lea, E., and A. Worsley. 2003. Benefits and barriers to the consumption of a vegetarian diet in Australia. *Public Health Nutr* 6 (5):505–11. doi:10.1079/PHN2002452.

Lin, C. K., D. J. Lin, C. H. Yen, S. C. Chen, C. C. Chen, T. Y. Wang, M. C. Chou, H. R. Chang, and M. C. Lee. 2010. Comparison of renal function and other health outcomes in vegetarians versus omnivores in Taiwan. *J Health Popul Nutr* 28 (5):470–5.

Mahajan, A., J. Simoni, S. J. Sheather, K. R. Broglio, M. H. Rajab, and D. E. Wesson. 2010. Daily oral sodium bicarbonate preserves glomerular filtration rate by slowing its decline in early hypertensive nephropathy. *Kidney Int* 78 (3):303–9. doi:10.1038/ki.2010.129.

McCance, R. A., and E. M. Widdowson. 1942. Mineral metabolism of healthy adults on white and brown bread dietaries. *J Physiol* 101 (1):44–85.

Moe, S. M., S. Abdalla, G. M. Chertow, P. S. Parfrey, G. A. Block, R. Correa-Rotter, J. Floege, C. A. Herzog, G. M. London, K. W. Mahaffey, D. C. Wheeler, B. Dehmel, W. G. Goodman, T. B. Drueke, and HCl Therapy to Lower Cardiovascular Events Trial Investigators Evaluation of Cinacalcet. 2015a. Effects of cinacalcet on fracture events in patients receiving hemodialysis: The EVOLVE trial. *J Am Soc Nephrol* 26 (6):1466–75. doi:10.1681/ASN.2014040414.

Moe, S. M., N. X. Chen, M. F. Seifert, R. M. Sinders, D. Duan, X. Chen, Y. Liang, J. S. Radcliff, K. E. White, and V. H. Gattone, 2nd. 2009. A rat model of chronic kidney disease-mineral bone disorder. *Kidney Int* 75 (2):176–84. doi:ki2008456 [pii]

Moe, S. M., G. M. Chertow, P. S. Parfrey, Y. Kubo, G. A. Block, R. Correa-Rotter, T. B. Drueke, C. A. Herzog, G. M. London, K. W. Mahaffey, D. C. Wheeler, M. Stolina, B. Dehmel, W. G. Goodman, J. Floege, and HCl Therapy to Lower Cardiovascular Events Trial Investigators Evaluation of Cinacalcet. 2015b. Cinacalcet, Fibroblast Growth Factor-23, and Cardiovascular Disease in Hemodialysis: The Evaluation of Cinacalcet HCl Therapy to Lower Cardiovascular Events (EVOLVE) Trial. *Circulation* 132 (1):27–39. doi:10.1161/CIRCULATIONAHA.114.013876.

Moe, S. M., J. S. Radcliffe, K. E. White, V. H. Gattone, 2nd, M. F. Seifert, X. Chen, B. Aldridge, and N. X. Chen. 2011a. The pathophysiology of early-stage chronic kidney disease-mineral bone disorder (CKD-MBD) and response to phosphate binders in the rat. *J Bone Miner Res* 26 (11):2672–81. doi:10.1002/jbmr.485.

Moe, S. M., M. P. Zidehsarai, M. A. Chambers, L. A. Jackman, J. S. Radcliffe, L. L. Trevino, S. E. Donahue, and J. R. Asplin. 2011b. Vegetarian compared with meat dietary protein source and phosphorus homeostasis in chronic kidney disease. *Clin J Am Soc Nephrol* 6 (2):257–64. doi:CJN.05040610 [pii]

Moorthi, R. N., C. L. Armstrong, K. Janda, K. Ponsler-Sipes, J. R. Asplin, and S. M. Moe. 2014. The effect of a diet containing 70% protein from plants on mineral metabolism and musculoskeletal health in chronic kidney disease. *Am J Nephrol* 40 (6):582–91. doi:10.1159/000371498.

Nitika, D. Punia, and N. Khetarpaul. 2008. Physico-chemical characteristics, nutrient composition and consumer acceptability of wheat varieties grown under organic and inorganic farming conditions. *Int J Food Sci Nutr* 59 (3):224–45. doi:10.1080/09637480701523249.

Sandberg, A. S., L. R. Hulthen, and M. Turk. 1996. Dietary Aspergillus niger phytase increases iron absorption in humans. *J Nutr* 126 (2):476–80.

Sandberg, A. S., T. Larsen, and B. Sandstrom. 1993. High dietary calcium level decreases colonic phytate degradation in pigs fed a rapeseed diet. *J Nutr* 123 (3):559–66.

Schlemmer, U., W. Frolich, R. M. Prieto, and F. Grases. 2009. Phytate in foods and significance for humans: Food sources, intake, processing, bioavailability, protective role and analysis. *Mol Nutr Food Res* 53 (Suppl 2):S330–75. doi:10.1002/mnfr.200900099.

Scialla, J. J., L. J. Appel, B. C. Astor, E. R. Miller, 3rd, S. Beddhu, M. Woodward, R. S. Parekh, and C. A. Anderson. 2011. Estimated net endogenous acid production and serum bicarbonate in African Americans with chronic kidney disease. *Clin J Am Soc Nephrol* 6 (7):1526–32. doi:10.2215/CJN.00150111.

Scialla, J. J., L. J. Appel, B. C. Astor, E. R. Miller, 3rd, S. Beddhu, M. Woodward, R. S. Parekh, C. A. Anderson, Disease African American Study of Kidney, and Group Hypertension Study. 2012. Net endogenous acid production is associated with a faster decline in GFR in African Americans. *Kidney Int* 82 (1):106–12. doi:10.1038/ki.2012.82.

Shinaberger, C. S., S. Greenland, J. D. Kopple, D. Van Wyck, R. Mehrotra, C. P. Kovesdy, and K. Kalantar-Zadeh. 2008. Is controlling phosphorus by decreasing dietary protein intake beneficial or harmful in persons with chronic kidney disease? *Am J Clin Nutr* 88 (6):1511–8. doi: 10.3945/ajcn.2008.26665.

Sprague, S. M., and S. M. Moe. 2012. The case for routine parathyroid hormone monitoring. *Clin J Am Soc Nephrol* doi:10.2215/CJN.04650512.

Taylor, L. M., K. Kalantar-Zadeh, T. Markewich, S. Colman, D. Benner, J. J. Sim, and C. P. Kovesdy. 2011. Dietary egg whites for phosphorus control in maintenance haemodialysis patients: A pilot study. *J Ren Care* 37 (1):16–24. doi:10.1111/j.1755-6686.2011.00212.x.

Tonelli, M., F. Sacks, M. Pfeffer, Z. Gao, and G. Curhan. 2005. Relation between serum phosphate level and cardiovascular event rate in people with coronary disease. *Circulation* 112 (17):2627–33.

Troesch, B., H. Jing, A. Laillou, and A. Fowler. 2013. Absorption studies show that phytase from Aspergillus niger significantly increases iron and zinc bioavailability from phytate-rich foods. *Food Nutr Bull* 34 (2 Suppl):S90–101.

Vucenik, I., and A. M. Shamsuddin. 2003. Cancer inhibition by inositol hexaphosphate (IP6) and inositol: From laboratory to clinic. *J Nutr* 133 (11 Suppl 1):3778S–3784S.

Williams, P. S., M. E. Stevens, G. Fass, L. Irons, and J. M. Bone. 1991. Failure of dietary protein and phosphate restriction to retard the rate of progression of chronic renal failure: A prospective, randomized, controlled trial. *Q J Med* 81 (294):837–55.

Zeller, K., E. Whittaker, L. Sullivan, P. Raskin, and H. R. Jacobson. 1991. Effect of restricting dietary protein on the progression of renal failure in patients with insulin-dependent diabetes mellitus. *N Engl J Med* 324 (2):78–84.

Section III

Food and Environmental Use and Regulation of Phosphorus

19 The Regulatory Aspects of Phosphorus Intake
Dietary Guidelines and Labeling

Mona S. Calvo and Susan J. Whiting

CONTENTS

Abstract 249
Bullet Points 250
19.1 History of Development and Application of
the Dietary Guidelines for Phosphorus Intake in Healthy Populations 250
    19.1.1 Biomarker Selection for Establishing Dietary Phosphorus Requirement 250
    19.1.2 How the Institute of Medicine Panel Set the RDA for Phosphorus in 1997 252
    19.1.3 How the European Food Safety Authority Set Dietary Reference Values for
    Phosphorus in 2015 252
19.2 Current Estimates of Dietary Phosphorus Intakes in North America and Europe 254
19.3 Dietary Sources of Phosphorus in North America and Europe 256
    19.3.1 Food and Supplement Sources of Phosphorus 256
    19.3.2 Phosphorus Food Additives 259
19.4 Regulatory Labeling of Phosphorus Content and Additives in Foods 261
19.5 Influence of High Phosphorus Intake on Bone Health and Other Health Risks 262
    19.5.1 Low Ca:P Intake Ratio: Impact on Bone Health 262
    19.5.2 Benefits from Dietary Patterns Low in Processed Foods and Phosphate
    Additives in CKD 262
    19.5.3 Association of Dietary Phosphorus with Variability in Levels of FGF23 in
    Vulnerable Populations 263
References 263

ABSTRACT

This chapter takes a close look at dietary factors that influence or contribute to higher serum phosphorus levels associated with greater incidence of morbidity and mortality in North America and Europe. There are dietary guidelines identifying how much phosphorus the general North American and European Union populations need to consume each day. Yet for a growing number of older individuals with failing kidneys, an estimated 26 million in America alone, these phosphorus guidelines, along with a basic lack of food labeling, a high phosphorus additive use in processing methods, and the predominant current dietary patterns, do not prevent a level of phosphorus that may be life threatening. The lack of coherent policies on phosphorus levels may also place others in the general healthy population at increased risk for cardiovascular, kidney, and bone disease because they facilitate an excess phosphorus intake. Total phosphorus intake when kidney function is impaired must be delicately balanced between what the body needs for maintenance and the inability to efficiently excrete phosphorus. This is a difficult task given the ubiquitous presence of phosphorus in foods of variable absorption efficiencies. The disrupted hormonal imbalance that occurs when phosphorus accumulates in serum and the adverse health effects of this imbalance that are discussed in Section I of this book underscore the ever-increasing need to reevaluate the safety of phosphorus intakes that far exceed our physiological requirements. With respect to maintaining renal function in a significant subpopulation worldwide, there is an immediate and pressing need to develop mandatory labeling, along with regulatory strategies, to identify the phosphorus content of packaged foods, to educate patients about the healthy dietary patterns that help limit phosphorus absorption, and to engage in dialogue with food manufacturers concerning the reduction of phosphate additive use in processing foods targeted to renal patients.

BULLET POINTS

- In North America, the recommended daily allowance (RDA) for phosphorus established by the Institute of Medicine (IOM) in 1997 is age specific and based on Estimated Average Requirement (EAR) values derived from studies using serum phosphorus as a biomarker. In contrast, the European Food Safety Authority (EFSA) set no requirement values for the European population in 2015, instead using an adequate intake estimate specific to age (AI) based on the calcium-to-phosphorus ratio (1.4:1) that reflects body tissue levels.
- Phosphorus intakes in industrialized countries exceed requirements by two- and three-fold in adult men and women.
- North American and European top contributing food sources of naturally occurring phosphorus include milk and milk products, meat, and grains and grain products, with animal-derived sources having the greatest density and bioavailability compared to plant sources with lower density and bioavailability.
- Less is known about the actual quantity and bioavailability of phosphorus contributed by phosphate food additives; however, their use in processed foods is growing and becoming widespread in industrialized countries, and mounting evidence stresses the need to label phosphorus content of foods to facilitate management of renal disease and prevent cardiovascular and other diseases in the general healthy population.
- In the absence of phosphorus content labeling on packaged processed foods, adoption of plant-rich healthy dietary patterns such as the DASH or Mediterranean diets may help to reduce the phosphorus intake of the typical Western diet and aid in correcting the disrupted hormone regulation in renal failure.

19.1 HISTORY OF DEVELOPMENT AND APPLICATION OF THE DIETARY GUIDELINES FOR PHOSPHORUS INTAKE IN HEALTHY POPULATIONS

19.1.1 BIOMARKER SELECTION FOR ESTABLISHING DIETARY PHOSPHORUS REQUIREMENT

To set population-based dietary recommendations, the first step is to find the average requirement of particular age/sex groups; this value is usually found in experimental dose-response studies, and as subject numbers may be small, the median value is chosen to represent the needs of 50% of the group (Otten et al. 2006). Such studies must have used accurate and sensitive methodology, involving selection of appropriate indicators of the nutrient's status. Selecting biomarkers for a nutrient normally involves understanding the nutrient's transport, storage, and functions. Ideally storage is best as it provides a measure of long-term gain or loss of a nutrient, for which transport is a measure of day-to-day availability. Testing for function of a nutrient is a way to determine the impact of low stores or transport on body needs. Phosphorus functions in the body as phosphate. It is transported in blood in organic compounds, but a small amount (~25% of total) is as the electrolytes monophosphate ($H_2PO_4^-$) and diphosphate (HPO_4^{-2}), which serve in maintaining acid–base balance (EFSA, 2015). This phosphorus is about 1% of the body's total. In cells, 14% of body phosphorus is found

The Regulatory Aspects of Phosphorus Intake 251

as phosphate molecules involved in almost every aspect of metabolism, as well as in cell regulation and signaling. Phosphate in cells is also found throughout membranes as phospholipids. The remaining 85% of body phosphorus is located in bones and teeth, where phosphate, along with calcium, provides the mineralization needed in these tissues (Otten et al. 2006).

In the case of phosphorus status, the indicators and biomarkers that have been used in nutrition studies are shown in Table 19.1. The Institute of Medicine's report on Dietary Reference Intakes (DRIs) for phosphorus reviewed methods to establish requirement levels for phosphorus (IOM, 1997). The panel concluded that studies involving phosphorus balance were not suitable for setting average requirement levels. Measuring serum levels of inorganic phosphorus, however, was deemed acceptable for determining adult requirements. Accretion of phosphorus into bones using factorial estimates that were based on published values for each component (as described later) serves as the indicator for children (IOM, 1997).

More recently, the European Food Safety Authority (EFSA) panel evaluated biomarkers and made different conclusions. In evaluating serum (plasma) inorganic phosphorus, several recent studies indicated that there was little association between changes in dietary intake of phosphorus and changes in serum phosphorus (ESFA, 2015). The panel noted that due to the tight renal

TABLE 19.1

Indicators/Biomarkers of Phosphorus Status Considered for Setting Dietary Requirements by the Institute of Medicine (IOM) in 1997 and by the European Food Safety Authority (EFSA) in 2015

Indicator/Biomarker	Etiology	Suitability in Setting EAR	Used in Setting Requirements?
IOM Report 1997			
Phosphorus balance	Urine + fecal excretion less than intake	Difficult to use as balance during growth and during old age not defined	IOM: No
Serum (plasma) inorganic phosphorus (Pi)	In adults, serum Pi related to P intake	Amount of dietary P needed to maintain serum Pi at lowest level of normal range	IOM: Yes, for adults but not children
P accretion	Amount of Pi incorporated into bones, teeth, and lean tissues during growth	Factorial method for estimation of P requirements in children	IOM: Yes, for children
EFSA Report 2015			
Serum (plasma) inorganic phosphorus	In adult serum Pi related to P intake	New data shows serum Pi not a reliable marker due to fluctuations after ingestion	EFSA: No
Urinary phosphorus	Kidney is main route of excretion but other factors (e.g. PTH influence)	Limited usefulness	EFSA: No
Serum regulating factors for Pi	PTH, FGF23, klotho are serum Pi-regulating and are elevated to promote Pi excretion	Role as biomarkers not well documented	EFSA: No

Note: GFR = glomerular filtration rate; PTH = parathyroid hormone; FGF23 = fibroblast growth factor-23.

regulation, fasting serum phosphorus concentration will show very modest fluctuations over a wide range of phosphorus intake. Serum phosphorus is usually measured in morning fasting samples that show changes on the order of 0.5 to 1.0 mg/dL with dietary restriction or phosphorus loading, requiring multiple serial measures of serum phosphorous throughout the day in order to detect significant changes due to dietary intake. (Portale et al. 1987; Calvo et al. 1990, 1991, 2014; Kemi et al. 2006). Previous decisions regarding the use of serum phosphorus had been based on an infusion experiment involving nonphysiologic amounts of phosphate, thus obscuring any effects of phosphorus absorption. The EFSA panel concluded that renal handling of dietary phosphorus was so well regulated that fasting serum inorganic phosphorus levels showed only minimal modification by dietary intakes. The ESFA panel also evaluated urinary phosphorus and serum levels of hormones important to maintenance of phosphorus balance and concluded none of these could be used for establishing phosphorus requirements. The EFSA panel concluded that there were no reliable biomarkers of phosphorus intake and status that could be useful for setting average requirement values for phosphorus.

19.1.2 How the Institute of Medicine Panel Set the RDA for Phosphorus in 1997

Phosphorus was in the first set of nutrients for which DRI values were set in 1997. In setting requirements for a population, one must examine the literature for studies that can be used to set the EAR. This population-based value is the amount of a nutrient that will meet the needs of 50% of a defined group, usually specified as age/sex.

In setting the EAR for young and middle-age adults (age 19–50 years), the IOM Panel used the published relationship between serum Pi and absorbed intake (Nordin, 1988) as expanded in the DRI report (IOM, 1997) to estimate intakes associated with the normal range of serum Pi. Then extrapolation from absorbed P to ingested P was calculated using data generated by the panel, assuming the efficiency of absorption was 62.5% in typical mixed diets not high in phytate. At the lower end of the normal serum Pi range for adults, of 0.87 mmol/L, an intake of 580 mg would meet the needs of 50% of the population and therefore was chosen as the EAR.

For older adults (age 51 years and older), the same EAR was set as there were no indications that absorption efficiency changes with age. The relationship between absorbed P and serum Pi remains constant until glomerular filtration rate (GFR) is reduced to below 20%. For infants and children, accretion of P in lean tissues and bone was estimated factorially using published studies through each stage of growth. Pregnancy and lactation are set based on the age of the woman, as hormones during these life stages improve efficiency of absorption and utilization.

The EAR is the level that meets the requirements of 50% of a group. To get to the RDA, one uses the following equation: $RDA = EAR + 2 SD_{EAR}$. The standard deviation of the EAR is an estimate of the variance in requirements and is set at 10% for micronutrients such as P where an actual level has not been determined. Solving this equation for adults, the RDA for both men and women is 700 mg per day. Values for EAR and RDA of all age/sex groups are shown in Table 19.2.

19.1.3 How the European Food Safety Authority Set Dietary Reference Values for Phosphorus in 2015

The EFSA panel, after reviewing all possible biomarkers for phosphorus status, concluded that there was insufficient evidence to set average requirements for phosphorus. In the absence of an average requirement, a recommended intake such as a recommended daily allowance (RDA) used in the United States and Canada, as well as other countries worldwide, or a Population Reference Intake (PRI) used in Europe, cannot be set. Instead, one sets an adequate intake (AI). Although an AI can be used in place of an RDA or PRI, the usefulness of an AI in dietary assessment is limited, as

TABLE 19.2

Dietary Reference Intake Values Set in 1997 for Phosphorus by the Institute of Medicine

Age Group	EAR mg/day	RDA mg/day
Infants		
0–6 mo	–	100[a]
7–12 mo	–	275
1–3 y	380	460
4–8 y	405	500
9–13 y	1055	1250
14–18 y	1055	1250
19–30 y	580	700
31–50 y	580	700
51–70 y	580	700
71 + y	580	700
Pregnancy		
≤ 18 y	1055	1250
> 18 y	580	700
Lactation		
≤ 18 y	1055	1250
> 18 y	580	700

[a] Infants have an adequate intake (AI) level based on breast milk composition.

TABLE 19.3

Adequate Intake (AI) Values Set in 2015 for Phosphorus by the European Food Safety Authority (EFSA)

Age Group	AI mg/day
Infants	
0–6 mo	–[a]
7–12 mo	160
1–3 y	250
4–10 y	440
11–17 y	640
18 + y	550
Pregnancy	550
Lactation	550

[a] Infants age 0 to 6 breastfed and intake not estimated.

prevalence of inadequacy cannot be found (Otten et al. 2006). The AI signals that the recommended intake value could not be set with much precision.

To derive the AIs for phosphorus, shown in Table 19.3, the ESFA panel used the calcium to phosphorus molar ratio in the whole body, which varies between 1.4:1 and 1.9:1. Having PRI values for calcium (and an AI value for infants) and choosing to use the lower bound of the range (i.e., 1.4:1), values for the AI for phosphorus were calculated. For example, for adults 18 years and over, the PRI of 1000 mg (25 mmol) for calcium was divided by 1.4 to obtain 18 mmol of P, which when converted to weight is 550 mg. Values were rounded down to the nearest 100 mg/day to obtain these estimates.

19.2 CURRENT ESTIMATES OF DIETARY PHOSPHORUS INTAKES IN NORTH AMERICA AND EUROPE

High serum Pi (> 5.5 mg/dL) has been implicated in the dysregulation of calcium and phosphorus homeostasis that is regulated by parathyroid hormone (PTH), 1,25-dihydroxyvitamin D (calcitriol), and fibroblast growth factor-23 (FGF23) and is associated with cardiovascular disease and increased mortality (Calvo and Uribarri 2013; Gutiérrez 2013b). The role of high dietary phosphorus intake in disease risk is unclear. Some evidence links phosphorus intakes in excess of physiologic requirements with increase in FGF23 (Antoniucci et al. 2006) and cardio-renal and bone morbidity and

TABLE 19.4

Mean (SE) Phosphorus and Calcium Intake (mg/d) from Food and Beverages Consumed per Individual by Gender and Age in the United States, NHANES 2013–2014[a]

Age Group	EAR[b] P mg/d	Phosphorus Intake (mg/d) Females	Phosphorus Intake (mg/d) Males	Calcium Intake (mg/dl) Females	Calcium Intake (mg/dl) Males
2–5 y	380	1016 (34.9)	1097 (37.1)	926 (45.1)	940 (33.6)
6–11 y	405–1055	1180 (19.4)	1388 (35.9)	960 (28.1)	1175 (41.5)
12–19 y	1055	1095 (37.4)	1604 (29.4)	842 (33.3)	1186 (35.4)
20–29 y	580	1191 (31.6)	1825 (53.0)	872 (32.8)	1284 (65.0)
30–39 y	580	1286 (29.9)	1681 (32.4)	912 (27.9)	1094 (30.1)
40–49 y	580	1217 (22.8)	1675 (44.5)	865 (23.6)	1092 (40.8)
50–59 y	580	1177 (23.1)	1589 (37.5)	828 (30.0)	1013 (36.7)
60–69 y	580	1154 (36.4)	1450 (26.4)	814 (30.4)	997 (41.1)
70+ y	580	1069 (25.1)	1377 (44.0)	809 (28.6)	940 (41.1)
20 y and over	580	1187 (12.2)	1625 (17.9)	852 (10.9)	1086 (18.2)

[a] *Data Source:* U.S. Department of Agriculture, Agricultural Research Service. 2016. Nutrient Intakes from Food and Beverages. Mean Amounts Consumed per Individual by Gender and Age, *What We Eat in America*, NHANES 2013–2014. (Nutrient intakes do not include phosphorus or calcium from dietary supplements or medications.)

[b] *EAR = Estimated Average Requirement.*

The Regulatory Aspects of Phosphorus Intake

increased mortality (Chang et al. 2014; Gutiérrez et al. 2015; Yamamoto et al. 2013; Itkonen et al. 2013, 2017) and in renal failure (D'Alessandro et al. 2015; Gutiérrez et al. 2011; Kalantar-Zadeh et al. 2010; Moore et al. 2015; Murgtaugh et al. 2012). In contrast, other studies found no direct association of disease risk with phosphorus intake (Chang et al. 2017; Ito et al. 2011; Kwak et al. 2014; Lee et al. 2014, 2015). Studies examining the effects of phosphate consumption with adequate calcium intake in young adults reported positive association between bone parameters and phosphorus intake, presumably reflecting greater need for bone growth (Teegarden et al. 1998; Whiting et al. 2002).

Phosphorus intake in the United States is monitored in the National Health and Nutrition Education Surveys (NHANES), which are nationally representative surveys conducted and analyzed in two-year waves since 2000. The most recent nutrient intake data release for NHANES 2013–2014 is shown in Table 19.4, which presents mean (SE) intakes of both phosphorus and calcium for survey participants over two years of age. The overall intake in women >20 years is twice the EAR, whereas that of men is nearly three-fold higher than the requirement guideline. As all the NHANES survey waves have shown, men consume more phosphorus than women.

Table 19.5 presents mean phosphorus intakes from different European countries in selected age groups for males and females. There is considerable variation from country to country likely due to differences in national surveys and nutrient content databases (Olza et al. 2017; EFSA, 2015). In general, the intake in men exceeds that of women and with the exception of 11- to 19-year-olds, both men and women far exceed the IOM requirement intake guideline (EAR).

There are many problems with the methods used in dietary survey estimates of nutrient intake, but the single most important issue for estimates of phosphorus intake lies with the incomplete

TABLE 19.5

Mean Phosphorus Intake (mg/d) from Different European Surveys According to Age and Country[a]

Age, years	Spain [b]	United Kingdom [c]	Finland [c]	France [c]	Germany [c]	Italy [c]	Netherlands [c]	Sweden [c]	Ireland [c]
1 – ≤3									
Female	~~	815	711	~~	641	641	~~	~~	~~
Male	~~	871	719	~~	699	924	~~	~~	~~
3 – ≤ 10									
Female	1206	991	1086	925	750	1155	1080	~~	~~
Male	1350	1076	1173	1033	808	1202	1146	~~	~~
10 – ≤ 18									
Female	1145	990	1264	922	1148	1226	1167	~~	~~
Male	1323	1231	1601	1243	1225	1494	1397	~~	~~
18 – ≤ 65									
Female	1108	1127	1239	1084	~~	1151	1279	1336	1302
Male	1247	1448	1614	1403	~~	1378	1671	1692	1767
65 – ≤ 75									
Female	1023	1145	1153	1050	~~	1098	1181	1310	~~
Male	1177	1498	1426	1372	~~	1311	1478	1558	1652
≥ 75									
Female	~~	1162	~~	1000	~~	1075	~~	1330	~~
Male	~~	1253	1280	1484	~~	1332	~~	1531	1484

[a] Age classifications were approximated due to differences in surveys.

[b] *Source:* Olza J et al., *Nutrients*, 9, 168, 2017.

[c] *Source:* EFSA Panel on Dietetic Products, Nutrition and Allergies (NDA). *EFSA J.*, 13, 4185, 2015.

information in the nutrient databases used by all countries (Table 19.5). To date, none include contributions from phosphorus added in processing (Calvo et al. 2014; Gutiérrez et al. 2013a). Recently, epidemiologists have documented the significant trend toward an increase in phosphorus intake in the United States (McClure et al. 2017). These investigators examined both the sources and trends in phosphorus consumption in a nationally representative sample of Americans ($n = 34{,}741$) 20 years and older using the combined waves of the NHANES surveys from 2001 to 2014. With data from the first 24-hour dietary recalls from the combined surveys they determined an overall increase in phosphorus consumption of 54 g or 4.01% increase from 2001 to 2014 (p-trend = 0.02) (McClure et al. 2017). These findings beg the important question as to what is the source of this increase in phosphorus consumption.

19.3 DIETARY SOURCES OF PHOSPHORUS IN NORTH AMERICA AND EUROPE

19.3.1 FOOD AND SUPPLEMENT SOURCES OF PHOSPHORUS

Total phosphorus intake as reported in nutrition surveys is largely based on reported serving sizes and food composition data derived from analytical or estimated phosphorus content, which often do not reflect that of products currently in the marketplace (Calvo and Park 1996; Calvo 1993). Examples of this are shown in Table 19.6, which lists the top food categories from NHANES 2011–2012 (Moshfegh et al. 2016). Those foods with an asterisk differ slightly in phosphorus contributions from the 2009–2010 survey. The examples of chicken and pizza are largely frozen products and were part of a government project that reanalyzed the nutrient content of specific foods whose consumption has markedly increased by the entire population, and the new data were included in the USDA Standard Release 29 (SR-29) database used in the 2011–2012 survey analysis (Moshfegh et al. 2016). These products are also known to have increased in consumption and in the use of phosphate additives in processing (Calvo and Park, 1996; Leon et al. 2013) and serve to underscore the importance of up-to-date chemical analysis needed for many commonly consumed processed foods.

TABLE 19.6

Top Contributing Food Categories to Phosphorus Intake in the United States and Europe

Country	Food Category	Contribution to Phosphorus Intake (%)	
United States	**Dairy Products**		
Data source:	Milk and flavored milk	11	
NHANES, 2011–2012	Cheese, ice cream, yogurt	9	
(Moshfegh et al. 2016)	**Bakery Products**		
	Breads, rolls, tortillas	5	
	Sweet bakery products, quick breads	5	
	Vegetables	5	
	Chicken[a]	5	
	Mexican Dishes	5	
	(Burritos, tacos, nachos)		
	Pizza[a]	5	
Europe		Men	Women
Adult men and women 18< 65	**Grains and Grain-Based Products**	20–29	19–38
Minimum and Maximum Percent	**Milk and Dairy Products**	19–35	21–39
Data source:	**Meat and Meat Products**	14–25	12–21
EFSA (NAD), 2015			

[a] Newly analyzed foods, notably frozen chickens and pizza processed with phosphorus containing additives from USDA SR-29.

The Regulatory Aspects of Phosphorus Intake

TABLE 19.7

Estimated Dietary Phosphorus Density (mg phosphorus/ kcal) by USDA Food Groups in NHANES: WWEIA 2001 to 2014 in Adults ≥ 20 y[a]

Food Group	Men	Women
Milk and Milk Products	1.322	1.292
Meat, Poultry, Fish, and Mixtures	0.848	0.863
Eggs	1.048	1.048
Legumes, Nuts, and Seeds	0.804	0.823
Grain Products	0.536	0.528
Fruits	0.305	0.305
Vegetables	0.537	0.595
Fats, Oils, and Salad Dressing	0.072	0.080
Sugar, Sweeteners, and Beverages	0.272	0.295
All Sources	0.627	0.640

Note: NHANES WWEIA: National Health and Nutrition Examination Survey: What We Eat in America.

[a]*Source:* McClure ST et al., *Nutrients*, 9, 95, 2017.

Food sources in Europe are similar for men and women and are shown in the lower half of Table 19.6. Consistent with the analyses by McClure et al. (2017), the greatest contributors to phosphorus intake are milk and dairy products, grains and grain-based products, and meat and meat products, which largely reflect naturally occurring phosphorus (Calvo and Uribarri, 2016; EFSA, 2015).

In contrast to the rise in phosphorus consumption from 2001 to 2014 NHANES, McClure et al. (2017) reported a slight decline in calorie intake, resulting in a significant overall 7.4% increase ($p < 0.01$) in phosphorus density of food sources consumed by men and women. Table 19.7 shows the estimated phosphorus density (mg P/kcal) for USDA food groups consumed by men and women illustrating higher phosphorus density in foods of animal origin (milk, meat, and eggs) and much lower density in foods of plant origin. This is an important finding because consumption of lower phosphorus density foods should help to manage phosphorus intake in chronic kidney disease.

Natural phosphorus in food is not the only source of phosphorus because phosphorus-containing fortificants, such as calcium phosphate, and phosphorus contained in multiple vitamin and mineral supplements usually taken daily may also contribute to total phosphorus intake. Fulgoni et al. (2011) illustrated how little is the phosphorus contribution from fortificants and dietary supplements to the total phosphorus intake at all percentiles of intake (shown in Figure 19.1). At each percentile of intake, less than 6% of the population failed to reach the EAR intake requirement for phosphorus and none reached the UL for phosphorus intake, discussed in Chapter 20. Multiple vitamin/mineral supplements most commonly label phosphorus content per serving, which is 109 mg/d, and relative to chemical analyses the mean percentage difference from the label was 15.4% in recent work from the Office of Dietary Supplements of the National Institutes of Health (Andrews et al. 2017). With respect to high phosphorus intake, dietary supplements and nutrient fortification of foods pose far less of a concern than the contributions from phosphate-containing additives or phosphorus density of the food source (Calvo and Uribarri, 2013).

The total amount of absorbed or biologically available phosphorus from food is significantly influenced by differences in food composition; in short, the source of the phosphorus matters. Phosphates in foods are found in cell membranes, proteins and structural components, and secretions of plant and animal cells that serve as food sources and from phosphate salts that are added to food during processing. These three sources of phosphorus shown in Figure 19.2 have very different physiologic digestion and absorption properties about which we have incomplete understanding.

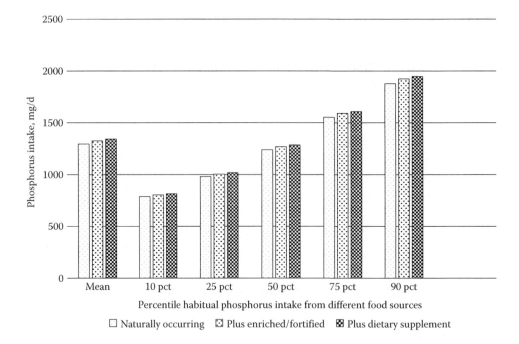

FIGURE 19.1 Usual intakes of phosphorus from naturally occurring food sources, + enriched/fortified foods and + dietary supplements from NHANES 2003–2006 U.S. participants ≥2 y. Distribution of habitual phosphorus intake (mg/d) across selected percentiles and the mean intake for naturally occurring foods alone ▢, plus enriched or fortified foods ▨, and plus dietary supplements ▨, are shown for NHANES 2003–2006 participants ≥2 y. (Figure is based on data from Fulgoni VL et al., *J Nutr.*, 141, 1847–54, 2011.)

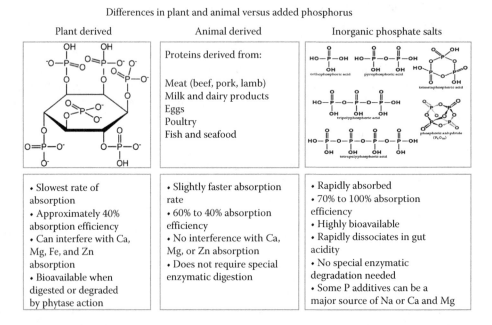

FIGURE 19.2 Food forms of phosphorus: physiological differences in plant and animal sources versus added phosphorus. The figure presents the physiological differences in phosphates from plant- and animal-derived foods compared to the predicted physiologic characteristics of phosphate salts added during food processing.

The Regulatory Aspects of Phosphorus Intake

Plant-derived phosphorus is largely present as phytate and has the slowest rate and lowest efficiency of phosphorus absorption unless the phytate can be degraded by nonhuman enzymes such as those from yeast that are used to leaven bread. In the acidic pH of the stomach phytate can chelate calcium and other essential cations, impairing their absorption. In contrast, natural phosphorus from animal food sources are absorbed slightly faster and with greater efficiency and show no interference with essential mineral absorption because dissociation of phosphate bound to animal protein does not require special enzymes not present in the human gut, such as phytase. Several studies have demonstrated the differences in bioavailability of phosphorus from plant and animal food sources (Karp et al. 2012a, b; Moe et al. 2011). For further information see Chapters 17 and 18.

Less is known about the physiologic digestion and absorption properties of phosphate salts added to food in processing. These inorganic phosphate salts differ in solubility and other chemical characteristics. Because these salts would dissociate rapidly in the acidic milieu of the gut, they are thought to be rapidly and efficiently absorbed; however, this understanding has been questioned recently (St-Jules et al. 2017). Consideration should be given to the widespread use of a variety of phosphate additives whose interaction with other food components and nutrients is largely unknown when exploring the physiologic effects of increased consumption of phosphate food additives. In studies exploring the possible adverse health effects of high phosphate additive consumption, variable and often spurious outcomes occur when the studies fail to consider the calcium or sodium content of the diets or fail to use serial sampling of blood after meals or use phosphate salt loads in lieu of commonly eaten foods containing phosphate additives whose phosphate content has been confirmed by chemical analyses (Trautvetter et al. 2016; Chang et al. 2017). Appropriately designed studies, although of short duration, have shown adverse hormonal changes that affect bone (Calvo et al. 1990; Gutiérrez et al. 2015) or reduction of serum Pi in CKD and ESRD by reducing the consumption of foods containing phosphate additives in renal patients, especially over long periods (six months) (De Fornasari et al. 2017; Moe et al. 2011).

19.3.2 PHOSPHORUS FOOD ADDITIVES

There has been a substantial increase in both the use of phosphate-containing additives and the amount or number per serving in a wide variety of foods over the last four decades (Calvo and Uribarri, 2016; Gutiérrez et al. 2015; EFSA, 2015), although there is little documentation available to the public about the extent of phosphate additive use in foods. Relevant to the safety of the growing use of phosphorus-containing food additives by food industries, the permissible limit for their use in most foods in the United States and Canada is set by "good manufacturing practices" (Calvo and Uribarri, 2016).

Early on, and even now, the safety of the permissible limits of phosphate additive use in food processing has been questioned in Europe (El-Shaarawy and Reith, 1976; Ritz et al. 2012), but it remains unclear whether permissible limits have been exceeded by their widespread use in food processing. The permissible limit in Europe, known as the Acceptable Daily Intake (ADI), has been set by the FAO/WHO Committee at 70 mg P/kg body weight (EFSA, 2015). Current estimates of phosphorus intake do not account for added phosphorus in processing that is considered to be "hidden phosphorus" (Uribarri and Calvo, 2003) and is a serious hazard for dialysis patients (Uribarri, 2009). Accuracy of nutrient databases for estimating phosphorus intake has long been questioned due these hidden sources of phosphorus (Oenning et al. 1988; Sullivan et al. 2007; Leon et al. 2013). Contributions of phosphate additives to total daily phosphorus intake are estimated to range from 300 to 1000 mg/day (Calvo and Park, 1996; EFSA, 2015). European estimations of the dietary intake of phosphorus from phosphate additives E338–343 and E450–452 were shown to exceed the ADI at the 97.5 highest percentile of intake in children 1 to 18 years in Italy, the United Kingdom, France, and Ireland, but not in adults. The intake in children ranged from 95.9 to 144 mg P/kg body weight per day, accounting for between 137% and 206% of the ADI (Vin et al. 2013).

There are about 28 commonly used phosphate-containing food additives out of the 48 declared GRAS (generally regarded as safe) ingredients used in the United States. Of these the most commonly

TABLE 19.8
Retail Food Products Containing One or More of Three Specific GRAS Phosphate Ingredients[a]

Food Category	Phosphoric Acid	Sodium Phosphate	Sodium Polyphosphate	Total Number
Cakes, cookies, and cupcake mixes	0	89	16	105
Breads	103	97	2	202
Breakfast sandwiches, biscuits, and meals	3	136	0	139
Cakes, cupcakes, and snack cakes	52	260	104	416
Canned and bottled beans	1	28	1	30
Chili and stews	1	45	17	63
Canned meat	2	65	16	83
Canned seafood	1	5	22	28
Canned vegetables	5	27	1	33
Cereal	0	629	81	710
Cheese	47	681	68	796
Cream	2	163	5	170
Dairy	13	158	35	206
Vegetable/lentil mixes	0	14	2	16
Deli products	27	758	50	835
Eggs and egg substitutes	0	9	14	23
Fish and seafood	4	40	272	316
Frozen dinners	28	994	143	1165
Frozen pizza	10	377	30	417
Frozen vegetables	0	33	2	35
Frozen meals	72	1068	307	1447
Frozen snacks	2	121	26	149
Sausage, hot dogs, and brats	0	330	11	341
Ice cream	112	154	7	273
Bacon, sausage, and ribs	0	280	3	283
Milk	0	92	43	135
Noodles	0	26	59	85
Other meats	0	79	4	83
Other pastry, croissants, and bakery products	16	29	25	70
Packaged deli meats, pepperoni, salami, and cold cuts	2	944	2	948
Packaged fruits and vegetables	25	93	13	131
Pancakes, waffles, and French toast	7	9	2	18
Pasta	30	330	67	374
Poultry, chicken, and turkey	0	137	14	151
Rice	0	47	9	56
Subs and sandwiches	21	88	5	114
Yogurt	3	12	0	15

GRAS: generally recognized as safe.

[a]*Source:* Calvo MS, Uribarri J. Phosphorus in the modern food supply: Underestimation of exposure, pages 47-76. In: *Clinical Aspects of Natural and Added Phosphorus in Foods.* Gutierrez OM, Kalatar-Zadeh K, Mehrota R (Eds.), 1st ed. 2016. Springer Science+Business Media.

used for a variety of different functions in food processing include phosphoric acid, sodium phosphate, and sodium polyphosphate (Calvo and Uribarri, 2013). These three ingredients were used to determine the extent of phosphate additive use in retail food products available across the United States in 2013 (Calvo and Uribarri, 2016). Table 19.8 shows the number of products containing

The Regulatory Aspects of Phosphorus Intake

261

one or more of these additives in retail food products. As shown, a number of foods contained two or more of these additives, and the frozen dinner food category, popular convenience foods, were shown to have the highest number of products with phosphorus-containing additives. Thus, there is a very wide distribution of phosphate additives in commonly consumed foods, a finding that has been confirmed by others (Leon et al. 2013). A high prevalence of phosphorus-containing additives was also reported for Australian retail foods (McCutcheon et al. 2015).

19.4 REGULATORY LABELING OF PHOSPHORUS CONTENT AND ADDITIVES IN FOODS

With the updating of the Nutrition Facts Panel by the U.S. Food and Drug Administration (FDA) in order to enable consumers to eat healthy foods, an opportunity arose for the nephrology community to communicate the need for mandatory labeling of the phosphorus content of foods. This was considered to be a compelling need given the evidence that both disease management and prevention of renal disease would benefit from the knowledge of how much phosphorus is in packaged foods. Regrettably, the FDA declined this request on the basis that nutrient content information appearing

(a)

Nutrition Facts
Serving size 1 cups (240g)
Serving per container 4

Amount Per Serving	
Calories 90	Calories from Fat 30
	% Daily Values*
Total fat 3.5g	**5%**
Saturated fat 0g	**3%**
Trans fat 0g	
Cholesterol 0mg	**0%**
Potassium 350mg	**10%**
Sodium 110mg	**5%**
Total carbohydrate 9g	**3%**
Dietary fiber 2g	**8%**
Sugars 6g	
Protein 6g	**12%**

Vitamin A 10%	•	Calcium 30%
Vitamin D 30%	•	Thiamin 6%
Riboflavin 40%	•	Vitamin B6 4%
Folate 10%	•	Vitamin B12 50%
Phosphorus 8%	•	Magnesium 8%
Zinc 10%	•	Copper 10%
Manganese 20%		

* Percent daily values are based on a 2,000 calorie diet. Your daily values may be higher or lower depending on your calorie needs.

	Calories	2,000	2,500
Total fat	Less than	65g	80g
Sat fat	Less than	20g	25g
Cholesterol	Less than	300mg	300mg
Sodium	Less than	2400mg	2400mg
Total carbohydrate		300g	375g
Dietary fiber		25g	30g

Soy milk
INGREDIENTS:
Filtered water, organic whole soybeans, organic evaporated cane juice, natural flavors, calcium carbonate, sea salt, sodium citrate, potassium citrate, carrageenan, vitamin A palmitate, ergocalciferol (vitamin D_2), DL-alpha tocopherol acetate (vitamin E) riboflavin (vitamin B_2), cyanocobalamin (vitamin B_{12}), zinc sulfate.

(b)

Nutrition Facts
Serving size 1 cups (240g)
Serving per container 4

Amount Per Serving	
Calories 50	Calories from Fat 40
	% Daily Values*
Total fat 4.5g	**7%**
Saturated fat 4g	**20%**
Trans fat 0g	
Cholesterol 0mg	**0%**
Potassium 65mg	**2%**
Sodium 65mg	**3%**
Total carbohydrate 2g	**1%**
Dietary fiber 1g	**4%**
Sugars 0g	
Protein 0g	**0%**

Vitamin A 10%	•	Calcium 10%
Vitamin D 30%	•	Folate 6%
Vitamin B12 50%	•	Magnesium 8%
Selenium 8%		

* Percent daily values are based on a 2,000 calorie diet. Your daily values may be higher or lower depending on your calorie needs.

	Calories	2,000	2,500
Total fat	Less than	65g	80g
Sat fat	Less than	20g	25g
Cholesterol	Less than	300mg	300mg
Sodium	Less than	2400mg	2400mg
Total carbohydrate		300g	375g
Dietary fiber		25g	30g

Coconut milk
INGREDIENTS:
Organic coconut milk (water, organic coconut cream), natural flavors, vanilla extract, calcium phosphate, magnesium phosphate, kosher sea salt, carrageenan, guar gum, REB A (stevia extract), monk fruit, vitamin A palmitate, vitamin D_2, L-selenomethionine (selenium), zinc oxide, folic acid, vitamin B_{12}

(c)

Nutrition Facts
Serving size 1 cups (240g)
Serving per container 8

Amount Per Serving	
Calories 110	Calories from Fat 20
	% Daily Values*
Total fat 2.5g	**4%**
Saturated fat 1.5g	**8%**
Trans fat 0g	
Cholesterol 15mg	**5%**
Potassium 410mg	**12%**
Sodium 130mg	**5%**
Total carbohydrate 13g	**4%**
Dietary fiber 0g	**0%**
Sugars 12g	
Protein 8g	**16%**

Vitamin A 10%	•	Calcium 50%
Vitamin D 25%	•	Vitamin B12 15%
Phosphorus 35%		

* Percent daily values are based on a 2,000 calorie diet. Your daily values may be higher or lower depending on your calorie needs.

	Calories	2,000	2,500
Total fat	Less than	65g	80g
Sat fat	Less than	20g	25g
Cholesterol	Less than	300mg	300mg
Sodium	Less than	2400mg	2400mg
Total carbohydrate		300g	375g
Dietary fiber		25g	30g

1% Low Fat Milk-Calcium Enriched
INGREDIENTS:
Low fat milk, tribasic calcium phosphate (calcium ingredient not in regular milk) carrageenan, guar gum, lactase enzyme, vitamin A palmitate and vitamin D_3

FIGURE 19.3 Examples of phosphorus content labeling currently allowed in the United States. Three different labeling options for voluntary labeling of phosphorus content in packaged foods (a), mandatory labeling of phosphate additives in the ingredient list (b), and both mandatory phosphate additive labeling and voluntary labeling of phosphorus content in the Nutrition Facts Panel (c).

on food labels is targeted to healthy populations and not to those with acute or chronic disease such as CKD and is not intended for the clinical management of existing diseases (Federal Register, 2016).

The new label provides little benefit to renal patients and will likely contribute to the confusion over adequate intakes since the daily value has been increased from 100 mg to 1250 mg P in the United States and Canada. The daily value (% DV) is the reference amount that is designed to help consumers make informed choices for a healthy diet and is based on the highest RDA value in all the age groups. With the current label or new label, there are only three options for manufacturers to list information about the phosphorus content. Figure 19.3 presents examples of product labels using these three options. The new label does allow the listing of phosphorus content as both %DV and in mg of P per serving size, but other label updates are not shown here. Voluntary or discretionary labeling is shown in Figure 19.3a and also lists the phosphorus content in mg. Label (b) shows the mandatory listing of phosphate additives in the ingredient list, and label (c) shows the options for both voluntary and mandatory labeling of ingredients (Calvo et al. 2014). Phosphate additives in the ingredient list are not always recognized by the concerned consumer, particularly if the words *phosphate* and *phosphorus* are not used, as is the case for the widely used modified food starches. For more information on the use of nutrition, labels in Europe see Chapters 21 and 22.

19.5 INFLUENCE OF HIGH PHOSPHORUS INTAKE ON BONE HEALTH AND OTHER HEALTH RISKS

19.5.1 Low Ca:P Intake Ratio: Impact on Bone Health

Table 19.4 shows the mean intakes of phosphorus and calcium across gender and age, clearly demonstrating an imbalance in the intake of the two minerals that is not consistent with dietary guidelines, which recommend an optional intake mass ratio of 1.1:1 (IOM, 1997). High phosphorus intake adversely affects bone and calcium metabolism (Takeda et al. 2012; Kemi et al. 2006), particularly when the calcium-to-phosphorus ratio (Ca:P) of the diet is low (Kemi et al. 2010; Adatorwovor et al. 2015). Evidence of the potential harm to bone was shown by significantly higher parathyroid hormone levels in the quartile with the lowest Ca:P molar ratio (0.5) in a cross-sectional study of Finish women, despite calcium intakes that met the RDA (Kemi et al. 2010).

Figure 19.4 shows the percentile distribution of Ca:P intake ratios for men and women 19 years and older determined for individual intakes in NHANES 2011–2012 (Calvo et al. 2014). Approximately 25% of the adult U.S. population is at risk for disrupted calcium and phosphorus regulation that could affect bone health with Ca:P mass intake ratios of 0.5 and lower. Calcium is a significantly underconsumed nutrient, whereas phosphorus consumption in Western countries exceeds intake guidelines, thus raising concern over the long-term impact on bone health.

19.5.2 Benefits from Dietary Patterns Low in Processed Foods and Phosphate Additives in CKD

In the absence of phosphorus content labeling, how can CKD and dialysis patients make healthy food choices that will slow the progression of their disease and reduce the intake of phosphorus? A number of studies have shown benefits from following specific dietary patterns such as the DASH diet (Dietary Approaches to Stop Hypertension) and the Mediterranean diet, both dominated by plant sources of phosphorus, rich in fruits, vegetables, and grains with some dairy, but little red meat and processed foods (Kelly et al. 2017; Reboholz et al. 2016; Gallieni et al. 2016; Asghari et al. 2016). A colorful visual tool—a phosphorus pyramid—has been developed to aid in the dietary management of CKD and dialysis patients (D'Alessandro et al. 2015). It is similar to the food intake guidelines for the Mediterranean and DASH diets, but also emphasizes avoidance of foods containing phosphorus additives. Plant protein intake was associated with the reduction in the level of FGF-23 in CKD patients, which is also consistent with the recommendations of the plant-rich DASH and Mediterranean diets (Scialla et al. 2012).

The Regulatory Aspects of Phosphorus Intake

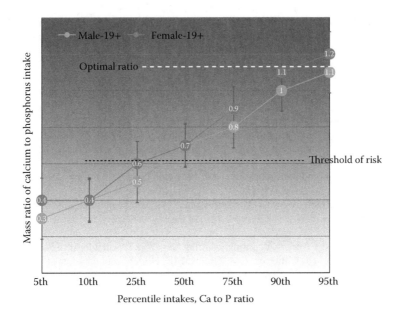

FIGURE 19.4 (See color insert.) NHANES, 2009–2010: Distribution of daily individual Ca to P intake ratios across selected percentiles of intake for men and women ≥19 y. Daily individual calcium-to-phosphorus (Ca:P) mass intake ratios for men (*n* = 2880) and women (*n* = 3038) age ≥19 y across selected percentiles of intake from day-1 dietary intake estimates of NHANES 2009–2010. (Reproduced from Calvo MS, Moshfegh AJ, Tucker KL, *Adv Nutr.*, 5, 104–13, 2014. With permission.)

19.5.3 Association of Dietary Phosphorus with Variability in Levels of FGF-23 in Vulnerable Populations

Low socioeconomic status is associated with higher serum phosphorus (Gutiérrez et al. 2010), possibly due to consumption of lower cost foods shown to be higher in phosphate-containing food additives (Leon et al. 2013). The association of higher serum Pi has been associated with higher FGF-23 levels, but Gutiérrez et al. (2010) found that the association was independent of race. Higher levels of FGF-23 are a well-established risk factor in cardiovascular disease (Scialla et al. 2012; Scialla 2015), with a recently recognized association with cause-specific mortality in the general urban population of Manhattan, but specifically affecting African Americans and Hispanics (Scialla et al. 2013; Souma et al. 2016). Associations between dietary factors and the level of FGF-23 have been established in individuals with African ancestry (Eckberg et al. 2015; Kosk et al. 2016). FGF-23 has been shown to differ across African populations by degree of industrialization, with those consuming the typical Western dietary pattern in the United States having the highest levels compared to individuals in less industrialized countries like Ghana (Eckberg et al. 2015; Yuen et al. 2016). Yeun and colleagues (2016) attribute this finding to the higher phosphate content of the Western diet and a greater consumption of highly processed foods.

REFERENCES

Adatorwovor, R, Roggenkamp, K, Anderson, JJB, Intakes of calcium and phosphorus and calculated calcium-to-phosphorus ratios of older adults: NHANES 2005-2006 data. *Nutrients.* 2015; 7:9633–9.

Andrews, KW, Roseland, JM, Gusev, PA, et al. Analytical ingredient content and variability of adult multivitamin/mineral products: National estimates for the dietary supplement ingredient database. *Am J Clin Nutr.* 2017; 105:526–39.

Antoniucci, DM, Yamahita, T, Portale, AA, Dietary phosphorus regulates serum fibroblast growth factor-23 concentration in healthy men. *J Clin Endocrinol Metab* 2006; 91:3144–9.

Asghari, G, Farhadnejad, H, Mirmiran, P, Dizavi, A, Yuzbashian, E, Azizi, F, Adherence to the Mediterranean diet is associated with reduced risk of incident chronic kidney diseases among Tehranian adults. *Hypertens Res.* 2016; 40:96–102. doi:10.1038/hr.2016.98.

Calvo, MS, Dietary phosphorus, calcium metabolism and bone. *J Nutr.* 1993; 123:1627–33.

Calvo, MS, Eastell, R, Offord, KP, Berstrahl, EJ, Burritt, MF, Circadian variation in ionized calcium and intact parathyroid hormone: Evidence for sex differences in calcium homeostasis. *J Clin Endocrinol Metab.* 1991; 72:69–76.

Calvo, MS, Kumar, R, Heath, H, Persistently elevated parathyroid hormone secretion and action in young women after ingesting high phosphorus, low calcium diets. *J Clin Endocrinol Metab.* 1990; 70:1334–40.

Calvo, MS, Moshfegh, AJ, Tucker, KL, Assessing the health impact of phosphorus in the food supply: Issues and considerations. *Adv Nutr.* 2014; 5:104–13.

Calvo, MS, Park, YM., Changing Phosphorus content of the U.S. diet: Potential for adverse effects on bone. *J Nutr.* 1996; 126 (4 Suppl):1168S–80S.

Calvo, MS, Uribarri, J, Contributions to total phosphorus intake: All sources considered. *Sem Dial.* 2013; 26:54–61.

Calvo, MS, Uribarri, J, Phosphorus in the modern food supply: Underestimation of exposure. *In: Clinical Aspects of Natural and Added Phosphorus in Foods.* Gutierrez, OM, Kalatar-Zadeh, K, Mehrota, R, (Eds.), 1st ed. 2016. New York, NY: Springer-Verlag New York (Available April 2017).

Chang, AR, Lazo, M, Appel, LJ, Gutierrez, OM, Grams, ME, High phosphorus intake is associated with all cause-mortality. Results from NHANES III. *Am J Clin Nutr.* 2014; 99:320–27.

Chang, AR, Miller, E, 3rd, Anderson, CA, et al. Phosphorus additives and albuminuria in early stages of CKD: Randomized controlled trial. *Am J Kidney Dis.* 2017; 69(2):200–9.

D'Alessandro, C, Piccoli, GB, Cupisti, A, The "phosphorus pyramid": A visual tool for dietary phosphate management in dialysis and CKD patients. *BMC Nephrol.* 2015; 16:9. doi:10.1186/147-2369-16-9.

De Fornasari, ML, Dos Santos Sens, YA, Replacing phosphorus-containing food additives with foods without additives reduces phosphatemia in End-Stage Renal Disease patients: A randomized clinical trial. *J Ren Nutr.* 2017; 27(2):97–1053.

Eckberg, K, Kramer, H, Wolf, M, Durazo-Arvizu, R, Tayo, B, Luke, A, Cooper, R, Impact of Westernization on fibroblast growth factor 23 levels among individuals of African ancestry. *Nephrol Dial Transplant.* 2015; 30:630–5.

EFSA Panel on Dietetic Products, Nutrition and Allergies (NDA). Scientific opinion on dietary reference values for phosphorus. *EFSA J.* 2015; 13(7):4185.

El-Shaarawy, MI, Reith, JK, On the phosphate problem. *Pahlavi Med J.* 1976; 7(2):195–213.

Federal Register Document Citation: 21 CFR 101.81 FR pages 3374-33999, Document No.2016-1186

Fulgoni, VL, 3rd, Keast, DR, Bailey, RL, Dwyer, J, Food, fortificants, and supplements: Where do Americans get their nutrients? *J Nutr.* 2011; 141:1847–54.

Gallieni, M, Cupisti, A, Editorial: Dash and Mediterranean diets as nutritional interventions for CKD patients. *Am J Kidney Dis.* 2016; 68(6):828–30.

Gutiérrez, OM, Sodium- and phosphorus-based food additives: Persistent but surmountable hurdles in the management of nutrition in chronic kidney disease. *Adv Chronic Kidney Dis.* 2013a; 20:150–6.

Gutiérrez, OM, The connection between dietary phosphorus, cardiovascular disease, and mortality: Where we stand and what we need to know. *Adv Nutr.* 2013b; 4:723–9.

Gutiérrez, OM, Anderson, C, Isakova, T, et al. Low socioeconomic status associates with higher serum phosphate irrespective of race. *J Am Soc Nephrol.* 2010; 21(11):1953–60.

Gutiérrez, OM, Luzuriaga-McPherson, A, Lin, Y, Gilbert, LC, Ha, SW, Beck, GR, Jr. Impact of phosphorus-based food additives on bone and mineral metabolism. *J Clin Endocrinol Metabol.* 2015; 100(11):4264–71.

Gutiérrez, OM, Wolf, M, Taylor, EN, Fibroblast growth factor-23, cardiovascular disease risk factors, and phosphorus intake in the health professionals' follow-up study. *Clin J Am Soc Nephrol.* 2011; 6:2871–8.

IOM (Institute of Medicine). 1997. *Dietary Reference Intakes for Calcium, Phosphorus, Magnesium, Vitamin D, and Fluoride.* Washington, DC: National Academy Press, pp. 454.

Itkonen, ST, Karp, HJ, Kemi, VE, et al. Association among total and food additive phosphorus intake and carotid intima-media thickness—A cross-secrtional study in a middle-aged population in Southern Finland. *Nutr J.* 2013; 12:94.

Itkonen, ST, Rita, HJ, Saamio, EM, et al. Dietary phosphorus intake is negatively associated with bone formation among women and positively associated with some bone traits among men—A cross-sectional study in middle-aged Caucasians. *Nutr Res.* 2017; 37:58–66.

Ito, S, Ishida, H, Uenishi, K, Murakami, K, Sasaki, S, The relationship between habitual dietary phosphorus and calcium intake, and bone mineral density in young Japanese women: A cross-sectional study. *Asia Pac J Clin Nutr.* 2011; 20:411–7.

The Regulatory Aspects of Phosphorus Intake

Kalantar-Zadeh, K, Gutekunst, L, Mehrota, R, et al. Understanding sources of dietary phosphorus in the treatment of patients with chronic kidney disease. *Clin J Am Soc Nephrol*. 2010; 5:519–30.

Karp, H, Ekholm, P, Kemi, V, Hironen, T, Lamberg-Allardt, CJ, Differences among total and in vitro digestible phosphorus content of meat and milk products. *J Ren Nutr*. 2012a; 22:344–9.

Karp, H, Ekholm, P, Kemi, VE, Itkonen, S, Hirvonen, T, Narkki, S, Lamberg-Allardt, CJ, Differences among total and in vitro digestible phosphorus content of plant foods and beverages. *J Ren Nutr*. 2012b; 22(4):416–22.

Kelly, JT, Palmer, SC, Wai, SN, Ruospo, M, Carrero, JJ, Campbell, KL, Strippoli, GF, Healthy dietary patterns and risk of mortality and ESRD in CKD: A meta-analysis of cohort studies. *Clin J Am Soc Nephrol*. 2017; 12(2):272–9.

Kemi, VE, Karkkainen, MU, Lamberg-Allardt, CJ, High phosphorus intakes acutely and negatively affect calcium and bone metabolism in a dose-dependent manner in healthy young females. *Br J Nutr*. 2006; 96:545–52.

Kemi, VE, Karkkainen, MU, Rita, HJ, Laaksonen, MM, Outila, TA, Lamberg-Allardt, CJ, Low calcium: Phosphorus ratio in habitual diets affects serum parathyroid hormone concentration and calcium metabolism in healthy women with adequate calcium intake. *Br J Nutr*. 2010; 103:561–8.

Kosk, D, Kramer, H, Luke, A, et al. Dietary factors and fibroblast growth factor-23 levels in young adults with African ancestry. *J Bone Miner Metab*. 2016. doi:10.1007/s00774-016-0804-5 (Epub ahead of print).

Kwak, SM, Kim, SJ, Choi, Y, et al. Dietary intake of calcium and phosphorus and serum concentration in relation to the risk of coronary artery calcification in asymptomatic adults. *Arterioscler Thromb Vasc Biol*. 2014; 34:1763–9.

Lee, AW, Cho, SS, Association between phosphorus intake and bone health in the NHANES population. *Nutr J*. 2015; 14:28.

Lee, KJ, Kim, KS, Kim, HN, Seo, JA, Song, SW, Association between dietary calcium and phosphorus intakes, dietary calcium: Phosphorus ratio and bone mass in Korean population. *Nutr J*. 2014; 13:114.

Leon, JB, Sullivan, CM, Sehgal, AR, The prevalence of phosphorus containing food additives in top selling foods in grocery stores. *J Ren Nutr*. 2013; 23(4):265–270.e2. doi:10.1053/j.jrn.2012.12.003.

McClure, ST, Chang, AR, Selvin, E, Rebholz, CM, Appel, LJ, Dietary sources of phosphorus among adults in the United States: Results from NHANES 2001-2014. *Nutrients*. 2017; 9:95. doi:10.3390/nu9020095.

Mc Cutcheon, J, Campbell, K, Ferguson, M, Day, S, Rossi, M, Prevalence of phosphorus-based additives in Australian food supply: A challenge for dietary education. *J Ren Nutr*. 2015; 25(5):440–4.

Moe, SM, Zidehsarai, MP, Chambers, MA, Jackman, LA, Radcliffe, JS, Trevino, LL, Donahue, SE, Asplin, JR, Vegetarian compared to meat dietary protein source and phosphorus homeostasis in chronic kidney disease. *Clin J Am Soc Nephrol*. 2011; 6:257–264.

Moore, LW, Nolte, JV, Gaber, AO, Suki, WN, Association of dietary phosphate and serum phosphorus concentrations by levels of kidney function. *Am J Clin Nutr*. 2015; 102:444–53.

Moshfegh, A, Kovalchik, AF, Clemens, JC, Phosphorus Intake of the U.S. Population: What We Eat in America, NHANES 2011-2012. *Food Surveys Research. Group Dietary Data Brief No.15. September 2016*.

Murgtaugh, MA, Filipowicz, R, Baird, BC, Wei, G, Greene, T, Beddhu, S, Dietary phosphorus intake and mortality in moderate chronic kidney disease: NHANES III. *Nephrol Dial Transplant*. 2012; 27:990–6.

Nordin, BEC, Phosphorus. *J Food Nutr*. 1988; 45:62–75.

Oenning, LL, Vogel, J, Calvo, MS, Accuracy of methods estimating calcium and phosphorus intake in daily diets. *J Am Diet Assoc*. 1988; 88:1076–80.

Olza, J, Arnceta-Bartrina, J, Gonzallez-Gross, M, Ortega, RM, Serra-Majem, L, Varela-Moreiras, G, Gil, A, Reported dietary intake, disparity between the reported consumption and the level needed for adequacy and food sources of calcium, phosphorus, magnesium and vitamin D in the Spanish population: Findings from the ANIBES study. *Nutrients*. 2017; 9:168. doi:10.339020168.

Otten, JJ, Hellwig, JP, Meyers, LD, (Eds.). *Dietary Reference Intakes: The Essential Guide to Nutrient Requirements*. Washington, DC: The National Academies Press, 2006.

Portale, AA, Halloran, BP, Morris, RC, Jr. Dietary intake of phosphorus modulates the circadian rhythm in serum concentration of phosphorus. Implications for the renal production of 1,25-dihydroxyvitamin D. *J Clin Invest*. 1987; 80:1147–54.

Reboholz, C, Crews, DC, Grams, ME, et al. DASH (Dietary Approaches to Stop Hypertension) diet and risk of subsequent kidney disease. *Am J Kidney Dis*. 2016; 68(6):853–61.

Ritz, E, Hahn, K, Kettler, M, Kuhlmann, MK, Mann, J, Phosphate additives in food—A health risk. *Dtsch Arztebl Int*. 2012; 109(4):49–55.

Scialla, JJ, Epidemiologic insights on the role of fibroblast growth factor 23 in cardiovascular disease. *Curr Opin Nephrol Hypertens*. 2015; 24(3):260–7.

Scialla, JJ, Appel, LJ, Wolf, M, et al. Plant protein intake is associated with fibroblast growth factor 23 and serum bicarbonate levels in patients with chronic kidney disease: The Chronic Renal Insufficiency Cohort study. *J Ren Nutr*. 2012; 22(4):379–88.

Scialla, JJ, Astor, BC, Isakova, T, Xie, H, Appel, LJ, Wolf, M, Mineral metabolites and CKD progression in African Americans. *J Am Soc Nephrol*. 2013; 24:125–35.

Souma, N, Isakova, T, Lipiszko, D, et al. Fibroblast growth factor 23 and cause-specific mortality in the general population: The Manhattan Study. *J Clin Endocrinol Metab*. 2016; 101(10):3779–86.

St-Jules, DE, Jagannathan, R, Gutekunst, L, Kalantar-Zadeh, K, Sevick, MA, Examining the proportion of dietary phosphorus from plants, animals and food additives excreted in urine. *J Ren Nutr*. 2017; 27(2):78–83.

Sullivan, CM, Leon, JB, Sehgal, AR, Phosphorus-containing food additives and the accuracy of nutrient databases: Implications for renal patients. *J Ren Nutr*. 2007; 17:350–54.

Takeda, E, Yamamoto, H, Yamanlo-Okuura, H, Taketani, Y, Dietary phosphorus in bone health and quality of life. *Nutr Rev*. 2012; 70:311–21.

Teegarden, D, Lyle, RM, McCabe, LD, et al. Dietary calcium, protein and phosphorus are related to bone mineral density and content in young women. *Am J Clin Nutr*. 1998; 68:749–54.

Trautvetter, U, Jahreis, G, Kiehntopf, M, Glei, M, Consequences of a high phosphorus intake on mineral metabolism and bone remodeling in dependence of calcium intake in healthy subjects—A randomized placebo-controlled human intervention study. *Nutr J*. 2016; 15:7.

Uribarri, J, Phosphorus additives in food and their effect in dialysis patients. *Clin J Am Soc Nephrol*. 2009; 4:1290–2.

Uribarri, J, Calvo, MS, Hidden sources of phosphorus in the typical American diet: Does it matter in nephrology? *Sem Dial*. 2003; 16(3):186–8.

Vin, K, Connolly, A, McCaffrey, T, Estimation of the dietary intake of 13 priority additives in France, Italy, the UK and Ireland as part of the FACET project. *Food Addit Contam Part A Chem Anal Control Expo Risk Assess*. 2013; 30(12):2050–80.

Whiting, SJ, Boyle, JL, Thompson, A, Mirwald, RL, Fukler, RA, Dietary protein, phosphorus and potassium are beneficial to bone mineral density in adult men consuming adequate dietary calcium. *J Am Coll Nutr*. 2002;21: 402–9.

Yamamoto, KT, Robinson-Cohen, C, de Oliveira, MC, et al. Dietary phosphorus is associated with greater left ventricular mass. *Kidney Int*. 2013; 83:707–14.

Yuen, SN, Kramer, H, Luke, A, et al. Fibroblast Growth Factor-23 (FGF-23) levels differ across populations by degree of industrialization. *J Clin Endocrinol Metab*. 2016; 101(5):2246–53.

20 Dietary Guidelines for Safe Levels of Phosphorus Intake in North America and Europe

Susan J. Whiting and Mona S. Calvo

CONTENTS

Abstract 267
Bullet Points 268
20.1 Introduction 268
20.2 Derivation of the Tolerable Upper Intake Level for Phosphorus 268
    20.2.1 Setting the UL for Phosphorus for Adults 19 to 70 years 268
    20.2.2 Setting the UL for Phosphorus for Other Age Groups 270
20.3 Scientific Opinion on a Safe Level of Phosphorus Intake from the European Food Safety Authority 270
    20.3.1 The EFSA's Opinion about an Upper Level of Safe Intake 270
    20.3.2 EFSA's Opinion Concerning the Use of Serum Phosphate as a Biomarker 271
20.4 Recent Data on Adverse Health Effects of High Phosphorus Intake in Healthy Adults 271
    20.4.1 High Phosphorus Intake and All-Cause Mortality 272
    20.4.2 High Phosphorus Intake and Risk of Cardiovascular Disease 272
    20.4.3 High Phosphorus Intake and Cancer 273
    20.4.4 High Phosphorus Intake and FGF23 Resistance 274
20.5 Future Research Needs Regarding the UL for Phosphorus 274
References 275

ABSTRACT

Many nutrients, including phosphorus (P), have had a tolerable upper intake level (UL) set as part of the Dietary Reference Intake process of the Food and Nutrition Board. These UL values are used in assessment and planning in the United States, Canada, and other countries who have adopted DRIs. A UL is deemed to be a safe intake, but as intake increases above the UL, risk for adverse effects increases also. The UL set in 1997 is 3000 mg/d for children 1 to 3 years, 4 to 8 years, and men and women 70 years and older; for all other age groups is it 4000 mg/d. It was set based on derived data that predicted intakes causing an increase in serum phosphorus above the normal range. In contrast, the European Food Safety Agency has repeatedly declined to set an upper level of safe intake. Recent advances indicate a need to revisit the UL for phosphorus intake. First, there is now greater concern about higher intakes in Western countries due to food additive use in food processing and the higher consumption of these convenience foods. Second, new health concerns have been recognized in the past two decades. A high serum phosphate level is associated with increased mortality, particularly in those with renal failure. In particular, in the general American population, phosphorus intake expressed as phosphorus density was associated with cardiovascular mortality. The mechanism for this effect may lie in serum phosphorus's effect to reduce calcitriol levels and increase secretion of fibroblast growth factor-23 (FGF23), which together are associated with left ventricular hypertrophy, a key risk factor in cardiovascular disease

(CVD). Other disease associations to high phosphorus intake are emerging. Thus the current UL for phosphorus, having been set in 1997 using outdated criteria and assumptions, needs re-examination in light of emerging evidence on the health risks of high phosphorus intakes.

BULLET POINTS

- The upper level (UL) of safe phosphorus intake for Canadian and American adults is 4000 mg/d and that for children 1 to 3 years, 4 to 8 years, and men and women 70 years and older is 3000 mg/d.
- No upper level of safe intake for phosphorus has been set by the European Food Safety Authority (EFSA).
- Growing evidence associates high phosphorus intake that is below the UL with all-cause mortality, cardiovascular disease, skeletal disorders, and cancer in renal failure and to a lesser degree in normal renal function, stressing the need to revisit the UL for phosphorus.
- High phosphorus intakes that are below the UL stimulate secretion of fibroblast growth factor-23 from bone, and this is thought to be a critical risk factor in cardiovascular disease, notably in renal failure.
- Intervention studies focused on lower dietary phosphorus intakes with adequate calcium intakes are needed to determine long-term effects on FGF23 levels associated with reduced risk of cardiovascular disease.

20.1 INTRODUCTION

The focal point of this chapter considers safety aspects of one of the four categories of Dietary Reference Intake (DRI) values for phosphorus: the tolerable upper intake level (UL). The DRIs were developed for over 35 micronutrients by the Food and Nutrition Board of the National Academies Institute of Medicine in conjunction with the U.S. and Canadian governments to help individuals optimize their health, prevent disease, and avoid consuming too much of a specific nutrient (IOM, 2006). The parameters used to develop the UL for phosphorus at critical life stages in the general healthy population and the appropriate use of this intake guideline in North America are discussed and compared to the intake guidelines set and used by the European Union to avoid consuming too much phosphorus. Additionally, recent examples of the growing evidence of adverse health effects associated with high phosphorus consumption and the changes in food sources thought to contribute to a high level of intake are discussed.

20.2 DERIVATION OF THE TOLERABLE UPPER INTAKE LEVEL FOR PHOSPHORUS

The DRI values for phosphorus were set by the Institute of Medicine (IOM) in 1997 and have not undergone any revisions since that time. These DRI values, shown in Table 20.1, apply to Canada and the United States and any other country that has adopted these DRIs (see Chapter 19). The processes of setting the DRIs for phosphorus are detailed in the book that was released by the IOM (1997), which also describes the rationale used at arriving at the UL for phosphorus intake (IOM, 1997). DRIs provide the daily reference values, intended for healthy people, for assessment and planning functions in nutrition. The four categories of DRI values include the Estimated Average Requirement (EAR), which is the median requirement; the recommended dietary allowance (RDA), which is the amount that meets the needs of almost all (97.5%) healthy persons in the population; the adequate intake (AI), which is set for infants age 0 to 1 year, and the tolerable upper intake level (UL), which is set at a level that poses no risk for adverse health effects.

20.2.1 Setting the UL for Phosphorus for Adults 19 to 70 years

To set the UL, the panel charged with determining the UL for phosphorus defined phosphorus excess as hyperphosphatemia (>1.5 mmol/L), especially in the extracellular fluid (ECF) (IOM,

TABLE 20.1
The 1997 Dietary Reference Intake Values for Phosphorus

Age Group	Estimated Average Requirement, EAR mg/day		Recommended Dietary Allowance, RDA or Adequate Intake, AI* mg/day		Tolerable Upper Intake Level, UL mg/day	
	M	F	M	F	M	F
0–6 mo	N/A	N/A	100*	100*	ND	ND
6–12 mo	N/A	N/A	275*	275*	ND	ND
1–3 y	380	380	460	460	3000	3000
4–8 y	405	405	500	500	3000	3000
9–18 y	1055	1055	1250	1250	4000	4000
		P 1055		P 1250		P 3500
		L 1055		L 1250		L 4000
19–50 y	580	580	700	700	4000	4000
		P 580		P 700		P 3500
		L 580		L 700		L 4000
51–70 y	580	580	700	700	4000	4000
> 70 y M	580	580	700	700	3000	3000

* Values with asterisk are AIs not RDAs.

N/A = not applicable (infant values are AIs that are based on the composition of breast milk); ND = not determined and stated that "source of intake should only be from food to prevent high levels of intake." M = males; F = females; P = pregnancy; L = lactation values

1997). In 1996 when the UL was undertaken for the first time, the signs and symptoms of health concerns resulting from hyperphosphatemia included changes in hormonal control of calcium (notably increased parathyroid hormone), evidence of ectopic calcification, with the kidney being particularly vulnerable, and increased skeletal porosity. Another possible adverse effect of excess phosphorus intake to consider was a reduction in calcium absorption, as well as the potential to reduce absorption of iron, copper, and zinc; however, it was noted that most of the evidence for mineral malabsorption was taken from animal studies and thus not directly applicable to humans. Extrapolating results from animal studies to the human situation presented a challenge as the phosphorus density of animal diets is much higher (4–6 mmol/100 kcal) compared to that of humans (2 mmol/100 kcal).

The four adverse effects of excess phosphorus intake identified by the IOM panel were further assessed for their appropriate use as criterion for setting the UL. Changes in hormonal control of calcium via increases in parathyroid hormone (PTH) release had been studied in both animal and human experiments. Human diets high in phosphorus and low in calcium produced sustained increases in PTH (Calvo et al., 1988, 1990); then again, the panel argued that low-calcium diets alone also stimulated PTH release. Accordingly, the panel was not convinced that high phosphorus, per se, was implicated in this adverse effect. An exception was made for infants ages 0 to 12 months. Infants were known to be sensitive to the dietary Ca:P ratio, developing hypocalcemia in the presence of excess serum phosphate (DeVizia and Mansi, 1992). For this age group, no UL was set; however, the panel cautioned that infants should receive only human milk or specially designed formula which would have the proper Ca:P ratio (IOM, 1997).

The second potential criterion for setting the UL was ectopic (metastatic) calcification, which occurs when the calcium and phosphate concentrations in the ECF exceed solubility, along with other factors promoting calcification such as an alkaline pH that can occur with elevated serum phosphate. The kidney is particularly vulnerable, as a drop in renal clearance will prevent phosphate excretion, further promoting supersaturation of phosphate and calcium and soft tissue calcification

(IOM, 1997). The IOM panel acknowledged the dangers of higher phosphorus intake and increased susceptibility to ectopic calcification in persons with end-stage renal disease (i.e., functioning tissue mass <20 % of normal). Although evidence of soft tissue calcification was not taken as the criterion for setting the UL, there was an adjustment for older adults (>70 years) based on the likelihood of their having poor renal function with advancing age (Lindeman et al., 1985).

Skeletal porosity was the third known problem of excess phosphorus intake examined by the IOM panel. Early studies in animals had shown bone lesions, but it was felt none of the reported situations in rabbits and bulls had application to human nutrition (IOM, 1997). Finally, the panel examined the effect of excess phosphorus intake on reducing calcium absorption, but concluded that calcium intake was the more important determinant. Despite their exhaustive assessment of the known literature, the IOM panel was unable to find a specific adverse effect related to excess phosphorus intake that could be used to set the UL for phosphorus. Instead, the panel chose to examine the intake of phosphorus that would cause serum to rise above the upper boundary of normal serum phosphate, defined as 1.5 mmol/L (IOM, 1997).

Data on dietary (ingested) phosphorus plotted against serum phosphate was inferred using data derived from Nordin (1988), data that in turn were based on values extrapolated from a phosphorus infusion study in young adults (Bijovet, 1969), not based on varying dietary phosphorus intakes. Examination of the plotted values revealed that an estimated intake of 3500 mg phosphorus would result in serum phosphorus concentrations at the upper boundary of the normal range; however, the panel did not use this as the cut-off for the No Observed Adverse Effect Level (NOAEL). Instead, the panel argued that even the upper boundary of serum phosphate was physiological, based on animal studies and on the situation in infants whose normal serum phosphate levels are higher than adults. Based on this reasoning, the panel defined the NOAEL as the amount of ingested phosphorus by an adult that would correspond to the higher values for serum phosphate in infancy, which was reported as 2.15 mmol/L (5th percentile, 1.88; 97.5th percentile, 2.42) (IOM, 1997). The amount of ingested phosphorus needed to reach this higher serum concentration was calculated to be 10.2 g (10,200 mg) phosphorus per day. An uncertainty factor (UF) of 2.5 was chosen based on the pharmacologic practice of relating intake to blood levels (Petley et al., 1995). In setting the UL for adults, the NOAEL (10,200 mg) was divided by the UF (2.5) to give a value of ~4,000 mg/day, shown in Table 20.1.

20.2.2 Setting the UL for Phosphorus for Other Age Groups

The IOM panel did not set a UL for infants; rather, they provided the following statement: "not possible to establish; source of intake should be from formula and food only" (IOM, 1997). For toddlers and children ages 1 to 8 years, the UL was set at 3000 mg per day using the same NOAEL as for adults, but increasing the UF to 3.3 to account for a smaller body size in this age range. For adolescents ages 9 to 18 years, the UL was set at the same level as for adults ages 19 to 70 years.

For adults over 70 years of age, the UL was lowered to 3000 mg, established through the use of a higher UF, one similar to that for children (UF = 3.3). This was done to account for a high prevalence of impaired renal function in older adults (Lindeman et al., 1985).

20.3 SCIENTIFIC OPINION ON A SAFE LEVEL OF PHOSPHORUS INTAKE FROM THE EUROPEAN FOOD SAFETY AUTHORITY

20.3.1 The EFSA's Opinion about an Upper Level of Safe Intake

In 2005, the EFSA published an opinion of its panel on Dietetic Products, Nutrition and Allergies (NDA) regarding an intake guideline for an upper level for phosphorus intake. Although the EFSA panel acknowledged that animal studies had found adverse effects of excessive amount of dietary

Dietary Guidelines for Safe Levels of Phosphorus Intake in North America and Europe   271

phosphorus, it concluded that evidence for humans, other than end-stage renal disease patients, was lacking (ESFA NDA, 2005). It did however, note the following:

> Observational data suggest that high phosphorus intakes might aggravate the effects of a state of secondary hyperparathyroidism in individuals with inadequate calcium intakes, or an inadequate vitamin D status.

20.3.2 EFSA's Opinion Concerning the Use of Serum Phosphate as a Biomarker

The EFSA panel on NDA recently issued a scientific opinion on dietary reference values for phosphorus (EFSA NDA, 2015). Unlike the IOM (1997), which set EAR and RDA values for phosphorus separate from those of calcium in 1997, the EFSA NDA panel chose to emphasize the importance of the dietary Ca:P ratio and to continue to use the molar equivalent values for calcium intake guidelines to set values for phosphorus intake. The EFSA 2015 panel found no evidence to the contrary and continues to use ideal Ca:P ratios in tissues to set values for phosphorus intake. Overall the EFSA NDA panel found no new compelling evidence to change the European dietary reference values (DRVs) for phosphorus that had been set in 1993. In examining criteria for assessing requirements for phosphorus, the EFSA panel rejected the use of serum phosphate as an indicator of adequacy using the Nordin (1988) equation as described earlier. Their contention was that dietary phosphorus would have only a relatively small effect on serum phosphate concentrations. New findings cast a different light on this argument. A recent study examining the association between dietary phosphorus intake and serum phosphate, using data from the Third NHANES nationally representative survey in the United States, found that an incremental intake of 500 mg phosphorus appeared to affect serum phosphate only by a factor of 1% (de Boer et al., 2009). What is now known as of 2015 that was not known previously is that regulatory hormones in addition to PTH and the active metabolite of vitamin D, such as FGF23 and klotho, regulate serum phosphate levels in persons with normal kidney function. Moreover, all these hormonal factors respond to changes in dietary phosphorus intake to rapidly increase or decrease renal phosphate excretion or modify skeletal resorption of calcium and phosphorus, adjusting serum phosphate to maintain it within a very narrow concentration range (Calvo et al., 2014). The EFSA panel concluded "because of fine renal regulation, fasting serum phosphate concentrations show only minimal modifications even in the presence of wide variations in intake" (EFSA NDA, 2015).

The EFSA declined to set an upper level of safe intake in 2005 and continues to maintain this decision in their recent scientific opinion on dietary reference values for phosphorus that was initially requested by the European Commission (EFSA NDA, 2005, 2015).

20.4 RECENT DATA ON ADVERSE HEALTH EFFECTS OF HIGH PHOSPHORUS INTAKE IN HEALTHY ADULTS

The UL for phosphorus was set almost two decades ago at a time when factors controlling phosphorus homeostasis were not completely understood (see Chapters 5, 6, and 7). For example, the roles of FGF23 and klotho and their negative influence on PTH and vitamin D activation were unknown. Recent data indicate a possible need for greater concern about higher phosphorus intake in Western countries, where intakes are high largely due to food additive use in processing and the higher consumption of processed and convenience foods (Calvo and Park, 1996; Kemi et al., 2009; Calvo and Uribarri, 2013 a, b; Takeda et al., 2014; Poti et al., 2015). What follows is a brief review of recent evidence supporting the need for more research examining the health impact of total phosphorus intakes in the general population. This discussion does not include the health risks for those with renal failure (see Chapters 8 and 9), nor a review of the effects of high phosphorus on bone metabolism (see Chapter 3).

20.4.1 High Phosphorus Intake and All-Cause Mortality

Studies have shown that high serum phosphate levels are associated with increased mortality, particularly in those with renal failure (see Chapter 4) (Ix et al., 2012). However, new data are emerging indicating that even those with apparently normal renal function can be adversely affected by phosphorus intakes that exceed the current RDA but are well below the current UL (Bates et al., 2012; Itkonen et al., 2013; Calvo and Uribarri, 2013a; Yamamoto et al., 2012; Chang et al., 2014).

In a follow-up study of the British National Diet and Nutrition Survey of people aged 65 years and older, both baseline plasma concentrations and phosphorus intake were found to predict all-cause mortality in older women, whereas only baseline plasma phosphate predicted all-cause mortality in older British men (Bates et al., 2012). Using follow-up mortality and cardiovascular disease (CVD) data of U.S. participants in NHANES III, Chang et al. (2014) analyzed the association of dietary phosphorus intake with these health outcomes. Close to 10,000 adults (nonpregnant) age 20 to 80 years who had complete mortality, dietary, and covariate data were included. The investigators excluded NHANES participants with indications of diabetes, cardiovascular disease (CVD), or kidney disease at the time of the survey. Follow-up for all-cause mortality and mortality from CVD was determined for 12 to 18 years. The main findings of this analysis are shown in Figure 20.1. All-cause mortality showed no relationship with total phosphorus intakes at or below 1400 mg/day. However, for those above 1400 mg/day, the hazard ratio (HR) was 1.89, indicating almost a two-fold risk of dying. This effect was not seen, however, when investigators examined phosphorus intake density (P intake per kcal) (HR = 1.05); neither phosphorus density nor total P intake was associated with CVD mortality. Notably, the adverse effect high phosphorus intake had on mortality was not due to differences in eating habits, serum phosphate, or body mass index.

20.4.2 High Phosphorus Intake and Risk of Cardiovascular Disease

Excess intake of phosphorus is a critical risk factor for CVD in chronic kidney disease, as well as in the general population (see Chapter 8). Dietary phosphorus has been shown to stimulate secretion of FGF23 from bone, the phosphaturic hormone that lowers 1,25-dihydroxvitamin D and inhibits PTH secretion (see Chapter 6). Both low active vitamin D (Bodyak et al., 2007) and high FGF23 (Faul et al., 2011) serum concentrations are associated with left ventricular hypertrophy (LVH), a key risk factor in CVD. Yamamoto et al. (2012) examined whether dietary phosphorus intake was associated with left ventricular mass in a multiethnic cohort of adults who were free of known CVD, using cardiac magnetic resonance imaging. In their analysis, higher estimated phosphorus

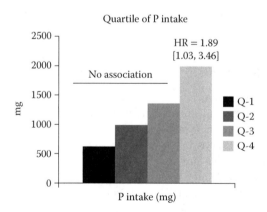

FIGURE 20.1 Four quartiles of phosphorus (P) intake. Using regression analysis, the authors found a significant increase in risk (HR, hazard ratio) for all-cause mortality in the fourth quartile (Q-4). (Adapted from Chang, A, R. et al., *Am J Clin Nutr.*, 99, 320–7, 2014.)

intake was positively associated with greater LVH. To better quantify the effect, the authors divided phosphorus intake into sex-specific quintiles (Q) of intake (mg): Q-1, 270 to 687 (M) 251 to 585 (F); Q-2, 688 to 917 (M) 586 to 775 (F); Q-3, 918 to 1166 (M) 776 to 1009 (F); Q-4, 1167 to 1553 (M) 1010 to 1345 (F); and Q-5, 1554 to 5032 (M) 1346 to 4069 (F). The increase in left ventricular hypertrophy over the quintiles of phosphorus was determined from the difference in weight from Q-1 (Figure 20.2) for each of the remaining quintiles with adjustment of the final regression model for demographic, dietary, and lifestyle factors, as well as for comorbidities. The LVH effect was significant for phosphorus intakes of quintiles 3, 4, and 5 (i.e., intakes above the RDA of 700 mg). This dietary phosphorus link was most significant in women, despite their lower phosphorus intakes, which suggests a possible gender difference for phosphorus health effects, a finding consistent with the earlier British study where phosphorus intake predicted all-cause mortality only in older women (Bates et al., 2012).

Further evidence for increased risk of CVD comes from work in Finland where Itkonen et al. (2013) showed that there was higher carotid intima-media thickness (IMT) among subjects with higher phosphorus intake. Moreover, there was a significant positive linear trend for phosphorus from food additives (determined from a Finnish-specific food frequency questionnaire) and IMT. In a cross-sectional study looking at the relationship between dietary intake and other cardiovascular risk factors for adults without a history of cardiovascular events, phosphorus intake was significantly correlated with both systolic and diastolic blood pressure. Crude and energy-adjusted phosphorus intake was a significant determinant of blood pressure (Mazidi et al., 2016). Thus, high dietary phosphorus intake merits further investigation due to its potential association with adverse cardiovascular health effects in the general population.

20.4.3 High Phosphorus Intake and Cancer

Clear evidence of a link between phosphorus intake and risk of diseases such as cancer that require long periods of follow-up are further confused by the changes in phosphorus content of the food supply over time. The significance of the association of phosphorus intake with cancer incidence are likely underestimated because nutrient composition databases do not measure food additive contributions, which have increased over time in the United States and EU (Calvo et al., 2014). Despite these obstacles, epidemiologic evidence is emerging demonstrating associations between

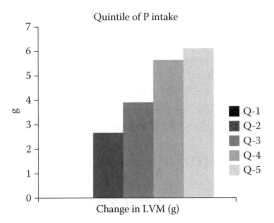

FIGURE 20.2 The change in mass (g) of the left ventricle (LV) by sex-specific quintiles of phosphorus (P) intake: Q-1, 270–687 (M) 251–585 (F); Q-2, 688–917 (M) 586–775 (F); Q-3, 918–1166 (M) 776–1009 (F); Q-4, 1167–1553 (M) 1010–1345 (F); and Q-5, 1554–5032 (M) 1346–4069 (F). There was a significant relationship in progressive hypertrophy by increased phosphorus intake. (Adapted from Yamamoto, K, T. et al., *Kidney Int.*, 83, 707–14, 2012.)

phosphorus intake and incident prostate cancer (Giovannucci et al., 2006; Tseng et al., 2005; Kesse et al., 2006; Mitrou et al., 2007; Wilson et al., 2015).

The most recent of these studies examined the joint association between calcium and phosphorus intake and risk of prostate cancer in a 24- year follow-up of the Health Professionals Study (Wilson et al., 2015). A total of 47,885 men were followed prospectively (1986–2010) for cancer incidence, metastases, and mortality and their relation to diet using information collected every four years after baseline. The authors used a semi-quantitative food frequency questionnaire (130 food items with a validated correlation of 0.63 for phosphorus intake compared to two weeks of + dietary records) to determine phosphorus intake. Quintiles of total phosphorus intake ranged from a mean 1079 ± 90 mg in Q-1 to 1783 ± 195 for Q-5. Even the lowest quintile far exceeds the RDA for adults. Wilson et al. (2015) found that high phosphorus intake was associated with increased risk of advanced-stage and high-grade prostate cancer, independent of calcium intake and other dietary factors after only zero to eight years from baseline measurement. These authors found similar increased risk of advanced and high-grade disease after 12 to 16 years of exposure to calcium intakes greater than 200 mg/d.

Experimental findings using rodent models demonstrate that both high dietary intakes and serum phosphate are linked to the development of cancer of the lung, skin, and bladder when clearly defined diets with known phosphorus contents are fed (Anderson, 2013; Camalier et al., 2013). A number of possible metabolic pathways through which high-phosphate diets may initiate cancer development in various organs and tissues are discussed in Chapter 2.

20.4.4 High Phosphorus Intake and FGF23 Resistance

Specific effects of high phosphorus intake, such as a rise in parathyroid hormone (PTH) release and decrease in plasma calcium concentration, are known. But relating these to possible adverse effects of high phosphorus intakes, especially effects on bone, have not been consistent. For example, dairy intake, which is high in phosphorus, is beneficial to bone health (Bonjour et al., 2013). It appears that concomitant calcium intake determines whether high phosphorus has adverse effects on bone.

To this end, Takeda et al. (2014) have examined this question using acute loading tests and found that FGF23 increases only after a high P-low Ca load but not after a high P-high Ca load. They postulated that increased serum FGF23 normally triggers the parathyroid gland to stop releasing PTH. However, a "resistance" to this effect can develop with prolonged intake of high-phosphorus diets, and this resistance may contribute to poor bone health. Kemi et al. (2009) showed that high total habitual dietary phosphorus intake increased serum PTH unfavorably and that consumers with the highest intakes of phosphorus showed the highest mean PTH levels, despite adequate calcium intakes. This finding underscores the importance of the dietary calcium-to-phosphorus intake ratio. In a cross-sectional study in middle-aged Caucasians with adequate calcium intakes, Itkonen et al. (2017) found negative associations of dietary phosphorus intake and bone formation in women and, in contrast, a positive association with bone features in men, suggesting a possible gender difference that may be related to differences in dietary intake.

20.5 FUTURE RESEARCH NEEDS REGARDING THE UL FOR PHOSPHORUS

This chapter shows that the current IOM UL for phosphorus was set using criteria and assumptions that are outdated and lack validity. Issues that need to be addressed include the following:

- **Determination of appropriate biomarkers of adverse health effects other than serum phosphate concentrations.** The EFSA NDA committee could find no compelling reason to use serum phosphorus as a biomarker, citing studies that showed serum phosphorus was only weakly influenced by phosphorus intakes (EFSA NDA, 2015). This would suggest the current IOM UL has a problem of validity.

Dietary Guidelines for Safe Levels of Phosphorus Intake in North America and Europe   275

- **Consideration of newly revealed hormone mechanisms regulating phosphorus homeostasis as potential biomarkers.** Since 1997, when the IOM's UL was set, there have been new discoveries regarding phosphorus handling in the body. Specifically, FGF23, a phosphaturic hormone, may contribute to PTH resistance in situations of high P-low Ca intakes (Takeda et al., 2014), findings that underscore the importance of an appropriate Ca:P intake ratio. Intervention studies targeting dietary phosphorus and adequate calcium intake are needed to determine if FGF23 can be lowered and the risk of CVD reduced (Scialla, 2015).
- **Further exploration by prospective studies to confirm early findings of the role of high phosphorus intake in the prevalence of all-cause mortality, CVD, and cancer in the general population.** This is especially important in Western countries with high phosphorus intakes. One recent prospective study has found high phosphorus intake (>1400 mg/day) to be associated with higher all-cause mortality than those ingesting <1400 mg in otherwise healthy adults (Chang et al., 2014). There was no association with cardiovascular mortality.
- **Determination of the mechanisms involved in high phosphorus intake (>RDA) association with increased mortality, cancer, and CVD risk in humans.** High phosphorus intakes have been identified as influencing CVD risk factors that include hypertrophy of the left ventricle (Yamamoto et al., 2012) and higher carotid IMT (Itkonen et al., 2013) and cancer risk (Wilson et al., 2015).
- **Measurement of total phosphorus intake based on methods that accurately account for the natural and added phosphorus in foods, dietary supplements, and commonly used medications.** Adverse effects of phosphorus intake are seen with dietary intakes above the RDA but below the current UL of 3,000 to 40,000 mg. Although intakes of phosphorus are underestimated due to lack of values for many processed foods, when contributions from food additives are included in phosphorus intake estimates, stronger links to cardiovascular abnormalities have been observed (Itkonen et al., 2013).

Overall, evidence is building that the UL for phosphorus needs reconsideration, with a concerted effort to assess food additive phosphorus intakes and a UL based on estimates of current additive contributions, analogous to the situation of the IOM setting ULs for vitamins such as vitamin E and folate, which are based on fortification and supplement levels.

REFERENCES

Anderson, J.J.B. 2013. Potential health concerns of dietary phosphorus: Cancer, obesity, and hypertension. *Ann NY Acad Sci* 1301:1–8.

Bates, C.J., Hamer, M. and Mishra, G.D. 2012. A study of relationships between bone-related vitamins and minerals related risk markers and subsequent mortality in older British people: The National Diet and Nutrition Survey of People Aged 65 years and over. *Osteoporosis Int* 23:457–66.

Bijovet, O.L.M. 1969. Relation of plasma phosphate concentration to renal tubular reabsorption of phosphate. *Clin Sci* 37:23–6.

Bodyak, N., Ayus, J.C., Achinger, S. et al. 2007. Activated vitamin D attenuates left ventricular abnormalities induced by dietary sodium in dahl salt-sensitive animals. *Proc Natl Acad Sci USA* 104:16810–5.

Bonjour, J.P., Kraenzlin, M., Levasseur, R. et al. 2013. Dairy in adulthood: From foods to nutrient interactions on bone and skeletal muscle health. *J Am Coll Nutr* 32:251–63.

Calvo, M.S., Kumar, R. and Heath, H. III. 1988. Elevated secretion and action of serum parathyroid hormone in young adults consuming high phosphorus, low calcium diets assembled from common foods. *J Clin Endocrinol Metab* 66:823–9.

Calvo, M.S., Kumar, R. and Heath, H. III. 1990. Persistently elevated parathyroid hormone secretion and action in young women after four weeks of ingesting high phosphorus, low calcium diets. *J Clin Endocrinol Metab* 70:1334–40.

Calvo M.S. and Park, Y.M. 1996. Changing phosphorus content of the U.S. diet: Potential for adverse effects on bone. *J Nutr* 126:1168S–1180S.

Calvo, M.S. and Uribarri, J. 2013a. Public health impact of dietary phosphorus excess on bone and cardiovascular health in the general population. *Am J Clin Nutr* 98:6–15.

Calvo, M.S. and Uribarri, J. 2013b. Contributions to total phosphorus intake: All sources considered. *Semin Dial* 26:54–61.

Calvo, M.S., Moshfegh, A.J. and Tucker, K.L. 2014. Assessing the health impact of phosphorus in the food supply: Issues and considerations. *Adv Nutr* 5:104–13.

Camalier, C.E., Yi, M., Yu, L.R. et al. 2013. An integrated understanding of the physiological response to elevated extracellular phosphate. *J Cell Physiol* 228: 1536–50.

Chang, A.R., Lazo, M., Appel, L.J. et al. 2014. High dietary phosphorus intake is associated with all-cause mortality: Results from NHANES III. *Am J Clin Nutr* 99:320–7. (erratum *Am J Clin Nutr* 105:1021–2.)

de Boer, I.H., Rue, T.C., and Kestenbaum, B. 2009. Serum phosphorus concentrations in the third national health and nutrition examination survey (NHANES III). *Am J Kidney Dis* 53:399–407.

DeVizia, B. and Mansi, A. 1992. Calcium and phosphorus metabolism in full-term infants. *Monatsschr Kinderheilkd* 140:S8–S12.

EFSA NDA Panel (EFSA Scientific Panel on Dietetic Products, Nutrition and Allergies). 2005. Opinion of the scientific panel on dietetic products, nutrition and allergies on a request from the commission related to the tolerable upper intake of phosphorus. *EFSA J* 233:1–19.

EFSA NDA Panel (EFSA Panel on Dietetic Products, Nutrition and Allergies). 2015. Scientific opinion on dietary reference values for phosphorus. EFSA J2015 13(7):4185–239. Available online: http://www.efsa.europa.eu/efsajournal

Faul, C., Amaral, A.P., Oskouei, B. et al. 2011. FGF23 induces left ventricular hypertrophy. *J Clin Invest* 121:4393–408.

Giovannucci, E., Liu, Y., Stampfer, M.J. et al. 2006. A prospective study of calcium intake and incident and fatal prostate cancer. *Cancer Epidemiol Biomarkers Prev* 15:203–10.

Institute of Medicine. 1997. *Dietary Reference Intakes for Calcium, Magnesium, Phosphorus, Vitamin D, and Fluoride.* Washington, DC: National Academy Press.

Institute of Medicine. 2006. *Dietary Reference Intakes: The Essential Guide to Nutrient Requirements.* Otten, J.J, Hellwig, J.P., Meyers L.D. (eds.). Washington, DC: National Academies Press.

Itkonen, S.T., Karp, H.J., Kemi, V.E. et al. 2013. Associations among total and food additive phosphorus intake and carotid intima-media thickness–A cross-sectional study in a middle-aged population in Southern Finland. *Nutr J* 12:94. Available online: http://www.nutritionj.com/content/12/1/94

Itkonen, S.T., Rita, H.J., Saarnio E.M., et al. 2017. Dietary phosphorus intake is negatively associated with bone formation among women and positively associated with some bone traits among men—A cross-sectional study in middle-aged Caucasians. *Nutr. Res.* 37: 58–66.

Ix, J.H., Katz, R., Kestenbaum, B.R. et al. 2012. Fibroblast growth factor-23 and death, heart failure, and cardiovascular events in community-living individuals: CHS (cardiovascular health study). *J Am Coll Cardiol* 60:200–7.

Kemi, V.E., Rita, H.J., Kärkkäinen, M.U. et al. 2009. Habitual high phosphorus intakes and foods with phosphate additives negatively affect serum parathyroid hormone concentration: A cross-sectional study on healthy premenopausal women. *Public Health Nutr* 12:1885–92.

Kesse, E., Bertrais, S., Astorg, P. et al. 2006. Dairy products, calcium and phosphorus intake, and the risk of prostate cancer: Results from the French prospective SU.VI.MAX (Supplementation en Vitamines et Mineraux Antioxydants) study. *Br J. Nutr* 95:539–545.

Lindeman, R.D., Tobin, J. and Shock, N.W. 1985. Longitudinal studies on the rate of decline in renal function with age. *J Am Geriatr Soc* 33:278–85.

Mazidi, M., Nematy, M., Heidari-Bakavoli, A.R. et al. 2016. The relationship between dietary intake and other cardiovascular risk factors with blood pressure in individuals without a history of a cardiovascular event: Evidence based study with 5670 subjects. *Diabetes Metab Syndr.* Dec 9.pii:S1871–4021(16)30217-x doi:1010161lj.dsx.2016.12.005. [Epub ahead of print]

Mitrou, P.N., Albanes, D., Weinstein, S.J. et al. 2007. A prospective study of dietary calcium, dairy products and prostate cancer risk (Finland). *Int J Cancer* 120:2466–73.

Nordin, B.E.C. 1988. Phosphorus. *J Food Nutr* 45:62–75.

Petley, A., Maxlin, B., Renwick, A.G. et al. 1995. The pharmacokinetics of nicotinamide in humans and rodents. *Diabetes* 44:152–5.

Poti, J.M., Mendez, M.A., Ng, S.W. et al. 2015. Is the degree of food processing and convenience linked with the nutritional quality of foods purchased by US households? *Am J Clin Nutr* 101(6):1251–62. doi:10.3945/ajcn.114.100925.

Scialla, J.J. 2015. Epidemiologic insights on the role of fibroblast growth factor-23 in cardiovascular disease. *Curr Opin Nephrol Hypertens*. 24(3):260–7.

Takeda, E., Yamamoto, H., Yamanaka-Okumura, H. et al. 2014. Increasing dietary phosphorus intake from food additives: Potential for negative impact on bone health. *Adv Nutr* 5:92–7.

Tseng, M., Breslow, R.A., Graubard, B.I. et al. 2005. Dairy, calcium and vitamin D intakes and prostate cancer risk in the National Health and Nutrition Examination Epidemiologic Follow-up Study cohort. *Am J Clin Nutr* 81:1147–54.

Wilson, K.M., Shui, I.M., Lorelei, A.M. et al. 2015. Calcium and phosphorus intake and prostate cancer risk: A 24-year follow-up study. *Am J Clin Nutr*. 101:173–83.

Yamamoto, K.T., Robinson-Cohen, C., de Oliveira, M.C. et al. 2012. Dietary phosphorus is associated with greater left ventricular mass. *Kidney Int* 83:707–14.

21 Phosphorus Food Additive Use in the European Union

Ray J. Winger

CONTENTS

Abstract 279
Bullet Points 280
21.1 Introduction 280
    21.1.1 Regulatory Authority Governing Food Additive Use in the EU 280
    21.1.2 General Principles of Food Additive Use in the EU 282
21.2 Focus on Phosphorus-Containing Food Additives Approved for Use in the EU 283
    21.2.1 Use of Phosphorus-Containing Food Additives in Processed Foods 283
    21.2.2 Food Sources of Approved Phosphorus Additives 284
        21.2.2.1 Existing Phosphorus Data on Raw Ingredients 284
        21.2.2.2 Processed Foods That are Problematic for CKD Patients 306
21.3 Consumption of Phosphorus-Containing Food Additives in Europe 307
    21.3.1 Acceptable Daily Intake for Europe 307
        21.3.1.1 Consumption of P-Containing Food Additives 308
        21.3.1.2 Limitations of ADIs 309
References 309

ABSTRACT

The European regulations on food additives apply universally across all European Union (EU) countries. The approved additives are provided in Regulation EU1129/2011 as a positive list defined for over 154 food categories. If the additives are defined for the foods described in this listing, then they are permitted for use in those foods (only) throughout the EU. Additives used in other countries that are not included in this list are forbidden in the EU, and food containing such additives cannot be legally sold. Many additives approved for some foods sold in the EU are not permitted in other foods sold. Unless an additive is approved specifically for a particular food, it may not be added to that food, even if it can be legally added to a different food.

Some phosphorus-containing food additives, such as riboflavin, lecithin, and the starches, are regulated separately. However, all the food phosphates (E338–E452) are combined into one group and all the nucleotides (E626–E635) into a second group for regulatory purposes. Apart from the nucleotides, phosphorus-containing food additives are quantified as P_2O_5 and this is used to establish maximum additive levels within foods. Each group of phosphorus-containing additives (i.e., phosphates and nucleotides) has a single maximum level assigned for each of the various food categories. This singular level means the maximum for any and all group additives used in combination, not a maximum for each additive.

The EU has defined an "Acceptable Daily Intake" (ADI) of 70 mg P/kg body weight/day for all phosphorus-containing food additives combined. This equates to 4.9 g P/day for a 70-kg man. Using consumption data from a small number of EU countries, it appears that phosphorus intakes for European adults are below the ADI, but a portion of children and adolescents may be exceeding their ADIs.

BULLET POINTS

- European food regulations apply universally across all EU countries and provide an important platform for fostering and facilitating internal EU free trade.
- Only those food additives that are listed in the regulations are allowed to be present in any foods sold within the EU, irrespective of their country of origin. If food additives are not listed in the regulations, they are not allowed in any food sold.
- Many food additives are restricted to specific foods and are not allowed to be used in other foods sold in the EU.
- The phosphorus-containing additives are regulated collectively as a single group. All maximum phosphorus contents are defined in terms of P_2O_5, allowing for easy comparison across the different additives. Maximum phosphorus levels in foods are defined for all phosphates, in combination, as a single group (not for the individual additives).
- The Acceptable Daily Intake (ADI) for phosphates in the EU is 70 mg P/kg body weight/ day, or equivalent to 4.9 g P/day for a 70-kg man. Note this is defined as phosphorus, not P_2O_5. In general, existing data suggest EU consumption for adults is below this threshold, whereas some children may exceed their ADI limits.

21.1 INTRODUCTION

21.1.1 Regulatory Authority Governing Food Additive Use in the EU

The use of food additives in the EU is regulated by the European Parliament and the Council of the European Union, based in Brussels, Belgium. Proposals for food regulations, routine amendments and updates to approved regulations, enforcement of regulations, and the management and implementation of EU policies are the responsibility and function of the EU's executive body, The European Commission, also based in Brussels.

The key EU Parliament regulations related to food additives, and the EU Commission regulations related to food additives in general, as well as those that contain phosphorus, are provided in Table 21.1. In general, the Parliament regulations define the philosophies, principles, policies, and key criteria related to food additives, whereas the EU Commission regulations provide a greater depth of technical details to complement or complete the Parliament's documents. For example, Parliament regulation 89/107/EEC is the definitive European regulation related to food additives. It provides policies, definitions, when a food additive can be used (or not), and some aspects of labeling and also establishes the annexes, which contain the lists of approved additives. However, Annex II, which contains the list of food additives approved in Europe, is empty. These lists of approved food additives and their maximum use in various foods were introduced as "Directives" in the 1990s, but it is the Commission regulation EU 1129/2011 that now is the definitive document that contains all of Annex II and thus completes a necessary component of the original regulation.

All EU countries are fully involved with the Parliament and Commission, and each country has their input to these regulations. Regulations are normally approved with unanimity, although consensus may apply in some instances. A fundamental platform for the EU is that of free trade among member states, so the agreement and implementation of regulations normally minimizes any constraint of trade. This can make the details associated with the regulatory process somewhat slow to accomplish, given the wide perspectives of the member states, as can be seen by the time scale from the original food additives regulation (1988). For this reason, the two-step process involving the Parliament (political, policy-based regulations) and the Commission (scientific, technical detail) is an effective way to provide timely and efficient regulations on foods.

Each of the member states (countries) within the EU is expected to comply with the regulations prepared and approved in Brussels. However, each member state can augment the European regulations to suit their own unique situation.

TABLE 21.1
European Regulations Related to Food Additives Containing Phosphorus

Regulation Number	Date Approved	Title	Comments
89/107/EEC[a]	December 21 1988	The approximation of the laws of the Member States concerning food additives authorized for use in foodstuffs intended for human consumption	
94/35/EC[a]	June 30 1994	Sweeteners for use in foodstuffs	
94/36/EC	June 30 1994	Colours for use in foodstuffs	
95/2/EC	February 20 1995	Food additives other than colours and sweeteners	
96/77/EC	December 02 1996	Laying down specific purity criteria on food additives other than colours and sweeteners	
EC 1333/2008	December 16 2008	On food additives	
EU 1130/2011[b]	November 11 2011	Establishing a Union list of food additives approved for use in food additives, food enzymes, food flavourings & nutrients	amending Annex III to EC 133/2008
EU 1129/2011	November 11 2011	Establishing a Union list of food additives	amending Annex II to EC 133/2008
EU 244/2013	March 20 2013	Use of tricalcium phosphate (E341(iii)) in nutrient preparations intended for use in foods for infants and young children	amending Annex III to EC 133/2008
EU 438/2013	May 13 2013	Use of certain food additives	amending Annex II to EC 133/2008
EU 1068/2013	October 30 2013	Use of diphosphates (E450), triphosphates (E451) and polyphosphates (E452) in wet salted fish	amending Annex II to EC 133/2008
EU 1069/2013	October 30 2013	Use of sodium phosphates (E339) in natural casings for sausages	amending Annex II to EC 133/2008
EU 298/2014	March 21 2014	Magnesium dihydrogen diphosphate for use as a raising agent and acidity regulator	amending Annex II to EC 133/2008 and the Annex to EU 231/2012
EU 601/2014	June 04 2014	The food categories of meat and the use of food additives in meat preparations	amending Annex II to EC 133/2008
EU 1084/2014	October 15 2014	Use of diphosphates (E450) as a raising agent and acidity regulator in prepared yeast based doughs	amending Annex II to EC 133/2008

[a] Regulations containing EEC and EC in the Regulation number were gazetted by the European Parliament and the Council of the European Union.

[b] Regulations containing EU in the Regulation number were gazetted by the European Commission.

As with almost all global food regulations, the EU differentiates between food additives and food processing aids. The definitions from regulation EC 1333/2008 are quite distinct as follows:

Food Additive (Article 3, #2(a)):
Any substance not normally consumed as a food in itself and not normally used as a characteristic ingredient of a food, whether or not it has nutritive value, the intentional addition of which to food for a technological purpose in the manufacturing, processing, preparation, treatment, packaging, transport or storage of such food results, or may be reasonably expected to result, in it or its by-products becoming directly or indirectly a component of such foods.

Processing aid (Article 3, #2(b)):
Shall mean any substance which:

1. is not consumed as a food by itself;
2. is intentionally used in the processing of raw materials, foods or their ingredients, to fulfil a certain technological purpose during treatment or processing, and;
3. may result in the unintentional but technically unavoidable presence in the final product of residues of the substance or its derivatives provided they do not present any health risk and do not have any technological effect in the final product.

In addition, this regulation defines "unprocessed food" (Article 3, #2(d)) as food that has not undergone any treatment resulting in a substantial change in the original state of the food, for which purpose the following in particular are not regarded as resulting in substantial change: dividing, parting, severing, boning, mincing, skinning, paring, peeling, grinding, cutting, cleaning, trimming, deep-freezing, freezing, chilling, milling, husking, packing, or unpacking.

21.1.2 General Principles of Food Additive Use in the EU

The principles are similar to most global jurisdictions, in that only food additives listed in the Community list (Annex II) may be added to food. In addition, Annex III provides a list of food additives that may be used as additives in other food additives, in food enzymes, and in food flavorings. If the additives are not on these lists, they are not allowed in food or any component part of food. For both these annexes, there are specific conditions of use specified.

The addition of food additives to foods in general is complicated by the variation in specific conditions from one food to another. To alleviate this complication, categories of foods have been defined (EU 1129/2011), and the individual food additives allowed within each food category have been identified, with their specific conditions of use.

Thus the annexes contain the name and E number for each food additive, the foods to which the food additive may be added, the conditions under which the food additive may be used, and, if appropriate, whether there are any restrictions on the sale of the food additive directly to the final consumer.

In many instances, the level of use of a food additive is numerically limited to a maximum level. However, often there is no maximum level fixed for a food additive (quantum satis), in which case it should be used at the lowest level necessary to achieve the desired effect.

Food additives are not approved for use in "unprocessed food," as defined earlier. Where there has been a successful argument for the use of food additives in unprocessed food, this has been specifically provided for in Annex II.

Finally, a "carry-over" principle exists under certain circumstances. If a food additive has been approved in Annex II in one of the ingredients of a compound food and the compound food itself is not referred to in Annex II, then the presence of the additive in the new compound food is acceptable. This is also true for a food to which a food additive (containing other food additives), food enzyme or food flavoring has been added, provided these components are in accordance with the regulations as defined in Annex III, and they have no technological function in the final food. However, there is a range of foods where the carry-over principle is expressly forbidden. These include unprocessed foods; honey; nonemulsified oils and fats; butter; unflavored versions of milk, cream, buttermilk, and fermented milk products; natural mineral water; coffee; unflavored leaf tea; sugars; and dry pasta.

In establishing the original list of approved food additives (Table 21.2), all additives that automatically had been approved and in use by 2009 were permitted under the new legislation. However, under EC1333/2008 the Commission is required to reassess all these permitted food additives by

TABLE 21.2
Complete List of Approved Phosphorus-Containing Food Additives in the European Union

E Number	Name	Group I	Group II	Regulated Combined
E 101	Riboflavins	–	√	–
E 322	Lecithins	√	–	–
E 338	Phosphoric acid	–	–	√
E 339	Sodium phosphates	–	–	√
E 340	Potassium phosphates	–	–	√
E 341	Calcium phosphates	–	–	√
E 343	Magnesium phosphates	–	–	√
E 442	Ammonium phosphatides	–	–	√
E 450	Diphosphates	–	–	√
E 451	Triphosphates	–	–	√
E452	Polyphosphates	–	–	√
E 541	Sodium aluminium phosphate acidic	–	–	–
E 626	Guanylic acid	√	–	√
E 627	Disodium guanylate	√	–	√
E 628	Dipotassium guanylate	√	–	√
E 629	Calcium guanylate	√	–	√
E 630	Inosinic acid	√	–	√
E 631	Disodium inosinate	√	–	√
E 632	Dipotassium inosinate	√	–	√
E 633	Calcium inosinate	√	–	√
E 634	Calcium 5'-ribonucleotides	√	–	√
E 635	Disodium 5'-ribonucleotides	√	–	√
E 1410	Monostarch phosphate	√	–	–
E 1412	Distarch phosphate	√	–	–
E 1413	Phosphated distarch phosphate	√	–	–
E 1414	Acetylated distarch phosphate	√	–	–
E 1442	Hydroxy propyl distarch phosphate	√	–	–

Source: Commission Regulation (EU) No 1129/2011.

2020. To that end, EC257/2010 defines the priorities and deadlines for the re-evaluation of these additives. The key phosphate additives are as follows:

- Riboflavin phosphate (December 31, 2015)
- Remaining food additives by December 31, 2018, with a priority on:
- Phosphoric acid and phosphates
- Dipolyphosphates and tripolyphosphates
- Ribonucleotides

21.2 FOCUS ON PHOSPHORUS-CONTAINING FOOD ADDITIVES APPROVED FOR USE IN THE EU

21.2.1 Use of Phosphorus-Containing Food Additives in Processed Foods

The phosphorus-containing additives approved for use in the EU is provided in Table 21.2. This table also identifies specific aspects of the use of these additives. Group 1 additives, when they are allowed to be added to foods, are allowed to be added to all foods in that category at *quantum satis* levels (i.e., no maximum quantity). Group II additives are permitted food colors authorized at *quantum satis* levels. The additives identified as "regulated combined" are groups of similar additives that may be regulated as a combined group. This includes the phosphates and ribonucleotides. This means these chemicals are regulated to a maximum level and that maximum level is for all of these individual food additives combined as a single group (either as phosphates or ribonucleotides).

There are 18 broad food categories, and most of these are divided into subunits. For example, "01" has the title "dairy products and analogues" and there are 17 subunits (categories) of food within that title. In total there are 154 categories of food defined in EU 1129/2011. Annex II, containing all the food additives allowed for each of these categories of foods, therefore, is a sizeable tome of some 145 pages.

Table 21.3 provides the complete set of food categories that allow P-containing food additives, the specific additives allowed, and the maximum quantities per food. Phosphates are defined in terms of P_2O_5 so that all quantities of the various chemicals are treated the same. Ribonucleotides have been defined in terms of guanylate. Maximum levels of the food additives for each category have been calculated in terms of P_2O_5 in quantities of mg per liter or mg per kilogram (wet or dry food product). For direct comparison to other conventions, these maximum levels have been calculated in Table 21.3 in terms of phosphorus (P).

Clearly, there is a wide range of levels of P-containing food additives used across the EU. In general, these maximum limits have been defined by usage and are justified by safety data to be safe for human consumption.

21.2.2 FOOD SOURCES OF APPROVED PHOSPHORUS ADDITIVES

21.2.2.1 Existing Phosphorus Data on Raw Ingredients

Advice on and analysis of renal diets relies heavily on composition databases derived from analytical research of a wide range of raw food ingredients, semiprocessed, and fully processed foodstuffs. Many European country composition databases are publicly available, and these are identified on the European Food Information Resource (EuroFIR, 2015). There is regular scientific analysis of foods from around the world, and the content of these databases is expanding.

It should be recognized, however, that the biological variation of nutrient content of raw food ingredients is inherently very large (often 40%–60%) due to a number of factors, including genotypes and varieties of the ingredient, geographic area, climate and environmental factors, agronomic practices (farming methods, fertilizers, etc.), and genetic "improvement" (normally meaning increased farming yields). There is evidence that concentrations of mineral elements in edible fruit and vegetable produce has declined over the last half-century through changes in crop genotypes, crop husbandry, environmental factors, geographical sampling strategies, portion analyzed, analytical methods, and interlaboratory variability (White and Broadley, 2009). Given that the modern food trade is global in nature, meaning the source of a given food ingredient could be from anywhere in the world, it is likely that a database-defined composition of a specific food item may vary significantly from the actual content.

In terms of phosphorus content, a variety of raw plant ingredients are particularly problematic for renal patients. Many plants, such as cereals and grains, legumes, nuts, and seeds, store their phosphorus as phytic acid. This chemical is not digested by humans and if present in foods will pass predominantly unabsorbed through the human digestive tract. Although this may seem to be an advantage for renal patients (Williams et al., 2013), phytic acid is a powerful chelating agent and especially binds calcium, zinc, iron, and magnesium present in the diet, rendering these minerals insoluble and unavailable to humans (Rimbach et al., 2008; Schlemmer et al., 2009). These cations are normally deficient in renal patients, so further reductions from the diet are undesirable. Fortunately, phytic acid is usually present in the husk and aleurone layers of many plants (the outside surfaces) as a protective measure for the plant, and selective removal of these layers during food processing will effectively remove phytic acid.

TABLE 21.3
Approved P-Containing Food Additives in the EU and Their Specific Use and Constraints (Annex II of EU 1129/2011)

No.	Food Category — Name	Food Additive Allowed — E Number	Food Additive Allowed — Name	Maximum Quantity Allowed — Quantity mg/L or mg/kg	Maximum Quantity Allowed — Expressed as	Maximum Quantity Allowed — Calculated as P (mg/L or mg/kg)	Comments
0	*All categories of foods*	338–452	Phosphoric acid, phosphates, di-, tri- and poly-phosphates	10,000	P_2O_5	4,366	only foods in dried powder form
01	*Dairy products and analogues*						
01.1	Unflavoured pasteurised and sterilised (including UHT) milk	338–452	Phosphoric acid, phosphates, di-, tri- and poly-phosphates	1,000	P_2O_5	437	only sterilised and UHT milk
01.3	Unflavoured fermented milk products, heat-treated after fermentation	Group 1	Lecithins, modified starches, ribonucleotides	quantum satis			
01.4	Flavoured fermented milk products including heat-treated products	Group 1	Lecithins, modified starches, ribonucleotides	quantum satis			
		Group 2	Riboflavins	quantum satis			
		338–452	Phosphoric acid, phosphates, di-, tri- and poly-phosphates	3,000	P_2O_5	1,310	
01.5	Dehydrated milk as defined by Directive 2001/114/EC	Group 2	Riboflavins	quantum satis			
		322	Lecithins	quantum satis			
		338–452	Phosphoric acid, phosphates, di-, tri- and poly-phosphates	1,000	P_2O_5	437	only partly dehydrated milk with less than 28% solids
		338–452	Phosphoric acid, phosphates, di-, tri- and poly-phosphates	1,500	P_2O_5	655	only partly dehydrated milk with more than 28% solids
		338–452	Phosphoric acid, phosphates, di-, tri- and poly-phosphates	2,500	P_2O_5	1,092	only dried milk and dried skimmed milk
01.6.2	Unflavoured live fermented cream products and substitute products with a fat content of less than 20%	1410	Monostarch phosphate	quantum satis			

(continued)

TABLE 21.3 (*Continued*)

Approved P-Containing Food Additives in the EU and Their Specific Use and Constraints (Annex II of EU 1129/2011)

	Food Category		Food Additive Allowed	Maximum Quantity Allowed			Comments
No.	Name	E Number	Name	Quantity mg/L or mg/kg	Expressed as	Calculated as P (mg/L or mg/kg)	
		1412	Distarch phosphate	quantum satis			
		1413	Phosphated distarch phosphate	quantum satis			
		1414	Acetylated distarch phosphate	quantum satis			
		1442	Hydroxy propyl distarch phosphate	quantum satis			
01.6.3	Other creams	Group 1	Lecithins, modified starches, ribonucleotides	quantum satis			
		Group 2	Riboflavins	quantum satis			only flavoured creams
		338–452	Phosphoric acid, phosphates, di-, tri- and poly-phosphates	5,000	P_2O_5	2,183	only sterilised, pasteurised, UHT cream and whipped cream
01.7.1	Unripened cheese excluding products falling in category 16	Group 1	Lecithins, modified starches, ribonucleotides	quantum satis			except Mozzarella, and unflavoured live fermented unripened cheese
		Group 2	Riboflavins	quantum satis			only unflavoured unripened cheese
		338–452	Phosphoric acid, phosphates, di-, tri- and poly-phosphates	2,000	P_2O_5	873	except Mozzarella
01.7.3	Edible cheese rind	Group 2	Riboflavins	quantum satis			
01.7.4	Whey cheese	Group 2	Riboflavins	quantum satis			
01.7.5	Processed cheese	338–452	Phosphoric acid, phosphates, di-, tri- and poly-phosphates	20,000	P_2O_5	8,732	
01.7.6	Cheese products (excluding products falling in category 16)	Group 1	Lecithins, modified starches, ribonucleotides	quantum satis			

(*continued*)

TABLE 21.3   (*Continued*)

Approved P-Containing Food Additives in the EU and Their Specific Use and Constraints (Annex II of EU 1129/2011)

No.	Food Category Name	E Number	Food Additive Allowed Name	Quantity mg/L or mg/kg	Expressed as	Calculated as P (mg/L or mg/kg)	Comments
		Group 2	Riboflavins	quantum satis			only flavoured unripened products
		338–452	Phosphoric acid, phosphates, di-, tri- and poly-phosphates	2,000	P_2O_5	873	only unripened products
01.8	Dairy analogues, including beverage whiteners	Group 1	Lecithins, modified starches, ribonucleotides	quantum satis			
		Group 2	Riboflavins	quantum satis			
		338–452	Phosphoric acid, phosphates, di-, tri- and poly-phosphates	5,000	P_2O_5	2,183	only whipped cream analogues
		338–452	Phosphoric acid, phosphates, di-, tri- and poly-phosphates	20,000	P_2O_5	8,732	only processed cheese analogues
		338–452	Phosphoric acid, phosphates, di-, tri- and poly-phosphates	30,000	P_2O_5	13,099	only beverage whiteners
		338–452	Phosphoric acid, phosphates, di-, tri- and poly-phosphates	50,000	P_2O_5	21,831	only beverage whiteners for vending machines
02	*Fats and oils and fat and oil emulsions*						
02.1	Fats and oils essentially free from water (excluding anhydrous milkfat)	322	Lecithins	30,000			except virgin oils and olive oils
02.2.1	Butter and concentrated butter and butter oil and anhydrous milkfat	338–452	Phosphoric acid, phosphates, di-, tri- and poly-phosphates	2,000	P_2O_5	873	only soured cream butter
02.2.2	Other fat and oil emulsions including spreads as defined by Regulation (EC) No 1234/2007 and liquid emulsions	Group 1	Lecithins, modified starches, ribonucleotides	quantum satis			

(*continued*)

TABLE 21.3 (*Continued*)

Approved P-Containing Food Additives in the EU and Their Specific Use and Constraints (Annex II of EU 1129/2011)

	Food Category		Food Additive Allowed	Maximum Quantity Allowed			Comments
No.	Name	E Number	Name	Quantity mg/L or mg/kg	Expressed as	Calculated as P (mg/L or mg/kg)	
		338–452	Phosphoric acid, phosphates, di-, tri- and poly-phosphates	5,000	P_2O_5	2,183	only spreadable fats
02.3	Vegetable oil pan spray	Group 1	Lecithins, modified starches, ribonucleotides	quantum satis			
		338–452	Phosphoric acid, phosphates, di-, tri- and poly-phosphates	30,000	P_2O_5	13,099	only water-based emulsion sprays for coating baking tins
03	*Edible ices*	Group 1	Lecithins, modified starches, ribonucleotides	quantum satis			
		Group 2	Riboflavins	quantum satis			
		338–452	Phosphoric acid, phosphates, di-, tri- and poly-phosphates	1,000	P_2O_5	437	
04	*Fruit and vegetables*						
04.2	Processed fruit and vegetables	Group 1	Lecithins, modified starches, ribonucleotides	quantum satis			
		101	Riboflavins	quantum satis			only preserves red fruit
04.2.2	Fruit and vegetables in vinegar, oil, or brine	Group 1	Lecithins, modified starches, ribonucleotides	quantum satis			
		101	Riboflavins	quantum satis			only preserves red fruit
04.2.3	Canned or bottled fruit and vegetables	101	Riboflavins	quantum satis			only preserves red fruit
04.2.4.1	Fruit and vegetable preparations excluding compote	Group 1	Lecithins, modified starches, ribonucleotides	quantum satis			
		Group 2	Riboflavins	quantum satis			only mostarda di frutta
		101	Riboflavins	quantum satis			only preserves red fruit
		338–452	Phosphoric acid, phosphates, di-, tri- and poly-phosphates	800	P_2O_5	349	only fruit preparations

(*continued*)

TABLE 21.3 (*Continued*)

Approved P-Containing Food Additives in the EU and Their Specific Use and Constraints (Annex II of EU 1129/2011)

	Food Category		Food Additive Allowed		Maximum Quantity Allowed			Comments
No.	Name	E Number	Name	Quantity mg/L or mg/kg	Expressed as	Calculated as P (mg/L or mg/kg)	
		338–452	Phosphoric acid, phosphates, di-, tri- and poly-phosphates	4,000	P_2O_5	1,746	only glazings for vegetable products
04.2.5.3	Other similar fruit or vegetable spreads	Group 2	Riboflavins	quantum satis			except crème de pruneaux
04.2.5.4	Nut butters and nut spreads	Group 1	Lecithins, modified starches, ribonucleotides	quantum satis			
		338–452	Phosphoric acid, phosphates, di-, tri- and poly-phosphates	5,000	P_2O_5	2,183	only spreadable fats excluding butter
04.2.6	Processed potato products	Group 1	Lecithins, modified starches, ribonucleotides	quantum satis			
		338–452	Phosphoric acid, phosphates, di-, tri- and poly-phosphates	5,000	P_2O_5	2,183	
05	*Confectionery*						
05.1	Cocoa and chocolate products as covered by Directive 2000/36/EC	Group 1	Lecithins, modified starches, ribonucleotides	quantum satis			
		442	Ammonium phosphatides	10,000			
05.2	Other confectionery including breath refreshening microsweets	Group 1	Lecithins, modified starches, ribonucleotides	quantum satis			
		Group 2	Riboflavins	quantum satis			
		338–452	Phosphoric acid, phosphates, di-, tri- and poly-phosphates	5,000	P_2O_5	2,183	only sugar confectionery, except candied fruit
		338–452	Phosphoric acid, phosphates, di-, tri- and poly-phosphates	800	P_2O_5	349	only candied fruit
		442	Ammonium phosphatides	10,000			only cocoa-based confectionery

(continued)

TABLE 21.3 *(Continued)*

Approved P-Containing Food Additives in the EU and Their Specific Use and Constraints (Annex II of EU 1129/2011)

	Food Category		Food Additive Allowed	Maximum Quantity Allowed			Comments
No.	Name	E Number	Name	Quantity mg/L or mg/kg	Expressed as	Calculated as P (mg/L or mg/kg)	
05.3	Chewing gum	Group 1	Lecithins, modified starches, ribonucleotides	quantum satis			
		Group 2	Riboflavins	quantum satis			
		338–452	Phosphoric acid, phosphates, di-, tri- and poly-phosphates	quantum satis	P_2O_5	#VALUE!	
05.4	Decorations, coatings and fillings, except fruit-based fillings covered by category 4.2.4	Group 1	Lecithins, modified starches, ribonucleotides	quantum satis			
		Group 2	Riboflavins	quantum satis			
		338–452	Phosphoric acid, phosphates, di-, tri- and poly-phosphates	5,000	P_2O_5	2,183	
		338–452	Phosphoric acid, phosphates, di-, tri- and poly-phosphates	3,000	P_2O_5	1,310	only toppings (syrups for pancakes, flavoured syrups for milkshakes and ice cream; similar products)
		442	Ammonium phosphatides	10,000			only cocoa-based confectionery
06	*Cereals and cereal products*						
06.2.1	Flours	338–452	Phosphoric acid, phosphates, di-, tri- and poly-phosphates	2,500	P_2O_5	1,092	
		338–452	Phosphoric acid, phosphates, di-, tri- and poly-phosphates	20,000	P_2O_5	8,732	only self-raising flour

(continued)

TABLE 21.3 (*Continued*)

Approved P-Containing Food Additives in the EU and Their Specific Use and Constraints (Annex II of EU 1129/2011)

| Food Category | | Food Additive Allowed | | Maximum Quantity Allowed | | | Comments |
No.	Name	E Number	Name	Quantity mg/L or mg/kg	Expressed as	Calculated as P (mg/L or mg/kg)	
06.2.2	Starches	Group 1	Lecithins, modified starches, ribonucleotides	quantum satis			
06.3	Breakfast cereals	Group 1	Lecithins, modified starches, ribonucleotides	quantum satis			
		Group 2	Riboflavins	quantum satis			only breakfast cereals other than extruded, puffed and/or fruit-flavoured breakfast cereals
		338–452	Phosphoric acid, phosphates, di-, tri- and poly-phosphates	5,000	P_2O_5	2,183	
06.4	Pasta	322	Lecithins	quantum satis			
06.4.2	Dry pasta	Group 1	Lecithins, modified starches, ribonucleotides	quantum satis			only gluten-free and/or pasta intended for hypoprotein diets in accordance with Directive 2009/39/EC
06.4.3	Fresh pre-cooked pasta	322	Lecithins	quantum satis			
06.4.4	Potato gnocchi	Group 1	Lecithins, modified starches, ribonucleotides	quantum satis			
06.4.5	Fillings of stuffed pasta (ravioli and similar)	Group 1	Lecithins, modified starches, ribonucleotides	quantum satis			
06.5	Noodles	Group 1	Lecithins, modified starches, ribonucleotides	quantum satis			
		Group 2	Riboflavins	quantum satis			

(*continued*)

TABLE 21.3 (*Continued*)
Approved P-Containing Food Additives in the EU and Their Specific Use and Constraints (Annex II of EU 1129/2011)

| Food Category | | Food Additive Allowed | | Maximum Quantity Allowed | | | Comments |
| | | | | | | Calculated as | |
No.	Name	E Number	Name	Quantity mg/L or mg/kg	Expressed as	P (mg/L or mg/kg)	
		338–452	Phosphoric acid, phosphates, di-, tri- and poly-phosphates	2,000	P_2O_5	873	
06.6	Batters	Group 1	Lecithins, modified starches, ribonucleotides	quantum satis			
		Group 2	Riboflavins	quantum satis			
		338–452	Phosphoric acid, phosphates, di-, tri- and poly-phosphates	12,000	P_2O_5	5,239	
06.7	Pre-cooked or processed cereals	Group 1	Lecithins, modified starches, ribonucleotides	quantum satis			
		Group 2	Riboflavins	quantum satis			
07	*Bakery wares*						
07.1	Bread and rolls	Group 1	Lecithins, modified starches, ribonucleotides	quantum satis			
		338–452	Phosphoric acid, phosphates, di-, tri- and poly-phosphates	20,000	P_2O_5	8,732	only soda bread
07.1.1	Bread prepared solely with the following ingredients: wheat flour, water, yeast or leaven, salt	322	Lecithins	quantum satis			
07.1.2	Pain courant français; Friss búzakenyér, fehér és félbarna kenyerek	322	Lecithins	quantum satis			
07.2	Fine bakery wares	Group 1	Lecithins, modified starches, ribonucleotides	quantum satis			

(*continued*)

TABLE 21.3 (Continued)
Approved P-Containing Food Additives in the EU and Their Specific Use and Constraints (Annex II of EU 1129/2011)

No.	Food Category — Name	Food Additive Allowed — E Number	Food Additive Allowed — Name	Maximum Quantity Allowed — Quantity mg/L or mg/kg	Expressed as	Calculated as P (mg/L or mg/kg)	Comments
		Group 2	Riboflavins	quantum satis			
		338–452	Phosphoric acid, phosphates, di-, tri- and poly-phosphates	20,000	P_2O_5	8,732	
		541	Sodium aluminium phosphate acidic	1,000	P_2O_5	437	only scones and sponge wares
08	*Meat*						
08.1.2	Meat preparations as defined by Regulation (EC) No 853/2004	338–452	Phosphoric acid, phosphates, di-, tri- and poly-phosphates	5,000	P_2O_5	2,183	only breakfast sausages; in this product, the meat is minced in such a way so that the muscle and fat tissue are completely dispersed, so that fibre makes an emulsion with the fat, giving this product its typical appearance
08.2	Processed meat						
08.2.1	Non-heat-treated processed meat	Group 1	Lecithins, modified starches, ribonucleotides	quantum satis			
		101	Riboflavins	quantum satis			
		338–452	Phosphoric acid, phosphates, di-, tri- and poly-phosphates	5,000	P_2O_5	2,183	
08.2.2	Heat-treated processed meat	Group 1	Lecithins, modified starches, ribonucleotides	quantum satis			
		338–452	Phosphoric acid, phosphates, di-, tri- and poly-phosphates	5,000	P_2O_5	2,183	except foie gras, foie gras entier, blocs de foie gras, Libamaj, libamaj egeszben, libamaj tombben

(continued)

TABLE 21.3 (*Continued*)

Approved P-Containing Food Additives in the EU and Their Specific Use and Constraints (Annex II of EU 1129/2011)

Food Category		Food Additive Allowed		Maximum Quantity Allowed			Comments
No.	Name	E Number	Name	Quantity mg/L or mg/kg	Expressed as	Calculated as P (mg/L or mg/kg)	
08.2.3	Casings and coatings and decorations for meat	Group 1	Lecithins, modified starches, ribonucleotides	quantum satis			
		Group 2	Riboflavins	quantum satis			except edible external coating of pasturmas
		101	Riboflavins	quantum satis			only edible external coating of pasturmas
		338–452	Phosphoric acid, phosphates, di-, tri- and poly-phosphates	4,000	P_2O_5	1,746	only glazings for meat
09	*Fish and fisheries products*						
09.1.1	Unprocessed fish	338–452	Phosphoric acid, phosphates, di-, tri- and poly-phosphates	5,000	P_2O_5	2,183	only frozen and deep-frozen fish fillets
09.1.2	Unprocessed molluscs and crustaceans	338–452	Phosphoric acid, phosphates, di-, tri- and poly-phosphates	5,000	P_2O_5	2,183	only frozen and deep-frozen molluscs and crustaceans
09.2	Processed fish and fishery products including mollusks and crustaceans	Group 1	Lecithins, modified starches, ribonucleotides	quantum satis			
		Group 2	Riboflavins	quantum satis			only surimi and similar products and salmon substitutes
		101	Riboflavins	quantum satis			only fish paste and crustacean paste
		338–452	Phosphoric acid, phosphates, di-, tri- and poly-phosphates	1,000	P_2O_5	437	only canned crustaceans products; surimi and similar products

(*continued*)

TABLE 21.3 (Continued)

Approved P-Containing Food Additives in the EU and Their Specific Use and Constraints (Annex II of EU 1129/2011)

No.	Food Category Name	E Number	Food Additive Allowed Name	Maximum Quantity Allowed — Quantity mg/L or mg/kg	Expressed as	Calculated as P (mg/L or mg/kg)	Comments
09.3	Fish roe	338–452	Phosphoric acid, phosphates, di-, tri- and poly-phosphates	5,000	P_2O_5	2,183	only fish and crustacean paste and in processed frozen and deep-frozen molluscs and crustaceans
		Group 1	Lecithins, modified starches, ribonucleotides	quantum satis			
		Group 2	Riboflavins	quantum satis			except Sturgeons' eggs (Caviar)
10	*Eggs and egg products*						
10.2	Processed eggs and egg products	Group 1	Lecithins, modified starches, ribonucleotides	quantum satis			
		338–452	Phosphoric acid, phosphates, di-, tri- and poly-phosphates	10,000	P_2O_5	4,366	only liquid egg (white, yolk or whole egg)
11	*Sugars, syrups, honey and table-top sweeteners*						
11.1	Sugars and syrups as defined by Directive 2001/111/EC	338–452	Phosphoric acid, phosphates, di-, tri- and poly-phosphates	10,000	P_2O_5	4,366	
11.2	Other sugars and syrups	Group 1	Lecithins, modified starches, ribonucleotides	quantum satis			
11.4.2	Table-top sweeteners in powder form	341	Calcium phosphates	quantum satis			
12	*Salts, spices, soups, sauces, salads and protein products*						
12.1.1	Salt	338–452	Phosphoric acid, phosphates, di-, tri- and poly-phosphates	10,000	P_2O_5	4,366	

(continued)

TABLE 21.3 *(Continued)*

Approved P-Containing Food Additives in the EU and Their Specific Use and Constraints (Annex II of EU 1129/2011)

	Food Category		Food Additive Allowed	Maximum Quantity Allowed			Comments
No.	Name	E Number	Name	Quantity mg/L or mg/kg	Expressed as	Calculated as P (mg/L or mg/kg)	
12.1.2	Salt substitutes	Group 1	Lecithins, modified starches, ribonucleotides	quantum satis			
		338–452	Phosphoric acid, phosphates, di-, tri- and poly-phosphates	10,000	P_2O_5	4,366	
		626–635	Ribonucleotides	quantum satis			
12.2.2	Seasonings and condiments	Group 1	Lecithins, modified starches, ribonucleotides	quantum satis			
		Group 2	Riboflavins	quantum satis			only seasonings, for example curry powder, tandori
		626–635	Ribonucleotides	quantum satis			
12.3	Vinegars	Group 1	Lecithins, modified starches, ribonucleotides	quantum satis			
12.4	Mustard	Group 1	Lecithins, modified starches, ribonucleotides	quantum satis			
		Group 2	Riboflavins	quantum satis			
12.5	Soups and broths	Group 1	Lecithins, modified starches, ribonucleotides	quantum satis			
		Group 2	Riboflavins	quantum satis			
		338–452	Phosphoric acid, phosphates, di-, tri- and poly-phosphates	3,000	P_2O_5	1,310	
12.6	Sauces	Group 1	Lecithins, modified starches, ribonucleotides	quantum satis			
		Group 2	Riboflavins	quantum satis			excluding tomato-based sauces

(continued)

TABLE 21.3 (*Continued*)

Approved P-Containing Food Additives in the EU and Their Specific Use and Constraints (Annex II of EU 1129/2011)

No.	Name	E Number	Name	Quantity mg/L or mg/kg	Expressed as	Calculated as P (mg/L or mg/kg)	Comments
		338–452	Phosphoric acid, phosphates, di-, tri- and poly-phosphates	5,000	P_2O_5	2,183	
12.7	Salads and savoury based sandwich spreads	Group 1	Lecithins, modified starches, ribonucleotides	quantum satis			
		Group 2	Riboflavins	quantum satis			
12.8	Yeast and yeast products	Group 1	Lecithins, modified starches, ribonucleotides	quantum satis			
12.9	Protein products, excluding products covered in category 1.8	Group 1	Lecithins, modified starches, ribonucleotides	quantum satis			
		Group 2	Riboflavins	quantum satis			
		338–452	Phosphoric acid, phosphates, di-, tri- and poly-phosphates	20,000	P_2O_5	8,732	only vegetable protein drinks
13	*Foods intended for particular nutritional uses as defined by Directive 2009/39/EC*						
13.1.1	Infant formulae as defined by Commission Directive 2006/141/EC (1)	322	Lecithins	1,000	P_2O_5	437	
		338	Phosphoric acid	1,000	P_2O_5	437	
		339	Sodium phosphates	1,000	P_2O_5	437	
		340	Potassium phosphates		P_2O_5	0	
13.1.2	Follow-on formulae as defined by Directive 2006/141/EC	322	Lecithins	1,000			
		338	Phosphoric acid		P_2O_5	0	
		339	Sodium phosphates	1,000	P_2O_5	437	

(*continued*)

TABLE 21.3 (*Continued*)
Approved P-Containing Food Additives in the EU and Their Specific Use and Constraints (Annex II of EU 1129/2011)

	Food Category		Food Additive Allowed		Maximum Quantity Allowed		Comments
No.	Name	E Number	Name	Quantity mg/L or mg/kg	Expressed as	Calculated as P (mg/L or mg/kg)	
		340	Potassium phosphates		P_2O_5	0	
13.1.3	Processed cereal-based foods and baby foods for infants and young children as defined by Commission Directive 2006/125/EC (2)	322	Lecithins	10,000			only biscuits and rusks, cereal-based foods, baby foods
		338	Phosphoric acid	1,000	P_2O_5	437	only processed cereal-based foods and baby foods, only for pH adjustment
		339	Sodium phosphates	1,000	P_2O_5	437	only cereals
		340	Potassium phosphates	1,000	P_2O_5	437	only cereals
		341	Calcium phosphates	1,000	P_2O_5	437	only cereals
		341	Calcium phosphates	1,000	P_2O_5	437	only in fruit-based desserts
		450	Diphosphates	5,000	P_2O_5	2,183	only biscuits and rusks
		1410	Monostarch phosphate	50,000			only processed cereal-based foods and baby foods
		1412	Distarch phosphate	50,000			only processed cereal-based foods and baby foods
		1413	Phosphated distarch phosphate	50,000			only processed cereal-based foods and baby foods
		1414	Acetylated distarch phosphate	50,000			only processed cereal-based foods and baby foods
13.1.4	Other foods for young children	322	Lecithins	10,000			
		338	Phosphoric acid		P_2O_5	0	
		339	Sodium phosphates	1,000	P_2O_5	437	

(*continued*)

TABLE 21.3 (Continued)

Approved P-Containing Food Additives in the EU and Their Specific Use and Constraints (Annex II of EU 1129/2011)

	Food Category		Food Additive Allowed	Maximum Quantity Allowed			Comments
No.	Name	E Number	Name	Quantity mg/L or mg/kg	Expressed as	Calculated as P (mg/L or mg/kg)	
		340	Potassium phosphates	1,000	P_2O_5	437	
		1410	Monostarch phosphate	50,000			
		1412	Distarch phosphate	50,000			
		1413	Phosphated distarch phosphate	50,000			
		1414	Acetylated distarch phosphate	50,000			
13.1.5.1	Dietary foods for infants for special medical purposes and special formulae for infants	338	Phosphoric acid	1,000	P_2O_5	437	only for pH adjustment
		339	Sodium phosphates	1,000	P_2O_5	437	
		340	Potassium phosphates	1,000	P_2O_5	437	
		341	Calcium phosphates	1,000	P_2O_5	437	
13.2	Dietary foods for special medical purposes defined in Directive 1999/21/EC (excluding products from food category 13.1.5)	338–452	Phosphoric acid, phosphates, di-, tri- and poly-phosphates	5,000	P_2O_5	2,183	
13.3	Dietary foods for weight control diets intended to replace total daily food intake or an individual meal (the whole or part of the total daily diet)	Group 1	Lecithins, modified starches, ribonucleotides	quantum satis			
		Group 2	Riboflavins	quantum satis			
		338–452	Phosphoric acid, phosphates, di-, tri- and poly-phosphates	5,000	P_2O_5	2,183	

(continued)

TABLE 21.3 (*Continued*)

Approved P-Containing Food Additives in the EU and Their Specific Use and Constraints (Annex II of EU 1129/2011)

	Food Category		Food Additive Allowed		Maximum Quantity Allowed			Comments
No.	Name	E Number	Name	Quantity mg/L or mg/kg	Expressed as	Calculated as P (mg/L or mg/kg)		
13.4	Foods suitable for people intolerant to gluten as defined by Commission Regulation (EC) No 41/2009 (4)	Group 1	Lecithins, modified starches, ribonucleotides	quantum satis			
		Group 2	Riboflavins	quantum satis			
		338–452	Phosphoric acid, phosphates, di-, tri- and poly-phosphates	5,000	P_2O_5	2,183	
14	*Beverages*						
14.1	Non-alcoholic beverages						
14.1.1	Water, including natural mineral water as defined in Directive 2009/54/EC and spring water and all other bottled or packed waters	338–452	Phosphoric acid, phosphates, di-, tri- and poly-phosphates	500	P_2O_5	218	only prepared table waters
14.1.2	Fruit juices as defined by Directive 2001/112/EC and vegetable juices	Group 1	Lecithins, modified starches, ribonucleotides	quantum satis			
14.1.3	Fruit nectars as defined by Directive 2001/112/EC and vegetable nectars and similar products	Group 1	Lecithins, modified starches, ribonucleotides	quantum satis			
14.1.4	Flavoured drinks	Group 1	Lecithins, modified starches, ribonucleotides	quantum satis			
		Group 2	Riboflavins	quantum satis			excluding chocolate milk and malt products
		338–452	Phosphoric acid, phosphates, di-, tri- and poly-phosphates	700	P_2O_5	306	

(*continued*)

TABLE 21.3 (*Continued*)

Approved P-Containing Food Additives in the EU and Their Specific Use and Constraints (Annex II of EU 1129/2011)

	Food Category		Food Additive Allowed	Maximum Quantity Allowed			Comments
No.	Name	E Number	Name	Quantity mg/L or mg/kg	Expressed as	Calculated as P (mg/L or mg/kg)	
		338–452	Phosphoric acid, phosphates, di-, tri- and poly-phosphates	500	P_2O_5	218	only sport drinks
		338–452	Phosphoric acid, phosphates, di-, tri- and poly-phosphates	4,000	P_2O_5	1,746	only whey protein containing sport drinks
		338–452	Phosphoric acid, phosphates, di-, tri- and poly-phosphates	20,000	P_2O_5	8,732	only vegetable protein drinks
		338–452	Phosphoric acid, phosphates, di-, tri- and poly-phosphates	2,000	P_2O_5	873	only chocolate and malt dairy-based drinks
14.1.5.2	Other	Group 1	Lecithins, modified starches, ribonucleotides	quantum satis			
		338–452	Phosphoric acid, phosphates, di-, tri- and poly-phosphates	2,000	P_2O_5	873	only coffee-based drinks for vending machines; Instant tea and instant herbal infusions
14.2.3	Cider and perry	Group 1	Lecithins, modified starches, ribonucleotides	quantum satis			
		Group 2	Riboflavins	quantum satis			excluding cidre bouche
		338–452	Phosphoric acid, phosphates, di-, tri- and poly-phosphates	1,000	P_2O_5	437	
14.2.4	Fruit wine and made wine	Group 1	Lecithins, modified starches, ribonucleotides	quantum satis			
		Group 2	Riboflavins	quantum satis			
		338–452	Phosphoric acid, phosphates, di-, tri- and poly-phosphates	1,000	P_2O_5	437	
14.2.5	Mead	Group 1	Lecithins, modified starches, ribonucleotides	quantum satis			

(*continued*)

TABLE 21.3 (*Continued*)
Approved P-Containing Food Additives in the EU and Their Specific Use and Constraints (Annex II of EU 1129/2011)

	Food Category	Food Additive Allowed		Maximum Quantity Allowed			Comments
No.	Name	E Number	Name	Quantity mg/L or mg/kg	Expressed as	Calculated as P (mg/L or mg/kg)	
		Group 2	Riboflavins	quantum satis			except whisky or whiskey
		338–452	Phosphoric acid, phosphates, di-, tri- and poly-phosphates	1,000	P_2O_5	437	
14.2.6	Spirit drinks as defined in Regulation (EC) No 110/2008	Group 1	Lecithins, modified starches, ribonucleotides	quantum satis			
		Group 2	Riboflavins	quantum satis			except: spirit drinks as defined in article 5(1) and sales denominations listed in Annex II, paragraphs 1–14 of Regulation (EC) No 110/2008 and spirits (preceded by the name of the fruit) obtained by maceration and distillation, London Gin, Sambuca, Maraschino, Marrasquino or Maraskino and Mistra
		338–452	Phosphoric acid, phosphates, di-, tri- and poly-phosphates	1,000	P_2O_5	437	except whisky, whiskey
14.2.7	Aromatised wine-based products as defined by Regulation (EEC) No 1601/91	Group 1	Lecithins, modified starches, ribonucleotides	quantum satis			
14.2.7.1	Aromatised wines	Group 2	Riboflavins	quantum satis			except americano, bitter vino
		101	Riboflavins	100			only americano, bitter vino

(*continued*)

TABLE 21.3   (*Continued*)

Approved P-Containing Food Additives in the EU and Their Specific Use and Constraints (Annex II of EU 1129/2011)

	Food Category		Food Additive Allowed		Maximum Quantity Allowed			Comments
							Calculated as	
No.	Name	E Number	Name	Quantity mg/L or mg/kg	Expressed as	P (mg/L or mg/kg)		Comments
		338–452	Phosphoric acid, phosphates, di-, tri- and poly-phosphates	1,000	P_2O_5	437		except whisky, whiskey
14.2.7.2	Aromatised wine-based drinks	Group 1	Lecithins, modified starches, ribonucleotides	quantum satis				
		Group 2	Riboflavins	quantum satis				except bitter soda, sangria, claria, zurra
		101	Riboflavins	100				only bitter soda
		338–452	Phosphoric acid, phosphates, di-, tri- and poly-phosphates	1,000	P_2O_5	437		
14.2.7.3	Aromatised wine-product cocktails	Group 1	Lecithins, modified starches, ribonucleotides	quantum satis				
		Group 2	Riboflavins	quantum satis				
		338–452	Phosphoric acid, phosphates, di-, tri- and poly-phosphates	1,000	P_2O_5	437		
14.2.8	Other alcoholic drinks including mixtures of alcoholic drinks with non-alcoholic drinks and spirits with less than 15% of alcohol	Group 1	Lecithins, modified starches, ribonucleotides	quantum satis				
		Group 2	Riboflavins	quantum satis				
		338–452	Phosphoric acid, phosphates, di-, tri- and poly-phosphates	1,000	P_2O_5	437		
15	*Ready-to-eat savouries and snacks*							
15.1	Potato-, cereal-, flour- or starch-based snacks	Group 1	Lecithins, modified starches, ribonucleotides	quantum satis				
		Group 2	Riboflavins	quantum satis				

(*continued*)

TABLE 21.3 *(Continued)*

Approved P-Containing Food Additives in the EU and Their Specific Use and Constraints (Annex II of EU 1129/2011)

No.	Name	E Number	Name	Quantity mg/L or mg/kg	Expressed as	Calculated as P (mg/L or mg/kg)	Comments
	Food Category		**Food Additive Allowed**	**Maximum Quantity Allowed**			**Comments**
		338–452	Phosphoric acid, phosphates, di-, tri- and poly-phosphates	5,000	P_2O_5	2,183	
15.2	Processed nuts	Group 1	Lecithins, modified starches, ribonucleotides	quantum satis			
		Group 2	Riboflavins	quantum satis			
		338–452	Phosphoric acid, phosphates, di-, tri- and poly-phosphates	5,000	P_2O_5	2,183	
16	*Desserts excluding products covered in categories 1, 3 and 4*	Group 1	Lecithins, modified starches, ribonucleotides	quantum satis			
		Group 2	Riboflavins	quantum satis			
		338–452	Phosphoric acid, phosphates, di-, tri- and poly-phosphates	3,000	P_2O_5	1,310	
		338–452	Phosphoric acid, phosphates, di-, tri- and poly-phosphates	7,000	P_2O_5	3,056	only dry powedered dessert mixes
17	*Food supplements as defined in Directive 2002/46/EC of the European Parliament and of the Council (5) excluding food supplements for infants and young children*						
17.1	Food supplements supplied in a solid form including capsules and tablets and similar forms, excluding chewable forms	Group 1	Lecithins, modified starches, ribonucleotides	quantum satis			
		Group 2	Riboflavins	quantum satis			

(continued)

TABLE 21.3 *(Continued)*

Approved P-Containing Food Additives in the EU and Their Specific Use and Constraints (Annex II of EU 1129/2011)

No.	Food Category Name	E Number	Food Additive Allowed Name	Maximum Quantity Allowed Quantity mg/L or mg/kg	Expressed as	Calculated as P (mg/L or mg/kg)	Comments
		338–452	Phosphoric acid, phosphates, di-, tri- and poly-phosphates	quantum satis			
17.2	Food supplements supplied in a liquid form	Group 1	Lecithins, modified starches, ribonucleotides	quantum satis			
		Group 2	Riboflavins	quantum satis			
		338–452	Phosphoric acid, phosphates, di-, tri- and poly-phosphates	quantum satis			
17.3	Food supplements supplied in a syrup-type or chewable form	Group 1	Lecithins, modified starches, ribonucleotides	quantum satis			
		Group 2	Riboflavins	quantum satis			
		338–452	Phosphoric acid, phosphates, di-, tri- and poly-phosphates	quantum satis			
18	*Processed foods not covered by categories 1–17, excluding foods for infants and young children*	Group 1	Lecithins, modified starches, ribonucleotides	quantum satis			

The bioavailability of phosphorus components of food is extremely variable. There has been very little research on P bioavailability, and conclusions about quantitative P absorption from the human gut are difficult to verify (See Chapter 17). However, it is clear that both the quantity and form of P are very important. The generally accepted norm is that P from plants is the least absorbed (around 40%—although if phytic acid is removed or destroyed, this value may be significantly higher), animal-derived P is more readily absorbed (40%–60%), and inorganic forms of P are almost completely absorbed (Noori et al., 2010; Moe et al., 2011; Winger et al, 2012).

21.2.2.2 Processed Foods That are Problematic for CKD Patients

Compositional databases contain limited current data on processed foods and the quantity of P in these foods, including fast foods, foods from restaurants and institutions. Where data are available they are in the form of total P and do not differentiate the addition of P from food additives. This is not surprising, given the huge variability in the preparation and manufacture of these foods among brands and competitors. The content of P in these foods is often considerably different and usually higher than would be estimated from compositional databases (Sarathy et al., 2008; Sullivan et al., 2007; Uribarri and Calvo, 2003; Benini et al., 2011; Lou-Arnal et al., 2014; Cupisti et al., 2012; Sherman and Mehta, 2009a, b; Sherman, 2007). Globally, there is no legal requirement to quantify the content of P on food labels.

P-containing food additives are used in a wide range of foods at varying concentrations. Consistent with food products across the world, the food classes typically containing these additives include dairy products, cereals, baked goods, processed meat and fish, formulated foods (such as soups, prepared meals, "fast foods"), snacks and sauces, and beverages (Vin et al., 2013; Lou-Arnal et al., 2014; McCutcheon et al., 2015). There is considerable variability in additive use and concentration across competitive brands of similar products, as the reason for using a P-additive can vary depending upon the processing and packaging methods and the form the food takes during storage and distribution to the consumer (such as dried, fresh, frozen, etc.). In Europe, the biggest sources of P across 10 countries were cereals and products, dairy and products, meat and products, fish and products, vegetables and beverages (alcoholic and nonalcoholic) (Welch et al., 2009).

European law (and most other countries in the world) mandates that ingredients and additives used in food preparation be clearly described in the ingredient lists on every food label (further described for North America in Chapter 19). Food additives may be classified in terms of E numbers, the unique numerical code that is prescribed for all approved additives in the EU. Although this labeling announces the presence of a P-containing additive in a food, the actual concentration used is not quantified in the nutrition panel. These so-called "hidden" sources of P can add 20 to 85 mg P/100 g food (Ritz et al., 2012; Gutierrez, 2013; Sarathy et al., 2008; Sullivan et al., 2007; León et al., 2013; Lou-Arnal et al., 2014; Karp et al., 2012a, b), but the true amount is complicated by lack of sufficiently comprehensive and up-to-date data.

Most studies on the relationship between bioavailable P in food diets and physiological levels of serum-P have not measured bioavailability of the P components in the diet, per se. They have tended to use high and low P diets, which may not be representative of real-life diets, to achieve significant differences in serum P. The fact that diets with high levels of added P do cause significant increases in blood P and changes in phosphorus regulating hormones justify the concern that food additives have a real impact on blood chemistry in humans (McCarty and DiNicolantonio, 2014; Bell et al., 1977; Calvo et al., 1990; Carrigan et al., 2014; Benini et al., 2011; Uribarri, 2009; Uribarri and Calvo, 2003; Itkonen et al., 2013). As more than 44% of the processed food, a significant part of all fast foods, and an unknown quantity of hospitality and institutional foods contain P additives (León et al., 2013; McCutcheon et al., 2015; Sullivan et al., 2007; Calvo and Uribarri, 2013) and the amounts are not quantified (but according to Table 21.3 could be quite significant), the appropriate advice for people with CKD is to avoid any food product with a P-containing food additive in the ingredient list (McCutcheon et al., 2015).

Recently, studies in Finland have proposed an in vitro measured "digestible P" measurement to better estimate bioavailable P in foods (Itkonen et al., 2012). The method, discussed in Chapter 17, has been used to evaluate wheat, rye and barley, meat and cheese, plant foods, and beverages and their products. There is a significant change in the digestible P in all products depending upon the processing methods and formulations used in their manufacture (Itkonen et al., 2012; Karp et al., 2012a, b). It is also noted that other food components have an impact on P absorption in the gut, as much as phosphate in food affects the absorption of other minerals (Schlemmer et al., 2009; Aguilar et al., 2012).

21.3 CONSUMPTION OF PHOSPHORUS-CONTAINING FOOD ADDITIVES IN EUROPE

21.3.1 Acceptable Daily Intake for Europe

The definition of Acceptable Daily Intake (ADI) involves both the dose (the exposure of the population to a food additive and its derivatives) and the incidence of an adverse health effect. The hazard may be acute toxicity (if any exists) or an estimate of a health risk following daily consumption over a lifetime (WHO, 2009). A science-based approach characterizes the risk in terms of exposure and hazard, including the daily intake across human population groups. The scientific assessment defines a No Observable Effect Level (NOEL) or a No Observable Adverse Effect Level (NOAEL) and also potential uncertainty associated with the published scientific literature and exposure data provided. A safety factor is then applied (typically for food additives this is a 100-fold factor) to create an ADI for the food additive. The ADI is defined as the amount of a food additive, expressed as mg/kg body weight, that can be ingested daily over a lifetime without incurring any appreciable health risk.

The WHO/FAO global organization, through the Codex Alimentarius Commission, has already reviewed many food additives in an attempt to harmonize global trade. However, actual laws need to be set by each country, or in the case of Europe, the European Parliament. In Europe, NOAEL in animals is used to define the hazard level of a food additive, as a surrogate for the actual threshold dose that produces an adverse effect in humans. Note that there may be changes in the animal model experiments that cause changes in the animals, where scientists believe these changes are not "adverse." This is the case with food additives, as they are normally tested at very high doses in order to generate any impact on the animals. In the absence of detectable abnormalities in animals, it may not be possible to define some changes (e.g., weight) as abnormalities and therefore the relevance of an endpoint may be questionable or debatable. However, a conservative approach is used in Europe. It is important to note that both short-term (acute) exposure and lifetime exposures are required for toxicology studies on test animals.

In some instances, available data may lead to a conclusion that the total potential intake from all sources does not represent a health hazard to consumers. In that instance, a quantifiable ADI may be considered unnecessary and the term "ADI not specified" is used.

Similarly, if there is insufficient or inadequate evidence to define a NOAEL, then a "temporary ADI" is allocated, for a defined period, when additional studies will have been conducted and the additive can be re-evaluated.

Sometimes, a "group ADI" is defined. This is the case for most phosphate compounds, for example. This single phosphate group contains all the phosphate additives from E338 to E452. In this instance, the single ADI covers all the compounds identified within the group (E338–E452), in combination, in any one food. This means the use of any of these compounds in the group is additive and the total when combined must not exceed the ADI.

The ADI is not a single, defined, and unchangeable quantity for any food additive. ADIs are often adjusted for different segments of the population, such as men and women, children, infants, elderly, sick and infirmed, and so forth. They are often re-evaluated, and new data may result in a change in the ADI. This is especially true when lifetime data from human exposure to additives becomes more available or toxicity testing evolves and becomes more relevant (Benford, 2000; WHO, 2009).

The ADI for phosphates (E338–E452) in Europe is 70 mg P/kg body weight/day (EU Commission, 2001). Thus, for a 70-kg man the ADI would be 4.9 g P per day.

21.3.1.1 Consumption of P-Containing Food Additives

The European Parliament and Council requires each member state to monitor the consumption and usage of food additives, and the Commission is required to submit a report on this exercise. A Commission report published in 2001 (EU Commission, 2001) was the first attempt to obtain dietary food additive intake in the EU. This report involved 10 member states (Austria, Denmark, Finland, France, Greece, Ireland, the Netherlands, Spain, Sweden, and the United Kingdom) and Norway. The data were compiled into three "tiers." Initially, additives were assessed in Tier 1 using theoretical consumption data combined with maximum permitted usage levels for children or adults. Any additives exceeding the ADI for either consumer group were moved to Tier 2, and these additives were assessed using actual national consumption data combined with maximum permitted usage level. Those additives still exceeding the ADI for either consumer group were moved to Tier 3 and then assessed using actual national consumption data and actual usage levels. All additives with *quantum satis* authorization were automatically moved to Tier 3, as they had no approved maximum level of use and could not be examined under Tier 1 or 2 criteria.

As this was a preliminary process designed to test the methodology and assess the data available, the results were considered "a very preliminary indication on the dietary intake of food additives." However, the terminology and definitions were maintained for future use within the EU.

Many of the phosphate-containing additives do not have an ADI. As a result, they were not assessed as part of this study. These included the following:

- E 101 Riboflavins
- E 322 Lecithins
- E 626–E 635 (ribonucleotides)
- E 1404–E 1442 (modified starches)

The phosphates (E 338–E 452) were all assessed for adults (body weight of 60 kg) using theoretical national consumption data and the maximum permitted use of each additive. The combined total consumption of these phosphate food additives was less than the ADI (which is 70 mg/kg body weight/day). These data are defined in terms of phosphorus (P), in contrast to the EU food regulations, which quantify usage in terms of P_2O_5. As a result, phosphates for adults were assigned as Tier 1.

In addition to this assessment, the phosphates were reviewed for young children (younger than three years old, 15 kg body weight), using actual national consumption data for UK and the Netherlands and the maximum permitted usage levels. The data indicated that phosphates were consumed between 53% and 172% of the ADI. In this instance, phosphates for children were moved to Tier 3.

Ammonium phosphatides (E 442) were assessed using the actual national consumption data from six member states. The ADI was 30 mg P/kg body weight/day, and the estimated usage (assuming maximum permitted levels) was between 1% and 11% of the ADI for all age groups.

The Commission's 2001 report did not provide any data related to the evaluations requiring actual national consumption and actual usage levels.

In 2005, the European Food Safety Authority (EFSA) published an opinion on the tolerable upper intake level of phosphorus in Europe (Becker et al., 2005). It summarized actual consumption data and phosphorus usage from five EU countries. The mean daily consumption ranged from 1112 to 1570 mg/person/day, with the 97.5% percentile consumption range from 1763 to 2601 mg/person/day. These data included phosphorus from all food sources, including food additives. More recently, EFSA has undertaken a toxicity review of phosphate additives (EFSA, 2013) following a request from the European Parliament. They concluded that the evidence from the single published review that they assessed did not make causal inferences between serum P levels and the observed adverse effects claimed in the review. It was not possible to attribute increased cardiovascular risk to intake of P in general, or food additives in particular.

In a major multinational, collaborative EU project, called "EPIC," over 36,000 people in 10 countries completed standardized 24-hour dietary recall interviews, which were then analyzed using comprehensive food composition databases for various nutrients, including phosphorus. Men consumed 1425 to 2070 mg/day, whereas the range for women was 1089 to 1478 mg/day (Welch et al., 2009).

Another EU collaborative study, FACET, reviewed "priority additives" in four European countries. The phosphate group (E338–343 and E450–452) exposure was below the ADI for adults and therefore confirmed the earlier study which classified them as Tier 1 for this group. However, using the Tier 2 criteria (actual consumption data combined with maximum permitted level) phosphate additive consumption exceeded the ADI for children between 1 and 18 years of age (Vin et al., 2013), which confirms the data from EU Commission (2001). It should be noted that Tier 2 criteria assumes the maximum use of additives in all foods that are allowed to contain them. When assessed using Tier 3 criteria (actual usage levels, not maximum levels) Vin et al., 2013 found *all* age groups, including children, were significantly below the ADIs.

21.3.1.2 Limitations of ADIs

Although estimates of consumption and additive usage are valuable in ascertaining risk and regulatory policy, there are serious limitations in the methodology. Collecting consumption data from consumers is unreliable and inaccurate. Using nutrient data tables to estimate food composition, albeit using data based upon sound scientific analyses, adds enormous errors to the results given the innate and global biological variability in foods. Indeed, being able to separate P contained in food additives from the natural P in foods themselves is questionable. The measurement of phosphorus in foods, in particular, is an extremely difficult analytical task, and different methods used over time and in different laboratories cause significant variability in the results. The underlying premise that a daily limit on any food additive or nutrient has no impact on human health over a lifetime is a scientific experiment yet to be conducted. We rely on several generations of animal experiments to justify that assumption, so how does that really compare to humans? In reality, the combination of these issues can be reflected in the results from published studies, such as Vin et al., 2013. The standard deviation of the mean for the phosphorus data in that paper was the same magnitude as the mean, effectively nullifying any statistical significance.

Of particular concern is the inability to assess the health impact of food phosphorus, in all its forms, upon susceptible members of the population, such as the renally impaired. There is unambiguous clinical evidence that food phosphorus has a direct and negative impact on the health of these consumers (Winger et al., 2012). However, although ADIs may focus on gender and age of consumers, there are no data for health-related population subgroups, where it is likely that these ADIs are overestimates for lifetime security.

REFERENCES

Aguilar MV, Mateos C, Meseguer I, Martinez-Para M, Calcium availability in breakfast cereals: Effect of other food components. *Eur Food Res Technol*. 2012; 235:489–495.

Becker W, Branca F, Brasseur D, Bresson J, Flynn A, Jackson AA, Lagiou P, Løvik M, Mingrone G, Moseley B, Palou A, Przyrembel H, Salminen S, Strobel S, van den Berg H, van Loveren H, Opinion of the scientific panel on dietetic products, nutrition and allergies on a request from the Commission related to the Tolerable Upper Intake Level of phosphorus. *EFSA J*. 2005; 233:1–19.

Bell RR, Draper HH, Tzeng DYM, Shin HK, Schmidt GR, Physiological responses of human adults to foods containing phosphate additives. *J Nutr*. 1977; 107:42–50.

Benford D, *The Acceptable Daily Intake: A Tool for Ensuring Food Safety*. 2000; Belgium: ILSI Europe, ILSI Press.

Benini O, D'Alessandro C, Gianfaldoni D, Cupisti A, Extra-phosphate load from food additives in commonly eaten foods: A real and insidious danger for renal patients. *J Ren Nutr.* 2011; 21(4):303–308.

Calvo MS, Kumar R, Heath H, Persistently elevated parathyroid hormone secretion and action in young women after four weeks of ingesting high phosphorus, low calcium diets. *J Clin Endocrinol Metab.* 1990; 70:1334–1340.

Calvo MS, Uribarri J, Contributions to total phosphorus intake: All sources considered. *Sem Dial.* 2013; 26(1):54–61.

Carrigan A, Klinger A, Choquette SS, Luzuriaga-McPherson A, Bell EK, Darnell B, Gutiérrez OM, Contribution of food additives to sodium and phosphorus content of diets rich in processed foods. *J Ren Nutr.* 2014; 24:13–19.

Cupisti A, Benini O, Ferretti V, Gianfaldoni V, Kalantar-Zadeh K, Novel differential measurement of natural and added phosphorus in cooked ham with or without preservatives. *J Ren Nutr.* 2012; 22:533–540.

EU Commission. Report from the Commission on Dietary Food Additive Intake in the European Union. 2001. http://ec.europa.eu/food/fs/sfp/flav_index_en.html

EuroFIR. Food Composition Databases. 2015. http://www.eurofir.org/?page_id=96#

EFSA. *European Food Safety Authority. Assessment of one published review on health risks associated with phosphate additives in food. EFSA J.* 2013; 11(11):3444, 27 pp. doi: 10.2903/j.efsa.2013.3444.

Gutierrez OM. Sodium- and phosphorus-based food additives: Persistent but surmountable hurdles in the management of nutrition in chronic kidney disease. *Adv in Chronic Kidney Disease.* 2013; 20(2):150–156.

Itkonen ST, Ekholm PJ, Kemi VE, Lamberg-Allardt CJE, Analysis of in vitro digestible phosphorus content in selected processed rye, wheat and barley products. *J. Food Composition and Analysis.* 2012; 25:185–189.

Itkonen ST, Karp HJ, Kemi VE, Kokkonen EM, Saarnio EM, Pekkinen MH, Karkkainen MUM, Laitinen EKA, Turanlahti MI, Lamberg-Allardt CJE, Associations among total and food additive phosphorus intake and carotid intima-media thickness—A cross-sectional study in a middle-aged population in Southern Finland. *Nutrition J.* 2013; 12:94–104.

Karp H, Ekholm P, Kemi V, Hirvonen T, Lamberg-Allardt C, Differences among total and in vitro digestible phosphorus of meat and milk products. *J. Ren Nutr.* 2012a; 22(3):344–349.

Karp H, Ekholm P, Kemi V, Itkonen S, Hirvonen T, Narkki S, Lamberg-Allardt C, Differences among total and in vitro digestible phosphorus content of plant foods and beverages. *J. Ren Nutr.* 2012b; 22(4):416–422.

León JB, Sullivan CM, Sehgal AR, The prevalence of phosphorus-containing food additives in top-selling foods in grocery stores. *J Ren Nutr.* 2013; 23(4):265–270.

Lou-Arnal LM, Arnaudas-Casanova L, Caverni-Múnoz A, Vercet-Tormo A, Caramelo-Gutiérrez R, Munguia-Navarro P, Compos-Gutiérrez B, Garcia-Mena M, Moragrera B, Moreno-Lopez R, Bielsa-Gracia S, Cuberes-Izquierdo M, Grupo de Investigación ERC Aragón. Hidden sources of phosphorus: Presence of phosphorus-containing additives in processed foods. *Nefrologia.* 2014; 34(4):498–506.

McCarty MF, DiNicolantonio JJ, Bioavailable dietary phosphorus, a mediator of cardiovascular disease, may be decreased with plant-based diets, phosphate binders, niacin, and avoidance of phosphate additives. *Nutrition.* 2014; 30:739–747.

McCutcheon J, Campbell K, Ferguson M, Day S, Rossi M, Prevalence of phosphorus-based additives in the Australian food supply: A challenge for dietary education? *J Ren Nutr.* 2015; 25(5):440–444.

Moe SM, Zidehsarai MP, Chambers MA, Jackman LA, Radcliffe JS, Trevino LL, Donahue SE, Asplin JR, Vegetarian compared with meat dietary protein source and phosphorus homeostasis in chronic kidney disease. *Clin J Am Soc Nephrol.* 2011; 6(2)257–264.

Noori N, Sims JJ, Kopple JD, Shah A, Coleman S, Shinaberger CS, Bross R, Mehrotra R, Kovesday CP, Kalantar-Zadeh K, Organic and inorganic dietary phosphorus and its management in chronic kidney disease. *Iran J. Kidney Dis.* 2010; 4(2):89–100.

Rimbach G, Pallauf J, Moehring J, Kraemer K, Minihane AM, Effect of dietary phytate and microbial phytase on mineral and trace element bioavailability—A literature review. *Curr Top Nutraceutical Res.* 2008; 6(3):131–144.

Ritz E, Hahn K, Ketteler M, Kuhlman MK, Mann J, Phosphate additives in food—A health risk. *Dtsch Arztebl Int.* 2012; 109(4):49–55.

Sarathy S, Sullivan C, Leno JB, Fast food, phosphorus-containing additives, and the renal diet. *J. Ren Nutr.* 2008; 18(5):466–470.

Schlemmer U, Frolich W, Prieto RM, Grases F, Phytate in foods and significance for humans: Food sources, intake, processing, bioavailability, protective role and analysis. *Mol Nutr Food Res.* 2009; 53:S330–S375.

Sherman RA, Dietary phosphate restriction and protein intake in dialysis patients: A misdirected focus. *Sem. Dial.* 2007; 20:16–18.

Sherman RA, Mehta O, Dietary phosphorus restriction in dialyses patients: Potential impact of processed meat, poultry, and fish products as protein sources. *Am J Kidney Dis.* 2009a; 54:18–23.

Sherman RA, Mehta O, Phosphorus and potassium content of enhanced meat and poultry products: Implications for patients who receive dialysis. *Clin J Am Soc Neph.* 2009b; 4:1370–1373.

Sullivan CM, Leon JB, Sehgal AR, Phosphorus-containing food additives and the accuracy of nutrient databases: Implications for renal patients. *J Ren Nutr.* 2007; 17(5):350–354.

Uribarri J, Phosphorus additives in food and their effect in dialysis patients. *Clin J Am Soc Nephrol.* 2009; 4:1290–1292.

Uribarri J, Calvo MS, Hidden sources of phosphorus in the typical American diet: Does it matter in nephrology? *Sem Dial.* 2003; 16:186–188.

Vin K, Connolly A, McCaffrey T, McKevitt A, O'Mahony C, Prieto M, Tennant D, Hearty A, Volatier JL, Estimation of the dietary intake of 13 priority additives in France, Italy, the UK and Ireland as part of the FACET Project. *Food Addit Contam Part A.* 2013; 30(12):2050–2080.

Welch AA, Fransen H, Jenab M, Boutron-Ruault MC, Tumino R, Agnoli C, Ericson U, Johansson I, Ferrari P, Engeset D, Lund E, Lentjes M, Key T, Touvier M, Niravong M, Larranaga N, Rodriguez L, Ocke MC, Peeters PHM, Tjønneland A, Bjerregaard L, Vasilopoulou E, Dilis V, Linscisen J, Nothlings U, Riboli E, Slimani N, Bingham S, Variations in intakes of calcium, phosphorus, magnesium, iron and potassium in 10 countries in the European Prospective Investigation into cancer and nutrition study. *Eur J Clin Nutr.* 2009; 63:S101–S121.

White PJ, Broadley MR, Biofortification of crops with seven mineral elements often lacking in human diets—Iron, zinc, copper, calcium, magnesium, selenium and iodine. *New Phytologist.* 2009; 182:49–84.

WHO. Principles and methods for the risk assessment of chemicals in food. *Environmental Health Criteria 240. 2009. Food and Agriculture Organization of the United Nations and the World Health Organisation.*

Williams C, Ronco C, Kotanko P, Whole grains in the renal diet—Is it time to reevaluate their role? *Blood Purif.* 2013; 36:210–214.

Winger R, Uribarri J, Lloyd L, Phosphorus-containing food additives: An insidious danger for people with chronic kidney disease. *Trends Food Sci Technol.* 2012; 24:92–102.

22 A European Perspective
Questionable Safety of Current Phosphorus Intakes in the General Healthy and Chronic Kidney Disease Populations

Kai M. Hahn, Markus Ketteler, and Eberhard Ritz

CONTENTS

Abstract 313
Bullet Points 314
22.1 Introduction 314
22.2 Contributing Factors to the European Trend of Higher Phosphorus Intakes 315
    22.2.1 Fast Food Contributions 315
    22.2.2 Contributions from Phosphate Additive Use in Processing 316
    22.2.3 Added Phosphates Contributing to Phosphorus Intake 317
22.3 European Union Regulation and Safety Assessment of Phosphate-Containing Food Additives 318
    22.3.1 European Union Regulation 318
    22.3.2 Events Leading to the European Commission Health Consumer Directorate Mandated Safety Review 319
22.4 European Union Recommendations and Actions Concerning Excess Phosphorus Intake as a Health Risk 321
    22.4.1 Mandated Re-Evaluation 321
    22.4.2 Further Data Needs for the EU Phosphate Additive Safety Re-Evaluation 322
    22.4.3 Food Industry Response to European Union Mandated Safety Assessment of Phosphate Additives 323
22.5 Phosphorus Sustainability Concerns 323
22.6 Conclusions 324
References 324

ABSTRACT

Phosphorus intake has long been a known risk factor for chronic kidney disease (CKD) patients and the dialysis population, but recent studies show this risk factor also exists in individuals with normal renal function. With the increase in the consumption of processed and convenience foods in the last decades, dietary phosphorus load has progressively increased and now far exceeds the nutrient requirements of men and women in Western cultures. The typical North American dietary pattern, characterized by a rise in processed food, fast food, and soft drink consumption, slipped across the Atlantic during the last decade, and Europe is now faced with the same high phosphorus intake. About 100,000 tons of phosphates are used for food applications in Europe every year. Food labels report the ingredients and food additives in packaged foods by either full name or by codification with E-numbers (e.g., E 450), but do not report the quantity of phosphorus that they contain. The compelling health need to quantify the phosphorus content of food that is addressed in this chapter has been ignored by the health authorities and politicians until now. Recently, efforts have been initiated to inform the European medical community and general public about the health risks of excess phosphorus intake per se and specifically about potential harmful contributions from phosphorus additives. These efforts led to the European Food Safety Authority (EFSA) mandate to scientifically assess the concerns raised related to phosphate additives in food. Against this background some considerable cooperation between the food industry and medical researchers has emerged. These and other efforts initiated by the European medical community are becoming even more important because phosphorus can be a health risk with its widespread addition to food, but it is also a limited natural resource and indispensible nutrient to humans, livestock, and agriculture which in excess can endanger the health of our environmental water resources. Growing awareness of the double-edge problem that excess phosphorus represents may hopefully lead to a more responsible and cautious use of phosphorus by the food industry, politicians, agriculturalists and the general population in Europe.

BULLET POINTS

- General aspects of phosphorus, notably its widespread use in food, is an increasing problem in Europe as well as the rest of the world.
- Excess phosphorus intake is not just a problem for people with kidney disease but also for healthy populations.
- Compelling evidence of the potential health risks from phosphate additives in food is growing.
- The EFSA has been mandated to re-evaluate all relevant toxicological information associated with phosphate additive use in the European Union by December 31, 2018.
- Cooperation between the food industry, the food safety regulators (EFSA), and health professionals is indispensable to solving the prospective increase in morbidity and mortality that epidemiology study findings predict with the current phosphorus intake levels and serum phosphate concentrations

22.1 INTRODUCTION

In the nephrological community there is little doubt about the devastating effects of high phosphorus intake and especially phosphate additives in food on cardiovascular risk and outcome of patients with chronic kidney disease (CKD). Moreover, there is mounting evidence that this health risk emanating from high phosphate intake is not just limited to people with failing kidneys. A growing number of epidemiologic studies show a strong association of blood phosphate concentrations, even in the normal range, with cardiovascular morbidity or mortality. Most of these studies come from the United States (Kestenbaum et al., 2005; Menon et al., 2005; Tonelli et al., 2005; 2014; Dinghra et al., 2007; Foley et al., 2009); however, the recent European LURIC study shows that imbalances of phosphate, fibroblast growth factor-23 (FGF23), and vitamin D significantly correlated with all-cause and cardiovascular mortality over 10 years follow-up (Brandenburg et al., 2014). One recent population study by McGovern et al. (2013) documented an increase of the cardiovascular event rate in CKD patients and in the normal British population at serum phosphate concentrations >1.25 mmol/L or 3.87 mg/dL, which is far lower than the currently accepted upper limit of the normal range. Interestingly, in individuals with normal renal function or CKD stages 1 to 2, a low phosphate concentration (as low as 0.75 mmol/L or 2.32 mg/dL) was associated with a survival benefit (McGovern et al., 2013). These and other studies led to the belief that the phosphate health risk is a cardiovascular risk factor and such phosphate health risks are not restricted to people with kidney disease.

A European Perspective

With the increase in the consumption of food and especially processed food items in the last decades, phosphorus consumption today far exceeds the nutrient requirements of men and women in the United States (Calvo and Uribarri, 2013). The problem is further compounded by the contributions from phosphate additives commonly added to bakery, processed meat or dairy products, and many other processed foods. Even if renal function (estimated glomerular filtration rate [eGFR]) is not impaired, an inappropriately high oral phosphate load may, in the long run, compromise kidney function, as observed in diabetes, hypertension, and advanced age.

22.2 CONTRIBUTING FACTORS TO THE EUROPEAN TREND OF HIGHER PHOSPHORUS INTAKES

22.2.1 FAST FOOD CONTRIBUTIONS

High phosphorus intake has recently become epidemic as a result of changing eating habits (dietary patterns) and the nature of the foods consumed (i.e., an incremental consumption of high-phosphate food). Fast food consumption has become a frequent occurrence in Europe, as well as in other Western and developed countries. In Europe, high-phosphorus fast food establishments began sprouting up in the 1970s, largely as North American burger chains, which are now widespread in the European Union and were soon followed by similar British and European franchises.

An important factor that drives the rapid growth in this sector is the use of franchising. In 2012, the 10 top-selling fast food chains in Europe had 22,202 outlets in 40 European countries. Fast food consumption continues to grow, with the fastest growth in the EU occurring in Eastern European countries, although, high consumption of fast food is also prevalent in Western Europe where Germany is a good example. According to *Food Service*, a renowned journal in brand gastronomy in central Europe, the six biggest fast food chains in Germany (McDonalds, Burger King, Subway, KFC, Pizza Hut, Nordsee) in 2013 had a total revenue of 4755 billion Euros. The leading fast food chain in Germany is McDonalds, accounting for a market share of 33% in 2013 (Food Service Europe and Middle East, 2013). McDonalds supersedes most of the chain's competitors in terms of seniority, level of brand recognition, and national penetration, due to its vast network of outlets and large-scale advertising campaigns. Stiftung Warentest, Germany's consumer goods testing organization, certifies that the McDonalds company offers "an uncommonly large and diverse product portfolio, with a plethora of supposedly healthier options and meal choices, as well as less harmful ingredients" (Stiftung Warentest, 2013). In this context, it appears that phosphorus additives are not considered harmful ingredients; however, phosphates are still used in standard McDonalds products in Europe, namely as leavening agents in buns, tortillas, and batter, but also in French fries and frappés. This information can only be found in the ingredient lists that are published by the company on the Internet (McDonalds, 2015). However, McDonalds Europe banned the usage of phosphates in cheese some time ago, so this might be a hint as to the rise of some healthy rethinking regarding the use of phosphates.

Fortunately, food patterns in Europe are beginning to change again, at least in Western Europe. There is an observed trend for quick business lunches or snacks to contain healthier foods, likely as a result of more health-conscious attitudes and behavior. Lower calorie food items with less processing and fewer added ingredients and even vegetarian or vegan options are increasingly offered and consumed. This new food-trend consumer is called "flexitarian" and his food choices are flexible but have to contain invariable fresh foods and ingredients. It is worth mentioning that this change of food patterns was launched after some serious incidents involving adulterated beef products with horse meat, which was partly drug contaminated (EFSA, 2013). These threats to public health scared consumers into paying more attention to proper food processing, the nature of the ingredient additions to their foods, and public demands for a higher level of transparency. This change in consumer behavior puts increasing pressure on the fast food chains to make their products safer and healthier. Consumers have become more aware of food additives in general, and this has affected the fast food industry, which underscores the importance of informing consumers about the health risks associated with high phosphorus intake.

22.2.2 Contributions from Phosphate Additive Use in Processing

According to information provided in 2007 by the phosphate industry, the vast majority of phosphates are used in fertilizers, detergents, and animal feed, and only 1% is used for food purposes. In Europe about 100,000 tons of phosphates per year are reported to be used for human food applications (Cefic.org, 2007).

Phosphates are among the most common food additives, in more than 20,000 products in the Food Scores Data Base of the Environmental Working Group (EWG.org, 2015). These additives can be used to extend conservation (shelf life), enhance color or flavor, leaven baked goods, reduce acidity, and improve moisture retention as well as tenderness in processed meats. The amount of consumed phosphorus additives is considerable when compared to the natural phosphorus content in food items due to their extensive use in a vast number of food categories. Personal consumption is estimated to have increased since 1990 from about 500 mg/day to more than 1000 mg/day (Calvo and Park, 1996; Sullivan et al., 2007; Uribarri, 2009). The absorption efficiency of inorganic phosphorus salts is very high and some are thought to be almost completely (>90%) absorbed in the intestine (Sherman and Mehta, 2009).

According to current regulations, the presence of phosphorus-containing additives must be reported on the food labels, but the food manufacturers are not required to give information about the quantity of phosphorus. Food labels report the additive ingredients either by their full name or with an abbreviation and code number (as the "E" = European series): for instance, from E 340 to E 349 are phosphorus-containing additives used as antioxidants and acidity regulators, where those from E 450 to E 458 serve as thickeners, emulsifiers, and regulators (for more information about the use of phosphate additives see Chapter 21). Hence, this extra phosphorus is sometimes also called "hidden phosphorus" because it does not usually appear in the nutrient composition databases and food composition tables (Benini et al., 2011; Cupisti et al., 2012). An example of how these additives are identified on a typical European food label is shown in Figure 22.1.

More than 300 food additives have been approved for use in Europe and given a uniform designation with an E number (see Chapter 21). According to the guidelines of the European Union, the E numbers of all food additives on packaged foods must be marked on the package. The EU ecoregulation further restricts the use of food additives for organically grown foods. Among additives containing phosphate, only calcium phosphate can be used in foods labeled as organic. The labeling requirement is, unfortunately, only qualitative and not quantitative. The consumer, or the patient, cannot determine how much phosphate is actually present in each item, as neither the overall phosphate content nor the quantity of added phosphate is shown on the label. Recent studies from the United States estimated that the extra burden of phosphorus coming from processed food may

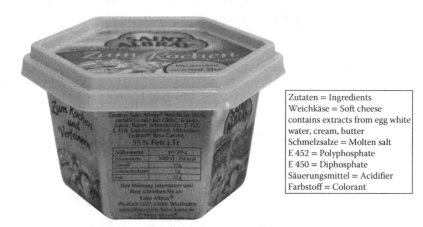

FIGURE 22.1 An example of how these additives are identified on a typical European food label.

A European Perspective   317

reach 700 to 800 mg per day (Leon et al., 2013; Carrigan et al., 2014). In kidney patients on dialysis, such a high content may impair the dialysis process and increase the costs of phosphate binder therapy, which is expected to remove no more than 200 to 300 mg of phosphorus per day (Daugirdas et al., 2011). Dietary phosphorus recommendations for end-stage renal disease patients on dialysis in Europe are restricted to 800 mg/d; thus it is clear that hidden intakes from phosphate additives can easily defeat any efforts to limit phosphorus intake in these patients. Indeed, potential contributions from phosphate additives alone could exceed the newly established EU Dietary Reference Values (DRV) for phosphorus intakes in healthy men and women (Adequate Intake level or AI = 550 mg P/d) (EFSA, 2015).

22.2.3 Added Phosphates Contributing to Phosphorus Intake

Apart from phosphates as natural constituents of processed and unprocessed food, the following sources of added phosphates shown next can be used according to EU regulatory and exposure perspectives. In addition, estimates of total phosphorus intake must give consideration to phosphorus ingestion from pharmaceuticals, water, and other nonfood sources:

1. **Phosphates used as excipients.** These phosphates can be used in pharmaceuticals according to the European Pharmacopoeia. Phosphates can serve as, for example, calcium phosphates: major components in tablets; as fillers and binders; or as a minor component in sachets as anticaking agents (Zahid, 1998).
2. **Phosphates used to treat drinking water.** According to Council Directive 80/778/EEC, the maximum permitted dosage level is 2.2 mg/L as phosphorus.
3. **Phosphate-processing aids.** Phosphate salts such as calcium phosphate can be used as an anticaking agent in food or food additive premixes. Regulation (EC) No 1333/2008 states that processing aids do not need to be labeled if they do not display any technological effect in the finished product.
4. **Phosphate-containing vitamins and mineral fortificants.** According to Regulation (EC) No 1925/2006, phosphates that are not used for technical purposes but for the fortification of food, including foods intended for particular nutritional uses as defined by the 2010 Revision on Directive 2009/39/EC, can be added to achieve a nutritional or health claim for phosphorus content. For more information about the allowed addition of phosphate as nutritional fortificants visit the following website: http://www.ec.europa.eu/food/committees/advisory/summary_20052010_en.pdf.

There are five approved health claims for phosphorus in the EU, which are described in Regulation 1924/2006 cited at: http://www.efsa.europa.eu/sites/default/files/event/documentset/corporate100601-p03.pdf. Four of the five phosphorus health claims are subsumed in Article 13 (1) of the regulation and deal with the role of phosphorus in energy metabolism and its function in cell membranes as well as in normal bone and teeth. These four health claims are nonrisk reduction claims targeted to the normal population. The fifth phosphorus health claim belongs to a different category described by Article 14 (1), and is specific for health claims featuring the reduction of disease or problems with child development. Here, the role of phosphorus is approved as necessary in normal growth and bone development in children. In addition, phosphates, when combined with minerals such as potassium, calcium, and magnesium, can be added to achieve a health claim for the specific nutrients combined with phosphorus. Caution should be exercised because when consumed daily, fortified food or dietary supplements may provide excessive amounts of phosphate over time.

5. **Organic food additives may contain inorganic phosphates.** Inorganic phosphate can serve as a minor constituent of some widely used organic (carbon-based) food additives. The most common examples of these are the widely used phosphorylated starches (E 1410–14414, E 1442) and ammonia caramel (E 150c).

6. **Phosphates lawfully added to unpackaged foods.** According to Regulation (EC) No. 1333/2008 phosphate food additives may be added to unpackaged, and thus nonlabeled, food, for example, phosphates used as leavening agents in fresh fine bakery items or for water-binding purposes in fresh sausages from the butcher.

7. **Phosphates used as food additives: E 338 to 341, E 343, E 450 to 452.** According to Regulation (EC) No 1333/2008, phosphates used as food additives need to be labeled as such on packaged food (e.g., phosphoric acid in cola beverages, sodium phosphate in individually wrapped processed cheese slices, or calcium phosphate in baking powder). High levels of phosphate exposure are to be expected particularly via consumption of processed cheese, meat, bakery, and food supplement products, which contain phosphate food additives.

8. **Other lawful additions of phosphate food additives.** Regulation (EC) No 1333/2008 allows the lawful addition of phosphate food additives to unpackaged or packaged food, for example, lecithins (E 322); ammonium phosphatides (E 442); ribonucleotides (E 626–635); riboflavin-5'-phosphate (E 101(ii)); sodium aluminum phosphate, acidic (E 541); and modified starches such as monostarch phosphate (E 1410), distarch phosphate (E 1412), phosphated distarch phosphate (E 1413), acetylated distarch phosphate (E 1414), hydroxypropyl distarch phosphate (E 1415). Under the conditions of this regulation, there is no mandatory requirement to label the phosphate ingredients, thus the term "hidden phosphorus" is appropriate, where nonmandatory labeling of phosphate ingredients makes it difficult to identify their content on the label.

Phosphate additives described in section 1, 7, and 8 fall under the pharma or food additive law in the EU and must be included in the ingredients section of the product label. However, this does not mean that the label conveys a complete and accurate accounting of all the added ingredients that contain phosphorus. First, all constituents that contain phosphate might be unrecognized because only the E number and their functional purpose (e.g., emulgator, stabilizer) is used and not their full name. Second (see section 8), other phosphate-containing constituents of food, as mentioned earlier, such as lecithin, ribonucleotides, or modified starches, may not appear to the average consumer to contain phosphate because phosphate is not given in the ingredient name. Finally, it is important to note that those fortificants mentioned in section 4 are by law not actually considered food additives. But this can be a problem if these nutritional additions contain phosphate and also contribute to the exposure scenario. Thus, it may be difficult or confusing for marketers, consumer, and even regulatory authorities to detect or evaluate the total phosphorus containing constituents in products as they are currently labeled.

22.3 EUROPEAN UNION REGULATION AND SAFETY ASSESSMENT OF PHOSPHATE-CONTAINING FOOD ADDITIVES

22.3.1 EUROPEAN UNION REGULATION

In the EU, phosphates are added for several technological purposes to a multitude of foodstuffs. There is a long history concerning the evaluation and use of phosphate food additives, which were reviewed by the Scientific Committee for Food (SCF) in 1990. The committee established a maximum tolerable daily intake (MTDI) of 70 mg P/kg body weight that translates to 4900 mg phosphorus per day in a 70-kg adult (SCF, 1991). The same level was proposed by the Joint FAO/WHO Expert Committee on Food Additives (JECFA) (SCF, 1991; JECFA, 1982). In 1992, the SCF defined the population reference intake for phosphorus as 550 mg/d for adults (SCF, 1993), which has remained the same after the 2015 revision (http://www.efsa.europa.eu/en/consultations/call/150310b.htm) and (http://www.efsa.europa.eu/de/efsajournal/pub/4185.htm). In the draft for this revision, the EFSA initially recommended 700 mg/d for adults, based on the equimolar ratio of calcium to phosphorus as it is found naturally in bone (http://www.efsa.europa.eu/en/consultations/call/150310b.htm), but

A European Perspective

later this basis was changed to reflect the ratio in all body tissues and the extracellular fluid which reduced this to 550 mg/d and even lower for children (see Chapter 20) (http://www.efsa.europa.eu/de/efsajournal/pub/4185.htm).

A concern with these recent changes is that the EFSA maintains their early position, declining to set an upper level (UL) of tolerable safe intake for phosphorus. In its 2005 opinion, EFSA was unable to establish a tolerable upper intake level of phosphorus, but the expert panel concluded that "normal healthy individuals can tolerate phosphorus intakes up to at least 3000 mg phosphorus per day without adverse systemic effects" (EFSA, 2005), which is consistent with the 1991 MTDI for total phosphorus intake, given that they are both very high thresholds. Both of these recommendations for upper safe levels of phosphorus intake are strongly disputed by many medical experts. This issue is addressed in Chapter 20, which describes the very high thresholds set for the Canadian and American phosphorus UL.

In total, more than 40 phosphate-containing food additives are currently permitted in the EU. In 2010, the EU passed Regulation (EU) No. 257 which defines a specific program for the re-evaluation of food additives in general. As all of the phosphate-containing additives were already permitted in the European Union before January 20, 2009, they are included in this program. As shown in Table 22.1, four additives have already been evaluated, six organic additives had a deadline for re-evaluation by the end of 2016, and the remaining additives (36 total) must be assessed for safety by the end of 2018, the latter including the vast majority of the inorganic phosphates.

22.3.2 Events Leading to the European Commission Health Consumer Directorate Mandated Safety Review

Against the background of the mounting evidence that phosphate is one of the major culprits for the excessive high risk of cardiovascular events in CKD patients and probably also in the general population, a group of German medical experts has launched a campaign to inform the general medical community. In 2012, an article regarding the health risks of phosphate intakes that exceed nutrient requirements and that questioned the safety of phosphate additives in food was published in the German medical journal *Deutsche Ärzteblatt* (Ritz et al., 2012). These experts concluded that there is critical need for a comprehensive labeling of phosphate additives in food—suggesting that ideally it could be done with a "traffic-light" scheme and a quantitative restriction of phosphate additives. The amount of added phosphate, whether low, medium, or high, should be indicated with a green, yellow, or red sign on the package, similar to what is currently done in Finland and the United Kingdom to indicate sodium chloride content. A nice example of such a "food traffic light" displaying the amount of fat, saturated fat, sugar, or salt in food has been developed by the Food Standard Agency (2007) in the UK (see Figure 22.2 or go to: http://food.gov.uk/multimedia/pdfs/publication/foodtrafficlight1107.pdf). In the *Deutsche Ärzteblatt* paper food governmental and quasi-governmental entities were approached for support in order to launch these measures. Industry, consumer protection organizations, medical societies, and this paper have gained substantial attention, not only in Germany, but also across Europe by professionals in the health promotion business. Since its publication, it has been downloaded and cited several hundred times, as well as receiving robust media coverage over the health concerns for excessive phosphorus intake. Meanwhile, government authorities are taking the health issue of consuming phosphate-loaded processed and ready-to-eat food seriously.

In March 2013, the Ritz et al. paper (2012) prompted the European Commission Health and Consumers Directorate to request scientific and technical assistance from the European Food Safety Authority (EFSA, Chrono #72038) concerning the safety of phosphate additives. In this mandate to EFSA, the EU Commission referenced the usage of phosphates as food additives only. In the course

TABLE 22.1

Phosphate Food Additives Required to be Reassessed According to EU No.257 and Their Scheduled Deadlines for Completion of the Safety Re-Evaluation

E-Number and Name of Food Additive	Organic	Inorganic	Assessment Deadline Date
E 101 (ii) RIBOFLAVIN-5′-PHOSPHATE	x		Finished
E 150a PLAIN CARAMEL*	x		Finished
E 150d SULPHITE AMMONIA CARAMEL*	x		Finished
E 322 LECITHINS	x		12/31/2016
E 338 PHOSPHORIC ACID		x	12/31/2018
E 339 (i) MONOSODIUM PHOSPHATE		x	12/31/2018
E 339 (ii) DISODIUM PHOSPHATE		x	12/31/2018
E 339 (iii) TRISODIUM PHOSPHATE		x	12/31/2018
E 340 (i) MONOPOTASSIUM PHOSPHATE		x	12/31/2018
E 340 (ii) DIPOTASSIUM PHOSPHATE		x	12/31/2018
E 340 (iii) TRIPOTASSIUM PHOSPHATE		x	12/31/2018
E 341 (i) MONOCALCIUM PHOSPHATE		x	12/31/2018
E 341 (ii) DICALCIUM PHOSPHATE		x	12/31/2018
E 341 (iii) TRICALCIUM PHOSPHATE		x	12/31/2018
E 343(i) MONOMAGNESIUM PHOSPHATE		x	12/31/2018
E 343(ii) DIMAGNESIUM PHOSPHATE		x	12/31/2018
E 442 AMMONIUM PHOSPHATIDES		x	12/31/2018
E 450 (i) DISODIUM DIPHOSPHATE		x	12/31/2018
E 450 (ii) TRISODIUM DIPHOSPHATE		x	12/31/2018
E 450 (iii) TETRASODIUM DIPHOSPHATE		x	12/31/2018
E 450 (v) TETRAPOTASSIUM DIPHOSPHATE		x	12/31/2018
E 450 (vi) DICALCIUM DIPHOSPHATE		x	12/31/2018
E 450 (vii) CALCIUM DIHYDROGEN DIPHOSPHATE		x	12/31/2018
E 451 (i) PENTASODIUM TRIPHOSPHATE		x	12/31/2018
E 451 (ii) PENTAPOTASSIUM TRIPHOSPHATE		x	12/31/2018
E 452 (i) SODIUM POLYPHOSPHATE		x	12/31/2018
E 452 (ii) POTASSIUM POLYPHOSPHATE		x	12/31/2018
E 452(iii) SODIUM CALCIUM POLYPHOSPHATE		x	12/31/2018
E 452 (iv) CALCIUM POLYPHOSPHATE		x	12/31/2018
E 541 SODIUM ALUMINIUM PHOSPHATE, ACIDIC		x	Finished
E 626 GUANYLIC ACID	x		12/31/2018
E 627 DISODIUM GUANYLATE	x		12/31/2018
E 628 DIPOTASSIUM GUANYLATE	x		12/31/2018
E 629 CALCIUM GUANYLATE	x		12/31/2018
E 630 INOSINIC ACID	x		12/31/2018
E 631 DISODIUM INOSINATE	x		12/31/2018
E 632 DIPOTASSIUM INOSINATE	x		12/31/2018
E 633 CALCIUM INOSINATE	x		12/31/2018
E 634 CALCIUM 5'-RIBONUCLEOTIDE	x		12/31/2018
E 635 DISODIUM 5'-RIBONUCLEOTIDE	x		12/31/2018
E 1200 POLYDEXTROSE*	x		12/31/2018
E 1410 MONOSTARCH PHOSPHATE	x		12/31/2016
E 1412 DISTARCH PHOSPHATE	x		12/31/2016
E 1413 PHOSPHATED DISTARCH PHOSPHATE	x		12/31/2016
E 1414 ACETYLATED DISTARCH PHOSPHATE	x		12/31/2016
E 1442 HYDROXYPROPYL DISTARCH PHOSPHATE	x		12/31/2016

A European Perspective 321

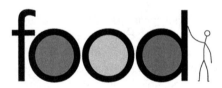
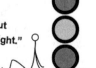

Do you want to eat more healthily?

The Food Standards Agency has developed a traffic light label that gives you independent expert scientific dietary advice to help you make healthier choices quickly and easily.

Look for products with **green**, amber or **red** coloured labels on the front of the pack. These show you at a glance if the food you are thinking about buying has **low**, medium or **high** amounts of fat, saturated fat, sugars and salt, helping you get a better balance.

"Healthy eating is all about getting the overall balance right."

using traffic lights
to make healthier choices

What the colours mean:

 means **HIGH**
indicating that the food is high in fat, sugars or salt

It's fine to eat this food occasionally or as a treat, but think about how often you choose it and how much of it you eat.

 means MEDIUM
making it an OK choice

Although going for green is even better!

 means it's **LOW**

Which makes it a healthier choice.

What if the traffic light panel has all three colours?

For a healthier choice try to pick products with more **greens** and ambers and fewer **reds**.

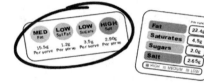

FIGURE 22.2 (See color insert.) A suggested system to warn the public about the content of phosphorus in food.

of the scientific discussion with EFSA, the need to also consider the exposure from phosphates coming from other sources as described earlier was also stressed. In November 2013, EFSA published a detailed 27-page statement (EFSA, 2013) in a direct response to the Ritz et al. review and concluded that: "Owing to the intrinsic limitations of the non-interventional design of the studies included, it is not possible at this point of time to make causal inferences for serum phosphate levels and the observed adverse effects."

22.4 EUROPEAN UNION RECOMMENDATIONS AND ACTIONS CONCERNING EXCESS PHOSPHORUS INTAKE AS A HEALTH RISK

22.4.1 Mandated Re-Evaluation

After much deliberation the EU Commission concluded that from the evidence reviewed it is not clear whether the increased cardiovascular risk observed in the observational studies submitted for review is attributable to differences in total dietary intake of phosphorus from all sources or only from phosphate additives (EFSA, 2013). As contributions from both sources do raise serum phosphate, EFSA made the following recommendations specific to these issues of determining causality and possible health risk of phosphate-containing additives lawfully used as food additives:

RECOMMENDATIONS

Phosphoric acid and phosphates (E 338–341; E 343) and polyphosphates (E 450–452) for use as food additives should be re-evaluated by EFSA with high priority by 31 December 2018, as set out in Regulation (EC) No 257/2010. In the context of this re-evaluation, the relevant and most up-to-date literature will be reviewed. Given that some of the published studies have shown inconsistent or contrasting results regarding the possible health risks associated with serum phosphate levels, a meta-analysis of a systematic review of the available literature should be performed.

In order to allow completion of the re-evaluation of phosphoric acid, phosphates, di-, tri- and polyphosphates (E 338–341; E 343 and E 450–452) for use as food additives within the set deadline, data relevant for the estimation of the human exposure to the relevant food additives should be submitted by interested parties to EFSA. To this end a dedicated call for data aimed at gathering information on usage levels will be launched in addition to the previous call for scientific data on miscellaneous food additives published by EFSA in 2012 (EFSA, 2013). According to information from EFSA, the aforementioned call for data will be open and launched in 2016–2017, and EFSA will welcome any scientific data and information that stakeholders can provide.

22.4.2 FURTHER DATA NEEDS FOR THE EU PHOSPHATE ADDITIVE SAFETY RE-EVALUATION

In the course of this re-evaluation process, it is among the responsibilities of the stakeholders to again highlight the need for a more holistic approach to the human exposure assessment of phosphorus intake in the EU that is beyond labeled food additives. Consideration should be given to potential hidden intake via drinking water, table water, and pharmaceuticals, but also through (unlabeled) processing aids and food additives. Special attention should also be paid to the usage of phosphate-containing minerals that serve as fortificants because they can contribute excessive amounts via fortified food or food supplements when consumed on a daily basis. This call for data (http://www.efsa.europa.eu/en/search/doc/3444.pdf) is aimed at gathering all relevant toxicological information on usage levels of phosphates in food in preparation for the re-evaluation. Therefore, it will be necessary to search the European scientific landscape and collect all available data that can help to illuminate the issue of health risks of phosphate additives, not only in CKD patients, but also in other population groups at risk and potentially even in the general population. Important relevant studies are already beginning to appear in the literature, such as the recent meta-analysis examining serum phosphate and progression of CKD and mortality among a large cohort of non-dialysis-dependent patients with CKD (Da et al., 2015).

A cautionary note warrants mention with respect to other regulatory issues governed by the EU. In this context, Professor Igor Pravst raised the question whether the phosphorus health claims approved in the EU for use on the label would lead to health risks. He concluded that phosphate-related health claims should be restricted (Pravst, 2011). Professor Pravst based his conclusions on a compelling argument illustrating how such health claims could lead to further addition of phosphate salts to foods that could result in serious health issues. To date, the overall phosphate content does not need to be labeled on the nutritional panel of packaged food unless phosphates are added for nutritional purposes. The presence of health claims requires that a minimum level of a nutrient be present in the food in order to justify the claim, thus potentially stimulating higher phosphorus content in products bearing a health claim.

Based on the abundance of phosphate in processed food and the postulated health risks, Ritz et al. (2012) called for a mandatory labeling of the phosphate content. This would best be done on the nutritional facts panel, as it is for other possible detrimental components like salt or saturated fatty acids.

22.4.3 FOOD INDUSTRY RESPONSE TO EUROPEAN UNION MANDATED SAFETY ASSESSMENT OF PHOSPHATE ADDITIVES

In general, the food industry responded positively to the EU safety assessment mandate for re-evaluation of phosphate additive use and is seriously considering the potential health risks described in the risk paper. Foremost among these was a June 2014 conference organized by Leatherhead Food Research, an organization based in the UK that delivers integrated scientific expertise and international regulatory advice to the global food, drink, and related industries. The conference goal was to explore possible alternatives to phosphate additive use in foods. It was revealed that phosphate alternatives are already in use or under development and are available for sensitive applications. Collaborative links were organized with universities or research institutes to investigate ongoing research that may offer future solutions. The final report from this conference is currently under review by the consortium partners, and a range of practical application study proposals will hopefully follow.

Leatherhead's call for alliance among food scientists and medical experts at this June meeting has already stimulated clinical studies examining the influence of varying phosphorus loads on serum phosphorus concentrations and hormonal regulators of phosphorus homeostasis in healthy young men and women. In this randomized placebo-controlled human eight-week-intervention study the investigators examined the consequences of a high phosphorus intake (1000 mg) on mineral metabolism and bone remodeling in dependence of different calcium intakes (0, 500, 1000 mg) in healthy subjects by measuring plasma-phosphate, renal excretion, and fecal phosphorus concentration (Trautvetter, 2016). As one could have expected, there was no change in fasting plasma phosphate-levels in these healthy adults, but there was an increase of FGF23 after four weeks, which normalized after eight weeks. These signs of a disturbed phosphate homeostasis, even in a healthy population without kidney injury, are indicative of possible health risks of a high phosphate burden in the long run.

Further studies are urgently needed; nevertheless, whether or not these and future study designs appropriately address EFSA's phosphate food additive safety assessment criteria remains to be determined.

22.5 PHOSPHORUS SUSTAINABILITY CONCERNS

Concern over the health effects of excess phosphorus intake is just one aspect of the phosphorus issues that are plaguing Europe and much of the world. An equally pressing concern is that of threatened sustainability of phosphorus sources used in agricultural applications that significantly affect food production. Phosphorus is an irreplaceable limited natural resource. The demand for phosphorus is growing, and in Europe there is no phosphorus depot to be mined.

The manyfold implications of phosphate needs were touched upon at the "First European Sustainable Phosphorus Conference," which was held in Brussels in 2013. Participants reached consensus to launch the European Phosphorus Platform ESPP (see: http://www.phosphorusplatform.eu/images/Conference/espc_programma_26022015.pdf), which brings together companies and stakeholders to continue dialogues, raise awareness, and trigger actions to address the phosphorus challenge that has implications for ensuring food security, geo-political stability, and environmental sustainability. Since then, some interesting projects have been launched, mostly regarding possibilities to reuse and sustain phosphorus like the Dutch Nutrient Platform which cooperates on a national level: http://www.nutrientplatform.org/english.html.

The second ESPP Conference was held in March 2016 in Berlin where leading experts and decision makers in the field of phosphorus management came together to exchange knowledge and experience and finally take action: https://ec.europa.eu/eip/agriculture/en/content/second-european-sustainable-phosphorus-conference-espc2. The presentations and discussions covered topics such as (1) EU policies on phosphorus management, (2) phosphorus global food security, (3) geo-political dependencies, and (4) planetary boundaries and more. Some presentations touched on the medical impact of phosphate in food, but the potentially dangerous consequences to humans of phosphate additive overuse were not discussed. This illustrates the need for more interaction between medical and nonmedical scientists. For more information on the sustainability of phosphorus, its impact on agriculture, animal husbandry, and interaction with human consumption and environmental health see Chapters 23 and 24.

22.6 CONCLUSIONS

The possible health risks of phosphate and especially phosphate additives in food have definitely raised the attention of the European health authorities, and a re-evaluation of phosphate additives will be completed by 2018. Until that time it will be necessary to collect and review all relevant data especially regarding phosphorus and the progression of CKD and cardiovascular disease. It is important that future and ongoing studies are designed to address EFSA's phosphate food additive safety assessment criteria. Maybe the problem of phosphate sustainability will help us recognize that it is time for a change and a chance for mutual efforts of the food industry and medical, food, and nutritional sciences to find substitutes for phosphate additives.

REFERENCES

Benini O, D'Alessandro C, Gianfaldoni D, Cupisti A. Extra-phosphate load from food additives in commonly eaten foods: A renal and insidious danger for renal patients. *J Ren Nutr* 2011;21:303–308.

Brandenburg VM, Kleber M, Vervloet MG, Tomaschitz A, Pilz S, Stojakovic T, Delgado G, Grammer T, Marx N, März W, Scharnagl H. Fibroblast Growth Factor (FGF23) and mortality: The Ludwigshafen Risk and Cardiovascular Health Study. *Atherosclerosis* 2014;237:53–59.

Calvo MS, Park YK. Changing phosphorus content of the U.S. diet: Potential for adverse effects on bone. *J Nutr* 1996;126:1168–1180.

Calvo MS, Uribarri J. Public health impact of dietary phosphorus excess on bone and cardiovascular health in the general population. *Am J Clin Nutr* 2013;98:6–15.

Carrigan A, Klinger A, Choquette SS, Luzuriaga-McPherson A, Bell EK, Darnell B, Gutiérrez OM. 2014. Contribution of food additives to sodium and phosphorus content of diets rich in processed foods. *J Ren Nutr* 24(1):13–19.

Cefic The European Chemical Industry Council 2007. http://www.cefic.org/Documents/Other/13-04-2007-Food-Phosphates-brochure-final.pdf.

Cupisti A, Benini O, Ferretti V, Gianfaldoni D, Kalantar-Zadeh K. Novel differential measurement of natural and added phosphorus in cooked ham with or without preservatives. *J Ren Nutr* 2012;22(6):533–540.

Da J, Xie X, Wolf M, Disthabanchongs, Wang, Zha Y, Lv J, Zhang L, Wang H. Serum phosphorus and progression of CKD and mortality: A meta-analysis of cohort studies. *Am J Kidney Dis* 2015;66(2):258–265.

Daugirdas JT, Finn WF, Emmett M, Chertow GM. Frequent Hemodialysis Network Trial Group: The phosphate binder equivalent dose. *Semin Dial* 2011;24(1):41–49.

Dinghra R, Sullivan LM, Fox CS, Wang TJ, D'Agostino RB Sr, Gaziano JM, Vasan RS. Relations of serum phosphorus and calcium levels to the incidence of cardiovascular disease in the community. *Arch Int Med* 2007;167:879–885.

European Food Safety Authority. Opinion of the scientific panel on dietetic products, nutrition and allergies on a request from the commission related to the tolerable upper intake level of phosphorus. *EFSA J* 2005;233:1–19.

European Food Safety Authority. Assessment of one published review on health risks associated with phosphate additives in food. *EFSA J* 2013;11(11):3444, 27pp.

EFSA NDA Panel (EFSA Panel on Dietetic Products, Nutrition and Allergies). Draft scientific opinion on dietary reference values for phosphorus. *EFSA J* 2015:51.

EWG Environmental Working Group is a non-profit, non-partisan organization dedicated to protecting human health and the environment. 2015. http://www.ewg.org/search/site/food%2520score%2520data%2520ba se%2520phosphate%2520additives.

A European Perspective

Foley RN, Collins AJ, Herzog CA, Ishani A, Kalra PA. Serum Phosphorus Levels associate with coronary Atherosclerosis in young adults. *JASN* 2009;20:397–404.

Food Standard Agency, 2007. (official food and health organization in the UK has created an example of a food traffic light). http://food.gov.uk/multimedia/pdfs/publication/foodtrafficlight1107.pdf

Food Service Europe and Middle East 03/2013 pg.014. http://www.food-service-europe.com/digital/epaper/

Joint FAO/WHO Expert Committee on Food Additives (JECFA), 1982. Evaluation of certain food additives and contaminants (Twenty-sixth report of the Joint FAO/WHO Expert Committee on Food Additives). *WHO Technical Report Series*, No. 683.

Kestenbaum B, Sampson JN, Rudser KD, Patterson DJ, Seliger SL,Young B, Sherrard DJ, Andress DL. Serum phosphorous level and mortality risk among people with chronic kidney disease. *JASN* 2005;16:520–528.

Leon JB, Sullivan CM, Sehgal AR. The prevalence of phosphorus-containing food additives in top-selling foods in grocery stores. *J Ren Nutr* 2013, 23(4):265–270.

McGovern AP, de Lusignan S, van Vlymen J, Liyanage H, Tomson CR, Gallagher H, Rafiq M, Jones S. Serum phosphate as a risk factor for cardiovascular events in people with and without chronic kidney disease: A large community based cohort study. *PLOS ONE* 2013;8(9):e74996.

Menon V, Greene T, Pereira AA, Wang X, Beck GJ, Kusek JW, Collins AJ, Levey AS, Sarnak MJ. Relationship of phosphorus and calcium-phosphorus product with mortality in CKD. *AJKD* 2005;46:455–463.

Pravst I. Risking public health by approving some health claims?- The case of phosphorus. *Food Policy* 2011;36:726–728.

Ritz E, Hahn K, Ketteler M, Kuhlmann MK and Mann J. Phosphate additives in food—A health risk. *Dtsch Aerztebl Int* 2012;109:49–55.

Scientific Committee for Food, 1991. First series of food additives of various technological functions. (Opinion expressed on18 May 1990). http://ec.europa.eu/food/fs/sc/scf/reports/scf_reports_25.pdf.

Scientific Committee for Food, 1993. Nutrient and energy intakes for the European Community. (Opinion expressed on December 1992). http://ec.europa.eu/food/fs/sc/scf/reports/scf_reports_31.pdf.

Sherman RA, Mehta O. Dietary phosphorus restriction in dialysis patients: Potential impact of processed meat, poultry and fish products as protein sources. *Am J Kidney Dis* 2009, 54:18–23.

Stiftung Warentest. Fastfood im Test. 2013. https://www.test.de/shop/test-hefte/test_09_2013/.

Sullivan C, Leon JB, Shegal AR. Phosphorus-containing food additives and the accuracy of nutrient databases: Implications for renal Patients. *J Ren Nutr* 2007;17:350–354.

Tonelli M, Sacks F, Pfeffer M, Gao Z, Curhan G. Relation between serum phosphate level and cardiovascular risk in people with coronary disease. *Circulation* 2005;112:2627–2633.

Trautvetter U. Consequences of a high phosphorus intake on mineral metabolism and bone remodeling in dependence of calcium intake in healthy subjects—A randomized placebo-controlled human intervention study. *Nutr J* 2016;15:7. doi:10.1186/s12937-016-0125-5.

Uribarri J. Phosphorus aditives in food and their effect in dialysis patients. *Clin J Am Soc Nephrol* 2009;4:1290–1292.

Zahid A. *Calcium Phosphates in Biological and Industrial Systems*, New York, NY: Springer, 1998.

23 Save the P(ee)!
The Challenges of Phosphorus Sustainability and Emerging Solutions

James J. Elser, Neng Iong Chan,
Jessica R. Corman, and Jared Stoltzfus

CONTENTS

Abstract 327
Bullet Points 328
23.1 Introduction 328
23.2 The First Dimension of the P Sustainability Challenge: The Supply of P 329
23.3 The Second Dimension of P Sustainability: The Fate of P 330
    23.3.1 Crop P Use and Loss of P from Farmlands 330
    23.3.2 Manure Fluxes 331
    23.3.3 Food Waste 332
    23.3.4 Fluxes from Humans 332
    23.3.5 Aquatic Eutrophication, Toxic Algae, and Dead Zones 333
23.4 Solutions 333
    23.4.1 Reduce Demand 333
    23.4.2 Continue to Improve Crop Varieties and Genetics 334
    23.4.3 Continue to Improve Fertilizer Practices 335
    23.4.4 Reduce P Needed for Animal Production 335
    23.4.5 Reduce Food Waste 335
    23.4.6 Recycle P from Rich Organic Systems 336
    23.4.7 Reduce Reliance on Crop-Based Biofuels 337
23.5 Conclusions 337
References 337

ABSTRACT

Phosphorus (P) is a chemical element that is essential for all living things, playing a central role in genetic molecules, energetic metabolism, cell membranes, and even bones. Because its geological abundance on Earth and its weathering rate from rocks are low and it has relatively low mobility in soils, P is often limiting to the growth of living things, including algae in lakes and oceans and plants in terrestrial ecosystems, including crops. To overcome these limitations, humanity has massively increased the extraction of P from geological deposits for the production of chemical fertilizers, allowing for the greatly increased yields of the Green Revolution. However, this amplification of the P cycle has damaged aquatic ecosystems due to losses of P from fields, livestock rearing, and human settlements that have triggered toxic algal blooms and dead zones in lakes and oceans. Increasing demand for P fertilizer has also led to increasing and wildly fluctuating prices for phosphate rock, raising concerns about the long-term supply of P for food production. These two dimensions, uncertainty about availability of affordable P and concerns about water quality impacts, comprise the P sustainability challenge. A variety of strategies are needed to address these dimensions. These include improvement in crop varieties for more efficient P utilization, enhanced efficiency of fertilizer use on the farm, reductions in food waste, shifts in diet toward less meat consumption, and development of P recycling pathways to recover P from organic waste streams (food waste, manure, human waste). By advancing these approaches at a sufficient scale, society may be able to sustain both the food and the water it needs for a healthy future.

BULLET POINTS

- Phosphorus is a chemical element essential for all living things, playing a key structural role in genetic material, energy processing, and cellular membranes. It also is a key ingredient in bones. Inputs of P as fertilizer are required for high crop yields, but production of fertilizer currently relies on mining from a finite number of geologic deposits that are located in just a few countries.
- Supplies of P in the environment are often limiting for growth; thus, large amounts of fertilizer are used to support modern agricultural systems, but much of this P is lost as non–point source pollution from fields and from animal rearing facilities as well as from cities and towns, causing undesirable eutrophication of inland and coastal waters.
- P for fertilizer production is mined from ancient deposits found in just a few countries; thus, concerns have arisen about the long-term security of phosphate rock supplies, especially in light of recent price increases and erratic fluctuations.
- Recent analyses suggest that long-term sustainability of P can be achieved via a combination of demand-based measures (diet, population size), improved agricultural approaches, and implementation of widespread recycling technologies, assuring a reliable and continuous source of fertilizer while reducing pollution of aquatic ecosystems.

23.1 INTRODUCTION

Phosphorus (P) is the 15th chemical element in the periodic table, forged by fusing the nuclei of two oxygen atoms in exploding stars during the earliest times of the universe. Only an exploding star could have been the site of such an event, as the fusion requires temperatures exceeding 1 billion degrees Kelvin. This information is important for a discussion of P sustainability because it makes clear that we cannot realistically "make" any more P if we should happen to "run out." Conversely, the physical stability of chemical elements means also that we cannot destroy P; instead, P atoms persist indefinitely, although their distribution in the environment may not always make them easy to access for use and reuse. Nevertheless, the indestructibility of P atoms means that indeed, in theory at least, P can be recycled and reused indefinitely.

Readers of this volume will know that P is essential for human health and indeed for the successful functioning of all living things. This is because P (as phosphate, PO_4) is a key player across major domains of biology. P is central to energetic metabolism (in the rapid cycling of ATP in photosynthesis and respiration), in gene regulation (phosphorylation), in key cell structures (such as phospholipids that make up cell membranes), and, perhaps most notably, in the structure of the key genetic molecules DNA and RNA, where P contributes ~9% of total molecular mass (Sterner and Elser 2002). Indeed, you could say that "phosphate holds your genes up." In vertebrate animals like humans, P has an additional central role: as a key component of the apatite mineral $(Ca_{10}(PO_4)_6(OH)_2)$ that makes up our bones. In vertebrates, >90% of the total body P is present in the bones at any one time (Sterner and Elser 2002). In contrast, in invertebrate animals and in bacteria, nucleic acids and especially RNA usually contain a preponderance of the biomass P.

The key role of P in supporting organism growth applies also to the key biota that make up our food system: crop plants, livestock, and soil microbes. However, P is released to the environment by slow processes of chemical weathering, building up in soil slowly over millennia. As a result, soils are often deficient in P as well as in other key nutrients, such as nitrogen (N) and potassium (K). To overcome this deficiency, farmers for millennia have used various means to augment soil fertility, applying manure (both livestock- and human-derived), guano, food and crop wastes, compost, and other nutrient-rich materials in a more or less closed system in a relatively low-intensity, local-scale food system.

With the dawn of industrial agriculture and the Green Revolution, fertilizer application has been taken to new heights. In ~1910, a means for industrial nitrogen fixation was invented (the Haber-Bosch reaction), using large amounts of natural gas to create chemical conditions needed to convert atmospheric N_2 to inorganic ammonia (NH_3). Although its first uses were to produce feedstock for explosives in World War I, the process was soon adopted for fertilizer production. However, soils are not only deficient in N but are also deficient in P. Thus, a large increase in the mining of phosphate rock was initiated and indeed has increased nearly continuously during the past century in support of the Green Revolution. The use of industrial fertilizers also allowed crop production to move further and further away from livestock and human populations. However, economically viable reserves of phosphate rock are geographically constrained (see Section 23.2) and prices of P rock have increased dramatically in recent years. This amplification of the P cycle has not come without costs. Indeed, considerable amounts of P escape the food system via erosion and leaching from farms, runoff from livestock rearing facilities, and point and nonpoint discharges of human sewage. These nutrient losses promote excessive growth of algae in rivers, lakes, and coastal oceans, including toxic cyanobacteria that can cause neurological and hepatic impairment as well as deoxygenated "dead zones" in lower water depths that impair freshwater and coastal fisheries.

We now have a sense of the two main dimensions of the P sustainability challenge: uncertainties regarding the long-term supply of affordable P to support global food production and increasing frequency and severity of P-induced aquatic eutrophication. These challenges are especially acute in light of the projected need to double food availability in order to achieve global food security in 2050 (Alexandratos et al. 2012). In the rest of this chapter we will describe the current state of the global P system, emphasizing the human flows that now dominate the global P cycle and that can result in undesirable impacts on water quality. We will finish with an overview of emerging ideas of how the global P cycle can be radically reconfigured to achieve a more sustainable P supply that can support future generations with abundant food, clean drinking water, and healthy aquatic ecosystems.

23.2 THE FIRST DIMENSION OF THE P SUSTAINABILITY CHALLENGE: THE SUPPLY OF P

Fertilizers are essential for sustaining high-level crop yields. By how much? Stewart et al. (2005) studied more than 350 crop growing seasons for corn, rice, wheat, soybean, and cowpea, concluding that 40% to 60% of crop yield is attributable to application of chemical fertilizers. This reliance on fertilizer is one of the three main components that support the Green Revolution, the others being development of high-yield crop varieties and expansion of arable land via irrigation. Although manure from free-ranging livestock does bring P to some croplands, the great majority of modern agricultural production ultimately relies on inputs of chemical fertilizers that are composed of a mixture of nitrogen (N) compounds (the N having been "fixed" from the atmosphere via the energy-intensive Haber-Bosch reaction), potassium (K), and phosphate (P). The P in these fertilizers is nearly entirely derived from mines, which access deposits of either igneous or sedimentary phosphates, the latter being the dominant geological form. These sedimentary deposits are ancient "phosphorites," the remains of biological deposition of P-rich sediments in shallow seas that built up over millions and millions of years. Thus, the phosphate rock we now rely so heavily on is a "fossil" resource.

Foreshadowed by Isaac Asimov in 1974 ("Life can multiply until all the phosphorus has gone and then there is an inexorable halt which nothing can prevent;" [Asimov 1974]), concerns have been expressed about the longevity of this phosphate rock supply, stimulated especially by the ~700%

increase in the price of phosphate rock during 2007–2008. Indeed, analyses based on global rock consumption rates and extant estimates of phosphate rock reserves (a "reserve" is the amount of a mined material that is confirmed to exist and that can be economically extracted using current technology and methods) led to an estimate of "peak phosphate" occurring within 30 to 50 years, with concomitant pressures on food security (Cordell et al. 2009). However, such concerns have been quelled to a degree by upward readjustments of the global reserve estimates by the International Fertilizer Development Center (Van Kauwenbergh 2010), which resulted in a massive (10-fold) increase in the phosphate rock reserves attributed to Morocco. However, technical aspects of this readjustment itself have been called into question (Edixhoven et al. 2014), and others have noted that this adjustment only delays the time horizon for emerging P scarcity (Ashley et al. 2011). Beyond the reserve estimates, another potential issue arises from the concentration of this essential commodity in just a few countries—Morocco (and its contested territory in Western Sahara) accounts for 85% of the current reserve estimates. This rarefied distribution presents a potential for market distortions such as those associated with petroleum. Indeed, in 2014 the European Union placed phosphate rock on its list of "critical materials," as there are essentially no phosphate rock deposits in Europe and thus European agriculture is entirely dependent on import of phosphate rock and phosphate fertilizers. In the United States, major phosphate mines are concentrated in Florida, and these likely have several decades of production remaining. These mines, however, are increasingly under pressure due to their environmental impacts (particularly the production of massive phosphogypsum stacks of mine waste), leading to local and regional opposition to mine expansion. Similar pressures can be seen elsewhere. For example, proposals to initiate seafloor mining of phosphate nodules off the coast of Namibia have been met by protests from the fishing industry. These emerging trends suggest that the extended postwar period of abundant and cheap phosphate fertilizer is coming to an end. An analysis of phosphate rock price dynamics indicates that it has undergone a "regime shift" in recent years (Elser et al. 2014) and has settled into a new, high-price state. This new regime implies difficulties for farmers in obtaining needed fertilizer to raise and maintain yields (especially in the developing world) but also (on the positive side!) opportunities for entrepreneurs to develop new technologies and approaches that can capture and recover P in the food and waste system to produce "next-generation" fertilizers that are recycled rather than mined.

23.3 THE SECOND DIMENSION OF P SUSTAINABILITY: THE FATE OF P

23.3.1 CROP P USE AND LOSS OF P FROM FARMLANDS

P is a limiting nutrient for plant growth because it is in high demand by rapidly growing crops but has a slow weathering rate and is prone to precipitate with cations in soil solution. The major forms of inorganic P that plants take up are $H_2PO_4^-$ and HPO_4^{2-} and these are only available when soil pH is around neutral. The inorganic P in soil solution seldom exceeds 10 µM even in more fertile soils (Marschner 2012). Phosphate moves from soil solution to plant roots primarily through diffusion and, thus, phosphate uptake is a relatively slow process in soils (Marschner 2012). Also, due to PO_4's chemical properties, fertilizer P is always 'fixed' with different soil cations immediately after fertilization. Thus, generally speaking, P is quite immobile in soils (Brady and Weil 2012).

Globally, due to local geological conditions, many soils have historically been P-deficient. Thus, large scale P fertilizer application is required in the majority of agricultural practices. However, the efficiency of crop P acquisition is relatively low (Figure 23.1): the average agricultural "phosphorus use efficiency," or PUE (the percentage of added P fertilizer that is removed in the annual harvest) is about 45% (Smil 2000). The rest of the added fertilizer remains in soils and may subsequently be made unavailable to plants due to chemical complexation, lost by erosion of soil particles, or leached out in solution. The accumulated P stores in soil forms a long-term P sink that is called "legacy P." Although legacy P is a potential source of P for future farming, it is also prone to be lost through runoff, percolation, and erosion. Particular soil management practices, such as conventional tillage,

Save the P(ee)!

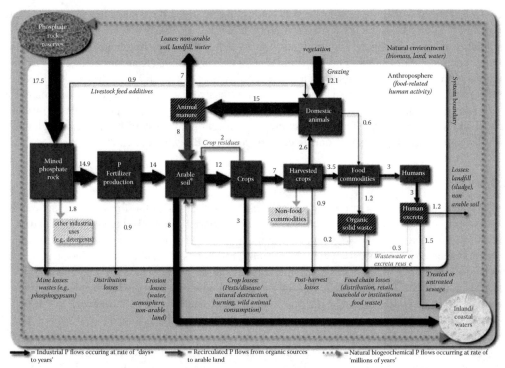

FIGURE 23.1 (See color insert.) Global flows of phosphorus (P) among major food system components. Flows are in units of million metric tons (MT) of P and arrows are approximately proportional to the size of the flux. Grey arrows represent recycling fluxes. The dotted arrow represents the natural geological cycle that operates over millions of years. (From Cordell, D et al., *Glob. Environ. Chang.*, 19, 292–305, 2009.)

in combination with factors like weather and landscape configuration, can elevate erosive P loss (Sharpley et al. 2000). Heavy rainfall after broadcast fertilization can lose considerable P through surface runoff (Tunney et al. 1997). A recent study (Fisher 2015) showed that substantial soil P can also be lost through subsurface flow due to preferential flow in soil macropores. Overall, the majority of P loss from farms is in particulate form. This P represents a "nonpoint" source, as it is coming from many diffuse sources. Large runoff volumes with relatively dilute P concentration from erosion and leaching of P from farmlands are notoriously costly and difficult to treat. It is estimated that nonpoint source inputs from agriculture contribute ~70% of the P entering the Gulf of Mexico (Alexander et al. 2008).

23.3.2 Manure Fluxes

There are numerable losses of phosphorus as it moves from our farming to food systems, including losses of P related to livestock production, food production, and human activities. Livestock production presents one of the greatest pressures on phosphorus cycling. Nearly a third of all arable land—and consequently fertilizer use associated with that land—is used just for producing animal feed (FAO 2006). Animal manure itself represents one of the largest of fluxes of P through any part of the global phosphorus cycle (Figure 23.1). The total flux of P in livestock manure actually exceeds P fertilizer use (Bouwman et al. 2009) (Figure 23.1). Fortunately, more than half of the P in manure is recycled back into the soils (Figure 23.1). Application of manure from dairy cows is often applied directly on the land, whereas that from poultry or pigs requires processing (Schoumans et al. 2015). However, substantial manure P is indeed "recycled" (returned to the land), although in recent times livestock manure is often used in lands adjacent to feedlots, lands that are already saturated with P. Therefore, the P is not used efficiently and is susceptible to soil erosion or other losses (Bateman et al. 2011; European Environment Agency 2012). P losses from fields can occur due to manure being applied to sloping, poorly drained, and/or frozen soils (Klausner et al. 1976) or due to extreme precipitation events that increase soil erosion rates (Carpenter et al. 2014). This loss can be substantial: for instance, in the United Kingdom, intensive livestock management can increase soil P losses up to 20% (Hooda et al. 2000). Unless practices change, phosphorus losses through livestock are likely to continue in the future; indeed, projections suggest a 54% increase in global P fluxes through livestock production during coming decades (Bouwman et al. 2013).

23.3.3 Food Waste

Food production represents the conversion of livestock and crops to the food items that we eat. Globally, about one-third of all food produced for human consumption is lost or wasted (Gustavsson et al. 2011). Production waste can occur at a number of points along the supply chain, including during shipment; at food processing plants; in restaurants, hotels, and other institutions; and within households—per capita waste tends to be much higher in developed versus developing countries (Gustavsson et al. 2011). As the waste in food production contains P, it can represent a substantial loss of P (Figure 23.1). In Sweden, P in organic waste represents nearly 40% of fertilizer P used to grow crops. Fortunately, much of this waste is recycled back into the system and only about 6% is lost (Neset et al. 2008). In the United States, P losses are similar; combined waste from food production and household processing represents ~7% of fertilizer P (Suh and Yee 2011). Animal bone matter, which is composed largely of phosphorus-containing mineral hydroxyapatite, represents a concentrated sink of P (hydroxyapatite, $Ca_5(PO_4)_3(OH)$, is 18.5% w/w P) that is often ashed and discarded in landfills. In the European Union, this sink may represent about ~12% of total fertilizer and feed P imports (Dawson and Hilton 2011).

23.3.4 Fluxes from Humans

Although much of the focus on P cycling is on agro-systems, urban systems, with their dense human populations and high demand for food imports and generation of wastes, are hotspots of P biogeochemistry (Chowdhury et al. 2013). In cities, P flows from humans, animals, and industry have increased by a factor of ~4.5 during the twentieth century (Morée et al. 2013). Urban areas can also be a substantial sink of P: ~30% and up to 80% of biodegradable waste is landfilled in developed and developing countries, respectively (UN-Habitat 2010). This sink of P is expected to increase due to increased waste generation with increased wealth in many areas (Kalmykova et al. 2012).

Household activities can be particularly important in cycling P in urban areas; in the Minneapolis-St. Paul region of Minnesota in the United States, approximately one-sixth of P exported is associated with household activities (Fissore et al. 2011). Households cycle P through consumption of human and pet foods and use of detergents, personal care products, paper, and wood materials (Fissore et al 2011; Kalmykova et al. 2012). Of these sources, human diets are the major importer of P into households (Fissore et al 2011; Kalmykova et al 2012). However, P consumption is often in excess, and nearly all of the P consumed is passed into the waste stream: 62% by urine; 35% by feces; and 3% by blood, sweat, and hair (Morée et al. 2013). This represents ~ 3 MMT P per year (Figure 23.1) (Smit et al. 2009,) or 1.5 g P per person per day (IWAR 2010). Phosphorus demand in a vegetarian diet is about half that of a meat-intensive diet (Cordell et al. 2009); indeed, estimates suggest that meat consumption accounts for over 70% of the global average P footprint (Metson et al. 2012). Based on expected changes in diet and human population growth, P demand by households is expected to increase by 68% to 141% by 2050 (Metson et al. 2012).

23.3.5 Aquatic Eutrophication, Toxic Algae, and Dead Zones

Phosphorus cycling is tied intimately to the health of aquatic ecosystems and, consequently, public health. When nutrients go into lakes, streams, and coastal regions due to the "leaky" parts of the phosphorus cycle described earlier (Cordell et al. 2009; Childers et al. 2011), they can cause eutrophication due to fertilization of excessive algal and cyanobacterial growth (Carpenter et al. 1998; Conley et al. 2009; Smith and Schindler 2009). A report from the late 1990s indicated nutrient-induced eutrophication accounted for 40% of the impaired lake area and 60% of the impaired river reaches in the United States, largely from impacts of nonpoint source inputs from agricultural systems (Carpenter et al. 1998). Often, these blooms contain noxious or toxic algal or cyanobacterial species; they can also lead to hypoxia and fish kills, shift food web dynamics, impair drinking water quality, and threaten livestock and human health (Johnson et al. 2010; Paerl et al. 2011). For instance, some cyanobacteria produce microcystin, a toxin to humans that can lead to liver damage when contaminated water or fish are consumed and can cause respiratory distress after prolonged time spent in or near contaminated surface waters (Funari and Testai 2008). This has considerable economic impact. In the United States, annual economic damages due to eutrophication of inland waters alone are estimated to be ~$2.8 billion (Dodds et al. 2009).

Although links between harmful cyanobacterial algal blooms and eutrophication are well recognized, connections between nutrient enrichment and the spread of human or wildlife diseases are also beginning to emerge (Johnson et al. 2010). For instance, in Belize, experimental results suggest phosphorus enrichment of wetlands promotes cattail growth, which provides habitat for *Anopheles vestitipennis* mosquito, an important vector of malaria-causing *Plasmodium* (Pope et al. 2005; Grieco et al. 2006; Rejmánková et al. 2006). Recent research also suggests eutrophication may influence the abundance, virulence, and survival of *Aspergillus* fungi, *Vibrio cholera*, and other pathogens (Bruno et al. 2003; Cottingham et al. 2003; Smith and Schindler 2009). Thus, the health impacts of P-induced eutrophication extend beyond the well-known direct impacts via impaired water quality.

23.4 SOLUTIONS

23.4.1 Reduce Demand

Societal demand for phosphorus is inevitable—it is a necessary component of all living things and, therefore, tied intimately to any agro-livestock system. However, P demand does not need to be as great as it currently is. Solutions toward a sustainable P system will include both demand-side and supply-side improvements, although as Figure 23.2 demonstrates, reducing our demand may be the most critical component. As hinted at in the previous sections, there are numerous ways in which P demand can be reduced.

The projection that we'll need to double food availability by 2050 is based on a continuation of current trends, including increasing affluence (with its implications for dietary choices) and larger populations. To avoid this enormous demand for P to produce our food, we can change behaviors that affect per capita P demand, limit population growth, or a combination of the two. Choices related to food consumption can play an especially significant role in reducing demand. Estimates based on food consumption suggest that the global demand for animal-based food products (e.g., meat, dairy, eggs) accounts for over 70% of the global average P footprint (Metson et al. 2012). Of the different types of animal-based foods, beef is the most P intense (Metson et al. 2012). Phosphorus is still necessary to grow plants for a plant-based diet; however, P needed to sustain a plant-based diet is roughly half of that needed for a meat-based diet (Cordell et al. 2009). Thus, shifting diets represent a significant contribution to scenarios for achieving long-term P sustainability (Figure 23.2). Switching to a vegetable-based diet has also been recognized as an effective way to reduce energy and water consumption (McMichael et al. 2007; Hanjra and Qureshi 2010); clearly, the benefits extend to phosphorus sustainability as well (and to human health).

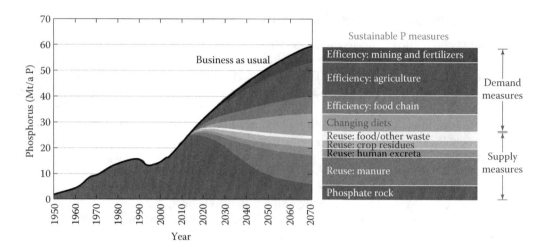

FIGURE 23.2 (See color insert.) A scenario from Cordell and White (2014) for achieving long-term P sustainability in which the food system no longer relies on use of "fossil P" (phosphate rock) for fertilizer production. Note that the "business-as-usual" scenario would result in more than a doubling of global P use by ~2100, with enormous implications for water quality and access to P fertilizers. In this scenario, achieving P sustainability requires a combination of demand-side (diet shifts, food chain efficiency, improved farm practices) and supply-side (implementation of large-scale P recycling from organic waste streams) measures.

Discussions about limiting population often conjure images of China's one-child policy or other oppressive measures that reduce individual freedoms and create the perception that people are the problem. There are, however, significant data that support the view that improved quality of life, especially among poor women in developing countries, leads to a lower fertility rate by choice (UN 2014). Improving access to education, alleviating poverty, empowering women to have a choice in when, or if they will have children, and decreasing the infant mortality rate all lead to smaller family sizes that could keep our global population below the upper forecasts of 10 to 11 billion people for 2050. Indeed, many developed countries actually have a negative fertility rate when immigration is excluded, indicating that improving the quality of life for the developing world could dramatically decrease population size below current projections.

23.4.2 Continue to Improve Crop Varieties and Genetics

Humans started plant domestication around 10,000 to 13,000 years ago (Purugganan and Gibson 2003). For example, humans domesticated bread wheat, which is a hexaploid, by hybridizing a tetraploid wheat and a diploid goatgrass. Transgenic technologies accelerate gains from crop breeding and allow more specific enhancement of desired phenotypes, such as those that enhance P acquisition. When plants are P deficient, they develop specific physical traits to acquire soil P. These traits include large root systems and altered root architecture, such as root morphology, topology, and distribution patterns; increases in root/shoot ratio, root branching, root elongation, and root hairs; and formation of specialized roots (Shen et al. 2011). These phenotypes regulated by specific genes, such as phosphate transporter genes, are potential candidates for genetic engineering. Since the 1990s, more than half-dozen phosphate transporter genes have been identified and isolated in plants and fungi. For example, the AVP1 gene in *Arabidopsis* was overexpressed in rice, tomato, and lettuce. Field trials show that these AVP1-enhanced crops have significantly improved root growth and PUE (Gaxiola et al. 2011). Such genetic engineering approaches for improving nutrient use efficiency are now in their infancy. However, although they offer considerable promise in enhancing food system sustainability, they must overcome societal objections to widespread deployment of genetically modified crops.

23.4.3 Continue to Improve Fertilizer Practices

Best management practices (BMPs) for fertilizer use include choosing high-PUE cultivars, using appropriate crop rotation, and improving water and soil management. Nevertheless, little is more important than using fertilizers appropriately in an integrated approach developed by the International Plant Nutrition Institute (IPNI) called the "4Rs" (Bruulsema et al. 2009). IPNI's 4Rs involve the following: giving the crop the right source of fertilizer, applying it at the right rate, at the right time, and in the right place. The right source of fertilizer targets that the specific nutrient needs for specific crops and provides P (and N) in the chemical forms most suitable for that particular crop in that particular soil (Mikkelsen et al. 2009). The right rate reduces the use of excess fertilizer so that less is wasted and enters the environment. Usually determining the right rate requires setting up a specific yield goal and using regular soil tests (Mikkelsen 2011). Fertilization at the right time involves knowing the nutrient availability of the soil and the crop physiological demand for nutrients during the germination and growing season. For example, germination and reproduction of crops both acquire large amount of P. Adding P before germination and a couple weeks before flower formation is critical for crop health and fruit quality but P fertilizer applied too late for these events goes wasted. Applying nutrients in the right place is also important, as plants do not move. Too much nutrient placed too close to plant roots may burn the roots. Fertilizer placed too far from the rooting zone cannot be accessed. Precision placement of fertilizers not only enhances root growth, it also reduces fertilizer lost through runoff or leaching. Appropriately integrating 4R nutrient stewardship on the farm will increase productivity and profit, as well as help reduce fertilizer demand and maintain environmental health. Together, changes in fertilizer practices, along with improved crops, represent an important component in scenarios for long-term P sustainability (Figure 23.2).

23.4.4 Reduce P Needed for Animal Production

Livestock and poultry are relatively inefficient in converting food intake to growth and especially in retaining P from their feed. One reason for this is that the P in animal feed grain is often in an unavailable form, as a molecule called "phytate" (or phytic acid), which poultry and nonruminant animals cannot access. Thus, the P footprint of livestock production can be reduced by lowering the recommended daily P requirement for farm animals by addition of phytase (an enzyme that liberates P from phytate) and/or by use of low-phytate corn in the animal's' diet; this may reduce up to half of annual P accumulation rates in livestock production (Perry et al. 1999; Tarkalson and Mikkelsen 2003).

23.4.5 Reduce Food Waste

As previously mentioned, approximately one-third of food produced globally is wasted. Completely eliminating this waste would thereby, all else being equal, reduce P demand by one-third! Although achieving 0% waste is highly impractical, there are a few specific areas to target. Figure 23.1 shows postharvest losses and food chain losses totaling 2.1 MT related to food waste. It's easy to blame food processors, restaurants, and grocery stores where the waste visibly accumulates; however, the average American throws away ~25% of the food she or he brings home (Buzby et al. 2014). This is important information when considering which intervention points are the most important, or logistically feasible, to address.

In developing countries, inadequate transportation and storage options can quickly lead to food spoilage, but improved access to refrigeration and local markets could eliminate much of this waste. For example, in Nogales, Mexico, where much of the produce from Mexico enters the United States, over 100 tons of produce per day is discarded because truck loads sit at the border for days waiting to be sold, only to have the produce spoil. Whereas this was previously dumped into the desert, new regulations require it be disposed of in approved landfills or other settings. Because landfill disposal

336   Dietary Phosphorus: Health, Nutrition, and Regulatory Aspects

is costly, several companies are pursuing composting or other alternatives that have potential for P recovery. In developed countries much of the waste occurs between the farm and grocery store, not because of rotting, but for aesthetic reasons. Misshapen, odd sized, or otherwise "ugly" fruits and vegetables never make it to the grocer's shelves. In France one grocery store chain is tackling this waste stream specifically by marketing the "ugly" produce at discounted prices and using them in juices, soups, and other prepared meals. Not only does this reduce waste, it has improved profits for both farmers and the stores.

According to the NRDC, another significant cause of food waste in the United States is the expiration date placed on food (Leib 2013). Although some foods can certainly spoil if stored too long, the sell by, best by, and born on dates often don't have a scientific basis or even a legal requirement. Items even approaching these dates are often discarded in favor of something fresher. Discount grocery store chains have appeared which cheaply buy expired or nearly expired packaged foods from retailers, then pass the savings on to their customers. When faced with large quantities of unsold food restaurants, grocers, and distribution companies can benefit from tax incentives through donations. Many cite concerns about legal liability if someone would become sick as one reason not to pursue this route, but the Bill Emerson Good Samaritan Food Donation Act, signed into law in 1996 eliminated that risk. Like other "Good Samaritan" laws, it protects businesses that are in good faith trying to do the right thing. Improved awareness about this law, coupled with a strong network of local food pantries and other nonprofit institutions, could prevent much of the institutional waste in the developed world.

Reducing food waste in homes will require a variety of cultural shifts from changing the way we buy food to how we cook. In addition to reducing the environmental impacts of food production by improving "food chain efficiency" (Figure 23.2), eliminating this waste will save consumers money! Awareness is growing as documentaries, news reports, and even satirical news outlets (e.g., *Last Week, Tonight* with John Oliver) shine a light on this problem that wastes both food and money. Much attention is given to feeding the future global population, but many of the waste reduction goals will also help feed Earth's current population, of whom ~1 billion are malnourished.

23.4.6 RECYCLE P FROM RICH ORGANIC STREAMS

All organic waste contains P that can be recovered, but rates of recycling of P within the food system are relatively low. Figure 23.1 estimates that 15 MT of P is available for recycling from animal manures alone, but only about 8 MT of P from manure is actually recycled. Human excreta, as well as food and yard waste, are all largely untapped sources of P. Manures, both human and animal, are already rich enough to use as fertilizer and indeed have been used throughout human history, returned to the farm soil in a closed cycle. However, with the rise of concentrated animal feeding operations (CAFOs) the supply of manure is no longer in the same location as the demand for the manure. Having a large supply of manure where it's not needed often results in overapplication and runoff into local water bodies. To address this imbalance, technologies (such as anaerobic bioreactors) are emerging that couple bioenergy production from manure with capture of manure P (and N) in concentrated forms that can be purified and economically shipped back to production areas (Rittmann et al. 2011). However, deployment of these approaches remains far from the scale needed to address the manure imbalances that now exist.

Organic waste created in cities often ends up in landfills but if diverted to composting, or other similar programs, a substantial amount of P could be recovered. Based on analyses of Metson et al. (2012), diverting food waste, wood chips, leaves, grass clippings, and other yard debris from landfills could lead to the recovery of 2.56 Gg P/year in the Phoenix metropolitan area annually. Recovery of P from cardboard and paper bound for the landfill would contribute another 1.13 Gg P/year (Metson et al. 2012). One study of the Twin Cities region suggested that the P recovered from its own organic waste could grow up to 50% of the required food for the existing population (Baker 2011). According to Figure 23.1, using the P inherent in all the major organic waste streams would reduce demand for mined P by ~15%. Coupled with the demand-side reductions listed earlier, organic waste streams could provide an even larger percentage of P needs (Figure 23.2), especially in areas currently underutilizing P fertilizers.

23.4.7 REDUCE RELIANCE ON CROP-BASED BIOFUELS

In an effort to improve national energy security and decrease greenhouse gas emissions, both the United States and EU have created targets for biofuel production and use. Unfortunately this directive has created a "food vs. fuel" competition for arable land, driven up prices of staple foods such as corn and soy, and increased demand for P fertilizers. For example, in 2009, 32% of all corn grown in the United States was for ethanol production and represented ~10% of all P fertilizer used in the United States that year (Jewett et al. 2010). Although biofuels will be an important step toward reducing dependence on fossil fuels and reducing emissions of carbon dioxide, they must be produced in a way that does not compete with the food system for land or nutrients. Research continues on algae- and bacteria-based biofuels that promise higher productivity in nonagricultural land, that could use nutrients from wastewater treatment plant effluent, and that can more easily recycle nutrients internally in the production system.

23.5 CONCLUSIONS

Phosphorus is "the stuff of life." As such, it plays a crucial role in the nutrition of all living things from humans to livestock to crops to bacteria. Because of this key role, enormous quantities of "fossil" P have been mobilized to produce the fertilizer needed for the Green Revolution. However, that mobilization has led to a number of unintended consequences, especially the undesirable proliferation of algae in inland and coastal waters, with their associated toxins, fish kills, and "dead zones." The massive mobilization of P has also placed increasing pressure on the P supply system itself, leading to higher and increasingly erratic prices for phosphate rock and P fertilizers. These dynamics are increasingly being recognized as a key sustainability challenge at the nexus of food, water, and energy (Jarvie et al. 2015). Addressing this sustainability challenge will require a variety of measures, including improvements in crops and in farming practices, protection of soil health, reduction in soil erosion, shifts in dietary patterns, dampened population growth, and development and widespread deployment of recycling pathways to recover P from various "waste" streams (crop, food, livestock, and human).

REFERENCES

Alexander, R., R. Smith, G. Schwarz, E. Boyer, J. Nolan, and J. Brakebill. 2008. Differences in phosphorus and nitrogen delivery to the Gulf of Mexico from the Mississippi River Basin. *Environ. Sci. Technol.* 42: 822–830.

Alexandratos, N., J. Bruinsma, and FAO. 2012. World Agriculture Towards 2030/2050: The 2012 Revision. *FAO.*

Ashley, K., D. Cordell, and D. Mavinic. 2011. A brief history of phosphorus: From the philosopher's stone to nutrient recovery and reuse. *Chemosphere* 84: 737–746.

Asimov, I. 1974. Asimov on Chemistry. New York City, New York: Doubleday.

Baker, L. 2011. Can urban P conservation help to prevent the brown devolution? *Chemosphere* 84: 779–784.

Bateman, A., D. van der Horst, D. Boardman, A. Kansal, and C. Carliell-Marquet. 2011. Closing the phosphorus loop in England: The spatio-temporal balance of phosphorus capture from manure versus crop demand for fertiliser. *Resour. Conserv. Recycl.* 55: 1146–1153.

Bouwman, A., A. Beusen, and G. Billen. 2009. Human alteration of the global nitrogen and phosphorus soil balances for the period 1970-2050. Global Biogeochem. *Cycles 23: n/a–n/a.*

Bouwman, L., K. Goldewijk, K. Van Der Hoek, A. Beusen, D. Van Vuuren, J. Willems, M. Rufino, and E. Stehfest. 2013. Exploring global changes in nitrogen and phosphorus cycles in agriculture induced by livestock production over the 1900-2050 period. *Proc. Natl. Acad. Sci.* 110, doi:10.1073/pnas.1206191109

Brady, N., and R. Weil. 2012. *The Nature and Properties of Soils*, 14th ed. India: Pearson Education.

Bruno, J., L. Petes, C. Harvell, and A. Hettinger. 2003. Nutrient enrichment can increase the severity of coral diseases. *Ecol. Lett.* 6: 1056–1061.

Bruulsema, T., J. Lemunyon, and B. Herz. 2009. Know your fertilizer rights. Crop. *Soils 13–18.*

Buzby, J. C., H. F. Wells, and J. Hyman. 2014. The estimated amount, value, and calories of postharvest food losses at the retail and consumer levels in the United States. *Econ. Inf. Bull.* 39.

Carpenter, S., E. Booth, C. Kucharik, and R. Lathrop. 2014. Extreme daily loads: Role in annual phosphorus input to a north temperate lake. *Aquat. Sci.* 77: 71–79.

Carpenter, S., N. Caraco, D. Correll, R. Howarth, A. Sharpley, and V. Smith. 1998. Nonpoint pollution of surface waters with phosphorus and nitrogen. *Ecol. Appl.* 8: 559–568.

Childers, D. L., J. Corman, M. Edwards, and J. J. Elser. 2011. Sustainability challenges of phosphorus and food: Solutions from closing the human phosphorus cycle. *Bioscience* 61: 117–124.

Chowdhury, R. B., G. A. Moore, A. J. Weatherley, M. Arora, C. Fissore, L. A. Baker, S. E. Hobbie, J. Y. King, J. P. McFadden, K. C. Nelson, I. Jakobsdottir, Y. Kalmykova, R. Harder, H. Borgestedt, I. Svanäng, a. L. Morée, a. H. W. Beusen, a. F. Bouwman, W. J. Willems, and J. V. D. M. H. G. Smit, A L, Bindraban, P S, Shroeder, J J, Conijin. 2013. A review of recent substance flow analyses of phosphorus to identify priority management areas at different geographical scales. *Ecol. Appl.* 5: 213–228.

Conley, D., H. Paerl, R. Howarth, D. Boesch, S. Seitzinger, K. Havens, C. Lancelot, and G. Likens. 2009. Controlling eutrophication: Nitrogen and phosphorus. *Science* 323: 1014–1015.

Cordell, D., J.-O. Drangert, and S. White. 2009. The story of phosphorus: Global food security and food for thought. *Glob. Environ. Chang.* 19: 292–305.

Cordell, D., and S. White. 2014. Life's bottleneck: Sustaining the world's phosphorus for a food secure future. *Annu. Rev. Environ. Resour.* 39: 161–188.

Cottingham, K. L., D. A. Chiavelli, and R. K. Taylor. 2003. Environmental microbe and human pathogen: The ecology and microbiology of Vibrio cholerae. *Front. Ecol. Environ.* 1: 80–86.

Dawson, C., and J. Hilton. 2011. Fertiliser availability in a resource-limited world: Production and recycling of nitrogen and phosphorus. *Food Policy* 36: S14–S22.

Dodds, W., W. Bouska, J. Eitzmann, T. Pilger, K. Pitts, A. Riley, J. Schloesser, and D. Thornbrugh. 2009. Eutrophication of U. S. freshwaters: Analysis of potential economic damages. *Environ. Sci. Technol.* 43: 12–19.

Edixhoven, J. D., J. Gupta, and H. H. G. Savenije. 2014. Recent revisions of phosphate rock reserves and resources: A critique. Earth Syst. *Dyn.* 5: 491–507.

Elser, J. J., T. J. Elser, S. R. Carpenter, and W. A. Brock. 2014. Regime shift in fertilizer commodities indicates more turbulence ahead for food security. *PLOS ONE* 9: e93998.

European Environment Agency. 2012. *European waters—Current status and future challenges: Synthesis.*

FAO. 2006. *Livestock's long shadow—Environmental issues and options.*

Fisher, M. 2015. Subsoil Phosphorus Loss: A complex problem with no easy solutions. *CSA News* 60: 4.

Fissore, C., L. A. Baker, S. E. Hobbie, J. Y. King, J. P. McFadden, K. C. Nelson, I. Jakobsdottir, Y. Kalmykova, R. Harder, H. Borgestedt, I. Svanäng, A. L. Morée, A. H. W. Beusen, A. F. Bouwman, and W. J. Willems. 2011. Carbon, nitrogen, and phosphorus fluxes in household ecosystems in the Minneapolis-Saint Paul, Minnesota, urban region. *Ecol. Appl.* 27: 619–639.

Funari, E., and E. Testai. 2008. Human health risk assessment related to cyanotoxins exposure. *Crit. Rev. Toxicol.* 38: 97–125.

Gaxiola, R., M. Edwards, and J. J. Elser. 2011. A transgenic approach to enhance phosphorus use effi-ciency in crops as part of a comprehensive strategy for sustainable agriculture. *Chemosphere* 84: 840–845.

Grieco, J., S. Johnson, N. Achee, P. Masuoka, K. Pope, E. Rejmánková, E. Vanzie, R. Andre, and D. Roberts. 2006. Distribution of Anopheles albimanus, Anopheles vestitipennis, and Anopheles crucians associated with land use in northern Belize. *J. Med. Entomol.* 43: 614–622.

Gustavsson, J., C. Cederberg, and U. Sonesson. 2011. *Global food losses and food waste, Food and Agriculture Organization of the United Nations.*

Hanjra, M., and M. Qureshi. 2010. Global water crisis and future food security in an era of climate change. *Food Policy* 35: 365–377.

Hooda, P., A. Edwards, H. Anderson, and A. Miller. 2000. A review of water quality concerns in livestock farming areas. *Sci. Total Environ.* 250: 143–167.

IWAR. 2010. *Phosphate recovery—Introduction to phosphate recycling.*

Jarvie, H. P., A. N. Sharpley, D. Flaten, P. J. A. Kleinman, A. Jenkins, and T. Simmons. 2015. The Pivotal Role of Phosphorus in a Resilient Water–Energy–Food Security Nexus. *J. Environ. Qual.* doi:10.2134/jeq2015.01.0030.

Jewett, E. B., D. M. Kidwell, C. B. Lopez, S. B. Bricker, M. K. Burke, M. R. Walbridge, P. M. Eldridge, R. M. Greene, J. D. Hagy, H. T. Buxton, and R. J. Diaz. 2010. Scientific Assessment of Hypoxia in U.S. Coastal Waters. Ann Arbor, MI: National Oceanic and Atmospheric Administration.

Johnson, P. T. J., A. R. Townsend, C. C. Cleveland, P. M. Glibert, R. W. Howarth, V. J. Mckenzie, E. Rejmankova, and M. H. Ward. 2010. Linking environmental nutrient enrichment and disease emergence in humans and wildlife. *Ecol. Appl.* 20: 16–29.

Kalmykova, Y., R. Harder, H. Borgestedt, and I. Svanäng. 2012. Pathways and management of phosphorus in urban areas. *J. Ind. Ecol.* 16: 928–939.

Van Kauwenbergh, S. J. 2010. World Phosphate Rock Reserves and Resources. *International Fertilizer Development Center.*

Klausner, S. D., P. J. Zwerman, and E. D.F. 1976. Nitrogen and phosphorus losses from winter disposal of dairy manure. *J. Environ. Qual.* 5: 47–49.

Leib, E. 2013. The Dating Game: How Confusing Food Date Labels. *Nat. Resour. Def. Counc. Rep.* R:13-09-A

Marschner, P. 2012. *Mineral Nutrition of Higher Plants*, Amsterdam, The Netherlands: Elsevier.

McMichael, A., J. Powles, C. Butler, and R. Uauy. 2007. Food, livestock production, energy, climate change, and health. *Lancet* 370: 1253–1263.

Metson, G. S., E. M. Bennett, and J. J. Elser. 2012. The role of diet in phosphorus demand. Environ. Res. Lett. *7: 044043.*

Mikkelsen, R. 2011. The "4R" nutrient stewardship framework for horticulture. *Horttechnology* 21: 658–662.

Mikkelsen, R., G. Schwab, and G. Randall. 2009. The four fertilizer rights: Selecting the right source. *Crop. Soils* 42: 28–32.

Morée, a. L., a. H. W. Beusen, a. F. Bouwman, and W. J. Willems. 2013. Exploring global nitrogen and phosphorus flows in urban wastes during the twentieth century. Global Biogeochem. *Cycles* 27: 836–846.

Neset, T., H. Bader, R. Scheidegger, and U. Lohm. 2008. The flow of phosphorus in food production and consumption—Link??ping, Sweden, 1870-2000. *Sci. Total Environ.* 396: 111–120.

Paerl, H., N. Hall, and E. Calandrino. 2011. Controlling harmful cyanobacterial blooms in a world experiencing anthropogenic and climatic-induced change. *Sci. Total Environ.* 409: 1739–1745.

Perry, T., A. Cullison, and R. Lowrey. 1999. *Feeds and Feeding*. Amsterdam, The Netherlands: Simon and Schuster

Pope, K., P. Masuoka, E. Rejmankova, J. Grieco, and S. Johnson. 2005. Mosquito habitats, land use, and malaria risk in Belize from Satellite Imagery. *Ecol. Appl.* 15: 1223–1232.

Purugganan, M., and G. Gibson. 2003. Merging ecology, molecular evolution, and functional genetics. *Mol. Ecol.* 12: 1109–1112.

Rejmánková, E., J. Grieco, N. Achee, P. Masuoka, K. Pope, D. Roberts, and R. Higashi. 2006. Freshwater community interactions and malaria, In S. Collinge and C. Ray [eds.], *Disease Ecology: Community Structure and Pathogen Dynamics*. Oxford University Press.

Rittmann, B. E., B. Mayer, P. Westerhoff, and M. Edwards. 2011. Capturing the lost phosphorus. *Chemosphere* 84: 846–853.

Schoumans, O., F. Bouraoui, C. Kabbe, O. Oenema, and K. van Dijk. 2015. Phosphorus management in Europe in a changing world. *Ambio* 44: 180–192.

Sharpley, A., B. Foy, and P. Withers. 2000. Practical and innovative measures for the control of agricultural phosphorus losses to water: An overview. *J. Environ. Qual.* 29: 1.

Shen, J., L. Yuan, J. Zhang, H. Li, Z. Bai, X. Chen, W. Zhang, and F. Zhang. 2011. Phosphorus dynamics: From soil to plant. *Plant Physiol.* 156: 997–1005.

Smil, V. 2000. Phosphorus in the environment: Natural flows and human interferences. *Ann. Rev. Energy Environ.* 25: 53–88.

Smit, A.L., P.S. Bindraban, J.J. Schröder, J.G. Conijn, and H.G. Van der Meer. 2009. *Phosphorus in agriculture: Global resources, trends and developments*. Report to the Steering Committee Technology Assessment of the Ministry of Agriculture, Nature and Food Quality, The Netherlands, and in collaboration with the Nutrient Flow Task Group (NFTG), supported by DPRN (Development Policy review Network) (No. 282). Plant Research International.

Smith, V., and D. Schindler. 2009. Eutrophication science: Where do we go from here? Trends Ecol. *Evol.* 24: 201–207.

Sterner, R. W., and J. J. Elser. 2002. *Ecological Stoichiometry: The Biology of Elements from Molecules to the Biosphere*. Princeton, NJ: Princeton University Press.

Stewart, W., D. Dibb, A. Johnston, and T. Smyth. 2005. The contribution of commercial fertilizer nutrients to food production. *Agron. J.* 97: 1–6.

Suh, S., and S. Yee. 2011. Phosphorus use-efficiency of agriculture and food system in the US. *Chemosphere* 84: 806–813.

Tarkalson, D., and R. Mikkelsen. 2003. A phosphorus budget of a poultry farm and a dairy farm in the southeastern U.S., and the potential impacts of diet alterations. *Nutr. Cycl. Agroecosystems* 66: 295–303.

Tunney, H., O. Carton, P. Brookes, and A. Johnston, eds. 1997. *Phosphorus Loss from Soil to Water*, UK: CAB INTERNATIONAL.

UN. 2014. *World Fertility Report 2013: Fertility at the Extremes*.

UN-Habitat. 2010. Solid waste management in the world's cities: Water and sanitation in the world's cities, U.N.H.S. Programme [ed.]. *Earthscan*.

24 The Effects of Changing Global Food Choices on Human Health and a Sustainable Supply of Phosphorus

Charles J. Ferro

CONTENTS

Abstract 341
Bullet Points 342
24.1 Phosphorus: An Element Key to Life on Our Planet 342
24.2 Phosphate in Evolution 342
24.3 The Phosphate Cycle 343
24.4 The Increasing Need For Chemical Fertilizers 343
24.5 Humans and Meat-Eating 344
24.6 Phosphate Additives 344
24.7 Phosphate Rock 345
24.8 Ways to Preserve Phosphate 347
24.9 What Next? 349
References 349

ABSTRACT

Phosphorus is one of the essential elements for life. On Earth it appears predominantly as phosphates at very low concentration. In evolutionary terms, this comparative scarcity may have given an evolutionary advantage to creatures able to efficiently conserve phosphate. In excess, phosphate has the potential to become a cause for disease, exemplified in the emerging evidence implicating it as a potential cardiovascular risk factor. There have been increasing concerns regarding this potential health problem caused by the increasing phosphate in human diets. Meat and dairy products, as well as the increasing use phosphate food additives, are the main sources of bioavailable phosphate in the diet. Public health campaigners are currently pushing for more information to be made available on the phosphate content of food, as well as regulation to reduce the amounts of phosphate containing food additives currently being used. The Paleoproterzoic era was characterized by an increase in the bioavailability of phosphate. This may have accelerated the oxygenation of the Earth's atmosphere and kickstarted the evolution and diversity of multicellular life forms. Currently the world has become dependent on mined phosphate rock for food production. This is a limited resource that is controlled by only a few countries. It is used poorly and often wasted, with phosphate fertilizers washing into water bodies causing eutrophication and algal blooms. Paradoxically, this is reducing the biodiversity of life on Earth through the extinction of hundreds of species. The unrestrained management of phosphate rock and our unrelenting dependency on it may lead to the

342   Dietary Phosphorus: Health, Nutrition, and Regulatory Aspects

paradoxical position in which phosphate rock becomes a resource to be fought over, whereas contemporaneously both health and environmental experts are advocating decreases in its current uses.

BULLET POINTS

- Phosphorus as an essential and relatively scarce element has been a key driver in the evolutionary process.
- The increasing world population and the rise of city dwelling has led to a loss in our ability to recirculate phosphate and placed an increasing reliance on mined phosphate rock for use in fertilizers.
- The increasing ingestion of phosphate from food, especially meat and dairy products, as well as the increasing use of phosphate in food additives and in agricultural production, is having a significant impact on the environment as well as human health.
- Phosphate rock is not a limitless resource, with the known high-quality, easily accessible reserves being controlled by only a handful of countries.
- Measures to reduce our dependence on phosphate rock are urgently needed for global food security and environmental sustainability.

24.1 PHOSPHORUS: AN ELEMENT KEY TO LIFE ON OUR PLANET

The formation of elemental phosphate from oxygen requires temperatures in excess of 1000 megakelvins (1,000,000,000 K) as well as tremendous quantities of energy. These intense settings are found only in large stars at least three times bigger than our Sun (Macia, 2005). In terms of abundance, phosphorus is only the 18th and 11th commonest element in the universe and on Earth, respectively. Of all the essential elements for life, phosphorus is the scarcest. This suggests that the quantity of phosphorus on Earth was not the key factor in defining its critical role in living organisms. The essential elements for life provide a minimal set of "building blocks" representing the valence states: hydrogen 1, oxygen and sulfur 2, nitrogen 3, carbon 4, and phosphorus 5 (Macia, 2005). This valence, as well as the reactive nature of phosphorus, is the key property that makes this element so central to life on Earth.

Phosphorus as an element is extremely reactive and not present as a free element naturally on Earth. Instead, phosphorus is mainly found as phosphates, based on the PO_4 group (Horiguchi and Kandatsu, 1959; Metcalf et al., 2009). Phosphates can form complex, tridimensional networks, including rings, cagelike structures, and planar arrangements, critical to its multiple biological roles. Phosphoric acid is an essential constituent of nucleic acids as it can simultaneously link two nucleotides and still doubly ionize (Westheimer, 1987). Different acids, including silicic, sulfuric, and arsenic acids, hydrolyze too quickly to be appropriate alternatives (Westheimer, 1987). In addition, phosphate has central roles in bone metabolism, glycolysis, regulation of biological processes including receptors and enzymes, as an acid–base buffer, and in the storage and release of energy. Phospholipids form membranes in all cells (Macia, 2005). Phosphate-containing cyclic nucleotides are indispensable components for hormones, nerve transmission, as well as immunity and inflammation. In living organisms, well over 2000 chemical reactions require phosphate (Razzaque, 2011).

24.2 PHOSPHATE IN EVOLUTION

The evolution of ecosystems in geological timescales is tightly linked to geological changes. At the start of life on Earth, phosphate was only found in rocks at low concentrations and anaerobic organisms were predominant (Falkowski et al., 2008; Papineau, 2010; Planavsky et al., 2010). At the start of the Proterozoic period (approximately 2.5 billion years ago) oxygen levels in the atmosphere increased from trace amounts to about 2% by volume—the Great Oxidation Event (Bekker et al., 2004). Organisms attained mitochondria and evolved the ability for effective oxidative metabolism. At the end of the Proterozoic period (approximately 0.5 billion years ago) oxygen levels rose again,

The Effects of Changing Global Food Choices on Human Health   **343**

this time to near present-day concentrations marking the appearance of multicellular organisms and a dramatic increase of organism diversity, often called the Cambrian Explosion (Papineau, 2010; Papineau, 2013). These phases of atmospheric change coincided with continental rifting and the exposure of widespread glacial deposits, which would have caused phosphate to flow into bodies of water (Papineau, 2010; Papineau, 2013). The effect on marine life might have been comparable to the flow of human and agricultural waste into bodies of water today, causing eutrophication and massive algal blooms (Geider et al., 2001; Bekker et al., 2004).

The relative rarity of phosphate would have provided an evolutionary advantage to organisms with efficient mechanisms to preserve it. Thus, in a manner perhaps analogous to salt, humans are better at facing situations of phosphate scarcity rather than disproportionate loads (Fouque, 2013). In today's developed and developing worlds, where dietary phosphate is available in excess, it may well have become a cause for disease. This is perhaps best exemplified by the increasing evidence linking excessive phosphate exposure to cardiovascular disease (Ferro et al., 2009). Whether our increasing exposure to phosphate is indeed harmful to health will be discussed by experts in other chapters in this book and will not be considered further here.

24.3 THE PHOSPHATE CYCLE

The phosphate cycle is unique among the essential elements as it takes millions of years and does not have a gaseous phase. Most soils and rocks contain phosphates but it is usually at very low concentrations (0.1%). Phosphate rock is rare and is accessible in very limited locations. It took millions of years to form from the remains of marine life buried on the sea floor. These remains mineralized and eventually came to the Earth's surface by tectonic uplift (Ashley et al., 2011). Rock erosion gradually and slowly returns phosphate to the soil. Plants extract phosphate from the soil and it then passes up again through the food chain (Ashley et al., 2011)

Initially, as humans moved from a nomadic existence to more permanent settlements and agriculture, crop production relied on soil phosphate supplemented by organic matter. This depended on the landscape, climate, and culture (Cordell et al., 2009) and included controlled burning and the use of manure. People lived close to where food was produced, and it was easy to use their excreta as fertilizer (Ashley et al., 2011). However, the Industrial Revolution in the late eighteenth century triggered the progressive worldwide migration of workers to cities. The health problems associated with this mass concentration of people and their waste led to the establishment of the principles of public health and sanitation leading to sewage systems and clean water supplies. The "Sanitation Revolution" led to the transition from land-based to water-based disposal of human waste and profoundly changed the developed world from a phosphate recycling society to a phosphate throughput society. However, in the developing world, rapid urbanization is still creating massive demands for the most basic of infrastructure in cities (Chinyama and Toma, 2013). Conventional urban water management systems struggle to deliver water and dispose of waste without adversely affecting the quality of life of the population and downstream environments (Chinyama and Toma, 2013).

24.4 THE INCREASING NEED FOR CHEMICAL FERTILIZERS

In 1840, Justus von Liebeg discovered that minerals (phosphate, nitrogen, and potassium) mediated the fertilizing actions of manure (Sherman, 1933; Rosenfeld, 2003). Food shortages and famines in Europe in the seventeenth and eighteenth centuries had precipitated the importation of organic fertilizers, such as crushed bones and guano. In addition, mined phosphate rock was being increasingly used and considered an unlimited resource. Its use in fertilizers grew rapidly, especially after World War II—the "Green Revolution." However, as already discussed, these rocks are not limitless and are essentially a biological resource that has taken 10 to 15 million years to form (Ashley et al., 2011). Indeed phosphate rock is very much a finite, nonrenewable commodity. Today, the world is heavily reliant on mined phosphate rock to maintain the current intensity of food production, especially the farming of meat (Ashley et al., 2011).

24.5 HUMANS AND MEAT-EATING

Human evolution and meat eating are intricately associated. Hunting and increasing carnivorousness are key developments that have made us human with bigger brains and smaller digestive tracts—the expensive tissue hypothesis. The killing and sharing of meat, especially large animals, led to the development of bipedalism, language, the ability to plan ahead, cooperation, and inevitably socialization and intelligence. The human gut has clearly evolved for an omnivore diet, with a preference for meat consumption. Through history, most of the population has had very limited access to meat. Indeed, their rulers and elite would see meat eating as a way of consolidating and demonstrating their power. Increased consumption of meat has been a significant feature of modern history starting in North America and Europe during the Industrial Revolution in the second half of the twentieth century. With spreading affluence this transition was repeated across Latin America and Asia in the second half of the twentieth century (Vaclav, 2002).

World meat consumption more than doubled from 1950 to 1975 and doubled again in the subsequent 25 years. By 2010, global meat production was nearly six times as high as in 1950 (Vaclav, 2002) leading to the rise of the mass-scale animal feed industry that relies mainly on grain and legumes to produce a variety of balanced foodstuffs. Unfortunately, it has also all too often led to widespread adoption of practices that increase productivity, but at the expense of animal welfare. Although overall the cost of meat has fallen in economic terms, environmentally it remains a high-cost product. Large animals especially, are very inefficient when it comes to converting feed into muscle and therefore require large amounts of cropland, water, and fertilizers (Vaclav, 2002). The phosphate cost of meat production is high and inefficient with significant losses during feed production and loss in animal excrement (Metson et al., 2012).

The average per capita phosphate consumption rose by 38% from 1961 to 2007 (Figure 24.1). There is, however, very large variation between countries with some countries such as Canada decreasing their phosphate footprint, whereas developing countries such as China increased its footprint by 400%, largely driven by an increased meat consumption (Metson et al., 2012). This has other major environmental implications, including increased gaseous emissions from livestock and water pollution from fertilizers.

24.6 PHOSPHATE ADDITIVES

Protein-rich foods, especially meat (200 mg/100 g) and dairy products (100–900 mg/100 g), are especially high in phosphate (European Food Safety Authority, 2013). Dietary phosphate intake in developed countries is estimated to be at least double (Welch et al., 2009) the nutritionally recommended intake of 600 to 700 mg/day (Institute of Medicine [U.S.] Standing Committee on the Scientific

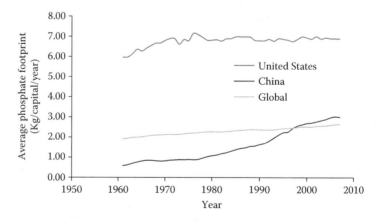

FIGURE 24.1 Average per capita phosphate footprint: global, China, and United States. (From Metson G et al., *Environ Res Lett*, 7, 044043, 2012.)

The Effects of Changing Global Food Choices on Human Health 345

Evaluation of Dietary Reference Intakes, 1997; European Food Safety Authority, 2013). The bioavailability of phosphate is also important and very much depends on the food sources. In plants, phosphate is mainly in the form of phytate. Humans, and indeed all mammals, lack the enzyme phytase, which is necessary to release phosphate from phytate. Thus, the phosphate found in plants is largely not in a readily bioavailable form. In contrast, phosphate in meat is readily bioavailable (Uribarri, 2007). Therefore, as already discussed, the increasing meat consumption in developed and developing countries has meant that the intake of readily bioavailable phosphate has also increased in parallel.

In addition to naturally occurring phosphate in food, a number of food additives contain phosphate in the form of inorganic salts. These are approved for widespread use in both the United States and the European Union (see Chapters 19, 21 and 22) (European Food Safety Authority, 2013). These additives are extensively used to break down protein, allowing more water binding, and as antimicrobial washes, acidifying agents, acidity buffers, emulsifying agents, stabilizers, and taste intensifiers, especially in processed foods. Indeed, the phosphate content of processed meat and poultry products is almost double that of the natural product because of the use of additives (Sherman and Mehta, 2009; Calvo and Uribarri, 2013; Uribarri, 2013). Phosphate additives are also found in very significant quantities in cola, other flavored drinks, and powdered milk and coffee (Ritz et al., 2012). Paradoxically, reducing the sodium intake of populations has led to an increase in phosphate ingestion with phosphate-based additives being used to replace some of the water-binding, emulsifying, and leavening roles of salt (Institute of Medicine Committee on Strategies to Reduce Sodium Intake Food and Nutrition Board, 2010).

Current estimates suggest that phosphate intake from additives has doubled to over 100 mg/day from 1990. Indeed, approximately 50% of phosphate intake in Western countries may now come from additives or "hidden phosphate" (Winger et al., 2012). Furthermore, the phosphate from food additives is generally much more readily bioavailable than the natural phosphate contained in food (Bell et al., 1977; Karp et al., 2007; Uribarri, 2009). However, food product labels provide little information on phosphate content (Lou-Arnal et al., 2014)((Calvo et al., 2014) and often underreport the amount of phosphate in their food and drink composition tables (Lou-Arnal et al., 2014; Moser et al., 2015). Over 50% of the top-selling foods in one U.S. Midwestern area supermarkets, especially refrigerated-frozen and packaged products, have phosphate-containing additives, increasing the phosphate quantity by 67 mg/100 g. As a whole, in this particular study, the authors found that products containing phosphate additives were significantly cheaper than those that did not (Leon et al., 2013). In the European Union, some phosphate additives are permitted at *quantum satis* levels in some food categories with little to no obligation on the manufacturers to display the phosphate content of these products (European Food Safety Authority, 2013).

There is currently no consensus of what constitutes a "safe" phosphate intake (European Food Safety Authority, 2013). Indeed, the Joint United Nations Food and Agriculture Organization and the World Health Organization considered it inappropriate to establish an acceptable daily intake because phosphate is an essential nutrient and an unavoidable constituent of food (European Food Safety Authority, 2013). However, as a direct consequence of increasing concerns on the potential public health implications of the increasing intake of readily bioavailable phosphate, the European Food Safety Agency has recently agreed to review the regulations concerning the use of phosphate food additives by the end of 2018 (European Food Safety Authority, 2013). In contrast, the United States and Canada have upper tolerable levels of phosphorus intake of 4000 mg for adults discussed in Chapter 20 (Institute of Medicine [U.S.] Standing Committeeon the Scientific Evaluation of Dietary Reference Intakes, 1997).

24.7 PHOSPHATE ROCK

Together, the Green and Sanitation Revolutions have meant that the once-closed loop of sustainable phosphate cycle (soil to plant to animal and back to soil) has not only been opened but massively sped up (discussed in Chapter 23). Large quantities of phosphate now literally flow from excavations to waterways. Unfortunately, this is all too often responsible for algal blooms and eutrophication (Vaccari, 2009; Elser and Bennett, 2011). In the United States alone, more than 100,000 miles of rivers and streams, nearly 2.5 million acres of lakes, reservoirs, and ponds and more than 800 square miles of bays and estuaries have poor-quality water because of nitrogen and phosphate pollution (United States Environmental Protection Agency, http://www2.epa.gov/nutrientpollution). In addition to the environmental effects, algal blooms have considerable health and economic implications with over US$1 billion lost to the U.S. economy every year due to their negative impact on tourism alone (United States Environmental Protection Agency, http://www2.epa.gov/nutrientpollution).

Approximately 70% of world phosphate production is from surface mining that in itself has a very significant environmental impact, making the process highly controversial.(Palmer et al., 2010) The phosphate content of currently mined rock ranges from <5% to 40%. The mined rock also has to be processed to remove impurities. In general, with the lower concentration of phosphate and lower-quality deposits, the more energy and chemicals are required to process it and the more waste is generated. Consequently, the costs of mining and processing phosphate rock increases significantly in relation to lower grade and lower quality deposit. Today, around 90% of the world's mined phosphate rock is used for agricultural and food production, predominantly for fertilizers (>80%) and to a lesser extent for animal feed and food additives (Neset and Cordell, 2012). The rest is used in detergents, metal processing, and other industrial applications.

It is currently far from clear as to how much phosphate rock is left. Consequently, evaluations of how long the Earth's phosphate rock reserves will last disagree enormously (Neset and Cordell, 2012). These predictions are heavily influenced by the country's own estimate and different methods of assessment. It is also important to consider other aspects than just the magnitude of reserves. These include the phosphate concentration of the rock, the quantity of impurities, the amount of contamination with toxic constituents including heavy metals, physical or legal accessibility, and the amount of energy needed for mining and processing. Indeed, it is becoming progressively clear that the phosphate rock that is left unexploited is of lower quality compared to older sources, with lower phosphate concentrations and higher levels of impurities, in addition to being much more awkward and difficult to mine (Cordell et al., 2009). These estimates often also assume a constant consumption rate and that demand will not grow (Neset and Cordell, 2012). The comparative scarceness of phosphate rock came to the fore globally in 2008 when the commodity price temporarily rocketed by over 800% (Figure 24.2). Current predictions as to when demand will exceed supply disagree extensively and vary from 40 to 400 years (Cordell et al., 2012).

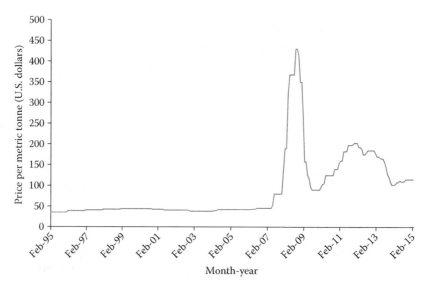

FIGURE 24.2 Phosphate rock commodity price in U.S. dollars (February 1995–February 2015). (Data obtained from Index Mundi www.indexmundi.com.)

The Effects of Changing Global Food Choices on Human Health

Furthermore, although about 30 nations currently produce phosphate rock, Morocco, China, and the United States are the biggest producers. Together, these three countries account for two-thirds of global production (Cordell et al., 2009; Ashley et al., 2011). Morocco alone accounts for over 30% of global exports. However, a significant proportion of Morocco's reserves are in Western Sahara, a territory Morocco is currently occupying in defiance of several resolutions from the United Nations (Neset and Cordell, 2012). There is also huge variability of dependence on imported phosphate rock. The European Union and Australia are practically totally reliant on imports of phosphate for agriculture (Neset and Cordell, 2012). Numerous farmers (especially in sub-Saharan Africa) are even now unable to afford to buy fertilizers to preserve harvests at current levels. These conditions could potentially lead to global instability.

It is obvious that at some point we will need to attain a state of global phosphate security. In essence this means that there is enough phosphate available to produce enough food to feed the increasing world population and at the same time not cause further extensive and irreversible damage to the environment and ecology of our plant (Shilton et al., 2012).

24.8 WAYS TO PRESERVE PHOSPHATE

Fortunately phosphate, unlike oil—another valuable biological commodity,—is not irrevocably lost after use. Unlike oil, though, the current utilization of phosphate is extremely inefficient. Only 80% of phosphate rock mined for use in fertilizers ends up being applied to the land. Of this, over 50% is lost through leaching and soil erosion into water bodies (McDowell, 2012; Neset and Cordell, 2012). Staggeringly, there is a massive loss of phosphate from mine to fork. In 2008, only 8% of the phosphate used in fertilizers and animal feed supplements ends up in food! The rest is lost as unused manure, rotten food, and processing inefficiencies. Overuse of phosphate fertilizers also leads to phosphate accumulation in soil (MacDonald et al., 2012). These losses present an obvious objective on which significant improvements can be made. An integrated approach to increasing the efficiency of phosphate use targeting every step of the chain is needed. This would need to include judicious use of fertilizers, genetically modified crops, and vegetative buffers around waterways (Metson et al., 2012). Losses of food from the minute it leaves the farm to the retail outlets, as well as losses from households themselves, also need to be targeted. It is estimated that up to 30% of purchased food is thrown out uneaten from households in the developed world (Neset and Cordell, 2012), which is a disgraceful situation given the millions of people who go to bed hungry every day.

In addition to optimizing use, there needs to be concerted moves to improve the recovery of phosphate from waste. These will need to include the recycling of human urine (Cordell et al., 2011; Metson et al., 2012). Considerable advances have already been made to check the discharge of phosphate into waterways to prevent pollution and eutrophication. These processes need to be enhanced and further developed to recover phosphate. This is all theoretically possible using current technology.

Nearly a third of the increase in phosphate requirements over the last decades has been due to changes in diet—mainly the demand for increased meat production (Metson et al., 2012). Reducing meat consumption is clearly a major potential way of lowering the world's dependence on phosphate rock. Indeed, a move to a less carnivorous diet is generally regarded as a vital part of any plan for future phosphate sustainability. Cordell and colleagues have estimated, based on global generic vegetarian and meat diets, that moving from a meat-based to a vegetarian-based diet could mean that phosphate consumption would be 50% lower in 2050 than in 2000. This could be a significant overestimate, and the report authors themselves recognize the very substantial limitations of their analyses (Cordell et al., 2009). However, this type of work does serve to highlight the significant gains that could theoretically be made.

There are huge differences between countries, however, with strong relationships between the use of phosphate and the wealth of a nation. Residents of less wealthy countries consume a lower amount of calories and less meat. Their diets consequently require less phosphate to produce (Metson et al.,

2012). In parallel with China's increasing wealth, its per capita phosphate requirement increased by 400% between 1961 and 2007. Despite this, China's per capita consumption of phosphate remained much lower during this period than most of North America and Europe (Figure 24.1) (Metson et al., 2012). Thus, changing the diet of a population will have very different potential impacts on global phosphate sustainability (Metson et al., 2012). Also, current models predict that the amount of phosphate needed to feed the world's population will increase by 68% to 141% between 2007 and 2050 (Metson et al., 2012). However, this will vary hugely from country to country. Developing countries will undoubtedly increase their phosphate consumption, whereas there is a very significant potential for developed countries to reduce their calorie and meat consumption with considerable public health and environmental paybacks (Metson et al., 2012). This is especially poignant with the recent report from the International Agency for Research on Cancer (part of the World Health Organization) that has classified processed meat as carcinogenic and red meat as probably carcinogenic to humans (Bouvard et al., 2015).

In addition to improvements in animal husbandry, attention needs to be drawn to pet ownership. A medium-sized dog will consume annually 164 kg of meat and 95 kg of cereal. This equates approximately to the use 0.84 hectares of agricultural land (Vale and Vale, 2009). This is a striking statistic especially when contrasted against the average citizen of Vietnam who has an ecological footprint of only 0.76 hectares or an Ethiopian with an even lower footprint of only 0.67 hectares. Measures such as feeding pets more leftovers, reducing waste, and the use of "greener" pet products also need to be part of the solution. Sustainable lifestyles require sacrifices, and even the family pet will need to contribute (Figure 24.3).

Developments in biotechnology also need to be optimally exploited. Pigs, like all mammals, cannot utilize phosphate from plant-derived phytate. To improve meat production yields they have to be fed phosphate supplements. Therefore, not surprisingly, pig waste is loaded with phosphate and is a significant contributor to phosphate pollution worldwide. The Enviropig was a transgenic pig experiment that synthesized phytase in its salivary glands secreting the active enzyme. The Enviropig could therefore use most of the phosphate from a plant-based diet, and not only did it not require any phosphate supplementation, but its feces contained 60% less phosphate when compared to conventional pigs (Forsberg et al., 2003). However, there are significant hurdles that need to be overcome regarding both regulatory safety assessments and public acceptance of genetically modified animals in the food chain and the use of genetically modified feed grains that contain phytase

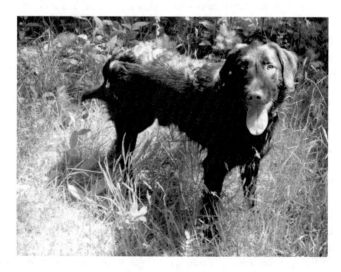

FIGURE 24.3 (See color insert.) In the struggle for global phosphate sustainability, even family pets will have to contribute.

The Effects of Changing Global Food Choices on Human Health

making the phytate bound phosphorus bioavailable and eliminating the need for phosphorus addition to the feeds (Forsberg et al., 2003; Blaabjerg et al., 2015). Sadly, at the time of writing there are currently no Enviropigs left. Their genetic material has been stored for a potential future comeback.

There is also a massive potential for recovering phosphate from human waste. Not only would this contribute to overall global phosphate sustainability and environmental protection but could have a significant impact on providing sanitation facilities for the 2.6 billion people currently without modern toilets (Neset et al., 2010; Cordell et al., 2011).

For any concerted effort targeting phosphate sustainability to be successful, it will almost certainly need to be linked with other strategies and sustainability efforts aimed at checking climate change (Neset and Cordell, 2012). Clear synergies could be gained from such approaches as well as significant public health benefits. Increased production/consumption of meat and processed food has a negative impact on human health; inevitably results in increased production of greenhouse gases; and requires considerably more fossil fuels, water, land, and nitrogen than similar levels of plant-based food production (Metson et al., 2012).

24.9 WHAT NEXT?

Phosphorus is an essential element for life, notwithstanding it being a comparatively rare element on Earth when compared to the other essential elements. This relative scarcity is likely to have provided a survival advantage in evolutionary terms to organisms that conserve it (Fouque, 2013). During the Paleoproterzoic era the "sudden" (albeit over hundreds of millions of years) increased bioavailability of phosphate was a key factor in the spectacular increase in the evolution of multicellular organisms and the emergence of new species. This process is now being mirrored over much shorter timeframes as phosphate literally flows into water bodies as a result of the increased use of phosphate fertilizers. This time, however, such a process is ironically leading to the extinction of hundreds of species and a reduction in the biodiversity of the planet through eutrophication and algal blooms.

Our current dependence on minded phosphate rock if unchecked will mean that the demand for phosphate might soon overtake supply potentially leading to global food insecurity. Without the development of worldwide sustainable phosphate strategies, we may find ourselves in the very strange situation where phosphate becomes a commodity to be fought over while simultaneously health and environmental experts are advocating decreases in its use for food processing and production.

REFERENCES

Ashley, K., Cordell, D. and Mavinic, D. (2011). A brief history of phosphorus: From the philosopher's stone to nutrient recovery and reuse. *Chemosphere*, 84, 737–746.

Bekker, A., Holland, H.D., Wang, P.L., et al. (2004). Dating the rise of atmospheric oxygen. *Nature*, 427, 117–120.

Bell, R.R., Draper, H.H., Tzeng, D.Y., Shin, H.K. and Schmidt, G.R. (1977). Physiological responses of human adults to foods containing phosphate additives. *J Nutr*, 107, 42–50.

Blaabjerg, K., Thomassen, A.M. and Poulsen, H.D. (2015). Microbial phytase addition resulted in a greater increase in phosphorus digestibility in dry-fed compared with liquid-fed non-heat-treated wheat-barley-maize diets for pigs. *Animal*, 9, 243–248.

Bouvard, V., Loomis, D., Guyton, K.Z., et al. (2015). Carcinogenicity of consumption of red and processed meat. *Lancet Oncol* , 16, 1599-1600.

Calvo, M.S., Moshfegh, A.J. and Tucker, K.L. (2014). Assessing the health impact of phosphorus in the food supply: Issues and considerations. *Adv Nutr*, 5, 104–113.

Calvo, M.S. and Uribarri, J. (2013). Public health impact of dietary phosphorus excess on bone and cardiovascular health in the general population. *Am J Clin Nutr*, 98, 6–15.

Chinyama, A. and Toma, T. (2013). Understanding the poor performance of urban sewerage systems. *Urban Planning Design Res*, 1, 43–49.

Cordell, D., Drangert, J.-O. and White, S. (2009). The story of phosphorus: Global food security and food for thought. *Global Environ Change*, 19, 292–305.

Cordell, D., Neset, T.S. and Prior, T. (2012). The phosphorus mass balance: Identifying 'hotspots' in the food system as a roadmap to phosphorus security. *Curr Opin Biotechnol*, 23, 839–845.

Cordell, D., Rosemarin, A., Schroder, J.J. and Smit, A.L. (2011). Towards global phosphorus security: A systems framework for phosphorus recovery and reuse options. *Chemosphere*, 84, 747–758.

Elser, J. and Bennett, E. (2011). Phosphorus cycle: A broken biogeochemical cycle. *Nature*, 478, 29–31.

European Food Safety Authority (2013). Assessment of one published review on health risks associated with phosphate additives in food. *EFSA J*, 11, 3444.

Falkowski, P.G., Fenchel, T. and Delong, E.F. (2008). The microbial engines that drive Earth's biogeochemical cycles. *Science*, 320, 1034–1039.

Ferro, C.J., Chue, C.D., Steeds, R.P., and Townend, J.N. (2009). Is lowering phosphate exposure the key to preventing arterial stiffening with age? *Heart*, 95, 1770–1772.

Forsberg, C.W., Phillips, J.P., Golovan, S.P., et al. (2003). The Enviropig physiology, performance, and contribution to nutrient management advances in a regulated environment: The leading edge of change in the pork industry. *J Anim Sci*, 81 (Suppl 2), E68–E77.

Fouque, D. (2013). The phosphorus-proteinuria interaction in chronic kidney disease. *Nephrol Dial Transplant*, 28, 493–495.

Geider, R.J., Delucia, E.H., Falkowski, P.G., et al. (2001). Primary productivity of planet earth: Biological derterminants and physcial constraints in terrestrial and aquatic habitats. *Glob Change Biol*, 7, 849–882.

Horiguchi, M. and Kandatsu, M. (1959). Isolation of 2-aminoethane phosphonic acid from rumen protozoa. *Nature*, 184, 901–902.

Institute of Medicine (U.S.) Standing Committeeon the Scientific Evaluation of Dietary Reference Intakes (1997). *Dietary reference intakes: Calcum, phosphorus, magnesium, vitamin D, and fluoride*. Washington, DC: National Academies Press (US).

Institute of Medicine Committee on Strategies to Reduce Sodium Intake Food and Nutrition Board (2010). *Strategies to reduce sodium intake in the United States*. Washington, DC: National Academies Press.

Karp, H.J., Vaihia, K.P., Karkkainen, M.U., Niemisto, M.J. and Lamberg-Allardt, C.J. (2007). Acute effects of different phosphorus sources on calcium and bone metabolism in young women: A whole-foods approach. *Calcif Tissue Int*, 80, 251–258.

Leon, J.B., Sullivan, C.M. and Sehgal, A.R. (2013). The prevalence of phosphorus-containing food additives in top-selling foods in grocery stores. *J Ren Nutr*, 23, 265–270 e262.

Lou-Arnal, L.M., Arnaudas-Casanova, L., Caverni-Munoz, A., et al. (2014). Hidden sources of phosphorus: Presence of phosphorus-containing additives in processed foods. *Nefrologia*, 34, 498–506.

MacDonald, G., Bennett, E. and Carpenter, S. (2012). Embodied phosphorus and the global connections of United States agriculture. *Environ Res Lett*, 7, 044024.

Macia, E. (2005). The role of phosphorus in chemical evolution. *Chem Soc Rev*, 34, 691–701.

McDowell, R.W. (2012). Minimising phosphorus losses from the soil matrix. *Curr Opin Biotechnol*, 23, 860–865.

Metcalf, W.W. and van der Donk, W.A. (2009). Biosynthesis of phosphonic and phosphinic acid natural products. *Annu Rev Biochem*, 78, 65–94.

Metson, G., Bennett, E. and Elser, J. (2012). The role of diet in phosphorus demand. *Environ Res Lett*, 7, 044043.

Moser, M., White, K., Henry, B., et al. (2015). Phosphorus content of popular beverages. *Am J Kidney Dis*, 65, 969–971.

Neset, T.-S.S., Drangert, J.-O., Bader, H.P. and Scheidegger, R. (2010). Recycling of phosphorus in urban Sweden: A historical overview to prepare a strategy for the future. *Water Policy*, 12, 611–624.

Neset, T.S. and Cordell, D. (2012). Global phosphorus scarcity: Identifying synergies for a sustainable future. *J Sci Food Agric*, 92, 2–6.

Palmer, M.A., Bernhardt, E.S., Schlesinger, W.H., et al. (2010). Science and regulation. Mountaintop mining consequences. *Science*, 327, 148–149.

Papineau, D. (2010). Global biogeochemical changes at both ends of the proterozoic: Insights from phosphorites. *Astrobiology*, 10, 165–181.

Papineau, D. (2013). High phosphate availability as a possible cause for massive cyanobacterial production of oxygen in the Paleoproterzoic atmosphere. *Earth Planetary Sci Letts*, 362, 225–236.

Planavsky, N.J., Rouxel, O.J., Bekker, A., et al. (2010). The evolution of the marine phosphate reservoir. *Nature*, 467, 1088–1090.

Razzaque, M.S. (2011). Phosphate toxicity: New insights into an old problem. *Clin Sci (Lond)*, 120, 91–97.

Ritz, E., Hahn, K., Ketteler, M., Kuhlmann, M.K. and Mann, J. (2012). Phosphate additives in food–A health risk. *Dtsch Arztebl Int*, 109, 49–55.

Rosenfeld, L. (2003). Justus Liebig and animal chemistry. *Clin Chem*, 49, 1696–1707.

Sherman, C.C. (1933). Theories of the nutrition of plants from Aristotle to Liebig. *Yale J Biol Med*, 6, 43–60.

Sherman, R.A. and Mehta, O. (2009). Phosphorus and potassium content of enhanced meat and poultry products: Implications for patients who receive dialysis. *Clin J Am Soc Nephrol*, 4, 1370–1373.

Shilton, A.N. and Blank, L.M. (2012). Phosphorus biotechnology. *Curr Opin Biotechnol*, 23, 830–832.

United States Environmental Protection Agency. Nutrient Pollution. http://www2.epa.gov/nutrientpollution. Retrieved 4th November 2015.

Uribarri, J. (2007). Phosphorus homeostasis in normal health and in chronic kidney disease patients with special emphasis on dietary phosphorus intake. *Semin Dial*, 20, 295–301.

Uribarri, J. (2009). Phosphorus additives in food and their effect in dialysis patients. *Clin J Am Soc Nephrol*, 4, 1290–1292.

Uribarri, J. (2013). Dietary phosphorus and kidney disease. *Ann N Y Acad Sci*, 1301, 11–19.

Vaccari, D.A. (2009). Phosphorus: A looming crisis. *Sci Am*, 300, 54–59.

Vaclav, S. (2002). Eating meat: Evolution, patterns, and consequences. *Popul Development Rev*, 28, 599–639.

Vale, R. and Vale, B. (2009). *Time to eat the dog: The real guide to sustainable living*. London: Thames and Hudson.

Welch, A.A., Fransen, H., Jenab, M., et al. (2009). Variation in intakes of calcium, phosphorus, magnesium, iron and potassium in 10 countries in the European Prospective Investigation into Cancer and Nutrition study. *Eur J Clin Nutr*, 63 (Suppl 4), S101–S121.

Westheimer, F.H. (1987). Why nature chose phosphates. *Science*, 235, 1173–1178.

Winger, R., Uribarri, J. and Lloyd, L. (2012). Phosphorus-containing food additives: An insidious danger for people with chronic kidney disease. *Trends Food Sci Technol*, 24, 92–102.

Index

A

ABD, *see* Adynamic bone disease (ABD)
aBMD, *see* areal bone mineral density (aBMD)
Acceptable Daily Intake (ADI), 259, 307, 345
Acid-ash hypothesis, 126–127, 136–137
Acidosis, 144, 202, 242
Acute alkalemia, 66
Additive-enhanced diet, 217
Additives, 344–345, *see also* Food additives containing phosphorus
    phosphate, 179, 283, 307, 323
    unpackaged foods, 318
ADHR, *see* Autosomal-dominant hypophosphatemic rickets (ADHR)
Adipocytes, 238
ad libitum high-protein diets, 103
Adolescence
    bone mass during, 187
    phosphorus in, 178–179
Adverse health effects, high phosphorus intake
    cancer and, 273–274
    cardiovascular disease (CVD), 272–273
    FGF23 resistance, 274
    mortality and, 272
Adynamic bone disease (ABD), 36
Albuminuria, 116, 117, 240
Alkaline diet, 126–127, 129
Ammonium phosphatides (E 442), 308, 318
Anemia risk, 7
Antibody-drug conjugate (ADC) approach, 20
Aortic calcifications, 37
Aquatic eutrophication, P sustainability, 333
areal bone mineral density (aBMD), 172
Atherosclerosis Risk in Communities (ARIC) study, 99, 115
Autosomal-dominant hypophosphatemic rickets (ADHR), 189, 192
Autosomal-recessive hypophosphatemia, 193

B

Best management practices (BMPs), 335
Bill Emerson Good Samaritan Food Donation Act, 336
Bioavailability
    challenges, 231
    quantitative P absorption, 306
    sources effect, on phosphorus metabolism in humans, 227–231
    in vitro determinations, *see* P bioavailability, *in vitro*
Biomarker
    determination, 274
    hormone mechanisms as, 275
    selection, 250–252
    serum phosphate as, 271
Biomaterials in tissue engineering, 159
Biomineralization, 75

Block Food Frequency Questionnaire, 55
Blood pressure, *see also* Cardiotoxicity
    dietary factors impact, 112–113
    nutritional epidemiology studies, limitations, 115–116
    phosphorus–blood pressure link, potential mechanisms, 118–120
    phosphorus intake and, 113–115
    protein intake and, 117–118
    serum phosphorus and intact PTH, 116
    trials, phosphorus intake dietary levels, 116–117
Blood urea nitrogen (BUN), 238
BMAD, *see* Bone mineral apparent density (BMAD)
BMC, *see* Bone mineral content (BMC)
BMPs, *see* Best management practices (BMPs); Bone morphogenetic proteins (BMPs)
Body phosphorus homeostasis
    alkali in bone, 66
    bone mineral, 64
    calciphylaxis, 67
    calcium-forming hydroxyapatite, 64–65
    calcium hydroxyapatite, 68
    calcium intestinal absorption, 68
    food phosphorus bioavailability, 67
    in healthy adult, 64–65
    kidney function and, 64, 67–68
    mean mineral composition, 65
    osseous calcifications, 65
    renal function, 66
    tumoral calcinosis, 67
    urinary phosphate excretion, CKD patients, 68
    vascular calcifications, 67
Bone-forming proteins, 33
Bone fragility in CKD
    parathyroid hormone (PTH) role, 36
    phosphorus role, 35–36
Bone health
    cell functions, activity of phosphorus ion, 157–159
    extraskeletal phosphorus fluxes, 159–160
    in mid-childhood, risk, 177–178
    phosphorus in relation to, 157
    in postmenopausal women and older men, 161–163
Bone loss, 235
Bone mineral apparent density (BMAD), 177
Bone mineral content (BMC), 172, 176
Bone morphogenetic proteins (BMPs), 33
Bone-specific alkaline phosphatase, 35

C

CAFOs, *see* Concentrated animal feeding operations (CAFOs)
Calcification inhibitors, 33
Calcific uremic arteriolopathy (CUA), 5
Calciphylaxis, 5, 67

353

Calcitriol, 168
 in HHRH, 190
 mitochondrial 1-alpha hydroxylase activity, 187
Calcium, 262
 balance, 129, 131
 and bone metabolism, 128, 129–132
Calcium-based binders, 89
Calcium-forming hydroxyapatite, 64–65
Calcium hydroxyapatite, 66, 68
Calcium oxalate stone formation
 and CaP, interaction between, 206
 precipitation and deposition, 206–207
 supersaturation, 203
Calcium phosphate (CaP), 257, 317
 CaOx and, interaction between, 206
 in gut, 204
 precipitation and deposition, 206–207
 precipitation product of, 203
 subepithelial deposits and intratubular plugs formed, 207–208
 supersaturation, 203
Calcium-sensing receptor (CSR), 188
Calcium stone formation, *see also* Calcium phosphate (CaP)
 amorphous calcium phosphate (ACP), 203
 CaOx and CaP, interaction between, 206
 components in Swedish patients, 202
 phosphate, renal handling, 203–206
 precipitation and deposition, 206–207
 recurrence, preventive considerations, 208–210
 supersaturation, 203
 in urinary tract, 202–203
Calcium-to-phosphorus ratio, 64–65
Cambrian Explosion, 343
Cancer
 cell–mediated angiogenesis, 8
 and dietary Pi, 14–15
 high phosphorus intake and, 273–274
 initiation and progression modulator, 15, 18
 preclinical models of, 15–16
 risk, 8, 16
Cardiotoxicity, *see also* Blood pressure
 dietary phosphorus, 94–95, 97
 endothelial function and arterial stiffness, 102–103
 FGF23 levels, 100, 102
 intake and mortality/cardiovascular outcomes, 97–100
 non-calcium-based binders, 104
 in nondialysis CKD patients, 104–105
 phosphorus and protein consumption, 103–104
 phosphorus binder therapy, 104
 serum phosphorus, 95–96, 101–102
 short-term dietary phosphorus interventions, 100–101
 sodium/hydrogen exchangers (NHE), 105
 urinary phosphorus, 96–97, 101
 vascular calcification, 103
Cardiovascular disease (CVD), 5–7
 clinical outcomes and surrogate markers of, 97–98
 high phosphorus intake, 272–273
 and mortality, 87–88
"Carry-over" principle, 282
Cell autonomous effects
 cell transport and sensing, 19
 cellular and molecular phenotype alteration, 19
 Pi availability and cell growth, 18–19

Slc20a1, 20
 Slc34a2, 20
Cell transport and sensing, Pi, 19
Cellular and molecular phenotype alteration, 19
Chemical fertilizers, phosphate for, 343
Childhood obesity, 177–178
Cholesterol and Recurrent Events (CARE) study, 95–96
Chronic health risks associated with phosphorus excess
 anemia risk, 7
 cancer risk, 8
 cardiovascular disease, 5–7
 chronic kidney disease, progression, 4
 mineral bone disease and soft tissue calcifications, 4–5
 mortality, 7
Chronic kidney disease (CKD), 235, 236
 diet, 241
 and ESRD, serum phosphorus levels in, 85
 hyperphosphatemia, 142
 impaired calcitriol production, 142
 mineral bone disorder, 85–86, 238
 nondialysis, cardiotoxicity in, 104–105
 phosphorus and progression, 86–87
 phosphorus homeostasis, 84
 processed foods and, 306–307
 progression, 4
 renal klotho deficiency, 142
 serum phosphate measurements, 85
Chronic Renal Insufficiency Cohort (CRIC) study, 216
Chronic Renal Insufficiency Standards Implementation Study (CRISIS), 96
CKD, *see* Chronic kidney disease (CKD)
CKD-MBD syndrome, 55, 56
Coconut milk, 261
Concentrated animal feeding operations (CAFOs), 336
Coronary Artery Risk Development in Young Adults (CARDIA) study, 96
Cow's milk–based HMF, 173–175
Cox proportional hazards modeling, 18
Crop-based biofuels, 337
Crop varieties and genetics improvement, P sustainability, 334
CSR, *see* Calcium-sensing receptor (CSR)
CUA, *see* Calcific uremic arteriolopathy (CUA)

D

DASH diet, 262
Dead zones, 333
Demineralization disorders, 168, *see also* mineralization
Dentin matrix protein 1(DMP-1), 75, 158, 193
Deoxygenated "dead zones", 329
Dietary acid–base balance and bone health
 calcium balance, 129, 131, 132–134
 Dietary Reference Intakes (DRI), 130, 132
 phosphate study, 129, 130
 phosphorus role, calcium and bone metabolism, 128, 129–132
 Revised Potential Renal Acid Load Food Lists, 129, 135–136
 urine calcium, 132–134
 urine pH and blood pH, 128, 129, 132
Dietary Approaches to Stop Hypertension (DASH), 112
Dietary factors, blood pressure and, 112–113

Index

355

Dietary inorganic phosphate (Pi), *see also* Inorganic phosphate (Pi)
  availability and cell growth, 18–19
  and cancer, 14–15, *see also* Cancer
  carcinogen-induced skin cancer, 16–17
  carcinogen-induced tumorigenesis, 17
  cell-based models identification, 16
  cell transport and sensing of, 19
  cellular and molecular phenotype alteration, 19
  oncogene-induced lung cancer, 17
Dietary phosphorus
  bioavailability, 241
  cardiotoxicity, 94–95, 97
  and intestinal P absorption and mortality, 57–58
  restriction, 236
Dietary Reference Intakes (DRI), 130, 132, 268
Dietary reference values (DRVs), 271
Digestible phosphorus (DP)
  in beverages, 225
  cereal, 224–225
  in dairy products, 226–227
  in meat and meat products, 225–226
  in plant-based foods, 223–224
1,25-Dihydroxyvitamin D (calcitriol), 254
DMP-1, *see* Dentin matrix protein 1 (DMP-1)
DP, *see* Digestible phosphorus (DP)
DRI, *see* Dietary Reference Intakes (DRI)
DRVs, *see* Dietary reference values (DRVs)
Dual-energy X-ray absorptiometry (DXA), 172, 177

E

Echocardiography, 96
Ectopic (metastatic) calcification, 269–270
Electroneutral sodium/hydrogen exchangers (NHE), 105
Endocrine regulation
  FGF23 regulation, *see* Fibroblast growth factor 23 (FGF23)
  phosphate and its regulators, 77–78
  phosphate homeostasis, 72
  phosphate regulation, hormonal feedback, 74–75
Endothelial dysfunction, 6, 55, 56
Endothelial function and arterial stiffness, 102–103
End-stage renal disease (ESRD), 49
  anemia risk, 7
  development of, 4
  serum phosphate measurements, 85
  serum phosphorus and blood pressure, 116
Enthesophyte, 192, 196
ESRD, *see* End-stage renal disease (ESRD)
European Commission Health and Consumers Directorate, 319–321
European food regulations
  approved phosphorus additives, 284
  CKD patients and processed foods, 306–307
  phosphorus-containing food additives, 282–284, 307–309
  regulatory authority governing, 280–282
European Food Safety Authority (EFSA), 250, 251, 270–271, 308–309, 314–315, 317–319, 345
  mandated re-evaluation, 321–322

European perspective, phosphorus intakes
  added phosphates contributing to phosphorus intake, 317–318
  EU phosphate additive safety re-evaluation, 322
  European Commission Health and Consumers Directorate, 319–321
  European Union regulation, 318–319
  fast food contributions, 315
  food industry response, 323
  mandated re-evaluation, 321–322
  phosphate additive use in processing, 316–317
  phosphorus sustainability concerns, 323–324
Extraskeletal phosphorus fluxes, 159–160

F

Fam20c, 75
Fast Food FACTS, 178
Ferric citrate, 89
Fertilizer
  application and P sustainability, 329
  practices improvement, P sustainability, 335
Fetus and neonate, phosphorus economy, 171–176
FGF23, *see* Fibroblast growth factor 23 (FGF23)
Fibroblast growth factor 23 (FGF23), 21, 235, 254
  cardiotoxicity, intake, 100
  gene, calcitriol transactivation of, 145
  genetic disorders, 75–76
  high phosphorus intake and, 274
  kidney function, 86
  levels, 102
  in neonates, 171–172
  osteocytes in bone, 73
  phosphate regulating hormones, 72–74
  and PTH in CKD, 77
  regulation, 76–77
  renal 1-alpha hydroxylase expression, 74
  renal phosphate cotransporters, 73
  serum levels, 34–35
  synthesis in bone, calcitriol induction of, 145–146
  urinary phosphate excretion, 73–74
Flexitarian, food-trend consumer, 315
Fluxes from humans, P sustainability, 332
Food additives containing phosphorus
  in Europe, 307–309
  labeled, 318
  lawful additions of, 318
  principles of, 282–283
  in processed foods, 283–306
  regulatory authority governing, 280–282
Food and Drug Administration (FDA), 261
Food chain efficiency, 336
Food frequency questionnaires (FFQs)
  dietary records, 95
  phosphorus intake and blood pressure, 115
Food phosphorus bioavailability, 67
Food Scores Data Base of the Environmental Working Group, 316
Food Service, journal, 315
Food waste, P sustainability, 332
Fortificants, 257
Framingham Heart Study (FHS), 87
Framingham Offspring Study, 96

356 Index

Frizzled-related protein 4 (FRP-4), 143
FRP-4, *see* Frizzled-related protein 4 (FRP-4)

G

Glomerular damage, phosphate and mortality, 55, 56
Glomerular filtration rate (GFR), 46, 252, 315
Grain-based foods, 236

H

Hazard ratios (HRs), 95
HDMF, *see* Human donor milk-based fortifiers
 (HDMF)
Hereditary hypophosphatemic rickets with hypercalciuria
 (HHRH), 190
HHRH, *see* Hereditary hypophosphatemic rickets with
 hypercalciuria (HHRH)
Hidden phosphorus, 316
Hidden P load, 49
High mineral demand and phosphate-wasting diseases,
 195–196
HMFs, *see* human milk fortifiers (HMFs)
Human donor milk-based fortifiers (HDMF),
 173–174
Human milk fortifiers (HMFs), 173–175
Humans and meat-eating, phosphate consumption, 344
Hydrolysis of phytate, 236
Hydroxyapatite in skeletal tissues, 47
25-Hydroxyvitamin D, 146–147
Hypercalciuria, in breastfed infant, 177
Hyperparathyroidism, 5, 190, 194, 196, 202
Hyperphosphatemia, 4, 32, 88–89
Hypertrophic chondrocytes, 187
Hypocalcemia, 4, 73, 144, 269
Hypophosphatasia (HPP), 157
Hypophosphatemia, 75
 defective mineralization and serious bone disorders,
 126
 phosphate-wasting disorders and, 190–193

I

IGF-I, 144, 160
Inorganic phosphate (Pi), 8, *see also* Dietary inorganic
 phosphate (Pi)
 availability and cell growth, 18–19
 cancer initiation and progression modulator, 18
 and carcinogen-induced skin cancer, 16–17
 cell-based models identification, 16
 cell transport and sensing of, 19
 cellular and molecular phenotype alteration, 19
 dietary form, 14–15
 intake, 216–217
 and oncogene-induced lung cancer, 17
 responsive endocrine factors, 20–21
 risk factor for cancer, 16
International Fertilizer Development Center, 330
International Plant Nutrition Institute (IPNI), 335
The International Study of Macro- and Micro-Nutrients
 and Blood Pressure (INTERMAP), 113
Intestinal phosphorus absorption, 160
Intestinal P uptake, 47
IPNI, *see* International Plant Nutrition Institute (IPNI)

J

JB6 cell model, 16

K

KDIGO, *see* Kidney Disease Improving Global Outcomes
 (KDIGO)
Kidney Disease Improving Global Outcomes (KDIGO), 88
Kidney function
 cardiovascular disease and mortality, 87–88
 CKD and ESRD, serum phosphorus levels in, 85
 FGF23, 86
 hyperphosphatemia treatment, 88–89
 mineral and bone disorders, 85–86
 phosphorous homeostasis, 84–85
 phosphorus and progression, 86–87
 serum phosphate, 85, 88
α-Klotho, 21–22, 39
 calcitriol induction of, 145
 expression, 35
 overexpression, 142

L

Lacto-ovo vegetarian, 238
Lanthanum carbonate, 118
Left ventricular hypertrophy
 functional association, 99
 phosphate and mortality, 55, 56
Legacy P, 330
Low fat milk, 261

M

Manure fluxes, P sustainability, 331–332
Matrix extracellular phosphoglycoprotein (MEPE), 143,
 158
Maximum tolerable daily intake (MTDI), 318
MDRD, *see* Modification of Diet in Renal Disease
 (MDRD)
Mean mineral composition, 65
Mediterranean-style diet and blood pressure, 112–113
MEPE, *see* Matrix extracellular phosphoglycoprotein
 (MEPE)
Mesenchyme-derived osteoblasts, 170
Metabolic acidosis on kidney, 243
Microbial-produced phytase, 238
Mineral and bone disorders, 85–86
Mineral bone disease and soft tissue calcifications, 4–5
Mineral homeostasis, 191
Mineralization, 64, 127, *see also* Demineralization
 disorders
Mineralization-induced maturation, 159
Modification of Diet in Renal Disease (MDRD),
 50, 97
Mortality, 7
 and high phosphorus intake, 272
 mechanisms, 55, 56
 nutritional P intake and P balance, assessment, 50–55
 observational studies, 55–59
 phosphate homeostasis in humans, 47–49
MTDI, *see* Maximum tolerable daily intake (MTDI)
Multi-Ethnic Study of Atherosclerosis (MESA), 99, 115

Index

357

N

N-acetyl β-D-glucosaminidase, 243
NaP-2A, 84
NaPi IIa cotransporter, 171, 187–189
NaPi IIB, *see* Sodium phosphorous cotransporter IIB
 (NaPi IIB)
National Health and Nutrition Education Surveys
 (NHANES), 87, 97, 255
Natural phosphorus in food, 257
Nephrocalcinosis, 4
Nephrolithiasis, 238
Next-generation fertilizers, 330
NOAEL, *see* No Observable Adverse Effect Level
 (NOAEL)
NOEL, *see* No Observable Effect Level (NOEL)
Non-calcium-based binders, 104
Nonhuman enzymes, 259
Nonskeletal adverse health effects
 cancer, diet, and phosphorus consumption, 14–16
 cell autonomous effects, 18–20
 phosphorus consumption on cancer, modulating effect,
  16–18
 phosphorus-responsive endocrine, paracrine and
  autocrine factors, 20–22
No Observable Adverse Effect Level (NOAEL), 270, 307
No Observable Effect Level (NOEL), 307
Nutritional epidemiology studies, limitations, 115–116
Nutritional P
 intake and P balance, assessment, 50–55
 overload, 49, 55, 56
 sources, 49
Nutrition Data System software, 113

O

Obesity, 177–178
Office of Dietary Supplements, 257
Oncogene-induced lung cancer, Pi, 17
OPG, *see* Osteoblasts secrete osteoprotegerin (OPG)
OPN, *see* Osteopontin (OPN)
Oral phosphate supplementation, 143
Oral phosphorus binders, 89
Organic food additives, 317
Organic matrix formation, 157
Organic phosphorus, 214–216, 237
Osseous calcifications, 65
Osteoblasts secrete osteoprotegerin (OPG), 170
Osteoclast lineage cells, 159
Osteocytes
 distribution and functions, 158–159
 and FGF23, 75
Osteogenic cells and phosphorus, 157–158
Osteomalacia, 157
Osteopontin (OPN), 17, 22
Osteoporosis treatment, 162
Oxidative stress, phosphate and mortality, 55, 56

P

Parathyroid hormone (PTH), 235, 254
 blood pressure and, 116
 bone fragility in CKD, 36
 calcium hormonal control, 269

gene deletion, 73
 phosphate regulating hormones, 72–74
 renal phosphate cotransporters, 73
 urinary phosphate excretion, 73–74
 vascular calcification, 34
P bioavailability, *in vitro*
 in beverages, 225
 cereal phosphorus digestibility, 224–225
 in dairy products, 226–227
 digestible phosphorus (DP), 223
 inductively coupled plasma mass spectrometry
  (ICP-MS), 223
 insoluble mineral, 223
 Itkonen method, 223
 in meat and meat products, 225–226
 in plant-based foods, 223–224
P-deficient farmlands, 330–331
Peak phosphate, 330
Pesco-vegetarian, 238
PHEX, *see* Phosphate-regulating neutral endopeptidase on
  chromosome X (PHEX)
Phosphate
 additives, 179, 283, 307, 323, 344–345
 for chemical fertilizers, 343
 cycle, 343
 in evolution, 342–343
 as excipients, 317
 global food insecurity, 349
 humans and meat-eating, 344
 pollution worldwide, 348
 preservation, 347–349
 replacement therapy, 194–195
 rock, 345–347
 salts, adjunct therapy of, 193–194
 vitamins and mineral fortificants containing, 317
Phosphate homeostasis
 animal proteins, 49
 assessments of, 169–170
 disturbances in, 189–190
 endocrine regulation, 72, *see also* Endocrine
  regulation
 end-stage renal disease (ESRD), 49
 GFR reduction, 49
 in health, 187–189
 hydroxyapatite in skeletal tissues, 47
 intestinal P uptake, 47
 nutritional P sources, 49
 organic P, 47
 P balance stimulation, 47–48
 serum P, 47
 urinary P excretion (UPE), 49
Phosphatemia, 55
Phosphate-regulating neutral endopeptidase on
  chromosome X (PHEX), 158, 191
Phosphate response elements (PRE), 194
Phosphate-wasting disorders
 alkaline phosphatase activity, 186
 autosomal-dominant hypophosphatemic rickets
  (ADHR), 192
 autosomal-recessive hypophosphatemia, 193
 combined phosphate therapy, limitations, 196
 comorbidities of, 192
 etiology and presentation, 190
 FGF23 in, 193, 196

358

Index

hypophosphatemia and, 190–193
management, 195–196
mineral demand and, 195–196
phosphate replacement therapy impact, 194–195
urinary, phosphate salts in therapy, 193
Phosphatonins, 186, 189
Phosphoethanolamine/phosphocholine phosphatase (PHOSPHO1), 157
PHOSPHO1, phosphatase enzyme, 170–171
Phosphorous homeostasis
bone-kidney link in, 160
extracellular, 161
kidney function, 84–85
mineralization-induced maturation, 159
osteocytes function, 158
Phosphorus
additives in food manufacturing industry, 216
in adolescence, 178–179
balance, 50–51, 214–217
binder therapy, 104, 317
bioavailability, 221–231, 258
bone fragility in CKD, 35–36
in bone modeling, 157
calcium and bone metabolism, 128, 129–132
depletion, 161, 162–163
dietary reference intakes (DRIs) for, 251
economy in fetus and neonate, 171–176
health claims, 317
inadequate supply and osteoporosis treatment, 162
insufficient intake, 161
key to life, 342
metabolism and bone, 170–171
metabolism in humans, 227–231
and osteoclast lineage cells, 159
and osteogenic cells, 157–158
physiology of, 186–187
preterm, metabolic bone disease of, 176–177
and protein consumption, 103–104
pyramid, 262
recommended daily allowance (RDA) for, 250, 252–253
recommended intake, 161
vascular calcification, 33–34
Phosphorus–blood pressure link, potential mechanisms, 118–120
Phosphorus depletion
in osteoporosis treatment with anabolic agents, 162–163
and skeletal muscle integrity and function, 161
Phosphorus homeostasis, 239
bone-kidney link in, 160
systemic, 214
Phosphorus intake, regulatory aspects of, 249–250
biomarker selection, 250–252
on bone health and other health risks, 262–263
dietary phosphorus intakes in North America and Europe, 254–256
European Food Safety Authority set dietary reference values, 252–254
food and supplement sources, 256–259
low Ca:P intake ratio, 262
in North America and Europe, 256–261
phosphorus food additives, 259–261
processed foods and phosphate additives in CKD, 262–263
RDA for, 252

regulatory labeling, 261–262
variability in levels of FGF -23 in vulnerable populations, 263
Phytate, 237–238, 335
Phytic acid, 237
Plant-based diets, 235–237
in CKD, effects of, 242–243
grain *vs.* synthetic feeds, 238–239
phytate, 237–238
protein on CKD-MBD in humans, 239–242
Plant-derived phosphorus, 259
Plant protein–based diet on urine parameters, 242
Plasma phosphate concentration, 66
Potential Renal Acid Load (PRAL), 127, 128, 135
PRAL, *see* Potential Renal Acid Load (PRAL)
Preclinical animal models, 15
Prescribed dietary P intake (PDP), 56
Preterm neonates
calcium absorption of, 176
metabolic bone disease of, 176–177
Priority additives, 309
Proliferating cell nuclear antigen (PCNA) labeling index, 17
Protein consumption and phosphorus, 103–104
Protein intake and blood pressure, 117–118
Proteinuria and GFR, 55, 56
P sustainability
aquatic eutrophication, 333
dead zones, 333
fluxes from humans, 332
food waste, 332
manure fluxes, 331–332
P-deficient farmlands, 330–331
solutions, 334–337
supply, 329–330
toxic algae, 333
PTH, *see* Parathyroid hormone (PTH)
PTH-independent phosphaturia, 189

R

Raine syndrome, 75
The Recommended Dietary Allowance (RDA), 94, 161
Renal calcitriol production, 142
control, 146
FGF23 synthesis in bone, 145–146
high dietary phosphorus upregulation, 143–144
low dietary phosphorus upregulation, 144–145
Renal osteodystrophy, 86
Renal phosphorus
reabsorption, 160
retention, 32
Renal tubular reabsorption, 156
Revised Potential Renal Acid Load Food Lists, 129, 135–136
Ribonucleotides, 284
Rich organic streams recycling, 336–337
Rickets, 75, 157
4Rs, fertilizer practices, 335

S

The "Sanitation Revolution", 343
Scientific Committee for Food (SCF), 318
Secreted frizzled-related proteins (SFRPs), 37–38
Serum parathyroid hormone (S-PTH), 17, 227–231

Index

Serum phosphate, 240
  as biomarker, 271
  homeostatic response, 84–85
  levels, endocrine regulators, 72
  measurements, 85
  monitoring, 88
Serum phosphorus, 47, 252, 263
  after controlled interventions on dietary P intake, 51–53
  blood pressure and, 116
  cardiotoxicity, 95–96
  levels among predialysis CKD, 54
  values, 101–102
Serum Pi, 17
Sex steroids, 178
SFRPs, *see* Secreted frizzled-related proteins (SFRPs)
Short-term dietary phosphorus interventions, 100–101
Skeletal and vascular adverse health effects
  bone fragility in CKD, pathophysiology, 35–36
  bone health and survival, 37–39
  vascular calcification, 32–35, 37–39
Skeletal muscle function, phosphorus depletion, 161
Skeletal porosity, 270
Skimmed, evaporated and lactose free (SEL) milk, 173
Skimmed, evaporated, lactose free and lyophilized (SELL) milk, 173
Slc20a1 and cell proliferation, 20
Slc34a2, cancer therapeutic target, 20
Small, integrin-binding, ligand N-linked glycoprotein (SIBLING) family, 171, 193
Sodium-dependent phosphate transporters, 19–20
Sodium excretion, 243
Sodium–hydrogen exchanger regulatory factor 1 (NHERF1), 168–169
Sodium/hydrogen exchangers (NHE), 105
Sodium phosphorous cotransporter IIB (NaPi IIB), 84, 168
Soft tissues calcification, 196
Soluble α-klotho (s-klotho), 145
Soy milk, 261
Surrogate of kidney dysfunction, 238
Swedish Apolipoprotein Mortality Risk (AMORIS) study, 17

T

12-O-Tetradecanoylphorbol-13-acetate (TPA), 16
Third National Health and Nutrition Examination Survey, 217
TIO, *see* Tumor-induced osteomalacia (TIO)
Tissue-nonspecific alkaline phosphatase (TNAP), 170
TmP, *see* Tubular maximum for phosphate (TmP)
TNAP, *see* Tissue-nonspecific alkaline phosphatase (TNAP)
Total phosphorus (TP), 223–224
  in beverages, 225
  cereal phosphorus digestibility, 224–225
  in dairy products, 226–227
  in meat and meat products, 225–226
  in plant-based foods, 223–224
Toxic algae, 333
Toxic cyanobacteria, 329
TP, *see* total phosphorus (TP)
Transcellular phosphate shifts, disorders, 66
Transient hyperphosphatasemia, 177
Tubular maximum for phosphate (TmP), 168

Tumoral calcinosis, 67
Tumor-induced osteomalacia (TIO), 192–193

U

Unpackaged foods, phosphate food additives in, 318
Unprocessed food, 282
Upper level (UL) of safe phosphorus
  for adults 19 to 70 years, 268–270
  all-cause mortality, 275
  biomarkers determination, 274
  European food safety authority (EFSA) opinion, 270–271
  high phosphorus intake, mechanisms, 275
  hormone mechanisms as biomarker, 275
  for other age groups, 270
  total phosphorus intake measurement, 275
Urinary phosphate excretion (UPE), 49, 50, 52, 190, 235
  CKD patients, body phosphorus homeostasis, 68
  intestinal phosphorus absorption, 95
Urinary phosphorus, 204
  cardiotoxicity, 96–97
  excretion, 101
  measurements, 95
Urine
  albumin, 243
  calcium, 132–134
  pH and blood pH, 128, 129, 132

V

Vascular calcification, 5
  body phosphorus homeostasis, 67
  bone-forming proteins, 33
  cardiotoxicity, 103
  dialysis patients with, 37
  FGF23 serum levels, 34–35
  inhibitors loss, 33
  klotho expression, 35
  osteoblastic transition, 33
  parathyroid hormone (PTH), 34
  phosphate and mortality, 55, 56
  phosphorus role, 33–34
  vascular smooth muscle cells (VSMCs) transition, 32–33
Vegetarian diets, 238
Ventricular hypertrophy, 235
Vitamin D metabolism, 21
  calcitriol's control, renal production, 146
  deficiency and skeletal muscle weakness, 162
  FGF23 synthesis in bone, calcitriol induction of, 145–146
  local bioactivation, 146–147
  metabolism and VDR activation, 146–147
  pro-aging actions, 142
  renal calcitriol production, 143–145
  renal α-klotho, calcitriol induction of, 145

X

X-linked hypophosphatemia (XLH), 75, 190–192, 196
  in children, 192
  rickets, 159

Y

Yale Rudd Center for Food Policy & Obesity, 178

PGSTL 09/27/2017